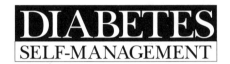

DIABETES
SELF-MANAGEMENT

Best-Ever Tips

1,001 TIPS
TO CONTROL YOUR DIABETES
AND KEEP YOU HEALTHY

DIABETES SELF-MANAGEMENT BOOKS
NEW YORK

Note to the reader:
The information contained in this book is not intended as a substitute for appropriate medical care. Appropriate care should be developed in discussion with your physician and the rest of your diabetes care team. This book has been published to help you with that discussion.

Library of Congress Cataloging-in-Publication Data
    Diabetes self-management best-ever tips : 1,001 tips to control your diabetes and keep you healthy.
    p. cm.
    Includes index.
    ISBN 0-9631701-9-8
    Diabetes—Popular works. 2. Diabetes—Miscellanea. 3. Self-care, Health—Miscellanea. I. Diabetes Self-Management Books.
    RC660.4.D558 2008
    616.4′62—dc22   2008014608

PROJECT EDITOR
James Hazlett

DESIGN AND ILLUSTRATION
Richard Boland

PROJECT DIRECTOR
Maryanne Schott Turner

SENIOR DTP MANAGER
Megan K. Coffey

DTP MANAGER
Delany Schucker

Diabetes Self-Management Books is an imprint of R.A. Rapaport Publishing, Inc., 150 West 22nd Street, New York, NY 10011.

Photographs contained in this book are for illustration purposes only. Photography credits: CORBIS/p358; GETTY IMAGES/p412; JUPITER IMAGES/p373, p490, p541; UNKNOWN/p219.

Printed in the United States of America
10 9 8 7 6 5 4 3 2 1

Contents

PREFACE 9

CONTRIBUTORS 10

BASIC INFORMATION

Tips 1–139 15

What Is Diabetes? 23
*Belinda O'Connell, M.S., R.D., C.D.E.,
and Laura Hieronymus, M.S.Ed., A.P.R.N.,
B.C.-A.D.M., C.D.E.*

What You Should Know About
Celiac Disease 26
Judy Giusti, M.S., R.D., L.D., C.D.E.

Sick Day Supplies 33
Make Sure You're Prepared
Margaret Hofacker, R.N., B.S.N., C.D.E.

Getting to Know Ketones 39
Richard Weil, M.Ed., C.D.E.

Understanding Hypoglycemia 43
*Belinda O'Connell, M.S., R.D., C.D.E.,
and Laura Hieronymus, M.S.Ed., A.P.R.N.,
B.C.-A.D.M., C.D.E.*

Managing Hyperglycemia 48
*Laura Hieronymus, M.S.Ed., A.P.R.N.,
B.C.-A.D.M., C.D.E., and Belinda O'Connell,
M.S., R.D., C.D.E.*

Diabetes in the Workplace 53
Deirdre J. Duke, R.N., M.S.N., J.D.

Your Diabetes Management Plan 57
Why It Pays to Have One
*Martha Funnell, M.S., R.N., C.D.E.,
and Michael Weiss*

Navigating Your Way to Optimal Health . . . 60
*Laura Hieronymus, M.S.Ed., A.P.R.N.,
B.C.- A.D.M., C.D.E., and Gregory Hood, M.D.*

Taking Diabetes to Heart 67
*Laura Hieronymus, M.S.Ed., A.P.R.N.,
B.C.-A.D.M., C.D.E., and Kristina
Humphries, M.D.*

DEALING WITH FEELINGS

Tips 140–194 75

Relaxation Techniques for
Stressful Times 79
Linda Wasmer Andrews

Spiritual Self-Care and the Use of Prayer . . . 83
Jacquelin Deatcher, A.P.R.N., B.C., C.D.E.

Body Image 86
How You See Yourself
Lisa Himmelfarb, C.S.W., R.D., C.D.E.

Overcoming Binge Eating Disorder 92
Lisa Himmelfarb, C.S.W., R.D., C.D.E.

Making Positive Changes 97
David Spero, R.N.

Understanding Depression
and Diabetes 101
Alisa G. Woods, Ph.D.

How Stories Can Heal 106
David Spero, R.N.

Diabetes and Your Marriage 111
Making Things Work
Paula M. Trief, Ph.D.

Eight Tips for Managing
Diabetes Distress 115
Lawrence Fisher, Ph.D.

How to Ask For Help—And Get It 118
Linda Wasmer Andrews

Getting a New Perspective on
Your Diabetes 121
Susan Shaw, C.Ht.

BLOOD GLUCOSE CONTROL

Tips 195–257. 127

HbA$_{1c}$ 132
What It is and Why It Matters
Mark Nakamoto

Blood Glucose Monitoring 137
What Do the Numbers Tell You?
*Virginia Peragallo-Dittko, A.P.R.N., M.A.,
B.C.-A.D.M., C.D.E.*

The Myth of Brittle Diabetes. 141
Gary Scheiner, M.S., C.D.E.

Strike the Spike 146
After-Meal Blood Glucose Highs
Gary Scheiner, M.S., C.D.E.

Take a Bite Out of Hypoglycemia. 153
10 Proven Strategies for Cutting Down
on Low Blood Glucose
Gary Scheiner, M.S., C.D.E.

Continuous Glucose Monitoring 160
Getting Started
Linda Mackowiak, M.S., R.N., C.D.E.

INSULIN AND INJECTION DEVICES

Tips 258–302. 167

Understanding Insulin. 171
*Laura Hieronymus, M.S.Ed., A.P.R.N.,
B.C.-A.D.M., C.D.E., and Patti Geil,
M.S., R.D., C.D.E.*

Rapid-Acting Insulin 177
Timing It Just Right
*Hope Warshaw, M.M.Sc., R.D.,
B.C.-A.D.M., C.D.E.*

Getting Down to Basals 182
Gary Scheiner, M.S., C.D.E.

Insulin Therapy for Type 2 Diabetes 187
*Virginia Peragallo-Dittko, A.P.R.N., M.A.,
B.C.-A.D.M., C.D.E.*

Insulin Delivery Devices. 191
*Stacy Griffin, Pharm. D., and Laura
Hieronymus, M.S.Ed., A.P.R.N.,
B.C.-A.D.M., C.D.E.*

DRUGS AND DIETARY SUPPLEMENTS

Tips 303–365. 199

Vitamins in Food and Supplements 204
Belinda O'Connell, M.S., R.D., C.D.E.

Minerals in Food and Supplements 211
Belinda O'Connell, M.S., R.D., C.D.E.

Antioxidants 219
Should You Supplement?
Robert A. Jacob, Ph.D.

Amylin. 224
Insulin's Partner
Wayne Clark

Exenatide 227
From the Gila Monster to You
Wayne Clark

Oral Medicine for Type 2 Diabetes. 230
*Patti Geil, M.S., R.D., C.D.E., and
Laura Hieronymus, M.S.Ed., A.P.R.N.,
B.C.-A.D.M., C.D.E.*

Blood Pressure Drugs 236
What Are the Options?
*Laura Hieronymus, M.S.Ed., A.P.R.N.,
B.C.-A.D.M., C.D.E., and Stacy Griffin,
R.Ph., Pharm.D.-C*

DIABETES COMPLICATIONS

Tips 366–463. 245

Keeping On Top of Neuropathy. 252
Wayne Clark

Dealing With Constipation 255
Judy Giusti, M.S., R.D., L.D., C.D.E.

Urinary Tract Infections 259
Treatment and Prevention
*Eduardo Randrup, M.D., and Neil Baum,
M.D.*

Cardiac Rehabilitation. 262
Linnea Hagberg, R.D.

Treating Heart Failure. 265
Wayne Clark

Stroke Rehabilitation. 270
Offering Hope and Help
Jeffrey Larson, P.T., A.T.C.

Say Yes to Intimacy. 274
Treatment Options for
Erectile Dysfunction
Donna Rice, B.S.N., R.N., C.D.E.

Sexual Wellness. 280
*Laura Hieronymus, M.S.Ed., A.P.R.N.,
B.C.-A.D.M., C.D.E., and Lawrence
Maguire, M.D.*

Protecting Your Kidneys 283
Robert S. Dinsmoor

Treating Gastroparesis 288
Kathryn Feigenbaum, R.N., M.S.N.,
C.D.E.

Diabetic Ketoacidosis 293
A Preventable Crisis
Jan Chait

FOOT HEALTH
Tips 464–532 299

Taking Steps Toward Healthy Feet 304
Laura Hieronymus, M.S.Ed., A.P.R.N.,
B.C.-A.D.M., C.D.E., and Belinda
O'Connell, M.S., R.D., C.D.E.

Wound Healing for Foot Ulcers 309
Jeffrey A. Stone, D.O., M.P.H.,
and Leon Brill, D.P.M.

Foot Care 315
Drugstore Do's and Don't's
J.C. Tanenbaum, D.P.M.

How to Choose Footwear 318
Roy H. Lidtke, D.P.M., C.Ped.

EXERCISE
Tips 533–594 327

Exercise Myths and Facts 332
Richard Weil, M.Ed., C.D.E.

Get Moving With Yoga 337
Gabrielle Kaplan-Mayer

The High Price of Inactivity 341
Richard Weil, M.Ed., C.D.E.

Improving Your Balance 345
Richard Weil, M.Ed., C.D.E.

Stretching 352
Richard Weil, M.Ed., C.D.E.

Biking 101 358
Marie Spano, M.S., R.D.

WEIGHT MANAGEMENT
Tips 595–620 365

How Hunger Happens 368
The Brain's Role in Obesity
Alisa G. Woods, Ph.D.

Strategies for Weight Management 373
Ann Goebel-Fabbri, Ph.D.

Bariatric Surgery 376
Lifestyle Changes for Before and After
Laurie Block, M.S., R.D., C.D.E.

NUTRITION AND MEAL PLANNING
Tips 621–679 383

Are You Label-Able? 388
Belinda O'Connell, M.S., R.D., C.D.E.,
and Laura Hieronymus, M.S.Ed.,
A.P.R.N., B.C.-A.D.M., C.D.E.

Sizing Up Your Servings 396
Belinda O'Connell, M.S., R.D., C.D.E.,
and Laura Hieronymus, M.S.Ed.,
A.P.R.N., B.C.-A.D.M., C.D.E.

Vegetarian and Vegan Meal Planning 400
Nancy Berkoff, R.D., Ed.D., C.C.E.

Trans Fat begone! 412
Julie Lichty Balay, M.S., R.D.

Extreme Makeover—Recipe Edition 416
Patti Geil, M.S., R.D., C.D.E., and
Laura Hieronymus, M.S.Ed., A.P.R.N.,
B.C.-A.D.M., C.D.E.

PREVENTIVE HEALTH
Tips 680–772 423

Lower Cholesterol to Lower Heart Risk . . . 429
Wayne Clark

Lifestyle Habits for a Healthy Heart 433
Heidi Mochari, M.P.H., R.D.

The Benefits of Tight Control 437
No End in Sight
Wayne Clark

Avoiding Eye Complications 440
A. Paul Chous, M.A., O.D.

Boning Up on Bone Health 445
Belinda O'Connell, M.S., R.D., C.D.E.

Emergency Preparedness 450
Just In Case
Judith Jones Ambrosini and Laura Laria

Getting the Sleep You Need 454
David Spero, R.N.

Diabetes and Your Skin 460
Protecting Your Outermost Layer
May Leveriza-Oh, M.D.

How to Avoid Errors in Diabetes Care 465
Patrick J. O'Connor, M.D., M.P.H.

WOMEN'S HEALTH

Tips 773–862. 473

Expecting the Best 478
Diabetes, Pregnancy, and
Blood Glucose Control
*Laura Hieronymus, M.S.Ed., A.P.R.N.,
B.C.-A.D.M., C.D.E., and Patti Geil,
M.S., R.D., C.D.E.*

Pregnant and Pumping 484
Great Expectations
*Laura Hieronymus, M.S.Ed., A.P.R.N.,
B.C.-A.D.M., C.D.E., and Patti Geil,
M.S., R.D., C.D.E.*

Managing Diabetes While
Breast-Feeding 490
Christine Bradley

Vaginitis. 493
What Every Woman Needs to Know
*Laura Hieronymus, M.S.Ed., A.P.R.N.,
B.C.-A.D.M., C.D.E., and Kristina
Humphries, M.D.*

Menopause 497
The Latest on Hormone Therapy
Helen L. Ross, M.D.

Top 10 Health Tips for
Women Over 65 503
*Helen L. Sloan, R.N., C.S., D.N.S.,
and Anne White Robinson, R.N., D.N.S.*

FOR PARENTS

Tips 863–1,001 513

Sending Your Kid to Camp 520
Karen Riley, R.N.

Preventing Obesity in Your Child 523
Nicholas Yphantides, M.D., M.P.H.

Be Aware of Hypoglycemia
Unawareness. 527
*Karen Kelly, R.N., B.S.N., C.D.E.,
and Amy Gilliland, R.N., M.S.N.*

When Kids Falsify Their Numbers 530
*Jean Betschart Roemer, R.N., M.N.,
C.P.N.P., C.D.E.*

Helping Young Children Succeed
With Diabetes Care 534
Alisha Perez, M.S., C.C.L.S.

Getting Eating Habits on a
Healthy Track 538
Amy Sullivan, R.D., L.D.N., C.D.E.

Dental Care for Kids 541
Brian S. Martin, D.M.D.

When Your Child Needs Surgery 544
Edward Scott Vokoun, M.D.

Getting Ready for College 547
*Amy Gilliland, R.N., M.S.N.,
and Linda Siminerio, R.N., Ph.D.,
C.D.E.*

QUIZZES

How Much Do You Know About
Blood Glucose Monitoring?. 554
*Virginia Peragallo-Dittko, A.P.R.N.,
M.A., B.C.-A.D.M., C.D.E.*

How Much Do You Know About
Storing Insulin? 556
*Virginia Peragallo-Dittko, A.P.R.N.,
M.A., B.C.-A.D.M., C.D.E.*

How Much Do You Know About
Handling Sick Days?. 558
Janice Woodrum, R.N., B.S.N.

How Much Do You Know About
Routine Medical Tests? 560
Robert S. Dinsmoor

How Much Do You Know About
Diabetes and Your Eyes? 562
A. Paul Chous, M.A., O.D.

How Much Do You Know About
Chronic Kidney Disease?. 564
Maria Karalis, M.B.A., R.D., L.D.

How Much Do You Know About
Heart Disease Risk? 566
Mark Nakamoto

INDEX 569

Preface

Regardless of whether you've had diabetes for many years or you were just diagnosed, dealing with diabetes is stressful.

And the information you need to manage your diabetes often seems overwhelming—lose weight, start exercising, tighten up your blood glucose control. And do it all at once, which is not only extremely difficult, it doesn't make any sense either.

The best way to get the information you need is to accumulate it, starting with the basics, then moving on to fill the gaps in your knowledge. This book is designed to help you do just that. Its purpose is to give you the information you need to sustain a lifetime of diabetes care, and we make it as accessible as possible.

We cover the 13 most asked-about areas of concern to someone with diabetes and start each of these sections with short tips, advice, and observations that we hope will add to the sum total of your knowledge about diabetes. You can go to any of the 100 articles in this book to dig deeper and understand more.

It's all in easy-to-understand everyday language. No medical jargon, and you won't have to plow through this book to get good ideas. With this book, you can cherry-pick your most important concerns and get the information you need quickly and easily.

I think you'll love this user-friendly book, and I hope you'll make it your first and last stop for all the right answers to controlling your diabetes. Read it in good health.

For the staff and the 70 contributors who made this book possible,

James Hazlett
Editor

Contributors

Judith Jones Ambrosini writes for www.Diabetes-Net.com and Diabetes Positive magazine and also writes for other diabetes-related publications. She is on the board of directors of the Diabetes Exercise and Sports Association and edits its quarterly newsletter, the DESA Challenge.

Linda Wasmer Andrews is a health and psychology writer based in Albuquerque, New Mexico.

Julie Lichty Balay, M.S., R.D., is a nutrition consultant and educator in New York City and Bergen County, New Jersey.

Neil Baum, M.D., is Clinical Associate Professor of Urology at Louisiana State University Medical School and Tulane University Medical School in New Orleans, Louisiana.

Nancy Berkoff, R.D., Ed.D., C.C.E., is a registered dietitian and certified chef based in Long Beach, California.

Laurie Block, M.S., R.D., C.D.E., is a nutrition consultant in La Jolla, California.

Christine Bradley is a lactation consultant in Utah.

Leon R. Brill, D.P.M., is the former chairman of the Department of Podiatric Surgery at Presbyterian Hospital of Dallas, Texas.

Jan Chait is a freelance writer who lives in Indiana.

A. Paul Chous, M.A., O.D., is a doctor of optometry specializing in diabetes education in Tacoma, Washington. He is the author of *Diabetic Eye Disease: Lessons From a Diabetic Eye Doctor.*

Wayne Clark is a freelance medical and science writer who lives in Maine.

Jacquelin Deatcher, A.P.R.N., B.C., C.D.E., is an adult nurse practitioner and Certified Diabetes Educator working in private practice in Alexander-Attica, New York.

Robert S. Dinsmoor is a freelance writer and a contributing editor at *Diabetes Self-Management.*

Deirdre Duke, R.N., M.S.N., J.D., is an employment attorney. She has previously worked as a clinical nurse specialist in diabetes and endocrinology and served on the editorial board of *Diabetes Self-Management.*

Kathryn Feigenbaum, R.N., M.S.N., C.D.E., is a clinical nurse specialist in endocrinology at the National Institutes of Health in Bethesda, Maryland. Her entry was prepared as part of her official duties as a government employee.

Lawrence Fisher, Ph.D., is a clinical psychologist and a professor in the Department of Family and Community Medicine at the University of California, San Francisco.

Martha Funnell, M.S., R.N., C.D.E., is a clinical nurse specialist at the Michigan Diabetes Research and Training Center and an adjunct lecturer in the Department of Medical Education at the University of Michigan Medical School in Ann Arbor, Michigan.

Patti Geil, M.S., R.D., C.D.E., is a diabetes educator and health consultant at Drs. Borders & Associates, PSC, in Lexington, Kentucky.

Amy Gilliland, R.N., M.S.N., is a pediatric diabetes educator at the Children's Hospital of Pittsburgh in Pittsburgh, Pennsylvania.

Judy Giusti, M.S., R.D., L.D., C.D.E., is a registered dietitian and Certified Diabetes Educator at the Joslin Diabetes Center in Boston.

Ann Goebel-Fabbri, Ph.D., is a clinical psychologist at the Joslin Diabetes Center in Boston.

Stacy Griffin, R.Ph., Pharm.D.-C., is a diabetes educator and a pharmacist at Central Baptist Hospital in Lexington, Kentucky.

Linnea Hagberg, R.D., is a registered dietitian and freelance writer based in Gloucester, Massachusetts.

Laura Hieronymus, M.S.Ed., A.P.R.N., B.C.-A.D.M., C.D.E., has more than 20 years of experience in diabetes care and education and is a Clinical Management Liaison for Amylin Pharmaceuticals, Inc.

Lisa Himmelfarb, C.S.W., R.D., C.D.E., is a clinical social worker, registered dietitian, and Certified Diabetes Educator who specializes in eating disorders. She maintains a private practice in New York City.

Margaret Hofacker, R.N., B.S.N., C.D.E., works for Cornell Cooperative Extension at the Martin Luther King, Jr., and Tri-Community Health Centers in Suffolk County, New York.

Gregory Hood, M.D., is a practicing internist and a diabetes care and education provider at Drs. Borders & Associates, PSC, in Lexington, Kentucky.

Kristina Humphries, M.D., is a practicing endocrinologist and a diabetes care and education provider at Drs. Borders & Associates, PSC, in Lexington, Kentucky.

Robert A. Jacob, Ph.D., is a retired nutrition research scientist whose specialty is the role of antioxidants and other micronutrients in health and disease. He was a member of the National Academy of Sciences panel that set the current recommended dietary allowances for antioxidant vitamins.

Gabrielle Kaplan-Mayer is a writer and educator based in Philadelphia. She is the author of the book *Insulin Pump Therapy Demystified.*

Maria Karalis, M.B.A., R.D., L.D., is the nutrition consultant for iKidney.com.

Karen Kelly, R.N., B.S.N., C.D.E., is a pediatric diabetes educator at the Children's Hospital of Pittsburgh in Pittsburgh, Pennsylvania.

Becky Klein, R.N., C.D.E., is a diabetes educator at HealthPartners Medical Group and HealthPartners Research Foundation in Minneapolis, Minnesota.

Laura Laria is a graphic designer and former contributor to the DESA Challenge, the newsletter of the Diabetes Exercise and Sports Association.

Jeffrey Larson, P.T., A.T.C., is the director of physical therapy at the Tioga Medical Center in Tioga, North Dakota, and a freelance medical writer.

May Leveriza-Oh, M.D., is a dermatologist in Boston.

Roy H. Lidtke, D.P.M., C.Ped., is a professor and director of the Gait Analysis Lab at Rosalind Franklin University of Medicine and Science. He also serves on the faculty of Rush University Medical Center and the Weil Foot and Ankle Institute, both in Chicago.

Linda Mackowiak, M.S., R.N., C.D.E., is a diabetes nurse specialist with 15 years experience in diabetes care. For the past seven years she has worked in the field of insulin pumps and glucose sensors and is currently employed by Abbott Diabetes Care.

Lawrence Maguire, M.D., is a practicing internist and a diabetes care and education provider at Drs. Borders & Associates, PSC, in Lexington, Kentucky.

Brian S. Martin, D.M.D., is Chief of Dental Services at the Children's Hospital of Pittsburgh in Pittsburgh, Pennsylvania, as well as an adjunct faculty member of the University of Pittsburgh School of Dental Medicine.

Heidi Mochari, M.P.H., R.D., is the nutrition director for the Preventive Cardiology Program of New York–Presbyterian Hospital.

Mark Nakamoto is a former associate editor at *Diabetes Self-Management.*

Belinda O'Connell, M.S., R.D., C.D.E., is a diabetes nutrition specialist in the Minneapolis, Minnesota, area and a freelance health and science writer.

Patrick J. O'Connor, M.D., M.P.H., is a clinician clinical physician at HealthPartners Medical Group and HealthPartners Research Foundation in Minneapolis, Minnesota.

Virginia Peragallo-Dittko, A.P.R.N., M.A., B.C.-A.D.M., C.D.E., is a diabetes nurse specialist and Director of the Diabetes Education Center at Winthrop–University Hospital in Mineola, New York.

Alisha Perez, M.S., C.C.L.S., is a former Certified Child Life Specialist in the Pediatric and Adolescent Unit at the Joslin Diabetes Center in Boston.

Eduardo Randrup, M.D., is a staff urologist at the Ochsner Clinic Foundation in New Orleans, Louisiana.

Donna Rice, B.S.N., R.N., C.D.E., is the Wellness Program manager at the Botsford Hospital Center for Health Improvement in Novi, Michigan.

Karen Riley, R.N., is a diabetes research nurse at the Children's Hospital of Pittsburgh in Pittsburgh, Pennsylvania, has been a camp nurse at Camp Crestfield in western Pennsylvania for more than 20 years, and is a past chairperson of the American Diabetes Association's diabetes camp project team.

Anne White Robinson, R.N., D.N.S., is an assistant professor emerita at the College of Nursing and Allied Health Professions at the University of Louisiana at Lafayette.

Jean Betschart Roemer, R.N., M.N., C.P.N.P., C.D.E., is a pediatric nurse practitioner in the Department of Diabetes, Endocrinology, and Metabolism at Children's Hospital of Pittsburgh.

Helen L. Ross, M.D., is a board-certified obstetrician/gynecologist and a member of the Department of Obstetrics and Gynecology at the University of Florida in Gainesville, Florida.

Gary Scheiner, M.S., C.D.E., is a Certified Diabetes Educator with a private practice near Philadelphia.

Susan Shaw, C.Ht., has had Type 1 diabetes for 37 years and is a certified hypnotherapist in Woodland Hills, California.

Linda Siminerio, R.N., Ph.D., C.D.E., is director of the Diabetes Institute at the University of Pittsburgh Medical Center in Pittsburgh, Pennsylvania.

Helen Sloan, R.N., C.S., D.N.S., is a gerontological nurse practitioner and assistant professor emerita at the College of Nursing and Allied Health Professions at the University of Louisiana at Lafayette.

Marie Spano, M.S., R.D., is a registered dietitian, exercise physiologist, and spokesperson for the International Society of Sports Nutrition.

JoAnn M. Sperl-Hillen, M.D., is a clinician at HealthPartners Medical Group and HealthPartners Research Foundation in Minneapolis, Minnesota.

David Spero, R.N., has been a registered nurse for 32 years and is a project director for the New Health Partnerships initiative of the Institute for Healthcare Improvement. He is the author of two books: *The Art of Getting Well: Maximizing Health When You Have a Chronic Illness* and *Diabetes—Sugar-coated Crisis: Who Gets It, Who Profits, and How to Stop It.*

Jeffrey A. Stone, D.O., M.P.H., is the medical director for the Hyperbaric Medicine Unit at the Institute for Exercise and Environmental Medicine at Presbyterian Hospital of Dallas, Texas, and a past president of the Texas Affiliate of the American Diabetes Association.

Amy Sullivan, R.D., L.D.N., C.D.E., is a clinical dietitian specializing in diabetes at the Children's Hospital of Pittsburgh in Pittsburgh, Pennsylvania.

J. C. Tanenbaum, D.P.M., is a podiatrist in private practice in the Houston, Texas, area and a diplomate of the American Board of Podiatric Surgery.

Paula M. Trief, Ph.D., is a professor in the departments of Psychiatry and Medicine at the State University of New York Upstate Medical University in Syracuse, New York.

Edward Scott Vokoun, M.D., is a Lieutenant Commander in the Department of Anesthesia at the Naval Medical Center in Portsmouth, Virginia. (The views expressed in his entry are his own and do not necessarily reflect the official policy or position of the Department of the Navy, Deparment of Defense, or the United States Government.)

Hope Warshaw, M.M.Sc., R.D., B.C.-A.D.M., C.D.E., is a dietitian and diabetes educator based in northern Virginia. She is the author of numerous books about diabetes nutrition management, including *Complete Guide to Carb Counting* and *Guide to Healthy Restaurant Eating.*

Richard Weil, M.Ed., C.D.E., is an exercise physiologist and a consultant to St. Luke's–Roosevelt Hospital Center in New York City.

Michael Weiss has had Type 1 diabetes for more than 20 years and is a past chair of the Board of Directors of the American Diabetes Association.

Janice Woodrum, R.N., B.S.N., is a Certified Diabetes Educator and former coordinator of the Diabetes Education Program at Miami County Medical Center in Paola, Kansas.

Alisa G. Woods, Ph.D., is a neurobiologist and science writer. She lives in Brooklyn, New York.

Nicholas Yphantides, M.D., M.P.H., is the Appointed Co-Chair of the San Diego County Childhood Obesity Task Force and the author of *My Big Fat Greek Diet: How a 467-Pound Physician Hit His Ideal Weight and How You Can Too.*

Basic Information

Tips 1–139 15

What Is Diabetes? 23

What You Should Know About Celiac Disease 26

Sick Day Supplies 33
Make Sure You're Prepared

Getting to Know Ketones 39

Understanding Hypoglycemia 43

Managing Hyperglycemia 48

Diabetes in the Workplace 53

Your Diabetes Management Plan 57
Why It Pays to Have One

Navigating Your Way to Optimal Health 60

Taking Diabetes to Heart 67

1

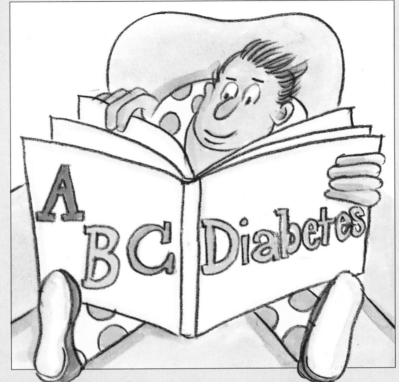

Basic Information Tips

1–139

1. In many cases of undiagnosed celiac disease, there are no symptoms at all.

2. Long-term complications of untreated celiac disease include osteoporosis, fertility problems, and benign or malignant tumors of the small intestine.

3. Celiac disease commonly shows up in children, but it has been diagnosed in people of all ages, mainly because not everyone with celiac disease experiences symptoms right away.

4. Since celiac disease is an inherited disease, all first-degree family members—parents, siblings, and children—of people with celiac disease should be screened.

5. If your doctor suspects celiac disease, you should continue to eat gluten-containing foods until after the biopsy.

6. The only treatment for celiac disease is a lifelong, 100% gluten-free diet.

7. In people with Type 1 diabetes, malabsorption of nutrients from undiagnosed celiac disease can lead to frequent, unexplained low or high blood glucose readings.

8. For people with diabetes and celiac disease, starting a gluten-free diet requires learning the carbohydrate content of new, gluten-free foods, so they can be introduced into a meal plan or so that insulin doses can be adjusted accordingly.

9. Since fiber is not digested or absorbed, you should subtract the grams of fiber from the total carbohydrate on the label if there are more than 5 grams of fiber per serving.

10. Keeping blood glucose levels close to normal requires learning how to balance food intake, physical activity, and the effects of any diabetes medicines your doctor may prescribe to lower your blood glucose level.

11. Because each person's situation is different, it is important to work with your diabetes care team to set individualized blood glucose goals that are right for you.

12. The best way to identify hyperglycemia is to routinely monitor your blood glucose levels on a schedule determined by you and your health-care team and to get regular HbA_{1c} tests, also on a schedule agreed on by you and your health-care team (usually two to four times a year).

13. Just because you feel OK doesn't necessarily mean your blood glucose level is well controlled.

14. No matter what type of diabetes you have or how you treat it, part of your hyperglycemia action plan will likely be more frequent blood glucose monitoring, at least temporarily, to help determine why your blood glucose is high and what you can do to avoid future episodes of hyperglycemia.

15. Reviewing the amount of carbohydrate in your meals and snacks may be helpful in determining the cause of hyperglycemia.

16. Carefully reading nutrition labels on food products and measuring portions will help you to meet your carbohydrate goals.

17. Meals that are high in fat may contribute to prolonged elevations in blood glucose after eating.

18. Working with a registered dietitian can be helpful in fine-tuning your meal-planning and carbohydrate-counting skills.

19. If your blood glucose level is high before

20. The expiration date on insulin packaging is for unopened, refrigerated vials, disposable pens, or pen cartridges.

21. Once opened, most vials of insulin last for 28 days, but many pens and pen cartridges are good for only 7, 10, or 14 days.

22. Pump users should change their infusion set and the insulin in the pump reservoir every 48 hours.

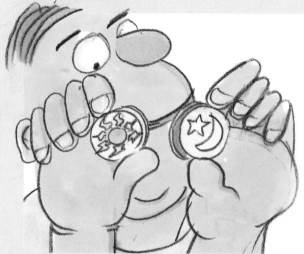

23. If you take pills, be sure you're taking them at the right time of day.

24. Some pills must be taken right before meals to work effectively; others do not.

25. You should be aware that if you switch to a different syringe or insulin pen or from one to the other, the injection technique may differ.

26. Store opened containers of medicines you are currently using at room temperature.

27. Unopened packages of pills can also be stored at room temperature.

28. Be careful not to place insulin in particularly cold areas of the refrigerator, where it may freeze.

29. If you use an insulin pump, review the set-up of your infusion set with your diabetes care team to assure accurate insulin delivery.

30. Pump users should have alternative methods of insulin delivery on hand

you exercise, it may go even higher during exercise.

should their pump malfunction or stop delivering insulin for any reason.

31. Tell your health-care team about any over-the-counter medicines or alternative therapies you use so that together you can determine whether those substances or practices are having an effect on your blood glucose control.

32. During periods of stress, the body releases so-called stress hormones, which cause a rise in blood glucose level.

33. If stress becomes chronic, hyperglycemia can also become chronic.

34. Work out a sick-day plan in advance with their diabetes care team.

35. Premenopausal women may experience higher-than-usual blood glucose levels about a week prior to menstruation.

36. Insulin adjustments are often necessary every 7–10 days during pregnancy.

37. Low testosterone levels may contribute to increased insulin resistance, which can contribute to hyperglycemia.

38. The only way you can truly know your blood glucose level is to check it with your meter.

39. You should discuss when and how often to monitor with your diabetes care team.

40. Keep in mind that even with your best efforts in managing your diabetes, you may still experience high blood glucose from time to time.

41. Since having diabetes often involves regular use of the health-care system and substantial medical costs, you will want to find out about a prospective employer's health benefits packages.

42. If your diabetes has no bearing on your ability to do the job, it would not be appropriate to bring it or any other personal medical information up during your interview.

43. If a new job will mean a big change in your daily schedule or activity level, speak to your doctor before you begin to discuss how and when any changes in your diabetes self-management regi-

men should be made. If possible, adopt your new schedule before you actually start your new job so you can see what effect, if any, it has on your blood glucose levels.

44. Wearing or carrying medical identification is always a good idea and no less so at work.

45. When you have diabetes, it is uncontrolled blood glucose levels that place you at the highest risk for heart disease.

46. Your cardiovascular risk factors should be assessed by your physician at least once a year.

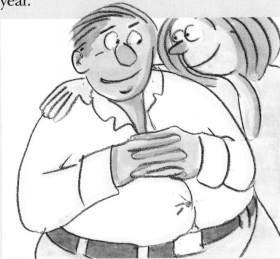

47. Carrying extra weight around your waist raises your risk of heart disease.

48. Smoking doubles your risk of developing heart disease.

49. If you haven't already worked with a dietitian to design an individualized meal plan, ask your diabetes care team for a referral to a registered dietitian.

50. Fat should make up no more than 30% of your total energy intake, and most of that fat should be monounsaturated or polyunsaturated.

51. Limiting the amount of saturated fat, *trans* fat, and cholesterol you eat can help to lower your blood cholesterol levels.

52. Before increasing your level of physical activity or starting a formal exercise plan, discuss your plans with your diabetes care team.

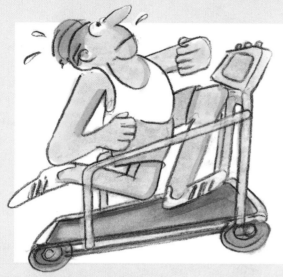

53. Performing at least 150 minutes of moderate-intensity aerobic activity a week and/or at least 90 minutes of vigorous aerobic exercise a week is recommended.

54. People with Type 2 diabetes are additionally encouraged to do resistance exercises targeting all major muscle groups three times weekly, as long as they have no medical reasons not to perform resistance exercise.

55. Increasing your physical activity while consuming fewer calories will help to make sure the weight you are losing is fat and not muscle.

56. If lifestyle changes alone don't bring your blood glucose, blood pressure, and blood cholesterol levels into target range, drug therapy may be necessary.

57. Remember, medication is not the enemy if it helps keep your "ABCs" in order.

58. Aspirin therapy is recommended in people with diabetes as a standard practice of care.

59. Regardless of sex, not everyone who has a heart attack has all the symptoms.

60. If you believe you are having a heart attack, don't delay: Get emergency help immediately.

61. People with diabetes have at least twice the risk of congestive heart failure as those without diabetes.

62. While having diabetes does increase your risk for heart disease, it doesn't make it inevitable.

63. Each person with diabetes and his diabetes care team should set individualized A1C goals. For most people with diabetes, the A1C target is below 7%.

64. Having diabetes may feel less overwhelming once you have an overall plan to guide you in your daily choices.

65. Your health-care providers should be a source of information, not just about diabetes in general but about your diabetes in particular and how it can best be managed.

66. The effect that diabetes will have on your life will become clearer—and will also probably change—over time.

67. If you're having a rough time or your feelings are keeping you from caring for yourself or doing the things you enjoy, consider seeking out support from others who have diabetes.

68. Ask your health-care providers for any money-saving tips they may have, and tell them if you cannot afford the drugs or other products they recommend.

69. Remember, no one knows what will fit into your life better than you do.

70. One common barrier to carrying out a diabetes plan is trying to make too many lifestyle changes at once.

71. If your heart isn't in making a particular change, you are unlikely to do it.

72. Rather than trying to ignore the parts of your plan that aren't working, examine them more carefully to see if you can figure out why they aren't working.

73. If something has happened in your life that has affected how you care for your diabetes, let your health-care provider know. Remember that your health-care providers are there to help you create a plan that will work for you, not to judge you on your ability to carry out a particular plan.

74. When you feel burned out by the demands diabetes puts on you, it's good to have people to turn to for support.

75. The clearer you can be about your needs, the more likely you are to have them met.

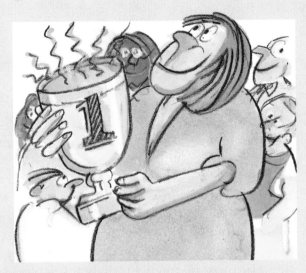

76. Celebrate your successes and learn from the things that do not work as well.

77. Give yourself credit for learning as much as you have about diabetes and for all of the efforts you make every day to stay in good health.

78. Understanding how and why diabetes develops can help you to be an active member of your diabetes-care team.

79. Blood glucose levels above normal are known to increase a person's chances of eventually developing heart disease and other complications of diabetes.

80. An individual's treatment may change over time as his degree of insulin resistance or ability to produce insulin changes.

81. Many people still make a fair amount of insulin when they are initially diagnosed with Type 2 diabetes, so their treatment may focus mainly on decreasing insulin resistance.

82. For most people, the need to use insulin to control their diabetes does not mean they lack willpower or the desire to take good care of their diabetes.

83. Diabetes is a chronic condition, meaning that once you are diagnosed, it's there to stay. But with regular medical care and optimal blood glucose control, you can live a long, healthy life.

84. If you have a history of diabetes and are visiting a physician for the first time, you should have a complete physical exam as well as a discussion about your current blood glucose control, the presence of any diabetes complications, and your ongoing diabetes care needs.

85. The primary goal of diabetes management is optimal blood glucose control. Self-monitoring of blood glucose helps you and your diabetes care team evaluate your overall blood glucose control and review the trends and patterns of your blood glucose levels during the course of the day.

86. Insulin users, especially those who take insulin multiple times a day, should monitor their blood glucose levels three times or more daily.

87. All people with diabetes should see a registered dietitian, preferably one with expertise in diabetes.

88. Keep in mind that as you age, your body and your diabetes treatment needs change.

89. Diabetes education should encourage you to set goals to achieve behavior change as well as address your specific needs.

90. See your doctor for a physical exam before starting an exercise program, especially if you haven't been active for a while.

91. Should you need to be admitted to the hospital for any reason, ask that a member of your diabetes care team be consulted regarding your treatment to ensure that you maintain the best possible blood glucose control.

92. Keeping your blood glucose levels as close as possible to their target ranges while you are in the hospital can reduce your chance of developing further illness or infection during your stay.

93. Using a food with added fat (such as a chocolate bar) is not recommended to treat hypoglycemia because fat may slow down the body's absorption of the carbohydrate.

94. All people with diabetes should receive a yearly influenza vaccine (flu shot). At least

one lifetime pneumonia vaccine is also recommended for adults with diabetes.

95. It is not uncommon for two or three different drugs to be used to reach blood pressure goals.

96. Cigarette smoking contributes to one of every five deaths in the United States and is the leading avoidable cause of premature death. If you are a smoker, you and your physician should discuss a plan for quitting.

97. The risk for retinopathy can be reduced with control of blood glucose and blood pressure levels.

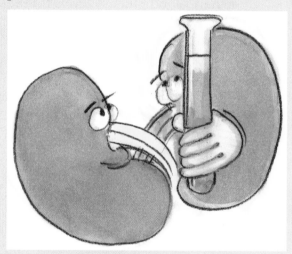

98. Nephropathy (diabetic kidney disease) is the most common cause of kidney failure in the United States and the greatest threat to life in adults with Type 1 diabetes. It is essential that people with diabetes undergo an annual test for the presence of microalbuminuria (the spilling of small amounts of the protein albumin into the urine, which indicates kidney damage).

99. If a person has nephropathy, early detection and treatment can improve his quality of life and delay or prevent the need for dialysis and renal transplantation.

100. Your physician should check your feet at each diabetes visit to assess any potential problems.

101. Your diabetes educator should give you guidelines for foot care to help prevent any injury and infection to your feet and legs due to loss of sensation from nerve damage.

102. The lower your HbA$_{1c}$, the better your chances of avoiding serious diabetes complications.

103. Controlling blood glucose is more than just managing the "highs"; it also involves preventing and managing "lows," or hypoglycemia.

104. Keeping blood glucose levels as close to normal as possible helps prevent damage to the blood vessels and nerves in the body.

105. For most people with diabetes, a blood glucose level of 70 mg/dl or less is considered low, and treatment is recommended to prevent it from dropping even lower. If you have symptoms of hypoglycemia and do not have your blood glucose meter available, treatment is recommended.

106. Recognizing emotional changes that may signal hypoglycemia is especially important in young children, who may not be able to understand or communicate other symptoms of hypoglycemia to adults.

107. When you take insulin or a drug that increases the amount of insulin in your system, not eating enough food at the times the insulin or drug is working can cause hypoglycemia.

108. Physical activity and exercise lower blood glucose level by increasing insulin sensitivity.

109. Being able to recognize hypoglycemia promptly is very important because it allows you to take steps to raise your blood glucose as quickly as possible.

110. Frequent episodes of hypoglycemia can blunt your body's response to low blood glucose.

111. If you have hypoglycemia frequently, you may need to raise your blood glucose targets, and you should monitor your blood glucose level more frequently and avoid alcohol.

112. In some cases, people who have had chronically high blood glucose levels may

experience symptoms of hypoglycemia when their blood glucose level drops to a more normal range.

113. Work with your diabetes care team to devise a plan for treating hypoglycemia that is right for you.

114. People at higher risk of developing hypoglycemia should discuss the use of glucagon with their diabetes educator, doctor, or pharmacist.

115. Avoiding all episodes of hypoglycemia may be impossible for many people, especially since maintaining tight blood glucose control brings with it a higher risk of hypoglycemia.

116. Learn how to count carbohydrates so you can keep your carbohydrate intake consistent at meals and snacks from day to day.

117. Have carbohydrate-containing foods available in the places you frequent, such as in your car or at the office, to avoid delays in treatment of hypoglycemia.

118. Always treat blood glucose levels of 70 mg/dl or less whether or not you have symptoms.

119. Although hypoglycemia can, at times, be unpleasant, don't risk your health by allowing your blood glucose levels to run higher than recommended to avoid it.

120. Ketones are formed when fat is burned for energy by the muscles. If you don't have glucose available for fuel (because you are on a low-carbohydrate diet, for example), you will form ketones when your muscles burn fat. Having measurable amounts of ketones in the urine (or blood) is cause for concern. The problem with high levels of ketones is that they are relatively strong acids, and because of their acidity, their presence in the blood can reduce the ability of oxygen to bind to hemoglobin, the molecule that transports oxygen to cells that need it.

121. If you're considering a low-carbohydrate, high-protein diet for weight loss or blood glucose control, check with your doctor or diabetes educator first.

122. People with Type 1 diabetes whose blood glucose level is over 250 mg/dl for two readings in a row or who are sick should always test for ketones.

123. Pregnant women with diabetes are usually advised to check their urine for ketones every morning before eating and additionally if their blood glucose level is above 200 mg/dl or if they are ill.

124. With just a little blood or urine, today's ketone-testing products can let you know whether you're producing ketones.

125. When you have diabetes, very high blood glucose or dehydration (and particularly the two together) can turn into an emergency situation requiring hospitalization.

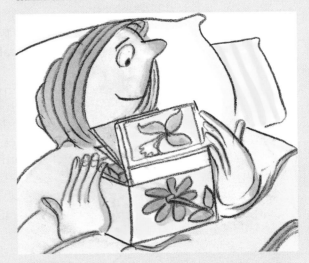

126. The idea behind a sick-day box is to have all of your sick-day supplies together in a place you can easily reach for when you do not feel like moving or cannot move very far. Work with your health-care team to personalize your sick-day box to cover all your health needs. Keep a list of names and important telephone numbers on a single page or file card in your sick-day box. A pen and pad of paper are among the most important items in your sick-day box. Every sick-day box should have a thermometer to check for fever.

127. Every person with diabetes should have individualized sick-day guidelines provided by or developed with the help of his health-care team before an illness occurs.

128. When you are ill, your sick-day plan may require you to monitor ketones or take fluids on a regular schedule—possibly as often as every hour or two.

129. Do not hesitate to call your health-care provider or the local emergency number if you believe you are headed for or are experiencing ketoacidosis or severe low blood glucose.

130. Plan ahead for sick days. Be sure you have back-up supplies for blood glucose monitoring because you may need to monitor more frequently when you are sick.

131. If you're not using individually wrapped ketone test strips, be sure to check expiration dates on the container for both the unopened as well as the opened strips.

132. All insulin users should have an extra package or two of syringes in their sick-day supplies, no matter what they usually use to deliver insulin.

133. If insulin injections or an insulin pump are part of your daily routine, always have at least an extra vial of unexpired insulin in the refrigerator. And discuss the need for a glucagon emergency kit with your health-care provider.

134. Because some foods may keep for less than a year, plan on checking your sick-day box every six months or so.

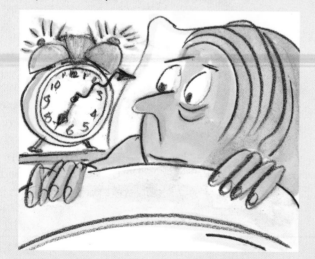

135. When sick, set your alarm to wake or alert you every 2–4 hours, so you can do any necessary blood glucose monitoring, ketone testing, or drinking of fluids.

136. Check blood glucose levels at least four times per day (at your usual mealtimes and bedtime) when you are sick.

137. Check your blood glucose more frequently when your results are higher than 240 mg/dl (and every two hours when your blood glucose is above 240 mg/dl and there are ketones in your urine or blood).

138. Check your blood or urine for ketones if you have nausea or your blood glucose level is above 240 mg/dl. If ketones are present, continue to check for them every two to four hours until they are gone and your blood glucose level is below 240 mg/dl.

139. Never omit your diabetes pills or insulin when you are not feeling well, unless instructed to by your health-care provider.

WHAT IS DIABETES?

by Belinda O'Connell, M.S., R.D., C.D.E.,
and Laura Hieronymus, M.S.Ed., A.P.R.N.,
B.C.-A.D.M., C.D.E.

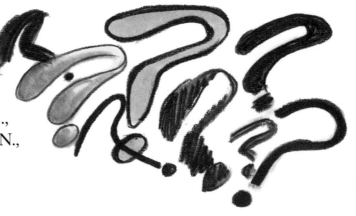

Most likely, you knew very little about diabetes before you learned that you had it. After your diagnosis, your next few doctor visits were probably a crash course in diabetes: learning how to check your blood glucose level, follow a schedule for taking pills, inject insulin and/or other diabetes medications (such as pramlintide or exenatide), adjust your eating habits, etc. Your doctor may also have mentioned what diabetes is and what causes it in this blitz of information, but with so much to learn at once, you may not remember what he said—or remember him saying anything at all on these topics.

It can be difficult to take in so much new information at one time, especially when you are just learning diabetes terminology and adjusting to the idea of having diabetes; many people find they miss a lot of the background information about the underlying causes of their diabetes. However, understanding how and why diabetes develops can help you to be an active member of your diabetes-care team.

The two main types

Diabetes mellitus, usually referred to as just diabetes, is characterized by a high blood glucose level. There are several different types of diabetes, each with a unique underlying cause. The most common forms are Type 1 diabetes and Type 2 diabetes. Both are considered chronic diseases, meaning that once diagnosed, they don't go away. Blood glucose levels that are higher than normal but not high enough to be diabetes are called prediabetes. For descriptions of other types of diabetes and related conditions, see "Types of Diabetes" on page 25.

Type 1 diabetes used to be called juvenile or insulin-dependent diabetes, and Type 2 diabetes was called adult-onset or non-insulin-dependent diabetes. The American Diabetes Association now favors the terms Type 1 and Type 2 diabetes, which are defined based on the underlying cause of the diabetes, not on a person's age at diagnosis or treatment method.

Type 1 diabetes

Type 1 diabetes occurs when the body's immune system launches an attack against the insulin-producing beta cells in the pancreas. Why the immune system does this is not completely understood, but it is thought that both genetics and some sort of environmental trigger are involved.

Certain combinations of genes make some people more likely to develop Type 1 diabetes, but having a genetic tendency alone is not enough: Not everyone at increased risk for Type 1 develops it. For instance, in identical twins (who by definition have the exact same genetic makeup), when one twin has Type 1 diabetes, the other twin also develops it only 50% of the time. It is believed that for a genetic tendency toward Type 1 to be "expressed," a person must be exposed to an environmental "trigger" that sets the autoimmune process in motion. Many potential triggers have been proposed, including viruses, bovine serum albumin (a protein in cow's milk), hormones, and environmental toxins, but none have been definitively proven to lead to Type 1 diabetes.

Once the process is set in motion, the immune system produces antibodies to beta cells and to insulin and begins to destroy them. (Under normal circumstances, antibodies seek out and flag harmful foreign substances within the body, such as bacteria or viruses, for destruction.) This process starts many years before diabetes is diagnosed. In fact, it's possible to identify people at risk of developing Type 1 diabetes by checking their blood for antibodies to beta cells and to insulin.

Over time, the quantity of insulin produced by the pancreas and the amount circulating in the bloodstream progressively decline. The resulting signs and symptoms of Type 1 diabetes, which include high blood glucose levels, weight loss, increased urination, hunger, and thirst, and large amounts of ketones in the blood and urine, generally occur only after a majority of the beta cells have been destroyed.

In the absence of insulin, glucose in the bloodstream cannot be transferred into cells as it normally would, resulting in high glucose levels in the bloodstream and a state of "starvation" within cells. The kidneys filter the excess glucose out of the blood, causing increased urination, thirst, and dehydration. Starving cells, no longer able to use glucose for energy, begin to use fat, resulting in loss of body fat and the production of ketones (chemical by-products of fat metabolism). If not treated (with insulin) in time, the combination of high blood glucose, high levels of ketones, and dehydration can lead to a very serious condition called diabetic ketoacidosis and, potentially, death.

Some people with Type 1 diabetes experience a "honeymoon" period after diagnosis, during which their pancreas regains the ability to produce insulin, and they require little or no injected insulin, but this generally lasts only a short time. Within a few months, most people have very little insulin-producing capacity and require an outside source of insulin.

Type 2 diabetes

Type 2 diabetes is much more common than Type 1 and has a stronger genetic link. (If one identical twin develops Type 2 diabetes, there is about a 90% chance that the other one will also.) Symptoms of high blood glucose are less pronounced in Type 2 diabetes compared to Type 1 diabetes; because of this, diagnosis often occurs many years after diabetes initially develops. However, the damage starts even in the absence of acute symptoms: Blood glucose levels above normal are known to increase a person's chances of eventually developing heart disease and other complications of diabetes.

Unlike Type 1 diabetes, Type 2 diabetes is not caused by an autoimmune attack. Instead, there are usually two underlying problems: insulin resistance and inadequate insulin production. Insulin resistance is when the cells of the body have a decreased response to insulin. Under normal circumstances, when blood glucose levels are high (after eating, for example), the pancreas releases insulin into the bloodstream. Insulin then interacts with muscle cells, fat cells, and other tissues, allowing them to transport glucose into the cells to be burned for energy or stored for use later.

In insulin resistance, these important messages do not get through. Remember playing "telephone" as a child, when one person would whis-

per a word to the person next to them, and that person would whisper what they heard to the next person, and so on down the line? By the time it got to the end of the line, the word had usually mutated to something completely unrecognizable. A similar breakdown in communication is thought to occur in insulin resistance, where the signal from insulin becomes garbled, and the cell does not respond normally, taking up much less glucose than normal.

When blood glucose levels remain high, the pancreas continues to secrete more insulin to compensate for its decreased effectiveness, and eventually, blood glucose returns to the normal range. Over time, however, the pancreas loses the ability to produce enough extra insulin to compensate for insulin's decreased effectiveness, and blood glucose levels remain high. At this point, a person might be diagnosed with diabetes or prediabetes, depending on his blood glucose level at the time of testing.

The liver also plays a key role in regulating blood glucose level. It releases glucose to the bloodstream when the blood glucose level is low, and it stores glucose when the level is high. When the blood glucose level is high, insulin has the important role of signaling the liver to turn off glucose production and start storing extra glucose. But if a person is insulin resistant, the liver does not respond normally to insulin, so it continues to release glucose to the bloodstream even if the blood glucose level is already elevated, making it even higher.

Treating Type 2 diabetes

Treating Type 2 diabetes involves treating both underlying problems (insulin resistance and inadequate insulin production). An individual's treatment may change over time as his degree of insulin resistance or ability to produce insulin changes. Many people still make a fair amount of insulin when they are initially diagnosed with Type 2 diabetes, so their treatment may focus mainly on decreasing insulin resistance. Ways to decrease insulin resistance include increasing physical activity, following a healthy meal plan, and losing weight (even losing as little as 10 pounds can make a difference, resulting in improvement in blood glucose levels). Certain drugs are also targeted to treat insulin resistance. Metformin (brand name Glucophage) decreases the amount of glucose made by the liver, and pioglitazone (Actos) and rosiglitazone (Avandia) make fat and muscle tissues more sensitive to insulin.

Other drugs address insulin deficiency by stimu-

TYPES OF DIABETES

Diabetes is not a single disease. It is a group of conditions that share the same primary symptom—consistently high blood glucose levels—but for different reasons. In the past, forms of diabetes were classified by the age at which it developed (juvenile or adult) or by the method of treatment (insulin or no insulin), but many cases of diabetes do not fall neatly into one of these categories. In 1997, the American Diabetes Association began to define diabetes based on its pathophysiology, or underlying cause. In 2003, modifications were made regarding the diagnosis of impaired fasting glucose. Diabetes classification includes four clinical classes:

Type 1 diabetes. The vast majority of cases of Type 1 diabetes are caused by the autoimmune destruction of pancreatic beta cells, which results in an inability to produce insulin and severe insulin deficiency. It is characterized by the rapid onset of symptoms, which include weight loss and increased thirst, urination, and hunger. A person's blood glucose level is often very high at diagnosis. Type 1 diabetes can occur at any age but is most commonly diagnosed in children and adolescents.

Type 2 diabetes. The two main underlying disorders in Type 2 diabetes are insulin resistance and relative insulin deficiency. It is believed that insulin resistance often occurs first, followed by declines in pancreatic function and insulin production. Type 2 diabetes can occur at any age, and cases of Type 2 in children continue to increase dramatically.

Prediabetes. This is a term for an intermediate state of glucose intolerance, where blood glucose level is higher than normal yet below the threshold for a diagnosis of diabetes. People who have prediabetes have a high risk of developing Type 2 diabetes in the future. Depending on how a person's blood glucose level is measured, prediabetes is sometimes called impaired glucose tolerance or impaired fasting glucose.

Syndrome X. Also known as insulin resistance syndrome or metabolic syndrome, this condition is associated with an increased risk of cardiovascular disease and diabetes. It consists of a group of symptoms, including insulin resistance, increased blood insulin levels, glucose intolerance, obesity, high blood pressure, and dyslipidemia, specifically low HDL ("good") cholesterol levels and high triglyceride levels. Diagnosis generally requires the presence of three of these symptoms or evidence of insulin resistance and two additional symptoms.

Gestational diabetes. High blood glucose that first occurs during pregnancy is called gestational diabetes. In most cases, blood glucose levels return to normal after delivery, but women who have had gestational diabetes are more likely to develop diabetes later in life.

MODY (Maturity Onset Diabetes of Youth). These relatively rare forms of diabetes, usually diagnosed in people under 25, are caused by genetic defects in beta-cell function.

Drug-induced diabetes. Several drugs and chemicals can cause glucose intolerance and diabetes. These include nicotinic acid (used to lower high triglycerides and raise HDL cholesterol), glucocorticoids (such as prednisone), thyroid hormone, thiazides (a type of blood pressure medicines), dilantin (an antiseizure drug), and beta-adrenergic agonists (used to treat asthma).

Genetic diseases. Several genetic diseases are associated with increased rates of diabetes, including Down syndrome. There also specific genetic defects in beta-cell function and insulin action that result in diabetes.

Infections and other diseases. Examples of diseases and disorders that can damage the pancreas and lead to diabetes include pancreatitis (inflammation of the pancreas), cystic fibrosis, and hemochromatosis (a genetic condition in which iron accumulates in the body). In addition, diseases that disturb levels of hormones such as growth hormone, thyroid hormone, or glucagon can cause insulin resistance or increased glucose production by the liver and potentially diabetes.

lating the pancreas to release more insulin or by slowing the digestion of carbohydrate in foods. Using one or more of these medicines and keeping carbohydrate intake moderate and spread out over the day can help the pancreas keep up with insulin needs. Ultimately, however, it is not unusual for many people with Type 2 diabetes to eventually need to take insulin injections to supply their bodies with enough insulin.

Many people with Type 2 diabetes see the progression to using insulin as a negative reflection on their ability to follow their meal plan, lose weight, or otherwise take care of their diabetes. But while there are always additional steps anyone could take to further improve their health, for most people, the need to use insulin to control their diabetes does not mean they lack willpower or the desire to take good care of their diabetes. It is simply a matter of disease progression and the decreased ability of their pancreas to continue producing supernormal levels of insulin. When the pancreas becomes less able to produce insulin, it also becomes less able to produce the hormone amylin. In some cases, you may need to take a drug called pramilintide, which is a synthetic form of this hormone, to help balance your blood glucose control.

Not just blood glucose

Diabetes is diagnosed based on blood glucose level, and keeping your blood glucose level in a near-normal range has been shown to prevent common complications of diabetes such as eye disease, kidney disease, and nerve disease. But blood glucose level is not the only concern in diabetes. High blood pressure and high blood fats (such as cholesterol and triglycerides) often occur along with high blood glucose and can also lead to complications, including heart disease. All of these concerns—blood glucose, blood pressure, and blood fats—should be addressed in a comprehensive diabetes treatment plan for good health today and to prevent diabetes-related complications down the road. □

WHAT YOU SHOULD KNOW ABOUT CELIAC DISEASE

by Judy Giusti, M.S., R.D., L.D., C.D.E.

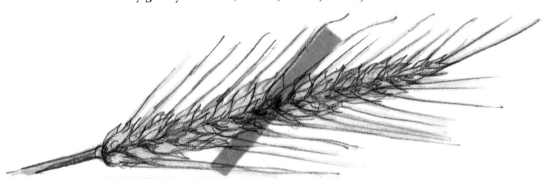

After years of living with Type 1 diabetes, you're a pro at counting carbohydrates and adjusting insulin doses. Over the past year, however, your diabetes has become difficult to control. You've experienced weight loss, frequent bouts of diarrhea, and fatigue. You've also had fluctuating blood glucose levels—both hypoglycemia and hyperglycemia—and needed frequent insulin adjustments. You don't know what's wrong, and what's worse, your doctor—make that doctors—can't explain your symptoms, either. They've suggested everything from irritable bowel disease to depression, but nothing seems to help.

Then one day, a friend mentions that a colleague of hers has a daughter who has Type 1 diabetes and celiac disease, or intolerance to gluten.

Her symptoms were similar to yours until her doctor put her on a special, gluten-free diet. Now she's fine—as long as she doesn't eat the wrong foods.

You've never heard of celiac disease before, but you're curious. What is this disease and what causes it? What foods are off-limits? Which are OK to eat? Most of all, how would giving up all gluten-containing foods affect your life and your diabetes control? Before you make another appointment with your doctor, you decide to do some research of your own.

What is celiac disease?

Celiac disease, sometimes called celiac sprue or gluten-sensitive enteropathy, is a hereditary, autoimmune disease in which the body launches

CARBOHYDRATE CONTENT
OF SELECTED GLUTEN-FREE FOODS

FOOD	SERVING SIZE	CARBOHYDRATE (grams)
Arrowroot flour	½ cup	57
Cornstarch	2 tablespoons	15
Cream of Rice cereal	½ cup, cooked	14
Grits	1 package, instant (137 grams)	20
Ground flaxseed	2 tablespoons	4
Millet flour	2 tablespoons	13
Potato flour	2 tablespoons	13
Potato starch	2 tablespoons	16
Puffed Rice cereal	1 cup	13
Brown rice	½ cup cooked	23
Rice flour, white	½ cup	63
White rice, long grain	½ cup cooked	22
White rice, medium grain	½ cup cooked	27
Corn taco shell	2 shells	14
Corn tortilla, medium	1	11
Rice bran bread	1 slice	12
White rice bread	1 slice	15
Corn pasta	½ cup cooked	16

an immune reaction when a person consumes gluten, a type of protein found in wheat, rye, barley, and possibly oats. For reasons still unknown to researchers, when people with celiac disease eat foods containing gluten, the immune system sees it as a toxin and launches an attack to prevent its absorption into the bloodstream. The effect of the attack is a flattening of the villi, the small, finger-like projections on the lining of the small intestine through which nutrients are absorbed. This leaves the intestinal surface smooth, with less surface area for absorbing nutrients. In addition, when the villi flatten out, the digestive enzymes normally present on the villi are destroyed, so food passes through the gut unabsorbed.

Common symptoms of malabsorption include gas, bloating, diarrhea, and weight loss. Other symptoms may include fatigue, anemia, irritability, or depression. In many cases of undiagnosed celiac disease, however, there are no symptoms at all.

Malabsorption of nutrients can create serious deficiencies of the fat-soluble vitamins A, D, E, and K; of folate and vitamin B_{12}, as well as of iron and calcium. In children, this can lead to delayed growth or short stature as well as delayed puberty. Long-term complications of untreated celiac disease include osteoporosis, fertility problems, and benign or malignant tumors of the small intestine. Vitamin and mineral supplements are an essential part of treatment when the intestinal damage, or villous atrophy, is first recognized.

Another autoimmune disease caused by gluten intolerance is dermatitis herpetiformis, which mainly involves the skin. A severe, itchy, blistering

MANUFACTURERS AND RETAILERS OF GLUTEN-FREE PRODUCTS

The companies listed here make and sell gluten-free foods. Orders can be placed online, by phone, or in some cases by mail. In addition, products made by Authentic Foods, Ener-G Foods, Gluten-Free Pantry, and Gillian's Foods are sold in select retail stores.

AUTHENTIC FOODS
1850 W. 169th Street, Suite B
Gardena, CA 90247
(310) 366-7612
www.authenticfoods.com

ENER-G FOODS, INC.
5960 First Avenue South
P.O. Box 84487
Seattle, WA 98124-5787
(800) 331-5222
www.ener-g.com

THE GLUTEN-FREE PANTRY
P.O. Box 840
Glastonbury, CT 06033
(800) 291-8386
www.glutenfree.com

ALLERGY GROCER
91 Western Maryland Parkway, Suite 7
Hagerstown, MD 21740
(800) 891-0083
www.allergygrocer.com

GILLIAN'S FOODS, INC.
82 Sanderson Avenue
Lynn, MA 01902
(781) 586-0086
www.gilliansfoods.com

skin rash shows up, usually on the elbows, knees, buttocks, and back; in severe cases, the rash can be on any skin surface. Dermatitis herpetiformis is diagnosed by a skin biopsy, but if an intestinal biopsy is also performed, damage to the villi is usually found, although to a lesser degree than that which occurs in celiac disease. Usually, there are no digestive symptoms of dermatitis herpetiformis, but it is treated with a gluten-free diet as well as with medication for the rash.

Celiac disease can be more difficult to diagnose than dermatitis herpetiformis because its symptoms often mimic other digestive diseases such as irritable bowel disease, Crohn's disease, ulcerative colitis, and intestinal infections. Complicating the matter is the fact that people with untreated celiac disease often develop lactose intolerance (the symptoms of which also include gas, bloating, and diarrhea) because of the damage to the intestinal villi. Lactose, the sugar in milk and other dairy products, is digested by the enzyme lactase, which is located on the villi. Usually, lactose intolerance disappears within about 2 to 12 months of starting a gluten-free diet. In some cases, however, a person remains lactose intolerant and must continue to avoid dairy products as well as gluten.

Once diagnosed, the only treatment of celiac disease is lifelong, complete elimination of gluten-containing foods from the diet. With gluten elimination, symptoms may disappear within a few days, but complete healing of the small intestine may take three to six months or, in some cases, up to two years. Eating even a small amount of gluten can make a person sick again. In a small percentage of people, a gluten-free diet does not improve symptoms; these people may need to be treated with steroids or immunosuppressive drugs.

Who gets this disease?

Celiac disease commonly shows up in children, but it has been diagnosed in people of all ages, mainly because not everyone with celiac disease experiences symptoms right away. In studies from several countries, including Scotland, England, the United States, and Canada, almost 50% of those with a new diagnosis of celiac disease did not experience symptoms. Several factors may influence the onset of symptoms in those genetically predisposed to the disease. It is believed that the longer an infant is breast-fed, the later the symptoms of celiac disease appear. (However, it is not known if breast-feeding can prevent celiac disease.) The age at which a person began eating gluten and how much gluten he consumes may also affect the onset of celiac disease. A bacterial or viral infection or the stress caused by pregnancy or surgery may trigger symptoms in susceptible individuals.

Since celiac disease is an inherited disease, all first-degree family members—parents, siblings, and children—of people with celiac disease should be screened. About 10% to 15% of first-degree family members will also have celiac disease. In addition, celiac disease often occurs in those with another autoimmune disorder, such as

NATIONAL SUPPORT GROUPS

Joining a support group can help you adjust to a gluten-free diet and give you the satisfaction of knowing you are contributing to celiac disease research. Benefits of membership may include newsletters, recipes, online message boards, updates from food manufacturers, and referrals to health-care professionals in your area. You do not have to be a member to access information from most groups' Web sites, and most also offer free pamphlets that can be ordered by phone or via the Internet.

CELIAC SPRUE ASSOCIATION (CSA)/
USA, Inc.
P.O. Box 31700
Omaha, NE 68131-0700
(402) 558-0600
www.csaceliacs.org
The Celiac Sprue Association has a network of over 100 chapters in the United States that provide educational services to people with celiac disease and their families. Membership costs $33 for the first year ($25 thereafter) and includes a copy of the group's newsletter, *Lifeline,* as well as several informational pamphlets. Some recipes and information sheets are posted on the Web site; additional pamphlets, videotapes, audiotapes, and cookbooks can be ordered online or by telephone.

CELIAC DISEASE FOUNDATION
13251 Ventura Boulevard, Suite 1
Studio City, CA, 91604-1838
(818) 990-2354
www.celiac.org
The Celiac Disease Foundation Web site offers general information about celiac disease, contact information for support groups throughout the United States, a list of recommended books, and news on both research and advocacy. Bene-

fits of the $35 annual membership fee include a quarterly newsletter and a handbook, Guidelines for a Gluten-Free Lifestyle.

GLUTEN INTOLERANCE GROUP OF
NORTH AMERICA
31214 124th Avenue SE
Auburn, WA 98092-3667
(253) 833-6655
www.gluten.net
This nonprofit organization has branches in several states and holds an annual education conference. Its Web site offers information about celiac disease and dermatitis herpetiformis, a recipe exchange, and several products including cookbooks for purchase. The group also hosts two summer camps for kids with gluten intolerance. Membership is $35 annually and includes a quarterly newsmagazine.

CANADIAN CELIAC ASSOCIATION
5170 Dixie Road, Suite 204
Mississauga, Ontario L4W 1E3
(905) 507-6208
(800) 363-7296
www.celiac.ca
The Web site offers basic information on celiac disease, dermatitis herpetiformis, and the essentials of a gluten-free diet. It also posts up-to-date alerts about Canadian foods found to contain gluten and provides links to the Canadian Food Inspection Agency and to Canadian and U.S. food manufacturers and celiac disease organizations. Select articles from *Celiac News,* a newsletter published three times a year, are posted on the Web site, and books, cookbooks, and pamphlets can be ordered by mail through a printable order form. Members get discounted prices on resource materials.

Type 1 diabetes, thyroid disease, Sjögren syndrome, rheumatoid arthritis, and Addison disease. Celiac disease is found in 5% to 7% of people who have Type 1 diabetes; some researchers recommend that all children with Type 1 diabetes be screened for celiac disease.

Women are about twice as likely to have celiac disease as men, and the disease is most common in people of European descent (the incidence is particularly high in Scandinavian countries, Italy,

and Ireland). It is less common in those of African or Asian heritage. In countries where there is greater awareness of the disease, there is increased diagnosis. In Central Europe, 1 in 200 people has celiac disease. In Italy, every child is screened for celiac disease by age six; approximately 1 in 250 Italians has the disease. In the United States, celiac disease is largely unrecognized and underdiagnosed. While only about 1 in 4,700 Americans is diagnosed with the disease, a recent study suggests

FOR FURTHER READING AND INFORMATION

The following books, cookbooks, newsletters, and Web sites offer additional information on celiac disease and living without gluten.

COOKBOOKS AND RESOURCE GUIDES

THE GLUTEN-FREE BIBLE
The Thoroughly Indispensible Guide to Negotiating Life Without Wheat
Jax Peters Lowell
Henry Holt and Company
New York, 2005

WHEAT-FREE, GLUTEN-FREE
200 Delicious Dishes to Make Eating a Pleasure
Michelle Berriedale-Johnson
Surrey Books
Chicago, 2002

GLUTEN-FREE DIET
A Comprehensive Resource Guide
Shelley Case
Case Nutrition Consulting
Regina, Saskatchewan, Canada 2002
Purchase via the Internet at www.glutenfreediet.ca, by calling (306) 751-1000, or by writing to Case Nutrition Consulting, 1940 Angley Court, Regina, SK S4V 2V2, Canada. *Gluten-Free Diet* is also available from online booksellers such as www.amazon.com.

THE GLUTEN-FREE GOURMET
Living Well Without Wheat
Bette Hagman
Henry Holt and Company, Owl Books
New York, 2000

THE GLUTEN-FREE GOURMET
BAKES BREAD
Bette Hagman
Henry Holt and Company, Owl Books
New York, 1999

THE GLUTEN-FREE GOURMET
COOKS FAST AND HEALTHY
Bette Hagman
Henry Holt and Company, Owl Books
New York, 2000

THE GLUTEN-FREE GOURMET
MAKES DESSERT
Bette Hagman
Henry Holt and Company
New York, 2002

WHEAT-FREE RECIPES AND MENUS
Delicious Dining Without Wheat or Gluten
Carol Fenster, Ph.D.
Savory Palate, Inc.
Centennial, Colorado, 2000

NEWSLETTERS AND INTERNET RESOURCES

CELIAC DISEASE FACT SHEET
National Digestive Diseases Information Clearinghouse
2 Information Way
Bethesda, MD 20892-3570
www.niddk.nih.gov/health/digest/pubs/celiac/index.htm

CELIAC.COM
Celiac Disease and Gluten-Free Diet Support Page
www.celiac.com
Started by an individual with celiac disease, this Web site offers online information sheets, articles, and studies on celiac disease. The site also has a section for frequently asked questions, recipes, and lists of safe and unsafe foods for people with celiac disease. For a subscription fee of $24.95, visitors can have online access to a quarterly newsletter, *Scott-Free Newsletter.* The cost to receive the print edition is $29.95.

---

that as many as 1 in 250 Americans may have undiagnosed celiac disease. Underdiagnosis of celiac disease is a serious concern, because the risk of long-term complications increases the longer it goes untreated.

Diagnosis

Several blood tests have been developed that can be used to screen people who are at risk for celiac disease. The tests detect the presence of certain *antibodies* that occur in higher numbers in the blood of people with celiac disease. Antibodies are produced by the body to recognize and fight off antigens or toxins. In people with celiac disease, there are elevated amounts of antigliadin, antiendomysium, and antireticulum antibodies. Recently, a blood test for the antibody to tissue transglutaminase (the specific part of endomysium to which the antibody reacts) was developed that is highly sensitive and accurate about 95% of the time,

CELIAC SPRUE RESEARCH FOUNDATION
www.celiacsprue.org
The mission of this California-based organization is to develop a pharmacological treatment for celiac disease. Members of the group's Scientific Advisory Board help evaluate, prioritize, and raise money for key drug development projects. The Web site offers information on current areas of research interest.

GLUTEN-FREE INFOWEB
www.glutenfreeinfo.com
The authors of this Web site maintain a list of food manufacturers who sell gluten-free products, including the date and content of manufacturers' letters responding to consumer inquiries about products. An extensive list of brand-name, gluten-free products by food type is also available, as are an online bookstore and links to state and national celiac disease support groups.

GLUTEN-FREE LIVING
www.glutenfreeliving.com
(914) 231-6361
A subscription to this quarterly magazine for people with celiac disease is $29 a year or $49 for two years. Subscribe online or over the phone.

UNIVERSITY OF MARYLAND CENTER FOR CELIAC RESEARCH
www.celiaccenter.org
The research center's Web site offers fact sheets, scientific articles, and updates on celiac disease research. The group sponsors a yearly fund-raiser walk in locations nationwide and participates in an annual international symposium for celiac disease researchers. Site users can find information about participating in trials for celiac disease research in their area.

making it helpful for screening at-risk groups. However, the gold standard for confirming a diagnosis of celiac disease if preliminary blood tests are positive is still an intestinal biopsy, in which a long, thin tube called an endoscope is threaded through the mouth and stomach to the small intestine to take a small tissue sample. If the biopsy reveals villous atrophy, a diagnosis of celiac disease is established. If your doctor suspects celiac disease, you should continue to eat gluten-containing foods until after the biopsy. It is much more difficult to diagnosis celiac disease if gluten has been removed from the diet and healing has already started.

Treatment

The only treatment for celiac disease is a lifelong, 100% gluten-free diet. Foods that contain gluten are any derivative or variation of wheat, rye, or barley, including bulgur, couscous, triticale, spelt, einkorn, farina, graham flour, semolina, and durum wheat. Until recently, people with celiac disease were told they could not eat oats, but some studies show that oats are not toxic to most people with celiac disease. However, since there is still a debate over this (and there is a strong possibility of gluten from other grains contaminating oats during harvesting, milling, or processing), it is probably best that people with celiac disease not consume oats.

Obvious foods to avoid on a gluten-free diet are most pizzas, breads, bagels, crackers, cookies, cakes, pies, gravies, and flour-based sauces. But there are many less obvious sources of gluten. Communion wafers contain gluten; cooking sprays may contain grain alcohol; malt and malt flavoring, found in cereals, syrups, and beer, are usually made from barley (although some malt products are made from corn). Many licorice candies contain gluten. For this reason, it is very important to read the ingredients list on the label of every food product you purchase and to scrutinize the fine print right down to the food colorings, seasonings, preservatives, and thickeners, many of which contain gluten.

Reading the label may not be enough, however, since some sources of gluten may not be listed on the label. Gum wrappers, for instance, are sometimes dusted with flour to prevent sticking. What's more, manufacturers sometimes change the way a product is made. Food that was gluten-free last month may have different ingredients this month. The only way to be sure about a product is to call or write the manufacturer. The manufacturer's name, address, and telephone number appear on the food label. When calling a manufacturer, have the lot number of the food in question available. Many manufacturers also provide lists of their gluten-free foods.

After a while, you will learn to recognize suspect foods and ingredients, but a general rule of thumb is, "If you don't know what's in it, don't eat it." In the United States, at least, the word "starch" on a food label indicates cornstarch, which is safe to eat. "Modified food starch" or "modified starch," on the other hand, could be made from corn, arrowroot, tapioca, or wheat. Hydrolyzed vegetable protein, textured vegetable protein, or hydrolyzed plant protein is usually made from wheat or wheat mixed with soy or corn. Vanilla and other flavoring extracts, prebasted turkeys, canned and dried soups, sauces, gravies, luncheon meats, caramel coloring, and soy sauce made from fermented wheat can all contain sources of gluten. Gluten is even used in nonfood items, such as some medicines, toothpastes, mouthwashes, and the glues on mailing labels and envelopes. Ask your pharmacist if any of your medicines contain gluten. Again, calling the manufacturer of a product to ask if it is totally gluten-free is a good habit to get into.

What to eat

By now you are wondering if there is anything that people with celiac disease *can* eat. Plain meats, fruits, vegetables, and most dairy products are all gluten-free, as long as they have not been breaded or cooked in the same pan with food that has been breaded. Likewise, corn, grits (made from corn), rice, potatoes, arrowroot, tapioca, beans, nuts, most soy products (except soy sauce), flaxseed, buckwheat (which is not actually a cereal but the seed of a flowering plant), sorghum, amaranth, quinoa, millet, and teff can be included in your meal plan. Packaged gluten-free cakes, cookies, waffles, pancakes, and pizza crust, as well as a wide variety of gluten-free baking mixes are available from specialty stores, some mainstream grocery stores, or from online or mail-order food companies. There are also bean, rice, and nut flours, which can be substituted in recipes that call for wheat flour. Mixing two or more types of flours when substituting for wheat flour gives the product a better texture. A gluten-free cookbook will give you tips for mixing flours and making conversions. These flours should be kept tightly sealed and stored in the refrigerator to prevent rancidity.

Since even a small amount of wheat, rye, or barley can set off a reaction, it's important to keep foods strictly segregated in households where those who don't have celiac disease consume those grains. If anyone in the household uses wheat flour in cooking or baking, be aware that it can remain in the air for up to 24 hours. It can also remain on hands that are not washed thoroughly. Cooking utensils that have touched foods containing gluten must be cleaned carefully before preparing gluten-free food. Difficult-to-clean items such as a flour sifter should not be used to sift both wheat flour and gluten-free flour.

Even using a toaster that has crumbs from a piece of wheat bread can contaminate gluten-free bread.

When ordering fried food in a restaurant, be sure to ask whether any foods that have a breaded coating have been cooked in the oil your food will be cooked in. Request that your food be cooked in a separate pan to be on the safe side.

There are several national organizations that provide information on celiac disease and foods to eat or avoid. A list of these organizations is provided on page 29. Joining a celiac support group in your area can provide you with emotional support, up-to-date information, and new meal ideas. Gluten-free cookbooks can help you find tasty recipes and provide you with tips on how to substitute gluten-free products in your favorite dishes.

Celiac disease with Type 1 diabetes

In people with Type 1 diabetes, malabsorption of nutrients from undiagnosed celiac disease can lead to frequent, unexplained low or high blood glucose readings. Insulin needs are frequently lower during the time before diagnosis. Once treatment of celiac disease has begun and nutrients are better absorbed, insulin doses may need to be adjusted. Treating celiac disease should make it easier to keep diabetes under control. A study published in the July 2002 issue of the journal *Diabetes Care* found that in children with Type 1 diabetes and celiac disease, 12 months of a gluten-free diet not only improved their growth but led to a significant reduction in HbA_{1c} level (indicating improved blood glucose control).

For people with diabetes and celiac disease, starting a gluten-free diet requires learning the carbohydrate content of new, gluten-free foods, so they can be introduced into a meal plan or so that insulin doses can be adjusted accordingly. In basic carbohydrate counting, one serving of carbohydrate is 15 grams of carbohydrate. For those who adjust their insulin doses based on the amount of carbohydrate they eat, it is important to know exactly how many grams of carbohydrate are in a serving of food. A registered dietitian can help you figure this out and make adjustments to your meal plan or insulin regime.

Nutrition software programs can also help you analyze foods and recipes for carbohydrate content per serving. The United States Department of Agriculture's nutrition Web site (www.nutrition.gov) is a good source of nutrition information. There are also books on carbohydrate counting that may be helpful. Don't forget to check the serving size on food labels and to assess how many servings you are actually eating. Since fiber is not digested or absorbed, you can subtract the grams of fiber from the total carbohydrate on the label if there are more than 5 grams of fiber per serving. When substituting new, gluten-free ingredients into your favorite recipes, add up the carbohydrate grams in each ingredient and divide by the number of servings the recipe yields. Write this information on your recipe cards so you will only have to do these calculations once.

Straying from a gluten-free diet—even just a little bit—can trigger the immune system reaction that damages your intestines, whether or not you experience symptoms. Just as adjusting to diabetes requires changing eating patterns and lifestyle habits, learning to prepare and enjoy gluten-free foods—and avoid gluten—can be a challenge at first, but it doesn't have to mean a lifetime of tasteless meals. The variety and availability of gluten-free foods is greater now than ever before, and food manufacturers and even restaurants are becoming increasingly sensitive to the needs of people with food intolerances. Moreover, omitting gluten may introduce you to a rich variety of "alternative" grains, nuts, and seeds that are not only flavorful, but also rich in vitamins, minerals, protein, and fiber. In the end, better health, higher energy, and improved blood glucose control are worth the effort of adjusting to your new meal plan. □

SICK-DAY SUPPLIES
Make Sure You're Prepared

by Margaret J. Hofacker,
R.N., B.S.N., C.D.E.

We all know how annoying it is to run out of tissues just as we come down with a cold or to find the box of throat lozenges empty when we have a sore throat. But these are minor inconveniences compared to discovering you're out of test strips, diabetes pills, insulin, or any of your other daily diabetes supplies when an illness or injury sets in. Not only are there no simple substitutions for your diabetes supplies—like paper towels instead of tissues or gargling with salt water or sipping tea instead of sucking on a lozenge—but there may be no more important time to check your blood glucose regularly and to have what you need to lower your blood glucose level than when you're ill.

Any illness, whether physical or emotional, can cause the body to release stress hormones, such as epinephrine, norepinephrine, cortisol, growth hormone, and glucagon. Stress hormones can be released if you have a headache, a virus, or a toothache; are recovering from a surgical procedure; or are experiencing anxiety or depression. The release of stress hormones helps to provide the body with the extra energy it needs to heal itself by stimulating the liver to release extra glucose into the bloodstream. This is normally a good thing, but we all know that too much of a good thing is often not a good thing.

In people who do not have diabetes, the pancreas can compensate for the extra glucose released by the liver by releasing more insulin into the bloodstream. In people who have diabetes, however, either the pancreas does not produce enough (or any) insulin or the insulin released cannot work effectively to open the cells up to accept glucose. The stress hormones themselves also counter the effects of insulin. The resulting high blood sugar level can lead to increased urination, which could lead to dehydration and imbalances of fluids and *electrolytes* (substances in the body that regulate the balance of water and chemicals). Diarrhea and vomiting can also lead to dehydration with fluid and electrolyte imbalances. When you have diabetes, very high blood sugar or dehydration (and particularly the two together) can turn into an emergency situation requiring hospitalization.

Although minor illnesses can turn serious more quickly and more easily in a person with diabetes, there are steps you can take to lower your chances of this happening. Keeping your blood sugar under control is one of the most important of these steps, and that means having the necessary supplies on hand when you need them. The best time to gather those supplies is, of course, while you're feeling well, and the best place to store them may be all together in one container or special place in your home. Some people call that container or place their "sick-day box."

What does a sick-day box look like? It can be an actual box or it can simply be a drawer or cabinet. Whatever you choose, remember that the whole idea behind a sick-day box is to have all of your sick-day supplies together in a place you can easily reach for when you do not feel like moving or cannot move very far. A sturdy, plastic, airtight container with a snap-on lid, which can be easily stored under a bed or in a nightstand or closet, works well. Before buying a box, read through this article, develop a sick-day plan with your diabetes team, and gather your supplies so you can better estimate the box size you'll need.

Work with your health-care team to personalize your sick-day box to cover all your health needs. For example, high blood pressure, which is quite common in people with diabetes, may require a person to pack low-sodium versions of the recommended food supplies in their box. The following supplies are recommendations that may come in handy, especially for people who live alone and those without access to a pharmacy that delivers.

The basics

Every person with diabetes should have individualized sick-day guidelines provided by or developed with the help of his health-care team before an illness occurs. (If your health-care provider has not given you written instructions to follow during an illness, ask about it at your next appointment.) These instructions could include the frequency, types, and amounts of fluids to drink; the amounts and types of foods to eat and when to eat them; how frequently to monitor your blood sugar level; how frequently to do ketone testing; when to call your health-care provider;

when to hold or alter the doses of your oral or injectable diabetes medicines; and when to go to the hospital. Even if you have sick-day guidelines, never hesitate to call your health-care provider if you are unsure of what to do.

Because illness can result in the release of stress hormones that raise blood sugar levels, people usually are told not to omit any diabetes medicine doses during an illness. In fact, there may be times when those who do not normally inject insulin will be asked to do so to help control their blood sugar. Your guidelines may include a *sliding scale,* instructions for administering Regular or rapid-acting insulin (aspart [NovoLog], lispro [Humalog], or glulisine [Apidra]) based on specific ranges of your blood glucose level, or they may include an *algorithm* (a formula) to help you figure out how much to increase or decrease your insulin doses.

Because your guidelines are specific for you, your set of instructions might say to go straight to the hospital if your blood sugar rises above a certain level, while someone else's may say to alter his insulin doses first. As your diabetes knowledge and expertise increases, your sick-day guidelines may change. Be sure to evaluate them periodically and change them as needed. In addition to a written sick-day plan, the following items are also useful to have on hand:

List of important telephone numbers. Rather than having to flip through a phone book or address book, keep a list of names and important telephone numbers on a single page or file card in your sick-day box. Some names and phone numbers you may want at your fingertips include those for your health-care provider, pharmacy, insulin pump manufacturer, podiatrist, dentist, hospital, local emergency services, police, medical insurance company, relatives or friends you can call on for help, a local certified home health agency, volunteer community services, and your church or synagogue.

Pen and paper. A pen and pad of paper are among the most important items in your sick-day box. They can be used for writing down information to report to your health-care provider and for writing down information given by your health-care provider.

Thermometer. Every sick-day box should have a thermometer to check for fever.

Tissues. These can wipe away nasal drips, blood from your monitoring sites, and any other type of drain-age.

Plastic bags. These can be used to dispose of tissues, used supplies, and vomit, as well as to store items for later use.

Hand sanitizer. This is a great item to have at your fingertips for those times when you are too weak, ill, or tired to get up to wash your hands. It will help prevent the spread of germs (bacterial and/or viral) to others.

Alarm clock or timer. When you are ill, your sick-day plan may require you to monitor ketones or take fluids on a regular schedule—possibly as often as every hour or two. But when you are feeling ill, you might be doing a lot of sleeping. You can set your alarm clock or timer to wake you up to check your blood sugar, inject your insulin, check your temperature, take your medicine, eat or drink fluids, or make any necessary phone calls.

An 8-ounce measuring cup. When you are sick, it is recommended that you drink 8 ounces (one cup) of liquid each hour. That amount is needed to help prevent dehydration, which could lead to an emergency hospitalization. An 8-ounce measuring cup can help to ensure you drink what you need.

Can opener. If you're unlucky enough to get sick during an electrical failure, a manual can opener can come in handy.

Food

When you are sick, you may not have much of an appetite. But to fight any infection or heal any wound, it is very important that you not only eat, but that you make nutritious food choices. The following items are all easily stored and can last a long time in your sick-day box, so consider including them in it.

Easily tolerated carbohydrates. These provide calories and energy and can help to prevent hypoglycemia. Examples are cooked cereal, powdered milk or milk shake mix, crackers, a jar of applesauce, and a can of creamed soup. Some of these items can be purchased sodium-free if you are on a salt-restricted diet.

Protein-rich foods. Protein is broken down in the digestive tract to its component *amino acids,* which the body's cells use to build and maintain tissues. When a person is sick, especially if there is not enough insulin to control blood sugar levels, the body breaks down stored fats and eventually even the stored protein in the muscles for energy. Easily stored protein-rich foods include prepackaged cheese and crackers, peanut butter, powdered milk, canned tuna, canned lentil soup, and vacuum-packed seeds and nuts.

Liquids

A vital part of your supplies, liquids are needed primarily to prevent dehydration, replacing fluids lost during breathing, perspiration, fever, vomiting, diarrhea, and excessive urination. Stocking a variety of types can help you prepare for a range of blood sugar levels. In general, liquids should be caffeine-free, because caffeine can raise blood sugar and upset your stomach.

Carbohydrate-containing liquids. These are necessary to provide calories and energy, particularly if you can't eat solid food, while helping you combat and prevent dehydration and hypoglycemia. Examples include regular soft drinks, boxes of regular gelatin, and boxed juices. Care should be taken not to drink too much, however, because these fluids can raise your blood sugar higher than desired.

Calorie-free liquids. Because sugary products can increase blood sugar, you also need to include carbohydrate-free products to prevent dehydration without raising blood sugar. So include items such as bottled water, diet soda, a can of broth, a box of sugar-free gelatin, packets or boxes of powdered sugar- free drinks, and decaffeinated tea and coffee bags.

Sports drinks, canned clear soups, and bouillon cubes. These can provide sodium and electrolytes and help prevent dehydration.

Medicines

Having an up-to-date list of your current medicines and doses can be very helpful. If you need to call your health-care provider or go to the hospital, you are likely to be asked for the names of your current medicines and their doses. When you are stressed or feeling ill, you can easily forget such information. Having such a list can also be a big help to your family members in case they need to speak on your behalf. Be sure to write down nonprescription medicines, vitamins, and supplements as well as prescription drugs.

Some drugs to keep in your sick-day box include the following (but check first with your health-care provider to determine which are the best choices for you):

Nonsteroidal pain and fever relievers. Medicines such as acetaminophen, ibuprofen, and aspirin are all good choices for your sick-day box. (If you are preparing a sick-day box for a child with diabetes, do not include aspirin. Aspirin should not be given to anyone under the age of 21 during a fever or viral illness because it increases the risk of a serious condition called Reye syndrome.)

Sugar-free cough drops, syrups, and throat lozenges. Depending on your choice, these can reduce coughing, decrease throat irritation, help rid your lungs of mucus, and help you breathe better, while not raising blood sugar.

SICK-DAY GUIDELINES

Each person with diabetes should have a set of guidelines, developed with the help of his health-care provider, for managing his diabetes during an illness. If you do not already have a set of sick-day guidelines, you can make a copy of these and ask your health-care provider to personalize them for you.

TRACKING YOUR HEALTH
■ Set your alarm to wake or alert you every 2–4 hours, so you can do any necessary blood glucose monitoring, ketone testing, or drinking of fluids.
■ Write down the date and time of symptoms and the results of all blood glucose monitoring and ketone tests.

BLOOD GLUCOSE MONITORING
■ Check blood glucose levels at least four times per day (at your usual mealtimes and bedtime).
■ Check more frequently when your results are higher than 240 mg/dl (and every two hours when your blood glucose is above 240 mg/dl and there are ketones in your urine or blood).

KETONE TESTING
■ Check your blood (with a Precision Xtra meter) or urine for ketones if you have nausea or your blood glucose level is above 240 mg/dl.
■ If ketones are present, continue to check for them every two to four hours until they are gone and your blood glucose level is below 240 mg/dl.
■ If your child has moderate to large amounts of ketones in his blood or urine, contact his health-care provider immediately or take him to the nearest emergency room.

MEDICATION PLAN
Any sickness can cause a rise in your blood glucose level. Never omit your diabetes pills or insulin when you are not feeling well, unless instructed to by your health-care provider.

Diabetes pills
■ Continue to take the following medicines:

_____

_____

Insulin injections
■ Continue injecting your usual doses of insulin at the usual times.
■ If your blood glucose level is over_____mg/dl and your ketones are over_____, inject supplemental doses of_____units of Regular/Humalog/NovoLog/Apidra every_____hours.
■ Inject additional Regular/Humalog/NovoLog/Apidra insulin according to the following scale when your blood glucose is greater than your before-meal goals.

BLOOD GLUCOSE RANGE	UNITS OF INSULIN

Antidiarrheal and antivomiting medicines. These should be considered since both diarrhea and vomiting can lead to dehydration, which can require an emergency room visit.

Diabetes supplies

When you're not feeling well or you're stressed out, it's easy to overlook symptoms of high or low blood sugar. That's why it's helpful to keep a list of the signs and symptoms of high and low blood sugar in your sick-day box, along with guidelines for treating high or low blood sugar. You or a family member can take it out to review and compare the list to your symptoms at any time. Do not hesitate to call your health-care provider or the local emergency number if you believe you are headed for or are experiencing ketoacidosis or severe low blood glucose.

Here are some other tools that will help you manage your diabetes while ill:
Blood glucose meter supplies. Be sure you have back-up supplies for blood glucose monitoring because you may need to monitor more frequently when you are sick. Your sick-day box is a good place to store a back-up meter if you have one. Include at least one container or box of unopened test strips, unopened control solution, lancets, batteries for your meter (if the batteries can be changed), and a logbook. An empty plastic medicine container or film canister can be

Insulin pumps
- Continue your basal dose of insulin. (You may need to temporarily increase or decrease your basal rate.)
- Give supplemental bolus doses as necessary.
- If two consecutive blood glucose readings are greater than 240 mg/dl and/or moderate to large amounts of ketones are in your blood or urine, take a supplemental bolus by syringe and then change your infusion set.

FLUIDS
- Drink 8 ounces (1 cup) of calorie-free liquids every hour you are awake. If there are ketones in your blood or urine, increase drinking to every half hour.
- If blood glucose levels are_____mg/dl or higher, drink calorie-free liquids instead of carbohydrate-containing liquids.
- If blood glucose levels are below_____mg/dl and you cannot eat solid foods, alternate drinking carbohydrate-containing and calorie-free liquids to replace your typical carbohydrate amounts at each meal.

FOODS
- Stick to your usual mealtimes as much as possible.
- Try to eat your usual food intake.
- If necessary, replace solid foods with easily tolerated carbohydrates.

OVER-THE-COUNTER DRUGS
The following are OK to take while ill:
Sore throat_____

Cough_____
Congestion_____
Runny nose/postnasal drip/
  sneezing_____
Fever_____
Nausea_____
Diarrhea_____

GETTING HELP
It's time to call your health-care provider at
(____)_____ when any of the following are true:
- You are unsure of what to do.
- You cannot tolerate any foods or fluids.
- You have been vomiting or have had diarrhea for more than two hours.
- You have trouble concentrating or staying awake.
- You cannot take your diabetes medicines.
- There are moderate to large amounts of ketones in your blood or urine.
- Your temperature is greater than 101°F.
- Your blood glucose level stays above 240 mg/dl (above 130 mg/dl during pregnancy) even after taking supplemental boluses of insulin.
- Your blood glucose level stays below 60 mg/dl.
- You have signs/symptoms of dehydration or ketoacidosis (nausea; sunken eyes; skin that remains tented up after being pinched; abdominal pain; difficulty breathing; fruity odor to breath; dry, cracked lips, mouth, or tongue; or difficulty concentrating).

stored for use as a small sharps container for lancets.

Ketone test strips. These are an absolute must for people with Type 1 diabetes, who are at higher-than-normal risk of developing ketoacidosis, a life-threatening condition, during an illness. If you have Type 2 diabetes, check with your health-care provider before investing in these strips. People with Type 2 diabetes are much less likely to develop dangerous levels of ketones in the blood.

If you have Type 1 diabetes, your health-care team will probably have you check your blood glucose level and urine or blood ketones every two to four hours and when you are vomiting or feeling nauseous. (Ketones can cause nausea.)

Depending on your other symptoms, your blood glucose level, and how high your ketone level is, your plan may call for taking more insulin, eating some carbohydrate, drinking water, or even calling for an ambulance.

When not enough usable insulin is present to allow glucose to enter the cells to be used for energy, the body breaks down fat for its energy needs. Ketone bodies are formed as by-products of this process. High levels of glucose, ketones, electrolytes, and water get passed into the urine. This is when dehydration and ketoacidosis can occur.

Most people use urine test strips for detecting ketones. If you're not using individually wrapped ketone test strips, be sure to check expiration dates on the container for both the unopened as well as the opened strips. People who have a MediSense Precision Xtra meter can use special strips designed for that meter to detect ketones in the blood.

Glucose tablets or gel. These can easily be stored in your sick-day box for treatment or prevention of low blood sugar.

Insulin supplies. All insulin users should have an extra package or two of syringes in their sick-day supplies, no matter what they usually use to deliver insulin (such as insulin pens or an insulin pump). Otherwise, you should think of what you normally use and stock up on those supplies. Pen users should include pen needles as well as alcohol prep pads. Having a sharps container for pump needles, syringes, or pen needles can help to safely get rid of them, preventing accidental sticks to anyone else in your home. It can help keep your nightstand tidy as well.

Insulin pump supplies. If you use an insulin pump, have one or two complete sets of supplies stored in your sick-day box. Include your backup pump if you have one, syringes (in case of pump malfunction or lack of pump supplies), infusion sets, reservoir syringes, alcohol wipes, antiseptic wipes, skin barrier, tape, adhesive remover, and batteries.

Insulin. If insulin injections or an insulin pump are part of your daily routine, always have at least an extra vial of unexpired insulin in the refrigerator. A vial of rapid-acting or Regular insulin is a necessity. If you're not feeling well, you may choose to keep your insulin close by and at room temperature. Be sure to keep your insulin away from temperature extremes however, because that can make it ineffective.

Glucagon. Discuss the need for a glucagon emergency kit with your health-care provider. Glucagon is usually advised for people who inject insulin. It can be used as an emergency treatment for low blood sugar when a person is unable to ingest food or drinks. If you use insulin, be sure to inform the people you live with or a neighbor who checks on you on how to administer glucagon and where it is stored prior to any emergency. Keep a copy of the instructions on how to prepare your glucagon injection in your sick-day box.

Keep it up to date

Once you've compiled your sick-day box, it's important to keep it up to date. If you change doctors, for example, remember to put the new provider's name and number on your list of important phone numbers. If you are prescribed a new drug or stop taking an old one, update your medicines list.

Be sure to check expiration dates of all medicines and supplies periodically. Check the expiration dates for both unopened and opened supplies. Because some foods may keep for less than a year, plan on checking your sick-day box every six months or so. If you live in an area that uses daylight saving time, you might use the days you "spring ahead" or "fall back" as reminders to check your box.

In addition to updating your supplies, remember to update your sick-day guidelines periodically with the help of your diabetes-care team. Your guidelines may change if, say, your diabetes treatment changes. They may also change as your knowledge of diabetes and experience managing your own diabetes increases.

With any luck, you won't need to use your sick-day box frequently. But don't try to economize by not maintaining one. The cost of occasionally throwing out some outdated test strips and insulin is nothing compared to the cost of treating the complications that can develop when an illness isn't properly treated in the first place. Besides, your health and comfort are worth it. □

GETTING TO KNOW KETONES

by Richard M. Weil, M.Ed., C.D.E.

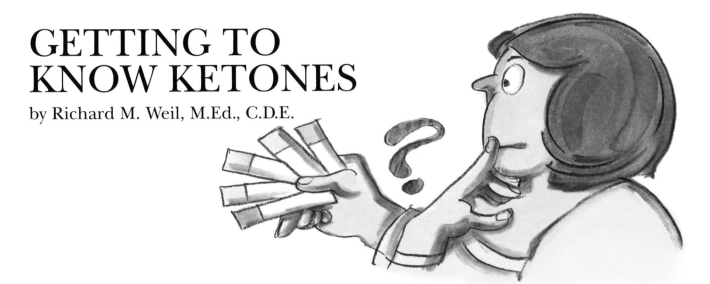

People with diabetes, particularly those with Type 1 diabetes, have been at least vaguely aware of the word *ketones* for a long time. With the recent resurgence of popular interest in low-carbohydrate diets, however, just about everyone seems to be talking about ketones these days. But does anyone really know what a ketone is? Are they a danger to your health (as in diabetic ketoacidosis), or a sign that you have lowered your carbohydrate intake enough to cause weight loss (as some people who follow low-carbohydrate diets believe)?

What are ketones?

Ketones are end-products of fat metabolism in the body. That is, they are formed when fat is burned for energy by the muscles. Chemically, they are acids known as *ketone bodies,* and there are three types: beta-hydroxybutyric acid, acetoacetic acid, and acetone. But you don't have to be a chemist to understand what role they play in the body.

To get to know ketones, it's helpful to understand how your body burns fuel. A simple analogy is that of an automobile. For a car engine to run, the engine must burn fuel (gasoline), and when the fuel is burned, exhaust (carbon monoxide) is created. The carbon monoxide is the end-product of gasoline combustion.

Your body also has an engine that must burn fuel to operate. The engine is muscle, and the fuel is fat, carbohydrate (glucose), and, in certain conditions, protein. When fat is burned, the "exhaust" is ketones, and when glucose is burned, the "exhaust" is lactic acid.

Fat is more desirable as a fuel than glucose because there are more calories in a gram of fat (9 calories per gram) than there are in a gram of glucose (4 calories per gram), so you get more energy per gram of fat burned. In a sense, you could call fat a high-test fuel. But there is one catch to burning fat: To burn it efficiently, with little "exhaust," you have to burn glucose at the same time. If you don't have glucose available for fuel (because you are on a low-carbohydrate diet, for example), you will form ketones when your muscles burn fat.

For most people, the ketones that form as a normal product of fat burning and weight loss are nothing to be concerned about because they are simply burned for energy by the body, and any excess are passed out of the body in the urine. In fact, while the brain normally uses glucose for energy, during exercise—and particularly during long-distance events like marathons, when glucose reserves may drop very low—the brain can use ketones for energy. Your liver makes extra ketones when glucose reserves are low so that your brain has enough energy.

For people with Type 1 diabetes, however, having measurable amounts of ketones in the urine (or blood) is cause for concern. Ketones in a person with Type 1 diabetes may be a sign that his diabetes is out of control, he is ill or has an infection, or he is under extreme stress. Because above-normal levels of ketones in the blood can lead to diabetic ketoacidosis, a life-threatening condition, people with Type 1 diabetes who have measurable ketones in their blood or urine should speak with their diabetes educator or doctor promptly.

Low-carbohydrate diets

Low-carbohydrate diets are sometimes called "ketotic" diets because they cause the body to burn mostly fat for energy (since the intake of carbohydrate is so low), which in turn causes the formation of ketones. Some people who follow low-carbohydrate diets periodically test their urine for ketones to see if fat-burning is indeed taking place. However, people who are losing weight on any diet might have a trace of ketones in their urine since a person who is losing weight is almost certainly burning and losing fat.

With all the talk of ketones, some people have gotten the mistaken impression that ketones are a sort of magic bullet that melts fat from the body, no matter how much a person eats. That's simply not the case. Ketones are only by-products of the metabolism of fat and are markers that show that you are burning fat. They have no active role in burning fat or weight loss. In fact, ketone levels in people who are on low-carbohydrate diets are just barely above baseline, indicating they have no role in producing weight loss. The reason people lose weight on low-carbohydrate diets is not because of ketones; it's because they have cut out a large food group from what they eat, and as a result, they end up eating fewer calories.

Another unproven belief about both ketones and low-carbohydrate diets is that they suppress appetite, and that's why people lose weight. Some scientists believe that the excess fat a person eats while on a low-carbohydrate diet has a satiating effect, causing people to eat less. Other experts believe that an elevated level of ketones causes a decrease in appetite, while still others believe that a high protein intake suppresses appetite. There are some studies in rats to suggest that elevated levels of protein during low-carbohydrate diets can cause a decrease in appetite, but so far, research on the effect of ketones and fat on appetite is inconclusive.

The jury is still out on the long-term safety and effectiveness of diets that are low in carbohydrates for the general population, although some nephrologists link a growing incidence of kidney stones to high-protein diets. (Low-carbohydrate diets tend to be high in protein.) Most diabetes experts, however, agree that a low-carbohydrate, high-protein diet is not worth the risk for people with diabetes because they have a high risk of developing kidney disease, and a high protein intake can be stressful on the kidneys in those with kidney disease.

Diabetes is the leading cause of kidney failure in the United States, accounting for approximately 43% of all Americans who start treatment for kidney failure each year. Between 10% and 21% of all people with diabetes will get some type of kidney disease. You may find it easier to control your blood sugar if you severely restrict your carbohydrate intake, but keep in mind that even in people without kidney disease, no one knows the effects

of a high-protein diet on the kidneys over the long term. If you're considering a low-carbohydrate, high-protein diet for weight loss or blood sugar control, check with your doctor or diabetes educator first.

Exercise and ketones

During exercise, both fat and glucose are burned for fuel by the muscles. If your glucose stores are low, fat will be your body's primary fuel. If you exercise and burn lots of fat without glucose, you will make ketones. People who are very lean and efficient at burning fat, people who are losing weight, and people who do lots of endurance exercise (like training for a marathon) use up their stores of glucose rather quickly, and when they do, they frequently develop ketones in the blood. The type of ketone they develop is acetone, and it's not unusual for their breath to smell fruity or like alcohol as the acetone leaves the body through their breath.

For people with diabetes, exercise typically lowers blood sugar. But sometimes exercise can raise blood sugar. This can happen when you are low on insulin. As you exercise, your liver converts stored glycogen into glucose to use for energy and pumps it into your bloodstream. If there's little insulin available, your muscles can't use the glucose and your blood glucose level will rise. If you have even a trace of ketones when you begin your exercise and your blood sugar rises as you exercise, the amount of ketones in your blood may rise as well, particularly if you have Type 1 diabetes. Although diabetic ketoacidosis as a result of exercise is very rare, it is possible, so precautions need to be taken. The American Diabetes Association guidelines for exercise, blood glucose, and ketones are as follows:

■ Avoid exercise if blood glucose levels are greater than 250 mg/dl and ketones are present.
■ Use caution if blood glucose levels are greater than 300 mg/dl and ketones are not present.

If your blood sugar level is higher than 250 mg/dl, you do not have ketones in your blood or urine, and you want to exercise, I recommend starting your workout then stopping after 15 minutes to see if your blood sugar level is rising or dropping. If it's dropping, it's OK to continue exercising. If it's rising, you should stop exercising and follow your doctor's recommendations for treating high blood sugar.

Diabetic ketoacidosis

As stated earlier, for most people, ketones are nothing to worry about. But when you have dia-

KETONE STRIPS

For people with Type 1 diabetes and pregnant women with diabetes, especially, monitoring ketone levels is an important part of staying healthy and preventing diabetic ketoacidosis, a potentially life-threatening state in which ketones build up in the blood and dehydration sets in. With just a little blood or urine, today's ketone-testing products can let you know whether you're producing ketones.

Checking your blood ketone levels with a Precision Xtra meter or CardioChek analyzer is very similar to checking your blood glucose: You simply place a drop of blood on the correct strip and wait for the meter to return a reading.

Urine reagent strips operate in a slightly different fashion. After a small amount of urine is placed on the reagent strip—either by holding the strip in the urine stream or by collecting urine in a clean container and dipping the strip into it—a chemical reaction takes place that changes the color of the strip. You then compare the strip color with the color chart that came with the ketone strips within the time limit specified by the strip manufacturer, generally 15 seconds. The color that matches shows the range within which your ketone level falls. The strip will continue to darken as it is exposed to air, so if you don't read the strip within the time limit, you should start over with a new strip.

Some urine reagent strips measure other substances besides ketones, such as glucose. However, testing urine for glucose is considered imprecise at best and is not recommended for diabetes self-care.

STRIP NAME	APPROXIMATE SHELF LIFE	PACKAGING	APPROXIMATE PRICE
BLOOD KETONE STRIPS			
CardioChek ketone test strips Polymer Technology Systems (877) 870-5610 www.ptspanels.com	70 weeks from manufacturing date	25 (loose in vial) 6 (loose in vial)	$70 $22
Precision Xtra blood ketone test strips Abbott Diabetes Care (888) 522-5226 www.abbottdiabetescare.com	12–18 months from manufacturing date	8 (individually wrapped)	$30–$35
URINE REAGENT STRIPS			
Chemstrip K Roche Diagnostics (800) 858-8072 www.roche-diagnostics.com	Two years from manufacturing date or 18 months from date of purchase	100 (loose in vial)	$16
Ketostix Reagent Strips Bayer Corporation Diagnostics (800) 348-8100 www.bayerdiabetes.com	One and a half years from manufacturing date	100 (loose in vial) 50 (loose in vial)	$21 $13

betes, particularly Type 1 diabetes, it may be a signal that your diabetes is out of control. Your body may make ketones when you are sick, have an infection, are injured, or are experiencing high levels of stress. They can appear in your urine (*ketonuria*) and in your blood (*ketonemia*).

The problem with high levels of ketones is that they are relatively strong acids, and because of their acidity, their presence in the blood can reduce the ability of oxygen to bind to hemoglobin, the molecule that transports oxygen to cells that need it. That means muscles and other organs might not function as well as they should. In addition, high levels of ketones for people with

Type 1 diabetes can lead to dehydration and diabetic ketoacidosis (sometimes called DKA). Diabetic ketoacidosis is rarely seen in people with Type 2 diabetes because their pancreases usually still produce some insulin, which means that the body is able to burn some glucose.

Testing for ketones

People with Type 1 diabetes have most likely been asked by a doctor or diabetes educator to test their urine for ketones at one time or another. The development of the Precision Xtra meter has also made it possible to check blood levels of ketones at home. Two other home analyzers, the CardioChek and the CardioChek/PA (which also measure blood cholesterol levels), can also measure blood ketone levels. It's a good idea to review ketone testing guidelines with your doctor or diabetes educator, but here are some general guidelines for who should test and when:

■ People with Type 1 diabetes whose blood glucose level is over 250 mg/dl for two readings in a row or who are sick should always test for ketones.

■ Pregnant women with diabetes are usually advised to check their urine for ketones every morning before eating and additionally if their blood glucose level is above 200 mg/dl or if they are ill.

■ Most adults with Type 2 diabetes don't need to worry about ketones, but check with your doctor or diabetes educator for specific instructions.

■ Most of the time, children with Type 2 diabetes don't need to check for ketones, but ask your doctor, especially if your child experiences unexplained weight loss or his blood sugar level consistently remains over 200 mg/dl.

Ketones are usually tested with urine test strips, which change color based on the presence and concentration of ketones in the urine. The results are usually expressed as "negative," "trace," "small," "moderate," or "large." If the test result is positive, you should call your doctor or diabetes educator. You may need to take extra insulin, and your health-care provider will instruct you on how much. You should also drink lots of water or other calorie-free beverages to flush out excess ketones, continue to check your blood glucose level every three hours, and continue to test for ketones if your blood glucose level is over 250 mg/dl.

If you are losing weight, you may have a small amount of ketones in your urine. This is OK for people with Type 2 diabetes, as long as their blood sugar level is in a normal range, but people with Type 1 diabetes should check with their doctor. The mild ketosis (the presence of small amounts of ketones in the body) that occurs in people on low-carbohydrate diets should not be confused with the life-threatening levels of ketosis that someone who has Type 1 diabetes can develop. Diabetic ketoacidosis is a serious medical emergency that requires immediate medical attention.

The Precision Xtra blood glucose meter can measure ketones in your blood with special strips that take a fingerstick blood sample, just like the procedure for blood glucose monitoring. The device has been carefully tested in studies and is very accurate. Blood testing for ketones is superior to urine testing because it measures beta-hydroxybutyric acid, the primary ketone that's formed in diabetic ketoacidosis, while urine testing measures acetoacetic acid. Urine testing can lead to a false negative result (which means it might show negative ketones when in fact you do have ketones), and there is a time delay to diagnosis of ketosis with urine testing since it takes some time for ketones to get from the blood to the urine. Another possible advantage to blood ketone testing is convenience. In a recent study of teenagers with Type 1 diabetes, teens preferred and were more likely to test their blood for ketones than they were to test their urine.

Here's what the results mean when testing blood for ketones:

■ Greater than 3.0 millimoles per liter (mmol/liter) is a serious metabolic condition and emergency medical care is necessary.

■ 1.6–3.0 mmol/liter is a high level of ketones and means you are at risk for diabetic ketoacidosis. Your doctor or diabetes educator should be contacted immediately.

■ 0.6–1.5 mmol/liter is a moderate level of ketones and probably indicates fat metabolism and weight loss, but not a deficiency of insulin. You should speak with your doctor or diabetes educator about what to do when ketones are in this range.

■ Below 0.6 mmol/liter is a normal blood level of ketones.

Ketogenic diets

While low-carbohydrate diets are usually discussed as tools for weight loss, that is not their only role. So-called ketogenic diets (diets that intentionally cause ketosis) have been used to treat epileptic seizures in children since the 1920's. The diets, which do not work in adults, are high in fat, low in protein, and virtually carbohydrate-free. The precise mechanism of how ketones work to prevent epilepsy is unknown, but for some children with difficult cases of epilepsy that do not fully respond to medication, the ketogenic diet is another treatment option. There are several centers in the United States that provide the diet. You can find out more at the following Web sites:

■ www.epilepsy.com/epilepsy/treatment_ketogenic_diet.html
■ www.stanford.edu/group/ketodiet

Ketogenic diets are also being tested for treatment of Parkinson disease. Some evidence suggests that ketones in the brain may help resolve some of the symptoms that people with Parkinson disease experience. Like epilepsy, the mechanism of action has not been discovered, and much more work needs to be done in this area.

Another piece of the puzzle

Understanding how your body works—and why it sometimes breaks down—puts you in the driver's seat when it comes to your health and diabetes care. Knowing about ketones is vital mainly for people with Type 1 diabetes, but it doesn't hurt for anyone to know what these substances are and what they can and can't do for you. □

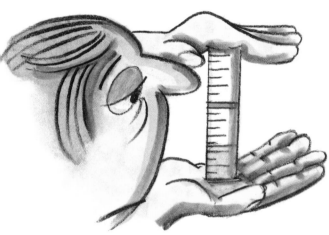

UNDERSTANDING HYPOGLYCEMIA

by Laura Hieronymus, M.S.Ed., A.P.R.N., B.C.-A.D.M., C.D.E., and Belinda O'Connell, M.S., R.D., C.D.E.

When you think about diabetes and blood glucose control, the first thing that comes to mind is probably avoiding high blood glucose levels. After all, the hallmark of diabetes is high blood glucose, or hyperglycemia. But controlling blood glucose is more than just managing the "highs"; it also involves preventing and managing "lows," or hypoglycemia.

Most people are aware that keeping blood glucose levels as close to normal as possible helps prevent damage to the blood vessels and nerves in the body. But keeping blood glucose levels near normal can carry some risks as well. People who maintain "tight" blood glucose control are more likely to experience episodes of hypoglycemia, and frequent episodes of hypoglycemia—even mild hypoglycemia and even in people who don't keep blood glucose levels close to normal—deplete the liver of stored glucose (called glycogen), which is what the body normally draws upon to raise blood glucose levels when they are low. Once liver stores of glycogen are low, severe hypoglycemia is more likely to develop, and research shows that severe hypoglycemia can be harmful. In children, frequent severe hypoglycemia can lead to impairment of intellectual function. In children and adults, severe hypoglycemia can lead to accidents. And in adults with cardiovascular disease, it can lead to strokes and heart attacks.

To keep yourself as healthy as possible, you need to learn how to balance food intake, physical activity, and any diabetes medicines or insulin you use to keep your blood glucose as close to normal as is safe for you without going too low. This article explains how hypoglycemia develops and how to treat and prevent it.

What is hypoglycemia?

Blood glucose levels vary throughout the day depending on what you eat, how active you are, and any diabetes medicines or insulin you take. Other things, such as hormone fluctuations, can affect blood glucose levels as well. In people who don't have diabetes, blood glucose levels generally range from 65 mg/dl to 140 mg/dl, but in diabetes, the body's natural control is disrupted, and blood glucose levels can go too high or too low. For people with diabetes, a blood glucose level of 70 mg/dl or less is considered low, and treatment is recommended to prevent it from dropping even lower.

Under normal circumstances, glucose is the

brain's sole energy source, making it particularly sensitive to any decrease in blood glucose level. When blood glucose levels drop too low, the body tries to increase the amount of glucose available in the bloodstream by releasing hormones such as glucagon and epinephrine (also called adrenaline) that stimulate the release of glycogen from the liver.

Some of the symptoms of hypoglycemia are caused by the brain's lack of glucose; other symptoms are caused by the hormones, primarily epinephrine, released to help increase blood glucose levels. Epinephrine can cause feelings of weakness, shakiness, clamminess, and hunger and an increased heart rate. These are often called the "warning signs" of hypoglycemia. Lack of glucose to the brain can cause trouble concentrating, changes in vision, slurred speech, lack of coordination, headaches, dizziness, and drowsiness. Hypoglycemia can also cause changes in emotions and mood. Feelings of nervousness and irritability, becoming argumentative, showing aggression, and crying are common, although some people experience euphoria and giddiness. Recognizing emotional changes that may signal hypoglycemia is especially important in young children, who may not be able to understand or communicate other symptoms of hypoglycemia to adults. If hypoglycemia is not promptly treated with a form of sugar or glucose to bring blood glucose level up, the brain can become dangerously depleted of glucose, potentially causing severe confusion, seizures, and loss of consciousness.

Who is at risk?

Some people are at higher risk of developing hypoglycemia than others. Hypoglycemia is not a concern for people who manage their diabetes with only exercise and a meal plan. People who use insulin or certain types of oral diabetes medicines have a much greater chance of developing hypoglycemia and therefore need to be more careful to avoid it. Other risk factors for hypoglycemia include the following:

■ Maintaining very "tight" (near-normal) blood glucose targets.
■ Decreased kidney function. The kidneys help to degrade and remove insulin from the bloodstream. When the kidneys are not functioning well, insulin action can be unpredictable, and low blood glucose levels may result.
■ Alcohol use.
■ Conditions such as gastropathy (slowed stomach emptying) that cause variable rates of digestion and absorption of food.

■ Having autonomic neuropathy, which can decrease symptoms when blood glucose levels drop. (Autonomic neuropathy is damage to nerves that control involuntary functions.)
■ Pregnancy in women with preexisting diabetes, especially during the first trimester.

A side effect of diabetes treatment

Hypoglycemia is the most common side effect of insulin use and of some of the oral medicines used to treat Type 2 diabetes. How likely a drug is to cause hypoglycemia and the appropriate treatment for hypoglycemia depends on the type of drug.

Secretagogues. Oral medicines that stimulate the pancreas to release more insulin, which include sulfonylureas and the drugs nateglinide (brand name Starlix) and repaglinide (Prandin), have the potential side effect of hypoglycemia. Sulfonylureas include glimepiride (Amaryl), glipizide (Glucotrol and Glucotrol XL), and glyburide (DiaBeta, Micronase, and Glynase).

Sulfonylureas are taken once or twice a day, in the morning and the evening, and their blood-glucose-lowering effects last all day. If you miss a meal or snack, the medicine continues to work, and your blood glucose level may drop too low. So-called sulfa antibiotics (those that contain the ingredient sulfamethoxazole) can also increase the risk of hypoglycemia when taken with a sulfonylurea. Anyone who takes a sulfonylurea, therefore, should discuss this potential drug interaction with their health-care provider should antibiotic therapy be necessary.

Nateglinide and repaglinide are taken with meals and act for only a short time. The risk of hypoglycemia is lower than for sulfonylureas, but it is still possible to develop hypoglycemia if a dose of nateglinide or repaglinide is taken without food.

Insulin. All people with Type 1 diabetes and many with Type 2 use insulin for blood glucose control. Since insulin can cause hypoglycemia, it is important for those who use it to understand how it works and when its activity is greatest so they can properly balance food and activity and take precautions to avoid hypoglycemia. This is best discussed with a health-care provider who is knowledgeable about you, your lifestyle, and the particular insulin regimen you are using.

Biguanides and thiazolidinediones. The biguanides, of which metformin is the only one approved in the United States, decrease the amount of glucose manufactured by the liver. The thiazolidinediones, pioglitazone (Actos) and rosiglitazone (Avandia), help body cells become more sensitive to insulin. The risk of hypoglycemia is very low with these medicines. However, if you take metformin, pioglitazone, or rosiglitazone along with either insulin or a secretagogue, hypoglycemia is a possibility.

Alpha-glucosidase inhibitors. Drugs in this class, acarbose (Precose) and miglitol (Glyset), interfere with the digestion of carbohydrates to glucose and help to lower blood glucose levels after meals. When taken alone, these medicines do not cause hypoglycemia, but if combined with either insulin or a secretagogue, hypoglycemia is possible. Because alpha-glucosidase inhibitors interfere with the digestion of some types of carbohydrate, hypoglycemia can only be treated with pure glucose (also called dextrose or *d*-glucose), which is sold in tablets and tubes of gel. Other carbohydrates will not raise blood glucose levels quickly enough to treat hypoglycemia.

Dipeptidyl peptidase-4 inhibitors. This drug class, which includes sitagliptin (Januvia), is used in Type 2 diabetes to block an enzyme that inactivates the hormone called *glucagon-like peptide-1* (GLP-1). GLP-1 levels are decreased in Type 2 diabetes. When used alone or with other oral agents that do not cause hypoglycemia, the risk is low. However, anytime this drug is used with a secretagogue, care is needed to avoid hypoglycemia.

Exenatide. Exenatide (Byetta) is an incretin mimetic used in the treatment of Type 2 diabetes that "mimics" GLP-1. This drug is typically used with specific types of oral agents. Exenatide does not cause hypoglycemia, but when added to drugs that have hypoglycemia as a side effect, such as secretagogues, care is need to avoid hypoglycemia.

Pramlinitide. Pramlintide (Symlin) is a synthetic form of amylin. Amylin is a naturally occurring hormone produced by the beta cells in the pancreas that works together with insulin to control blood glucose levels. While pramlintide does not cause hypoglycemia alone, when it is used with insulin, your premeal insulin dose may need to lowered to avoid hypoglycemia.

Striking a balance

Although hypoglycemia is called a side effect of some of the drugs used to lower blood glucose levels, it would be more accurate to call it a potential side effect of diabetes treatment—which includes food and activity as well as drug treatment. When there is a disruption in the balance of these different components of diabetes

treatment, hypoglycemia can result. The following are some examples of how that balance commonly gets disrupted:

Skipping or delaying a meal. When you take insulin or a drug that increases the amount of insulin in your system, not eating enough food at the times the insulin or drug is working can cause hypoglycemia. Learning to balance food with insulin or oral drugs is key to achieving optimal blood glucose control while avoiding hypoglycemia.

Too much diabetes medicine. If you take more than your prescribed dose of insulin or a secretagogue, there can be too much insulin circulating in your bloodstream, and hypoglycemia can occur. Changes in the timing of insulin or oral medicines can also cause hypoglycemia if your medicine and food plan are no longer properly matched.

Increase in physical activity. Physical activity and exercise lower blood glucose level by increasing insulin sensitivity. This is generally beneficial in blood glucose control, but it can increase the risk of hypoglycemia in people who use insulin or secretagogues if the exercise is very vigorous, carbohydrate intake too low, or the activity takes place at the time when the insulin or secretagogue has the greatest (peak) action. Exercise-related hypoglycemia can occur as much as 24 hours after the activity.

Increase in rate of insulin absorption. This may occur if the temperature of the skin increases due to exposure to hot water or the sun. Also, if insulin is injected into a muscle that is used in exercise soon after (such as injecting your thigh area, then jogging), the rate of absorption may increase.

Alcohol. Consuming alcohol can cause hypoglycemia in people who take insulin or a secretagogue. When the liver is metabolizing alcohol, it is less able to break down glycogen to make glucose when blood glucose levels drop. In addition to causing hypoglycemia, this can increase the severity of hypoglycemia. Alcohol can also contribute to hypoglycemia by reducing appetite and impairing thinking and judgment.

Hypoglycemia unawareness

Being able to recognize hypoglycemia promptly is very important because it allows you to take steps to raise your blood glucose as quickly as possible. However, some people with diabetes don't sense or don't experience the early warning signs of hypoglycemia such as weakness, shakiness, clamminess, hunger, and an increase in heart rate. This is called "hypoglycemia unawareness." Without these early warnings and prompt treatment, hypoglycemia can progress to confusion, which can impair your thinking and ability to treat the hypoglycemia.

If the goals you have set for your personal blood glucose control are "tight" and you are having frequent episodes of hypoglycemia, your brain may feel comfortable with these low levels and not respond with the typical warning signs. Frequent episodes of hypoglycemia can further blunt your body's response to low blood glucose. Some drugs, such as beta-blockers (taken for high blood pressure), can also mask the symptoms of hypoglycemia.

If you have hypoglycemia frequently, you may need to raise your blood glucose targets, and you should monitor your blood glucose level more frequently and avoid alcohol. You may also need to adjust your diabetes medicines or insulin doses. Talk to your diabetes care team if you experience several episodes of hypoglycemia a week, have hypoglycemia during the night, have such low blood glucose that you require help from someone else to treat it, or find you are frequently eating snacks that you don't want simply to avoid low blood glucose.

Treating lows

Anyone at risk for hypoglycemia should know how to treat it and be prepared to do so at any time. Here's what to do: If you recognize symptoms of hypoglycemia, check your blood glucose level with your meter to make sure. While the symptoms are useful, the numbers are facts, and other situations, such as panic attacks or heart problems, can lead to similar symptoms. In some cases, people who have had chronically high blood glucose levels may experience symptoms of hypoglycemia when their blood glucose level drops to a more normal range. The usual recommendation is not to treat normal or goal-range blood glucose levels, even if symptoms are present.

Treatment is usually recommended for blood glucose levels of 70 mg/dl or less. However, this may vary among individuals. For example, blood glucose goals are lower in women with diabetes who are pregnant, so they may be advised to treat for hypoglycemia at a level below 70 mg/dl. People who have hypoglycemia unawareness, are elderly, or live alone may be advised to treat at a blood glucose level somewhat higher than 70 mg/dl. Young children are often given slightly higher targets for treating hypoglycemia for safety reasons. Work with your diabetes care team to devise a plan for treating hypoglycemia that is right for you.

To treat hypoglycemia, follow the "rule of 15": Check your blood glucose level with your meter, treat a blood glucose level under 70 mg/dl by consuming 15 grams of carbohydrate, wait about 15 minutes, then recheck your blood glucose level with your meter. If your blood glucose is still low (below 80 mg/dl), consume another 15 grams of carbohydrate and recheck 15 minutes later. You may need a small snack if your next planned meal is more than an hour away. Since blood glucose levels may begin to drop again about 40–60 minutes after treatment, it may be a good idea to recheck your blood glucose level approximately an hour after treating a low to determine if additional carbohydrate is needed.

The following items have about 15 grams of carbohydrate:
- 3–4 glucose tablets
- 1 dose of glucose gel (in most cases, 1 small tube is 1 dose)
- ½ cup of orange juice or regular soda (not sugar-free)
- 1 tablespoon of honey or syrup
- 1 tablespoon of sugar or 5 small sugar cubes
- 6–8 LifeSavers
- 8 ounces of skim (nonfat) milk

If these choices are not available, use any carbohydrate that is—for example, bread, crackers, grapes, etc. The form of carbohydrate is not important; treating the low blood glucose is. (However, many people find they are less likely to overtreat low blood glucose if they consistently treat lows with a more "medicinal" form of carbohydrate such as glucose tablets or gel.)

If you take insulin or a secretagogue and are also taking an alpha-glucosidase inhibitor (acarbose or miglitol), carbohydrate digestion and absorption is decreased, and the recommended treatment is glucose tablets or glucose gel.

Other nutrients in food such as fat or resistant starch (which is present in some diabetes snack bars) can delay glucose digestion and absorption, so foods containing these ingredients are not good choices for treating hypoglycemia.

If hypoglycemia becomes severe and a person is confused, convulsing, or unconscious, treatment options include intravenous glucose administered by medical personnel or glucagon by injection given by someone trained in its use and familiar with the recipient's diabetes history. Glucagon is a hormone that is normally produced by the pancreas and that causes the liver to release glucose into the bloodstream, raising the blood glucose level. It comes in a kit that can be used in an emergency situation (such as when a person is unable to swallow a source of glucose by mouth). The hormone is injected much like an insulin injection, usually in an area of fatty tissue, such as the stomach or back of the arms. Special precautions are necessary to ensure that the injection is given correctly and that the person receiving the injection is positioned properly prior to receiving the drug. People at higher risk of developing hypoglycemia should discuss the use of glucagon with their diabetes educator, doctor, or pharmacist.

Avoiding hypoglycemia

Avoiding all episodes of hypoglycemia may be impossible for many people, especially since maintaining tight blood glucose control brings with it a higher risk of hypoglycemia. However, the following tips may help to prevent excessive lows:

■ Know how your medicines work and when they have their strongest action.

■ Work with your diabetes care team to coordinate your medicines or insulin with your eating plan. Meals and snacks should be timed to coordinate with the activity of your medicine or insulin.

■ Learn how to count carbohydrates so you can keep your carbohydrate intake consistent at meals and snacks from day to day. Variations in carbohydrate intake can lead to hypoglycemia.

■ Have carbohydrate-containing foods available in the places you frequent, such as in your car or at the office, to avoid delays in treatment of hypoglycemia.

■ Develop a plan with your diabetes care team to adjust your food, medicine, or insulin for changes in activity or exercise.

■ Discuss how to handle sick days and situations where you have trouble eating with your diabetes team.

■ Always check your blood glucose level to verify any symptoms of hypoglycemia. Keep your meter with you, especially in situations where risk of hypoglycemia is increased.

■ Wear a medical alert identification tag.

■ Always treat blood glucose levels of 70 mg/dl or less whether or not you have symptoms.

■ If you have symptoms of hypoglycemia and do not have your blood glucose meter available, treatment is recommended.

■ If you have hypoglycemia unawareness, you may need to work with your diabetes care team to modify your blood glucose goals or treatment plan.

■ Check your blood glucose level frequently during the day and possibly at night, especially if you have hypoglycemia unawareness, are pregnant, or have exercised vigorously within the past 24 hours.

■ Check your blood glucose level before driving or operating machinery to avoid any situations that could become dangerous if hypoglycemia occurred.

■ Check the expiration date on your glucagon emergency kit once a year and replace it before it expires.

■ Discuss alcohol intake with your diabetes care team. You may be advised not to drink on an empty stomach and/or to increase your carbohydrate intake if alcohol is an option for you. If you drink, always check your blood glucose level before bed and eat any snacks that are scheduled in your food plan.

Don't risk your health

Although hypoglycemia can, at times, be unpleasant, don't risk your health by allowing your blood glucose levels to run higher than recommended to avoid it. Meet with your diabetes care team to develop a plan to help you achieve the best possible blood glucose control safely and effectively. Think positive, and learn to be prepared with measures to prevent and promptly treat hypoglycemia should it occur. □

MANAGING HYPERGLYCEMIA

by Laura Hieronymus, M.S.Ed., A.P.R.N., B.C.-A.D.M., C.D.E.,
and Belinda O'Connell, M.S., R.D., C.D.E.

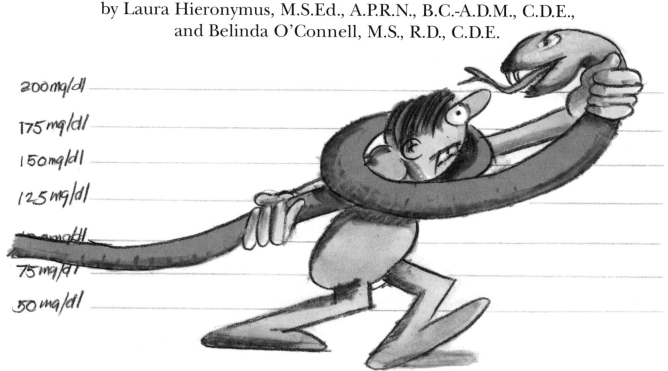

200 mg/dl

175 mg/dl

150 mg/dl

125 mg/dl

75 mg/dl

50 mg/dl

When you were diagnosed with diabetes, your doctor probably told you that your blood glucose levels were too high. Indeed, high blood glucose, or *hyperglycemia,* is the hallmark of diabetes. Regardless of your knowledge of diabetes at that time, you may have wondered what the significance of high blood glucose levels was for you. The answer is that hyperglycemia is linked to the development of long-term diabetes complications, which include nephropathy (kidney disease), retinopathy (eye disease), neuropathy (nerve damage), foot and skin problems, heart and blood vessel disease, and tooth and gum disease. That's why individual treatment plans for people with diabetes focus on preventing hyperglycemia and keeping blood glucose levels as close to the normal range as possible. Keeping blood glucose levels close to normal requires learning how to balance food intake, physical activity, and the effects of any diabetes medicines your doctor may prescribe to lower your blood glucose level. For some people, the balancing act also involves learning to avoid *hypoglycemia,* or low blood glucose.

Blood glucose goals

In healthy people who don't have diabetes, blood glucose levels typically run in the range of 65–110 mg/dl and may rise to 120–140 mg/dl one to two hours after eating. A diagnosis of diabetes is made when a person's fasting blood glucose level is above 126 mg/dl on two separate occasions or when a person has symptoms of diabetes (such as excessive thirst and urination) and his nonfasting blood glucose level is greater than 200 mg/dl on two separate occasions.

Until recently, a diagnosis of prediabetes, a condition in which blood glucose levels are high but not high enough for a diagnosis of diabetes, was made when a person's fasting blood glucose level was between 110 mg/dl and 126 mg/dl. More recently, an international expert committee on diabetes recommended diagnosing prediabetes when a person's fasting blood glucose level is 100 mg/dl, and the American Diabetes Association (ADA) has adopted this recommendation.

On the basis of research showing that maintaining near-normal blood glucose levels significantly reduces the risk of diabetes-related complications, both the ADA and the American College of Endocrinology (ACE) have established recommended goals for blood glucose control for most adults with diabetes. (See "Blood Glucose Targets" on page 49.) These goals may be modified for certain populations. For example, the goals for blood glucose control are typically lower for women with diabetes who are pregnant. For children and the elderly, particularly those who take insulin as part

BLOOD GLUCOSE TARGETS

Both the American Diabetes Association (ADA) and the American College of Endocrinology (ACE) have published recommendations for blood glucose control goals for healthy, nonpregnant adults with diabetes. Why two sets of targets? While both are based on studies showing the benefits of intensive blood glucose control, the differences reflect the differing membership in the two organizations. Members of the ACE are endocrinologists, physicians who specialize in endocrine disorders, including diabetes. ADA recommendations are approved by committees of medical professionals that include endocrinologists as well as nurses, dietitians, and physicians with specialties other than endocrinology or diabetes.

	AMERICAN DIABETES ASSOCIATION RECOMMENDATIONS	AMERICAN COLLEGE OF ENDOCRINOLOGY RECOMMENDATIONS
HbA_{1c}	less than 7%	6.5% or lower
Fasting or before-meal plasma glucose levels	90–130 mg/dl	less than 110 mg/dl
Plasma glucose levels after meals	less than 180 mg/dl	less than 140 mg/dl

of their treatment plan, the goals may be higher for safety reasons. Because each person's situation is different, it is important to work with your diabetes care team to set individualized blood glucose goals that are right for you.

Two significant studies that paved the way toward today's blood glucose goals are the Diabetes Control and Complications Trial (DCCT) and the United Kingdom Prospective Diabetes Study (UKPDS). Both demonstrated that the closer blood glucose levels are kept to normal, the less likely a person with diabetes is to develop complications.

DCCT. The DCCT followed 1,441 people with Type 1 diabetes for an average of about seven years. The subjects were divided into two groups: the "conventional" treatment group, and the "intensive" treatment group. While the group that was treated intensively did not achieve normal, nondiabetic blood glucose levels, they were able to achieve an average blood glucose level of 155 mg/dl. The conventionally treated group's blood glucose level averaged 231 mg/dl. During the study period, the intensively treated group had an approximate 60% reduction of risk for neuropathy, nephropathy, and retinopathy. Intensive therapy not only delayed the onset of complications but it also slowed the progression of complications in those who already had them, regardless of age, sex, or duration of diabetes.

UKPDS. The UKPDS examined the effects of varying levels of blood glucose control in 5,102 individuals with Type 2 diabetes, who were followed for an average of 10 years. The intensively treated group achieved an average blood glucose level of 150 mg/dl, while the conventionally treated group's average blood glucose levels were approximately 177 mg/dl. In this study, intensive blood glucose control resulted in a 25% reduction of risk for neuropathy, nephropathy, and retinopathy. Furthermore, the study concluded that for every percentage drop in glycosylated hemoglobin (HbA_{1c}, a measure of long-term blood glucose control), there was a 35% reduction in the risk of complications.

As these studies make clear, it is worth the effort to take steps to control your blood glucose, but how do you do that? And how do you know if you have hyperglycemia in the first place?

Identifying hyperglycemia

The best way to identify hyperglycemia is to routinely monitor your blood glucose levels on a schedule determined by you and your health-care team and to get regular HbA_{1c} tests, also on a schedule agreed on by you and your health-care team (usually two to four times a year). That's because hyperglycemia may not cause any symptoms until blood glucose levels are much higher than recommended ranges. So just because you feel OK doesn't necessarily mean your blood glucose level is well controlled.

When they do occur, symptoms of hyperglycemia may include frequent urination, hunger, dry mouth, thirst, blurred vision, numbness or tingling in the hands and feet, decreased sexual function, and fatigue. All of these symptoms should prompt immediate action, starting with checking your blood glucose level with your meter to see if it's high. What you do next will depend in large part on how you normally treat your diabetes.

Because regimens for treating diabetes vary widely, there is no "one size fits all" plan for treating hyperglycemia. If you currently treat your Type 2 diabetes with meal planning and exercise, for example, you may be instructed to add several minutes to your usual exercise routine or to decrease your carbohydrate intake at your next meal when your blood glucose level is high. If you have Type 1 diabetes and use an insulin pump, you may be instructed to take more insulin (possibly via syringe or insulin pen), and your diabetes care team will teach you how to determine how much insulin to take based on your blood glucose level. It's extremely important to work with your diabetes care team to develop an individualized hyperglycemia action plan for you.

No matter what type of diabetes you have or how you treat it, part of your hyperglycemia action plan will likely be more frequent blood glucose monitoring, at least temporarily, to help determine why your blood glucose is high and what you can do to avoid future episodes of hyperglycemia. Indeed, prevention is the best and most effective way to treat hyperglycemia.

Many variables, some of which are described here, can upset the delicate balance that is necessary for the best diabetes control. When dealing with diabetes, you will inevitably experience some if not all of the following issues.

Food

If you eat more food than is balanced with your physical activity and, in some cases, diabetes medicines, your blood glucose level may rise above your goal range. Carbohydrate-containing foods directly affect your blood glucose level after eating, so reviewing the amount of carbohydrate in your meals and snacks may be helpful in determining the cause of hyperglycemia. Carefully reading nutrition labels on food products and measuring portions will help you to meet your carbohydrate goals. On packaged foods, the total carbohydrate per serving is listed on the Nutrition Facts panel of the label. Meals that are high in fat

may contribute to prolonged elevations in blood glucose after eating. Working with a registered dietitian, preferably one with experience in diabetes management, can be helpful in fine-tuning your meal-planning and carbohydrate-counting skills.

If you experience hyperglycemia in spite of sticking to your meal plan most of the time, it may indicate that the medicines included in your diabetes regimen need adjusting. If this is the case, undereating will not help lower your blood glucose level; you should consult your physician.

Exercise

Exercise usually lowers blood glucose levels because it improves your cells' sensitivity to insulin and helps cells burn glucose for energy. But if your blood glucose level is high before you exercise, it may go higher during exercise. When you begin exercising, your liver pumps out extra glucose to fuel your muscles. If your body has too little insulin circulating in the bloodstream to allow the cells to use the extra glucose, your blood glucose level will rise. High blood glucose levels with exercise can also be a sign that you are working too hard and your body is under stress. If this is the case, you need to slow down and gradually work up to a more strenuous level of activity.

For people with Type 1 diabetes, the ADA advises avoiding exercise if fasting blood glucose levels are above 250 mg/dl and ketones are present in blood or urine; caution should be used if blood glucose levels are above 300 mg/dl and no ketones are present. People with Type 2 diabetes may wish to consult their diabetes care team for individual recommendations.

Medication

Insulin and diabetes pills are taken to lower blood glucose levels, so forgetting a dose, taking the wrong dose, or taking the right dose at the wrong time can contribute to hyperglycemia. If you develop hyperglycemia, here are some questions you may want to ask yourself regarding your medicine(s):

■ *Did you take the proper dose?* Double-check to make sure your dose was accurate. Sometimes different doses of the same oral diabetes medicine or insulin are prescribed at different times of day. Did the correct dose coincide with the correct time?

■ *Could you have forgotten to take your medicine?* It is only human to forget things from time to time, even parts of your daily routine. If you think you may have forgotten to take your medicine, ask yourself if you specifically remember taking it. Can you backtrack to determine if you took it? If you seem to forget to take your medicine regularly, look for patterns: Are you having difficulty remembering a certain dose? If so, you may want to brainstorm some ways to remember it, such as setting an alarm for dose time or posting a note to yourself in a place you can't miss. Insulin pumps generally have a review screen that allows you to see whether doses have been delivered.

■ *Has the medicine expired?* Check the expiration date on your medicine to see if it is still good. Most pills have a long shelf life, but insulin does not. In addition, the expiration date on the insulin packaging is for unopened, refrigerated vials, disposable pens, or pen cartridges. Once opened, most vials of insulin last for 28 days, but many pens and pen cartridges are good for only 7, 10, or 14 days. Pump users should change their infusion set and the insulin in the pump reservoir every 48 hours. These limits should be noted in the insulin package insert. If you're not sure how long your opened container of insulin will last, ask a member of your diabetes care team or your pharmacist or call the manufacturer's customer service number.

■ *Is your technique for taking your medicine adequate?* If you take pills, be sure you're taking them at the right time of day. Some pills must be taken right before meals to work effectively; others do not. If you take insulin by pen or syringe, review your injection technique with your diabetes care team. You should be aware that if you switch to a different syringe or insulin pen or from one to the other, the injection technique may differ.

■ *Are you storing your medicine properly?* Insulin, as well as oral medicines, can lose potency if exposed to heat, cold, or moisture. Your best bet is usually to store opened containers of medicines you are currently using at room temperature. Unopened pills can also be stored at room temperature. Insulin that has not been opened should be stored in the refrigerator. Be careful not to place insulin in the particularly cold areas of the refrigerator—typically the meat compartment and at the backs of the main shelves—where it may freeze.

■ *Is your insulin being delivered adequately?* If you use an insulin syringe or insulin pen, do you always use the same size needle? Some people find that a change in the needle length can disrupt their control. If you use an insulin pump, review the set-up of your infusion set with your diabetes care team to assure accurate insulin delivery. If you order pump supplies by mail, double-check your order when it arrives to make sure you received the correct supplies. Using a different size catheter or a different tubing length than usual may change the amount of priming necessary. (All pump users should have alternative methods of insulin delivery on hand should their pump malfunction or stop delivering insulin for any reason.) In addition, check your injection or infusion sites periodically. If toughening or scarring of the skin is present, this may affect absorption of your insulin.

■ *If you use an insulin pump, is the battery power sufficient?* Avoid going to sleep at night or becoming preoccupied with other things when your battery is low. Be attentive to low battery warning alarms, and change your batteries promptly when they sound. Don't wait until you've used the last drop of energy in your battery.

■ *Are you taking any other medicines that could affect your blood glucose level?* Certain types of drugs—including prescription drugs, over-the-counter drugs, and herbal preparations—may contribute to hyperglycemia. Common prescription drugs that have a tendency to increase blood glucose levels include corticosteroids (used to treat inflammation) and thiazide diuretics (used to treat high blood pressure).

Any time you receive a prescription for a new drug, whether for a diabetes-related condition or not, ask your doctor if it may have any effects on your blood glucose levels. In addition, tell your health-care team about any over-the-counter medicines or alternative therapies you use so that together you can determine whether those substances or practices are having an effect on your blood glucose control.

Stress

During periods of stress, the body releases so-called stress hormones, which cause a rise in blood glucose level. In the short term, this gives the body the extra energy it needs to cope with the stress. But if a person doesn't have adequate insulin circulating in his bloodstream to enable his cells to use the extra energy, the result will be hyperglycemia. And if stress becomes chronic, hyperglycemia can also become chronic. Stress hormones may be released during physical, mental, and emotional stresses.

Physical stress. Injury, illness, infection, and surgery are some examples of physical stresses that often cause hyperglycemia. In fact, hyperglycemia may be a clue that an otherwise symptomless infection is present. Resolving hyperglycemia caused by physical stress generally involves both treating the underlying cause and treating the hyperglycemia itself with changes to the usual diabetes treatment regimen.

Because everyone can expect to be ill at some point, people with diabetes are encouraged to work out a sick-day plan in advance with their diabetes care team. Your sick-day plan should have specifics on what to eat and drink when you're sick, over-the-counter products that are safe to use, as well as details on taking your usual medicines and adding supplemental insulin if needed. It should also indicate when to call your health-care provider.

Mental and emotional stresses. Psychological stresses such as difficulties with relationships, job pressures, financial strain, and even concerns about self-worth can contribute to hyperglycemia. If these issues become overwhelming, decreased attention to the diabetes treatment plan may also contribute to hyperglycemia. Learning stress-reduction techniques may help over the long term, and your diabetes care team may be able to help you identify other resources that can help you deal with feelings of overwhelming stress.

Hormones

Hormones other than stress hormones can affect blood glucose levels, as well. Premenopausal women may experience higher-than-usual blood glucose levels about a week prior to menstruation, when levels of progesterone, estrogen, and other hormones involved in ovulation are changing. In addition, some women find that they have a tendency to eat more during this phase of the menstrual cycle, which may further increase blood glucose levels. It can be useful to track your menstrual cycle along with your blood glucose levels to determine whether your cycle is affecting your blood glucose levels and to learn to make adjustments to your diabetes regimen when needed.

During perimenopause, which can last for several years before the complete cessation of menstruation, the menstrual cycle becomes less and less consistent. This can upset the balance of blood glucose control due to the unpredictability of hormonal levels.

Pregnancy hormones also affect blood glucose control. In fact, insulin adjustments are often necessary every 7–10 days during pregnancy, especially during the second and third trimesters, to adjust for changes in hormone levels as well as for the weight increases that come with pregnancy. Because hyperglycemia can contribute to a number of complications during pregnancy, close monitoring of blood glucose control is essential during and ideally before pregnancy.

In men with diabetes, low testosterone levels may contribute to increased insulin resistance, which can contribute to hyperglycemia. However, while testosterone replacement therapy has become a topic of great interest among both consumers and medical professionals, few studies have examined the long-term effects of testosterone replacement. Men concerned about low testosterone should seek individual guidance from their doctors.

Other causes

Some people with diabetes allow their blood glucose levels to run higher than recommended because they are afraid of developing hypoglycemia (low blood glucose). This fear is certainly normal, since hypoglycemia can cause a person to lose bodily control, but a better response to this fear is to learn to prevent episodes of hypoglycemia while keeping your blood glucose levels in the best possible control. If fear is causing you to let your blood glucose level run high, talk with your diabetes care team to work out a plan that will help you avoid both lows and highs.

Another potential cause of hyperglycemia is the intentional or deliberate omission of insulin doses. This behavior is often linked to the presence of an eating disorder. Omitting needed insulin allows blood glucose levels to run high enough to cause the body to eliminate glucose through the urine and therefore decrease calorie absorption. This practice can enable a person to control his weight and, over time, to lose weight, which may be the desired result. However, repeated omission of insulin can lead to diabetes complications, worsen existing complications, and even lead to coma and death. If you or someone you know is intentionally omitting insulin doses as a means of weight control, it is urgent that you seek help from your diabetes care team or a qualified mental health professional. Eating disorders can be treated; left untreated, they can cause devastating health consequences.

Severe hyperglycemia

Managing hyperglycemia is important both to avoid long-term complications and to avoid the acute hyperglycemic states known as ketoacidosis and hyperosmolar hyperglycemia. These disorders can occur in people with Type 1 diabetes as well as those with Type 2 diabetes, although the risk of ketoacidosis is higher among people with Type 1 and the risk of hyperosmolar hyperglycemia is higher among elderly people with Type 2.

Ketoacidosis is characterized by high blood glucose levels (over 250 mg/dl), the presence of ketones in the blood or urine, and dehydration. In hyperosmolar hyperglycemia, blood glucose levels are typically extremely high (over 600 mg/dl), and small amounts of ketones may be detectable in blood or urine. Emergency care in the hospital may be needed to reverse ketoacidosis or hyperosmolar hyperglycemia.

Infection, which, as noted earlier, causes the release of stress hormones, is the most common precipitating factor in the development of both problems. An interruption in insulin delivery from a pump or taking inadequate amounts of insulin by pen or syringe is also a common underlying factor in the development of ketoacidosis. Other factors that may lead to acute hyperglycemia are stroke, alcohol abuse, pancreatitis, heart attack, trauma, and certain drug therapies.

Preventing episodes of severe hyperglycemia involves knowing the causes and symptoms of hyperglycemia, monitoring blood glucose levels often enough to catch hyperglycemia in its early stages, and having a plan to deal with hyperglycemia should it occur. The fact that infection is what commonly leads to ketoacidosis and hyperosmolar hyperglycemia underscores the importance of discussing sick-day management with your diabetes care team before you become sick.

Staying in check

The only way you can truly know your blood glucose level is to check it with your meter. You should discuss when and how often to monitor with your diabetes care team. A diabetes educator can help you determine the type of equipment that is best for you, as well as make sure you are familiar with how the equipment works. More important, with your doctor's help, your diabetes educator can help you learn to self-manage your diabetes by working through the challenges of managing hyperglycemia.

Keep in mind that even with your best efforts in managing your diabetes, you may still experience high blood glucose from time to time. But if your blood glucose levels remain higher than your treatment goals on a regular basis despite your attempts to follow your diabetes treatment plan, talk to your physician. You may need to update your plan to meet your diabetes control needs. □

DIABETES IN THE WORKPLACE
by Deirdre J. Duke, R.N., M.S.N., J.D.

Nearly 21 million Americans age 20 or older have diabetes. Many of those people are currently employed or intend to enter or reenter the workforce in the future. While a few jobs, such as flying commercial airplanes, are still off-limits to people who use insulin to treat their diabetes, for the most part, having diabetes should not limit a person's job or career possibilities. It can, however, mean that a person needs certain accommodations to fulfill his job duties while also taking care of his diabetes.

Whether you are entering or reentering the workforce or just changing jobs, how you present yourself and your diabetes (if you present it at all) can make a big difference in making a smooth job transition. Here are some thoughts to keep in mind when conducting a job search or when integrating your diabetes care into your current job responsibilities.

Job selection

In general, people with diabetes who are seeking a job have the same concerns as anyone else: Will the work interest me? What does the job pay? How are the hours? Do I have the education, skills, and experience that the employer is looking for?

Having diabetes can enter into the job selection process if the position that interests you would require major changes in your diabetes management routine or lifestyle. For example, working evening or night shifts, working weekends, working primarily outside, driving extensively or commuting for long hours, or performing significantly more or less physical activity than you currently do could affect your diabetes control. Before committing to a job that requires big changes like these, it is advisable to talk with your physician or diabetes educator about how your diabetes management routine could be adjusted to accommodate such changes.

Since having diabetes often involves regular use of the health-care system and substantial medical costs, you will want to find out about a prospective employer's health benefits packages. Examples of benefits that should be evaluated include medical and dental insurance, short- and long-term disability insurance, prescription drug and vision care discounts, medical reimbursement accounts (often called flexible spending plans), pension, and employee fitness and wellness programs. Some employers may offer you a written summary of their benefits, and others may be able to give you written materials if you ask. If not, you may have to ask for specifics such as premium costs, deductibles, copayments for doctor visits, drugs, and emergency room visits, and any other items of particular interest to you. (However, it is not necessary to specify if or how you expect to be using medical or other benefits.)

The job interview

The "rules" for job interviewees are pretty standard whether or not a person has diabetes: Arrive punctually for your interview, be well rested, and dress appropriately. Before your interview, learn what you can about the company from sources such as the Internet, newspaper, local public library, or people you know who work there. You may also want to prepare some questions in advance, either about the company or about the position for which you are interviewing. Showing that you understand company culture and what the company is trying to accomplish will help you to convince the interviewer that you would fit in well within the organization and make a positive contribution if you were hired.

There are some standard rules for interviewers, too. For one thing, it is unlawful for any employer subject to federal or state disability discrimination laws, such as the federal Americans With Disabilities Act (ADA) or Rehabilitation Act, to ask job applicants about their medical history, current state of health, or disabilities, if any, unless a particular physical ability (such as a certain level of visual acuity) is required for the position. This means that in most cases, an employer cannot ask you whether you have diabetes or whether you use insulin or other prescription drugs. In addition, with the exception of a few safety-sensitive jobs, an employer also cannot require an applicant to undergo a medical examination before it makes a conditional job offer. Employers can ask job candidates whether they can perform the essential functions of a job with or without a reasonable accommodation. A reasonable accommodation is defined under the Americans With Disabilities Act as a change or adjustment that an employer can make that would enable a disabled person to perform the essential functions of his job.

If your diabetes has no bearing on your ability to do the job, it would not be appropriate to bring it or any other personal medical information up during your interview. However, if, because of your diabetes, you would need an accommodation to do a job, such as permission to eat at your desk, extended or combined meal or break periods to ensure adequate time for meals and blood glucose monitoring, or a private location for monitoring or injections, the interview process is an appropriate time to identify and discuss your concerns. Most employers are receptive to making reasonable adjustments of various kinds to support their workers, whether for medical reasons, personal issues, or otherwise.

The job offer

In some cases, your employer may simply ask when you can start after you've accepted a job offer, but in others, a job offer is conditional until the employer has checked your references, done a criminal background check, or checked your driving record, for example. After you have accepted a conditional job offer, your new employer may ask you about your health and medical history and may require you to submit to a preemployment physical exam—as long as all applicants are treated alike. Employers are legally permitted to—and for certain safety-sensitive jobs, must—require physical examinations, obtain health histories, and/or do drug screenings on newly hired employees. Employers may inquire about health information at this stage of hiring as long as their questions are job-related and consistent with business necessity. Generally, health information is stored in confidential employee medical files that are maintained separately from employee personnel files.

If your employer does not ask about your health history or require a preemployment physical, you are not obliged to reveal your diabetes. However, if your workplace has an employee health department, you may want to disclose your medical diagnosis and health history so that on-site health-care professionals can provide you with timely emergency or medical care should you become ill or injured on the job or experience severe hypoglycemia. The employee health office may also be able to provide you with information or guidance about job accommodations and other programs such as wellness, dietary counseling, corporate fitness, and health screening, that may be available.

Adjusting to a new job

Before you start your new job, think through your new work routine and what it will mean for your diabetes care regimen. If starting work will mean a big change in your daily schedule or activity level, speak to your doctor before you begin to discuss how and when any changes in your diabetes self-management regimen should be made. (Even if you can't get in for an appointment, your doctor should be able to advise you over the phone or by e-mail.) If possible, adopt your new schedule before you actually start your new job so you can see what effect, if any, it has on your blood glucose levels and so you can identify any problems you may have carrying out your diabetes regimen.

If you usually inject insulin into your arm or leg and your new job involves increased walking or repetitive arm or leg motions, speak to your doctor about whether to change your insulin injection sites. Injecting insulin into a limb then exercising that limb can accelerate the rate at which insulin is absorbed into your bloodstream, possibly resulting in hypoglycemia.

For the first day on your new job, try to be well rested, and give yourself extra time to get dressed and arrive at work. Pack your meals, snacks, and diabetes supplies the night before, and be sure to include some glucose tablets, LifeSavers, or similar source of carbohydrate so that you are prepared to treat hypoglycemia promptly if necessary. Once you become familiar with your new surroundings and dining options, you may be able to purchase snacks or meals at or close to work.

Wearing or carrying medical identification is always a good idea and no less so at work. If you become ill at work and are not able to communicate your needs, medical ID can help you to receive prompt and appropriate medical treatment.

After you are oriented to your work area, find a secure place such as a desk drawer or locker to store your self-care supplies. It may also be helpful to remind your employer of any previously discussed work accommodations that you may need to be successful in your new role.

Starting a new job can be exciting, but it's also stressful, and stress can cause changes in your blood glucose level. Increases or decreases in your activity level at work can also affect your blood glucose level. Monitoring your blood glucose level more frequently for the first week or two at your new job will help you see whether adjustments in your diabetes self-care regimen are in order.

Disclosing your diabetes

Legally speaking, your employer must limit its disclosure of information about your diabetes (and any other disability) and any job accommodations that are made for you to people who must know about them from a practical standpoint. Your employer cannot disclose this information unless it must to ensure your safety in an emergency, process any claims you file for worker's compensation, implement an accommodation that will

JOB AND WORKPLACE RESOURCES

The following resources can help you learn about your rights as an employee and determine what sort of accommodations might help you at your job.

DIABETESATWORK.ORG
www.diabetesatwork.org
This Web site is aimed mainly at employers and has tools for assessing the effects of diabetes on the workplace and for helping employees with diabetes care for their health.

EQUAL EMPLOYMENT OPPORTUNITY COMMISSION
www.eeoc.gov/facts/diabetes.html
(800) 669-4000 (calling this number connects you directly with the nearest EEOC field office)
TTY: (800) 669-6820
The document "Questions and Answers About Diabetes in the Workplace and the Americans With Disabilities Act (ADA)" explains the provisions of the Americans With Disabilities Act of 1990 and how it applies to people with diabetes.

FAMILY MEDICAL LEAVE ACT OF 1993
(866) 4-USWAGE (487-9243)
TTY: (877) 889-5627
www.dol.gov/esa/whd/fmla
The Web site of the Department of Labor spells out the provisions of the Family Medical Leave Act of 1993 as well as those of many other federal laws that regulate employment in the United States.

JOB ACCOMMODATION NETWORK
(800) 526-7234
www.jan.wvu.edu
The Job Accommodation Network is a free consulting service that provides information about accommodation methods, devices, and strategies for disabled workers.

enable you to do your job, or respond to a subpoena or court order. If your coworkers become aware of and question any accommodations you receive, such as being permitted to eat at your desk or take extended meals or breaks, your employer can only state that it is permitting these things to provide assistance or for business necessity.

Whether to share information about your diabetes with your coworkers is a personal choice. It may be advisable to inform at least a few people if there's a possibility that you could develop hypoglycemia during work hours and need assistance treating it. Informing others may also be a good idea if you work in a remote location or on an evening or night shift where there are few employees and the employee health office is closed.

Dealing with difficulties

If, in the course of performing your job, you encounter difficulties that relate to your diabetes, talk to your supervisor immediately. It's possible that certain work procedures or the work environment (such as lighting, computer software, seating, etc.) can be changed in a way that enables you to do your job. For information on accommodation methods, devices, and strategies, contact the Job Accommodation Network (contact information is on page 55). Don't wait until you receive disciplinary warnings or a poor evaluation from your supervisor to speak up about work-related problems.

If you find you are not able to perform the job for which you were hired in spite of one or more accommodations, ask your employer about being transferred to another position for which you are qualified. Keep in mind, however, that your employer does not have to permit you to continue working if he feels that you pose a direct threat to your own safety or the safety of others because of the effect your diabetes has on your work performance. If you need assistance exploring other job opportunities within the company, contact the human resources department. Some companies even provide employees with career counseling to help them move to jobs outside the company.

Attendance and leave policies

Any employee would be wise to familiarize himself with his employer's policies regarding working hours, lateness, sick leave, personal days, vacation, leaves of absence, and anything else covered in an employer's personnel policy. If any policies are unclear, ask your supervisor or someone in the human resources department for clarification.

Most employers require some sort of notice if you will be absent for the day, and some specify who you must speak to—usually your immediate supervisor but in some cases the human resources department or employee health department. How much notice is required may depend on your position and whether the employer must find someone to take your place during your absence. In general, policies regarding when you must call in if you're sick or can't make it to work for some

other reason are in place to ensure the smooth running of the operation. Making an effort to observe those policies can go a long way toward maintaining good relations with your employer.

If you will be out for more than one day, maintain regular contact with your employer, and let your supervisor know when you expect to return to work. In some cases, you may be required to produce documentation such as a note from your doctor confirming an illness, or you may have to obtain a health clearance from either your doctor or the employee health department showing you are well enough to return to work following a prolonged absence. If you need to miss work for an extended period due to health reasons, speak with your manager and employee health or human resources department to find out which leave programs and benefits, such as short-term disability, you may be eligible for and to ensure that you, your employer, and your doctor complete all the necessary paperwork. If you are able to do some work but cannot return right away to your usual job following an absence, ask your employer if it has a light-duty work program.

If you have worked for your employer for one year or more, have worked 1,250 hours in the year immediately preceding the onset of a serious health condition, and must be out of work for an extended period or for even just part of your normal work week, you may be eligible for a leave of absence under the Family and Medical Leave Act of 1993 (FMLA) if your employer has at least 50 employees within 75 miles of the main office. If you are eligible for an FMLA leave, you can take up to 12 weeks of unpaid leave, during which time your employer must maintain your existing group health coverage. (Some employers continue to pay their employees' salaries during FMLA leave.) The FMLA allows employees to take leave on an intermittent basis or to work reduced hours in some cases. If an eligible employee returns to work at the end of an FMLA leave (or earlier), a covered employer must restore that person to the same job he had or to an equivalent one.

Parting impressions

Most people change jobs at some point, and parting impressions are as important as initial ones. If you leave a job, be sure to provide your employer with proper notice, and express your appreciation for the opportunity to have been employed there, even if you're happy to leave. You never know when you might consider returning to work there or when you might need to ask your employer for a job reference, so be sure to leave on good terms. □

YOUR DIABETES MANAGEMENT PLAN

WHY IT PAYS TO HAVE ONE

by Michael A. Weiss and Martha M. Funnell, M.S., R.N., C.D.E.

Whether you have had diabetes for years or are newly diagnosed, you know that dealing with this condition can be a challenge. For one thing, diabetes never goes away. Although there are numerous medicines and other therapies available for treating diabetes, none of them are cures. Diabetes is always present, and almost everything you do, including ordinary activities like eating or taking a walk, affects your blood glucose level.

Another key characteristic of diabetes is that the primary responsibility for managing it rests with you and not with your health-care providers. Managing diabetes requires making decisions and performing various tasks several times a day. Your doctor or diabetes educator can't possibly be there with you each time you have to make a choice about what and how much to eat, what physical activity to perform, and how much insulin or medicine to take. You will have your health-care providers' input and guidance for managing your diabetes, but only you can perform the daily tasks necessary for keeping yourself healthy. No one can make you use a meal plan or get the regular physical activity that could make you feel better today and possibly prevent serious complications down the line. Similarly, no one can force you to take medicines or monitor your blood glucose. When it comes down to it, you must take care of your diabetes for yourself, by yourself.

Another defining feature of diabetes is the number of decisions you have to make each day. It is easier to make these decisions if you develop an overall plan. While medicines, meal planning, physical activity, and blood glucose monitoring form the basis of most diabetes plans, each person's plan is different. Your plan needs to combine what you know about yourself with what you and your health-care team know about diabetes. So along with caring for the physical side of diabetes, your plan needs to take into account the amount of stress you face, your emotional response to diabetes, and the other demands and priorities in your life.

The chronic nature of diabetes, along with the need to make so many daily decisions, can make living with diabetes feel overwhelming at times, but it may feel less so once you have an overall plan to guide you in your daily choices. This article provides an outline for making and using a plan for managing your diabetes. The basic steps are to learn more about diabetes and how it affects you physically, emotionally, and practically; establish your goals for blood glucose, blood pressure, and cholesterol and determine what you are willing to do to meet these goals; develop a self-management strategy with the help of your health-care team; give your plan a trial run and see what's working and what's not; and seek out support to help you stay the course.

Learning more

Most people know little about diabetes before they're diagnosed and even less about the impact it will have on their lives. A good way to start learning is to take a diabetes education class in your community. Inquire at your local hospital or visit www.diabetes.org, the Web site of the American Diabetes Association, to find classes in your area. Your health-care providers should also be a source of information, not just about diabetes in general but about your diabetes in particular and how it can best be managed. But managing diabetes is about more than just learning about an illness. To create a workable plan, you also need to know about yourself and how your priorities, cultural and religious beliefs, personality, genetics, likes, and dislikes affect how you care for yourself and your diabetes.

The effect that diabetes will have on your life will become clearer—and will also probably change—over time. Most people react to a diagnosis of diabetes with shock or fear, often followed by anger or sadness. Feelings like these can make it difficult to take steps to learn about your condition and how to manage it. Because your feelings can affect what steps you take to care for yourself, your plan needs to take your feelings into account and include strategies for dealing with them. Your health-care professionals can help you identify such strategies.

If you're having a rough time or your feelings are keeping you from caring for yourself or doing the things you enjoy, consider seeking out support from others who have diabetes and have gone through what you're going through. Many hospitals and clinics that provide diabetes education also have diabetes support groups that meet regularly. Some communities also have diabetes support groups that operate independently of any hospital or organization. The people in your group can provide both emotional support and practical information about living with diabetes that may be helpful to you. Another option is to seek the counsel of your clergy or to make an appointment with a mental health-care provider who has experience working with people with diabetes (or at least with people with other chronic illnesses).

Diabetes doesn't just affect you physically and psychologically; it can have a noticeable financial impact as well. Even when you have insurance coverage, the co-payments for frequent health-care appointments and multiple drugs can add up quickly. Your financial situation may also influence decisions about what foods you eat and where and how you exercise. Ask your health-care providers for any money-saving tips they may have, and tell them if you cannot afford the drugs or other products they recommend.

Establish your goals

When you are first diagnosed with diabetes, your doctor will probably offer you a plan of action. However, as you learn more about diabetes and as you experience its effects on your life, you will probably want to take on a greater role in designing your own plan. On the other hand, your attitude may be "tell me what to do and I'll do it." Either way, let your health-care providers know how involved you want to be in the decision-making process.

One of the first decisions you need to make is what your target blood glucose goals will be. Although the American Diabetes Association and the American Association of Clinical Endocrinologists have established target levels for the general population with diabetes, your goals may be different. Even if you choose to work toward maintaining near-normal blood glucose levels, there are many reasons it may make sense to set interim goals as you work toward your ultimate targets. For one, you may be just learning how to care for yourself. For another, if your blood glucose levels have been very high, it will take time and effort to bring your blood glucose down into your target range.

Other areas of decision-making include your meal plan, exercise plan, whether weight loss is part of your plan, blood cholesterol and blood pressure control, and strategies for coping with stress and the emotional side of diabetes. Your health-care providers can offer advice about the various options, and you need to tell them what actions you are willing and able to take at this time. Remember, no one knows what will fit into your life better than you do.

Keep in mind that the more flexibility you want in your daily routine, the more work you will probably need to do. If you wish to have more flexibility in your food choices or the timing of your meals, you will probably have to make more daily decisions, monitor your blood glucose more often, or take more injections. That is the trade-off, and only you can decide if greater flexibility is worth the extra work to you.

Create a self-management plan and try it out

Once you have learned about diabetes and established your treatment goals, you are ready to work on creating a self-management plan or fine-tuning the one you are currently using.

As you carry out your plan, note what works and what doesn't. You will probably need to make changes as you go along. One common barrier to carrying out a diabetes plan is trying to make too many lifestyle changes at once. If that seems to be the case for you, you may need to prioritize the items in your plan or scale back in some areas. For example, if your original plan was to exercise every day and you haven't exercised once since then, try revising your goal to exercising twice a week or to whatever you feel confident you'll actually do. In fact, every time you set a goal, ask yourself how confident you feel about achieving it. If your answer is "not very confident," revise your plan until you've come up with an action you're sure you will do. Breaking large goals into smaller steps often makes them more manageable.

It's also common to try to make a particular lifestyle change because your health-care provider or family is encouraging you to do so. If your heart isn't in it, however, you are unlikely to do it. But that doesn't mean that all is lost. Rather than trying to ignore the parts of your plan that aren't working, examine them more carefully to see if you can figure out why they aren't working. Maybe you need to focus on another area of your diabetes right now or talk with your health-care team about an alternative approach.

DIABETES RESOURCES

It helps to know some basics about diabetes when creating your diabetes management plan. The following resources can help get you started.

AMERICAN DIABETES ASSOCIATION COMPLETE GUIDE TO DIABETES, 4TH EDITION
This book is a reference for a wide range of topics related to diabetes care, including managing blood glucose levels, traveling, exercising, and dealing with insurance. This edition also includes a searchable CD-ROM that contains the full contents of the book. The book and CD-ROM combination can be purchased by visiting the American Diabetes Association's online store at http://store.diabetes.org or by calling (800) 232-6733.

DIABETES SELF-MANAGEMENT ANSWER BOOK: 501 TIPS AND SECRETS TO KEEP YOU HEALTHY
This guide covers various aspects of diabetes care in a question-and-answer format. The questions are arranged by topics such as daily living, blood glucose monitoring, weight loss, and successful aging. To purchase the book, call (800) 664-9269 or visit www.diabetesselfmanagement.com/answerbook.

NATIONAL INSTITUTE OF DIABETES AND DIGESTIVE AND KIDNEY DISORDERS (NIDDK)
The NIDDK is a component of the National Institutes of Health that conducts and supports research on diabetes and a number of other conditions. The institute's Web site, www.niddk.nih.gov, has a variety of information about diabetes, including basic facts about diabetes, links to diabetes research and clinical trials, and Spanish-language publications about diabetes.

THINK LIKE A PANCREAS: A PRACTICAL GUIDE TO MANAGING DIABETES WITH INSULIN
Written by Gary Scheiner, M.S., C.D.E., a certified diabetes educator who also has Type 1 diabetes, this book covers the ins and outs of using insulin to control blood glucose levels. Chapters cover topics such as mastering the basics of an insulin regimen, calculating basal and bolus doses, and adjusting to a new lifestyle. The book is available by visiting www.integrateddiabetes.com or calling (877) SELF-MGT (735-3648).

Make sure your concerns get addressed at your doctor appointments by making a list of questions or topics you'd like to discuss before each appointment. This includes dealing with the emotional side of diabetes as well as the physical side. If something has happened in your life that has affected how you care for your diabetes, let your health-care provider know. Be sure to tell your doctor at the start of the visit that you have some things to discuss. Remember that your health-care providers are there to help you create a plan that will work for you, not to judge you on your ability to carry out a particular plan.

Seek out support

Once you have diabetes, you have it for life, which means that you need to care for it every single day. There may be times when you feel burned out by the demands diabetes puts on you. When this happens, it's good to have people to turn to for support. For many people, family members and close friends are the people they turn to first. The people close to you may be able to offer emotional support, if that's what you need most, or practical help with carrying out diabetes tasks. It makes it easier for both you and them if you are able to tell them exactly what you would like in the way of help. Maybe you need someone to listen without judging or offering advice, or maybe you want a friend or family member to perform a specific activity, such as accompanying you to a doctor appointment. The clearer you can be about your needs, the more likely you are to have them met.

Your health-care providers can also be a source of support. They, too, may be available to just listen, or they may be able to refer you to resources you weren't aware of. It can also be helpful to talk to other people who are living with diabetes, either in a support group or online, through a message board or chat room devoted to diabetes.

While you never want to forget your ultimate goals, whatever they may be, it often feels less overwhelming to focus on the choices and steps you will make today. Some days will be better than others, and you will probably feel disappointed and discouraged from time to time. Celebrate your successes and learn from the things that do not work as well. Don't forget to give yourself a pat on the back, too, every now and then. You've taken on a responsibility that you never wanted and that most people don't have to deal with. Give yourself credit for learning as much as you have about diabetes and for all of the efforts you make every day to stay in good health. □

NAVIGATING YOUR WAY TO OPTIMAL HEALTH

by Laura Hieronymus, M.S.Ed., A.P.R.N., B.C.-A.D.M., C.D.E., and Gregory Hood, M.D.

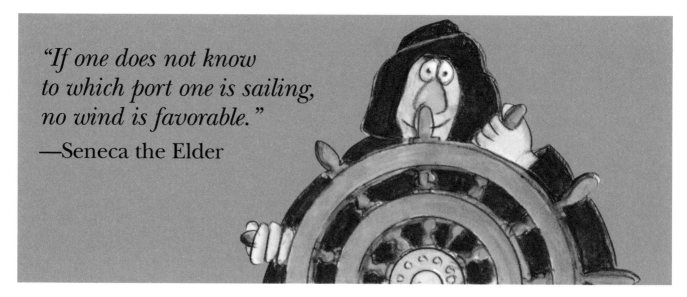

"If one does not know to which port one is sailing, no wind is favorable."
—Seneca the Elder

Diabetes is a chronic condition, meaning that once you are diagnosed, it's there to stay. While this idea can be daunting and even overwhelming at times, the good news is that with regular medical care and optimal blood glucose control, you can live a long, healthy life. With the proper training in diabetes self-management, you will become the navigator of your daily care, while your physician and other health-care professionals act as both the compass that helps guide you in the right direction and the crew that helps to troubleshoot any changes in course.

Charting the course

When you choose a destination, a map can be the most useful tool to get you there. In diabetes management, guidelines that are based on research studies and practical experience act like a map for health-care professionals to help them provide the safest, most effective plan for their patients with diabetes. Every year, the American Diabetes Associ-

ation (ADA) publishes a supplement to the medical journal *Diabetes Care* that includes updated "Standards of Medical Care in Diabetes." While this publication is written for health-care professionals, you should also be aware of these standards so that you can work with your diabetes care team to chart your course toward optimal diabetes health.

Diagnosing diabetes

All adults 45 years of age and over should be screened for diabetes, and if the results are normal, the screening test should be repeated every three years. However, people who have additional risk factors for diabetes may need to be tested at a younger age, more frequently, or both. These risk factors include being overweight, having a first-degree relative with diabetes (a parent, child, or sibling), having high blood pressure or abnormal blood lipid (cholesterol and triglyceride) levels, having had gestational diabetes (diabetes that occurs during pregnancy) or having delivered a baby that weighed more than nine pounds, as well

Basic Information

as being a member of an ethnic group that has a high rate of diabetes.

A fasting plasma glucose test is the preferred method for diagnosing diabetes in most people, although a different test is preferred for women who are pregnant. It is necessary to fast for at least eight hours before having blood drawn for this test to get an accurate result. A fasting plasma glucose level of 126 mg/dl or higher, with a repeat test with similar results on a different day, confirms the diagnosis.

Other acceptable criteria for a diagnosis of diabetes include a combination of symptoms of diabetes (see "Symptoms of Diabetes" on this page) and a casual (nonfasting) plasma glucose level of 200 mg/dl or higher. Again, it is recommended that the blood test be repeated to confirm diagnosis.

A third test, called the oral glucose tolerance test, can also be used to diagnose diabetes. In this test, a person's fasting plasma glucose level is measured before he drinks a solution that contains a specific amount of glucose. Subsequent blood tests are then done one, two, and usually three hours after the glucose solution is consumed. A plasma glucose level of 200 mg/dl or greater at the two-hour mark indicates diabetes. The oral glucose tolerance test is not routinely used to diagnose either Type 1 or Type 2 diabetes. However, it is sometimes used in diagnosing impaired glucose tolerance, which indicates prediabetes, a strong risk factor for developing diabetes, and the oral glucose tolerance test should be used to diagnose gestational diabetes.

Diabetes care

A complete medical evaluation is necessary to diagnose the type of diabetes a person has, to determine whether complications of diabetes are already present at diagnosis, and to decide on treatment methods and a plan for ongoing diabetes care. If you have a history of diabetes and are visiting a physician for the first time, you should have a complete physical exam as well as a discussion about your current blood glucose control, the presence of any diabetes complications, and your ongoing diabetes care needs.

The best care for diabetes management involves a team approach. Typical team members include (but aren't necessarily limited to) physicians (whose coproviders may include nurse practitioners or physician assistants), nurses, dietitians, pharmacists, and mental health professionals, all of whom should have experience working with people with diabetes. It's best if your team members

SYMPTOMS OF DIABETES

The following are some common symptoms of diabetes. However, not all people with diabetes have symptoms before diagnosis. That is why regular screening for adults 45 and older and for anyone with risk factors for diabetes (such as being overweight and having a family history of diabetes) is so important.

- Frequent urination
- Dry mouth or extreme thirst
- Hunger
- Blurry vision
- Fatigue
- Numbness or tingling in the hands and feet
- Decreased sexual function
- Sores that have trouble healing
- Weight loss

can work together to offer you the most up-to-date diabetes management plan possible.

Blood glucose control

The primary goal of diabetes management is optimal blood glucose control, since the complications of diabetes are directly linked to high blood glucose levels. Learning how to monitor your blood glucose levels and learning what the results mean are therefore essential parts of your diabetes treatment plan. Self-monitoring of blood glucose helps you and your diabetes care team evaluate your overall blood glucose control and review the trends and patterns of your blood glucose levels during the course of the day.

General recommendations for how often you should monitor may vary with the type of diabetes you have, your treatment plan, and the extent to which your health insurance plan will reimburse you for monitoring supplies. Insulin users, especially those who take insulin multiple times a day, should monitor their blood glucose levels three times or more daily. People with Type 2 diabetes who use insulin less frequently, use other diabetes medicines, or manage their diabetes with meal-planning and physical activity alone should monitor their blood glucose levels as recommended by their diabetes care team to keep tabs on their level of blood glucose control. (To get a sense of what you're aiming for, see "Blood Glucose Targets" on page 62.)

If you are meeting your blood glucose target levels, you should have a glycosylated hemoglobin (HbA_{1c}) test at least twice a year. The HbA_{1c} test is a blood test that gives a measure of your diabetes control over the preceding two to three months. If you have had a recent change in your diabetes treatment plan, or if your blood glucose levels are regularly outside of the recommended ranges, you should have an HbA_{1c} test every three months. (To see how HbA_{1c} test results correlate with blood glucose monitoring results, see "What Does My HbA_{1c} Mean?" on page 63.)

Tools for management

When it comes to diabetes self-management, knowledge is the best tool you can have. Knowing the steps you can take and the contingencies you should plan for will help keep you healthy and keep the sailing smooth.

Nutrition. When you have diabetes, it is important to understand the relationship between food and blood glucose control. All people with diabetes should see a registered dietitian, preferably one with expertise in diabetes. You and your dietitian should discuss and customize a meal plan for you, taking your health and your personal goals into consideration. Your dietitian can show you how to monitor the effects of the foods you eat on your blood glucose levels.

If you are interested in losing weight, a dietitian can provide suggestions that will help you do so in a safe, nutritionally sound manner while still focusing on blood glucose control to prevent the complications of diabetes. If you have high blood pressure or abnormal blood lipid levels, which are common among people with diabetes, your meal plan should address those issues as well. If you have any diabetes complications, the dietitian may also recommend some changes in your meal plan that can help slow their progression.

Keep in mind that as you age, your body and your diabetes treatment needs change, so your nutrition status and caloric needs will need to be reevaluated. Periodic follow-up visits with the dietitian are key to maintaining your diabetes health.

Diabetes education. In addition to covering your medical visits, most health plans, including Medicare, provide some coverage for diabetes self-management education and training. All people with diabetes should receive diabetes education from a diabetes educator, preferably at an American Diabetes Association–recognized education service, which must meet a set of national standards. Certified diabetes educators (C.D.E.'s) are health-care professionals, such as doctors, nurses,

BLOOD GLUCOSE TARGETS

The ADA has established the following targets for most adults with diabetes. Pregnant women have their own set of recommended targets, and senior citizens and children may also have different, individualized goals. Lower targets may be recommended for certain people who are at lower risk for hypoglycemia (low blood glucose), while those with frequent or unrecognized hypoglycemia may have higher blood glucose targets for safety purposes. Your diabetes care team may also recommend that you monitor your blood glucose level at times besides before and after meals.

TIME	GOAL
Premeal	90–130 mg/dl
Postmeal (1–2 hours after eating)	less than 180 mg/dl

dietitians, pharmacists, exercise physiologists, psychologists, and social workers, who specialize in the care and treatment of people with diabetes. They can help you learn how to stay healthy with diabetes.

Diabetes education can take place in group or individual sessions. Initially, the educator should cover topics such as what diabetes is; tools for managing the condition, including meal planning, physical activity, diabetes drugs, blood glucose monitoring, and common lab tests that should be done periodically; potential complications related to diabetes; and coping skills. Special training is also available for women with diabetes who are planning to become pregnant or are currently pregnant.

Individualized training that considers your age, career, and culture as well as your medical status can be essential to your success in managing diabetes. Diabetes education should encourage you to set goals to achieve behavior change as well as address your specific needs. If you feel your individual needs have not been addressed, let your educator know what areas you need help with.

Physical activity. The benefits of physical activity for people with diabetes include improvement in blood glucose levels, weight control, and, when moderate-to-intense aerobic physical activity is done regularly, reduction of cardiovascular disease risk. Research has also shown that resistance training exercises (such as weight lifting) can be helpful in the management of Type 2 diabetes (though lifting heavy weights may not be appropriate for people with certain diabetes complications).

See your doctor for a physical exam before starting an exercise program, especially if you haven't been active for a while. Your physician may recommend a graded exercise test with electrocardiogram (ECG) monitoring to evaluate the effect of physical activity on your heart.

While physical activity can have a positive effect on blood glucose control, there are times when it should be avoided. If you have Type 1 diabetes and your blood glucose levels are above 250 mg/dl and you detect ketones in your urine, or if your blood glucose levels are above 300 mg/dl (even if there are no ketones in your urine), you should not exercise until your blood glucose levels have been brought into your target range. If your blood glucose level is less than 100 mg/dl and you use insulin or a drug that stimulates the pancreas to release more insulin (such as glyburide, glipizide, or glimepiride), you should have a carbohydrate-containing food or beverage to raise your blood glucose level before you exercise. Your diabetes care team can help you determine a safe way to include physical activity in your diabetes care plan.

Mental health care. The day-to-day necessity of dealing with a chronic illness can add stress and strain to one's life, and your diabetes care team should address these issues with you. If you're having trouble coping, they may recommend that you see a psychologist (or other mental health care professional) to talk about issues such as your attitude toward having diabetes, your expectations for managing the condition, your general and health-related quality of life, and the financial, social, and emotional resources at your disposal. If needed, including a mental health professional in your diabetes care team is recommended, because emotional well-being is an important part of your personal diabetes management.

Sick-day plan. Physical stressors, such as illness, trauma, or surgery, can disrupt your blood glucose control, leading to very high blood glucose levels. This, in turn, can trigger serious conditions such as *diabetic ketoacidosis* (in which poisonous acids called ketones build up in the blood) or *nonketotic hyperosmolar state* (in which high blood glucose levels cause severe dehydration). You and your diabetes care team should determine a sick-day plan in advance that spells out what to do if one of these stressors occurs. Your sick-day plan may call for more frequent blood glucose monitoring,

WHAT DOES MY HbA$_{1c}$ MEAN?

The glycosylated hemoglobin (HbA$_{1c}$) test gives a snapshot of a person's blood glucose control over the previous 2–3 months. The lower your HbA$_{1c}$, the better your chances of avoiding serious diabetes complications. The ADA's recommended HbA$_{1c}$ goal for people with diabetes in general is less than 7%, while individuals should pursue an HbA$_{1c}$ level as close to normal (less than 6%) as possible. (Less stringent targets may be recommended for certain populations.) Here's how HbA$_{1c}$ test results relate to blood glucose monitoring results (when using a meter that gives plasma glucose levels):

HbA$_{1c}$ TEST RESULT	AVERAGE PLASMA GLUCOSE LEVEL
6%	135 mg/dl
7%	170 mg/dl
8%	205 mg/dl
9%	240 mg/dl
10%	275 mg/dl
11%	310 mg/dl
12%	345 mg/dl

monitoring of ketones in the blood or urine, and ongoing communication with your physician to help you manage your diabetes during an illness. Should you need to be admitted to the hospital for any reason, ask that a member of your diabetes care team be consulted regarding your treatment to ensure that you maintain the best possible blood glucose control. Keeping your blood glucose levels as close as possible to their target ranges while you are in the hospital can reduce your chance of developing further illness or infection during your stay.

Hypoglycemia plan. Knowing how to deal with hypoglycemia (low blood glucose) is important for people whose diabetes treatment plans include insulin or diabetes drugs that increase the body's own production of insulin, such as glyburide, glipizide, or glimepiride. Learn to identify your particular signs and symptoms of hypoglycemia, which may include weakness, shakiness, a sweaty or clammy feeling, fast heart rate, confusion, dizziness, changes in vision, and lack of coordination. Treatment to raise blood glucose is usually called for in adults with diabetes if blood glucose levels fall below 70 mg/dl. Usually, 15–20 grams of pure glucose (the amount found in 3–5 glucose tablets) is the recommended treatment, although any form of carbohydrate in the appropriate amount is acceptable. Using a food with added fat (such as a chocolate bar) however, is not recommended to treat hypoglycemia because fat may slow down the body's absorption of the carbohydrate.

Your diabetes care team will recommend that you check your blood glucose 15 minutes after treatment to assure that your blood glucose level has returned to the recommended range. If it hasn't, treating again is generally recommended. Your physician may also prescribe a glucagon emergency kit if you are at risk for severe hypoglycemia. When a person develops severe hypoglycemia, he may lose consciousness and be unable to treat himself. Glucagon is a hormone that causes the liver to release glucose into the bloodstream, raising blood glucose levels. It must be injected and should be given by someone, such as a family member, friend, or coworker, who has been trained to administer it.

Immunizations. Influenza and pneumonia are especially dangerous in people with chronic medical conditions such as diabetes. Therefore, all people with diabetes who are at least six months old should receive a yearly influenza vaccine (flu shot). Your physician may ask you some questions to confirm that the vaccine will be safe for you. For example, the vaccine is usually not given to people who are allergic to eggs or egg products.

At least one lifetime pneumonia vaccine is also recommended for adults with diabetes. In some cases, the vaccine needs to be repeated. Check with your diabetes care team for specific recommendations regarding a pneumonia vaccine for you.

Preventing cardiovascular disease

Cardiovascular disease is the cause of death in at least 65% of adults with diabetes. Type 2 diabetes is an independent risk factor for macrovascular disease (disease of the large blood vessels, including the heart's blood vessels), and cardiovascular complications may already be present when diabetes is diagnosed.

Risk factors for cardiovascular disease include dyslipidemia (abnormal levels of blood lipids such as cholesterol and triglycerides), high blood pressure, smoking, a family history of developing heart disease at an early age, and the presence of the protein albumin in the urine.

TARGET LIPID LEVELS FOR ADULTS WITH DIABETES

Both lifestyle changes and drug therapy may be recommended to achieve these cholesterol and triglyceride levels.

LIPID	GOAL LEVEL
LDL cholesterol	less than 100 mg/dl
LDL cholesterol in people with cardiovascular disease	less than 70 mg/dl
HDL cholesterol (men)	higher than 40 mg/dl
HDL cholesterol (women)	higher than 50 mg/dl
Triglycerides	less than 150 mg/dl

You can lower your risk of cardiovascular disease by controlling your cholesterol, triglyceride, and blood pressure levels with diet, exercise, and drug therapy if necessary; by stopping smoking if you smoke; and by taking aspirin if your physician recommends it.

Lipid management. Abnormal lipid, or blood fat, levels contribute to higher rates of cardiovascular disease, particularly in people who have Type 2 diabetes. You and your physician should discuss lifestyle measures you can take, such as following an eating plan that focuses on reduction of saturated fat, dietary cholesterol, and *trans* fat intake as well as weight loss (if necessary); increased physical activity; and, if you smoke, smoking cessation. These measures can help lower low-density lipoprotein (LDL, or "bad") cholesterol, raise high-density lipoprotein (HDL, or "good") cholesterol, and lower triglycerides (see "Target Lipid Levels for Adults With Diabetes" above). Keeping blood glucose levels close to the normal range can also improve lipid levels, particularly high triglyceride levels.

If you do not meet your goals with lifestyle changes alone, your physician will likely recommend drug therapy. The first priority is to lower LDL cholesterol to a target level of less than 100 mg/dl, and a class of drugs called *statins* is the first choice for this job (except during pregnancy). If you already have cardiovascular disease, a reduction in LDL to a level of less than 70 mg/dl is an option that is widely recommended to stave off cardiovascular events. Lipid levels are usually measured once a year in people with diabetes, although they may be measured more or less often depending on a person's cardiovascular risk.

Controlling high blood pressure. High blood pressure, defined as blood pressure greater than or equal to 140/90 mm Hg, affects the majority of people with diabetes. In people with Type 1 diabetes, it is often the result of underlying nephropathy (kidney disease). In people with Type 2 diabetes, high blood pressure contributes to high rates of cardiovascular disease.

Because high blood pressure is so common and can do a lot of damage to your internal organs, your blood pressure should be measured at every routine diabetes visit. If your systolic blood pressure (the top number) is greater than or equal to 130 mm Hg or your diastolic blood pressure (the bottom number) is greater than or equal to 80 mm Hg, you will need to take steps to lower these values. You should also have your blood pressure measured again on another day to confirm that it is elevated.

The goal for blood pressure for adults with diabetes is less than 130/80 mm Hg. If your blood pressure exceeds this level, your diabetes care team will likely recommend that you reduce your sodium intake and increase your intake of fruits, vegetables, and low-fat dairy products; avoid excessive alcohol consumption; increase your level of physical activity; and make an effort to lose weight if you're overweight.

You may also be prescribed blood-pressure–lowering drugs if lifestyle measures don't produce the desired change or if your blood pressure is higher than a certain cutoff. People with a systolic blood pressure of 130–139 mm Hg or a diastolic blood pressure of 80–89 mm Hg are usually advised to start with lifestyle and behavior changes alone, and if target blood pressure levels are not reached in three months, to begin drug therapy. People with a systolic blood pressure greater than 140 mm Hg or a diastolic blood pressure 90 mm Hg or higher are usually advised to start blood-pressure–lowering drug therapy right away, in addition to lifestyle and behavior changes.

Taking care to lower blood pressure gradually to avoid any complications is a goal for elderly people. If medicine is necessary, your physician will likely prescribe either an angiotensin-converting enzyme (ACE) inhibitor or an angiotensin receptor blocker (ARB). It is not uncommon for two or three different drugs to be used to reach blood pressure goals. It is important to be aware that ACE and ARB therapy, as well as some other antihypertensive drugs, should not be used during pregnancy.

Smoking cessation. Cigarette smoking contributes to one of every five deaths in the United States and is the leading avoidable cause of premature death. Smoking is related to the early development of cardiovascular disease as well as the microvascular complications of diabetes (such as eye and kidney disease). If you are a smoker, you and your physician should discuss a plan for quitting. Counseling or other forms of treatment should be a routine part of your diabetes care.

Aspirin therapy. If you are over 40 years old, your physician will recommend aspirin therapy to prevent cardiovascular events, including stroke and heart attack, unless there is a reason for you not to use it. Research has shown reductions of 20% in strokes and 30% in heart attacks with aspirin therapy. Although doses of 75 to 325 mg a day have been studied, there is no evidence to support a specific dose, so using the lowest possible dose may help reduce side effects.

Everyone with diabetes should consider aspirin therapy except those under the age of 21 because of an increased risk of a rare but potentially deadly disorder called Reye syndrome, which is associated with viral infection and aspirin use in this age group. The beneficial effects of aspirin therapy have also not been studied in people younger than 30.

Preventing other complications

Retinopathy (diabetic eye disease) is the leading cause of new cases of blindness in adults under age 65. Uncontrolled blood glucose levels damage small blood vessels in the eye, weakening the blood vessel walls and allowing fluid or blood to leak into the retina, which is the light-sensitive part of the eye that sends visual signals to the brain. The presence of retinopathy is strongly related to how long a person has had diabetes. In people with Type 1 diabetes, retinopathy rarely appears before the fifth year of having the condition; however, the risk for retinopathy is greater for people with Type 1 than for those with Type 2 diabetes.

High blood pressure and nephropathy (kidney disease) are also associated with an increased risk of retinopathy. The risk for retinopathy can be reduced with control of blood glucose and blood pressure levels.

The following are current recommendations for adults regarding eye examinations:

■ Adults with Type 1 diabetes should have an initial dilated and comprehensive eye examination within three to five years of the onset of diabetes.
■ Adults with Type 2 diabetes should have an initial dilated and comprehensive eye examination shortly after the diagnosis of diabetes because retinal changes may already have occurred by the time diabetes is diagnosed.
■ All people with diabetes should have the eye examination repeated annually.
■ Women with diabetes who are planning a pregnancy should be counseled on the risk of the development and/or progression of diabetic retinopathy. Pregnant women should have an eye examination during the first trimester of pregnancy and follow-up exams as recommended.

Nephropathy (diabetic kidney disease) is the most common cause of kidney failure in the United States and the greatest threat to life in adults with Type 1 diabetes. One-third of people with Type 1 diabetes develop kidney disease within 15 years of diagnosis. Diabetes damages the small blood vessels in the kidneys, impairing their ability to remove impurities from the blood. People with severe kidney damage must have a kidney transplant or rely on dialysis to filter waste from their blood.

Intensive diabetes management with the goal of achieving near-normal blood glucose levels has been shown to reduce the risk and slow the progression of kidney disease in people with Type 1 and Type 2 diabetes. Optimal control of blood pressure is another recommendation to reduce risk for nephropathy. It is essential that people with diabetes undergo an annual test for the presence of *microalbuminuria* (the spilling of small amounts of the protein albumin into the urine, which indicates kidney damage). This should be done in everyone who has had Type 1 diabetes for five years or more and in everyone with Type 2 diabetes starting at diagnosis. Testing for microalbuminuria should also occur during pregnancy.

If microalbuminuria is detected, optimal blood glucose control, as well as controlling blood pressure levels using either angiotensin-converting enzyme (ACE) inhibitors or angiotensin receptor blockers (ARBs) can slow the progression to kidney damage. In this situation, your dietitian will recommend restricting protein intake to about 10% of calories daily, or 0.8 grams per kilogram of body weight per day (the current adult recommended dietary allowance for protein), which may also slow the decline of kidney function. If a person has nephropathy, early detection and treatment can improve his quality of life and delay or prevent the need for dialysis and renal transplantation.

MONITORING FOR CONTROL AND COMPLICATIONS

This list provides a summary of recommendations for various types of monitoring related to diabetes health. To individualize your diabetes management plan, the frequency and type of monitoring may be modified by your diabetes care team to best meet your needs.

These should be checked at every visit to your primary health-care provider:
■ Blood pressure
■ Feet (to identify any loss of sensation)

This should be checked every 3–6 months:
■ Glycosylated hemoglobin (HbA_{1c}) level

These tests should be done annually:
■ Dilated eye exam
■ Lipid level test
■ Microabuminuria test (to test for kidney disease)
■ Serum creatinine measurement to estimate glomerular filtration rate (GFR) (to test for kidney disease)

Neuropathy (diabetic nerve disease) is one of the most common and most challenging complications of diabetes. Elevated blood glucose levels can cause damage to the peripheral nervous system (*peripheral neuropathy*), which affects the sensory nerves that reach the arms, legs, hands, and feet. Neuropathy is a major contributing factor in foot and leg amputations among people with diabetes. Damage can also be done to the autonomic nerves (*autonomic neuropathy*), which control blood pressure, heart rate, digestion, and sexual function, as well as other internal organ processes. Studies have shown that intensive control of blood glucose can reduce the development and progression of nerve damage in Type 1 and Type 2 diabetes by as much as 60%.

Although most neuropathies are detected based on symptoms, your physician should screen you annually for peripheral neuropathy with tests such as those for sensation (feeling); pressure, temperature, and vibration perception; and reflexes. Your physician should also check your feet at each diabetes visit to assess any potential problems. While there have been several advances in therapies to treat neuropathy, there is no known direct treatment for the underlying causes of neuropathy at this time (though stabilizing blood glucose levels is an important first step). Treatment of peripheral neuropathy currently focuses on pain management. Your diabetes educator should give you guidelines for foot care to help prevent any injury and infection to your feet and legs due to loss of sensation from peripheral neuropathy. Treatment of autonomic neuropathy also focuses on relief of symptoms and is based on each individual's condition.

Setting sail

With the ADA's standards of care serving as a map to guide you, you can control your diabetes destiny. The sailing may not always be smooth, but if you stay on course with self-care, optimal blood glucose control, continuing diabetes education, and regular visits to and communication with your diabetes care providers, good health and prevention of diabetes-related complications can be your charted destination.

Bon voyage. □

TAKING DIABETES TO HEART

by Laura Hieronymus, M.S.Ed., A.P.R.N., B.C.-A.D.M., C.D.E., and Kristina Humphries, M.D.

Keep your heart with all diligence;
for from it flow the springs of life.
—Proverbs 4:23

It is well documented that the risk of heart disease is 2–4 times higher in people with diabetes as compared to the general population. In fact, the risk is so high that two in three people with diabetes die from heart disease or stroke. However, when you have diabetes, it is *uncontrolled* blood glucose levels that place you at the highest risk for heart disease. Uncontrolled blood glucose levels and related complications may contribute to the development of fatty deposits on the insides of your blood vessels. This is referred to as *atherosclerosis*, the "hardening of the arteries" that can reduce the amount of blood flow to the heart, brain, and limbs.

What this means for people with diabetes is that they may develop heart disease at an earlier age than others and that their chance of having a heart attack is as high as that of a person without diabetes who has already had a heart attack. While women who don't have diabetes see their risk of heart disease increase dramatically after menopause, women with diabetes have an increased risk even before menopause, because diabetes cancels out the protective effects of higher levels of estrogen. Also, heart attacks in people with diabetes tend to be more serious, being more likely to result in death.

Assessing your risk factors

In addition to uncontrolled blood glucose levels, there are other risk factors for heart disease that

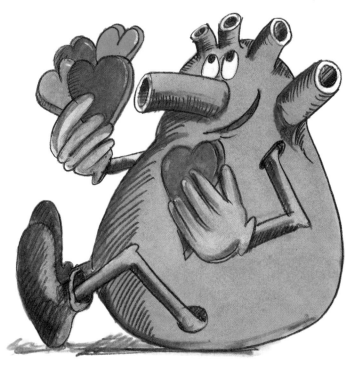

are common among people with diabetes. Since many of them can be treated effectively, your cardiovascular risk factors should be assessed by your physician at least once a year. Timely diagnosis allows you to develop a plan with your diabetes care team to prevent or treat existing heart disease. The following factors contribute to heart disease risk:

Genetics. Heart disease tends to run in families, and so does diabetes. When you have diabetes, your risk for heart disease may be higher if a family member has had a heart attack at a younger age (before 55 years old for men and before 65 years old for women).

Central weight. Carrying extra weight around your waist raises your risk of heart disease. You may have heard central weight distribution referred to as an "apple-shaped" weight pattern (as opposed to "pear-shaped," where extra weight is concentrated in the hips and legs). Your risk further increases if you are obese. For that reason, the National Heart, Lung, and Blood Institute now recommends taking both body-mass index and waist circumference into consideration when assessing a person's risk of heart disease. Men who are both obese and have a waist circumference of 40 inches or larger, and women who are obese and have a waist circumference of 35 inches or larger are at very high risk of developing cardio-vascular disease.

Abdominal fat is associated with an increase the body's production of low-density lipoprotein (LDL, or "bad") cholesterol. A high level of LDL cholesterol or a high proportion of small, dense LDL cholesterol particles raises the risk of heart disease.

High blood pressure. Chronic high blood pressure affects the majority of people with diabetes. High blood pressure is a major risk factor for atherosclerosis and heart disease and can contribute to other blood vessel problems in diabetes, as well.

Dyslipidemia. Having high total blood cholesterol, high LDL cholesterol, high triglycerides, and low HDL cholesterol raises the risk of heart disease. Cholesterol and triglycerides are collectively called *blood lipids*, and any combination of abnormal lipid levels is called *dyslipidemia*. People with Type 2 diabetes very often have high triglycerides, low HDL cholesterol, and a high proportion of small, dense LDL cholesterol particles, which are more harmful than normal LDL cholesterol particles.

Smoking. Smoking doubles your risk of developing heart disease. Smoking causes narrowing of the blood vessels and deprives them of oxygen, an important nutrient to the circulatory system.

Diabetes ABCs

In an effort to draw public attention to the connection between diabetes and heart disease and stroke, the American Diabetes Association and the American College of Cardiology have joined together in an educational initiative that focuses on the acronym "ABC." The letters stand for "A1C," "Blood Pressure," and "Cholesterol."

People with diabetes are encouraged to be aware of their A1C (also called HbA_{1c} or glycosylated hemoglobin) level, blood pressure level, and cholesterol levels. It is hoped that increased awareness of these numbers, what they mean to a person's health, and what a person's target numbers are for good health will lead to more discussion with health-care providers and more action taken to bring levels into target range.

To read more about the ABCs, how often they should be measured, and recommended goals for most people with diabetes, see "ABCs of Diabetes" on page 69.

Modifying your lifestyle

The benefits of the healthy lifestyle habits that are recommended for the management of diabetes extend to your heart health, as well. A healthy lifestyle includes healthy eating, getting regular physical activity, maintaining a healthy weight, and stopping smoking if you smoke.

Healthy eating. Good nutrition is vital for anyone, and for people with diabetes it is an important part of their treatment plan. If you haven't already worked with a dietitian to design an individualized meal plan, ask your diabetes care team for a referral to a registered dietitian. It is best to work with a dietitian who specializes in diabetes.

The good news is that you can tackle blood glucose, blood pressure, and blood lipid levels head-on with the right nutrition intake. Common recommendations include increasing the amount of fiber in your meal plan, which may help lower blood cholesterol. Foods such as oat bran, oatmeal, whole-grain breads and cereals, dried beans and peas (such as kidney beans, pinto beans, and black-eyed peas), fruits, and vegetables are all good sources of fiber.

Monitoring your fat intake can also be important for cholesterol control. Fat should make up no more than 30% of your total energy intake, and most of that fat should be monounsaturated or polyunsaturated. Limiting the amount of saturated fat, *trans* fat, and cholesterol you eat can help to lower your blood cholesterol levels.

Efforts to control your blood pressure may include reducing your sodium (or salt) intake.

Physical activity. Performing regular physical activity or exercise can improve blood glucose control, help control weight, improve your overall well-being, and reduce your risk for heart disease. To achieve these results, performing at least 150 minutes of moderate-intensity aerobic activity a week and/or at least 90 minutes of vigorous aerobic exercise a week is recommended. The activity should be distributed over at least three days of

ABCs OF DIABETES

The American Diabetes Association and the American College of Cardiology have teamed up to raise public awareness of the "ABCs of diabetes," namely A1C, blood pressure, and cholesterol. To have a good sense of your risk of cardiovascular disease and other diabetes complications, you need to "know your numbers."

A

The A1C, or HbA_{1c}, test is a measure of blood glucose control over the previous 2–3 months. Your doctor will likely recommend that you have an A1C test at least twice a year. It is usually done in a laboratory setting, which may or may not be located within your health-care provider's office. Small changes in A1C can make a big difference in your risk for diabetes-related complications. For example, lowering your A1C level by just one percentage point can reduce your risk for all complications by 30% to 35% and cut your risk of heart attack by 18%. Each A1C percentage point above 7.0% doubles your risk of complications.

For most people with diabetes, the A1C target is below 7%. However, even lower levels reduce the risk for complications even more, so each person with diabetes and his diabetes care team should set individualized A1C goals. Certain populations (including children, pregnant women, and elderly people) require special considerations.

Monitoring your blood glucose levels at home between doctor visits helps you know if what you are doing is working to keep your blood glucose levels controlled. The blood glucose targets for most people using a standard, plasma-calibrated blood glucose meter are as follows:
- Before meals, 90–130 mg/dl
- 1 to 2 hours after the start of a meal, less than 180 mg/dl

B

Your blood pressure should be checked at every medical appointment. For most people with diabetes, the recommended blood pressure target is blood pressure below 130/80 mm Hg.

C

People with diabetes are advised to have a blood test to measure triglycerides, low-density lipoprotein (LDL) cholesterol, and high-density lipoprotein (HDL) cholesterol at least once a year. The goals for most people are as follows, but these numbers may be modified based on your individual risk profile:
- LDL ("bad") cholesterol, under 100 mg/dl
- Triglycerides, under 150 mg/dl
- HDL ("good") cholesterol for men, above 40 mg/dl
- HDL ("good") cholesterol for women, above 50 mg/dl

the week, with no more than two consecutive days without physical activity. People with Type 2 diabetes are additionally encouraged to do resistance exercises targeting all major muscle groups three times weekly, as long as they have no *contraindications,* or medical reasons not to perform resistance exercise.

Before increasing your level of physical activity or starting a formal exercise plan, discuss your plans with your diabetes care team. Your health-care providers may want to conduct certain medical tests prior to exercise, especially if you have been sedentary. In addition, you and your diabetes care team should talk about how to control your blood glucose levels during exercise and when to make adjustments to your usual diabetes regimen. (For more about physical activity, see "Staying Active" on page 70.)

Healthy weight. The goals you set with your diabetes care team for staying active and eating healthfully should help you to achieve and maintain a healthy weight. If you need to lose weight, a sensible, gradual weight loss plan is most likely to result in permanent weight loss. Increasing your physical activity while consuming fewer calories will help to make sure the weight you are losing is fat and not muscle.

Stopping smoking. If you smoke, quitting is highly recommended because of the detrimental effects smoking has on the blood vessels and heart. That is not to say it is easy. The first step is deciding that you are willing to quit, then working with your diabetes care team to decide on a plan that will work for you.

Medication

If lifestyle changes alone don't bring your blood glucose, blood pressure, and blood cholesterol levels into target range, drug therapy may be necessary. Some people are reluctant to take drugs, particularly if they are experiencing no symptoms or don't feel bad on a day-to-day basis. But while high blood glucose, high blood pressure, and cholesterol disorders may cause no or few symptoms in the early stages, over time they can do real damage to your internal organs, which will cause symptoms, so it is important to treat them early.

Regularly monitoring your A1C level, blood pressure, and blood lipids will provide you and your diabetes care team with the information needed to make decisions about your need for drug therapy. Remember, medication is not the enemy if it helps keep your "ABCs" in order.

Aspirin therapy is recommended in people with diabetes as a standard practice of care. It has been shown to reduce the risk of heart attack by 30% and the risk of stroke by 20%. However, aspirin therapy is not for everyone, so you should consult your physician before you start to take aspirin regularly. Your physician will take into consideration your age, your heart disease risk factors, other drugs you might be taking, and your heart health history in making a recommendation regarding aspirin therapy.

Symptoms of heart disease

Angina, or pain that occurs when a blood vessel to the heart is narrowed and blood flow is reduced, is a common sign of heart disease. The pain can vary in severity from one episode to the next and can include chest discomfort or pain that radiates to your shoulders, arms, jaw, or back, especially during exercise. The pain may go away when you rest or take a medicine that your physician prescribes for the angina. Angina does not typically cause permanent damage to the heart muscle, but it is a symptom of diminished blood flow to the heart and a warning of an increased risk of having a heart attack.

When a blood vessel that flows to the heart becomes blocked and blood flow to the heart is inhibited, a heart attack occurs. If not enough blood reaches a part of the heart muscle, permanent damage will result.

Men and women tend to have somewhat different symptoms when having a heart attack. Common symptoms of a heart attack in men include the following:
■ Chest pain, pressure, or discomfort
■ Pain or discomfort in the arms, back, jaw, neck, or stomach
■ Shortness of breath
■ Sweating
■ Nausea and sometimes vomiting
■ Dizziness or a feeling of light-headedness

STAYING ACTIVE

Engaging in regular physical activity is good for just about anyone. So is engaging in regular exercise, but exercise and physical activity are not exactly the same thing. Before beginning a program of physical activity that is more vigorous than brisk walking, make an appointment with your diabetes care provider to talk about your plans and any precautions you should take with regard to choice and intensity of activity.

The 1996 report of the Surgeon General, entitled *Physical Activity and Health,* offers the following definitions for the various forms of physical activity and exercise:
■ Physical activity is defined as bodily movement produced by the contraction of skeletal muscle that requires energy expenditure in excess of resting energy expenditure. Brisk walking is the most popular form of physical activity.
■ Exercise is a subset of physical activity. It is planned, structured, and repetitive bodily movement performed to improve or maintain one or more components of physical fitness (such as strength, stamina, flexibility, or ratio of fat to muscle).
■ Aerobic exercise consists of rhythmic, repeated, and continuous movements of the same large muscle groups for at least 10 minutes at a time. It includes activities such as walking, bicycling, jogging, swimming, and water aerobics. Many sports, such as soccer, can include aerobic exercise, as well.
■ Resistance exercise training consists of activities that use muscular strength to move a weight or work against a resistive load. Examples include weight lifting, exercises using weight machines, exercises using body weight such as pushups, and exercises using large latex bands or rubber tubing.

Common symptoms of a heart attack in women include these:
■ Unusual fatigue
■ Sleep disturbances
■ Shortness of breath
■ Diffuse discomfort
■ Depression
Regardless of sex, not everyone who has a heart attack has all the symptoms. In fact, some people,

particularly those with diabetes, may have very subtle symptoms or none at all. This is usually because of nerve damage caused by diabetes, which may result in lack of pain during a heart attack.

If you believe you are having a heart attack, don't delay: Get emergency help immediately. Keep in mind that treatment is most effective if given within an hour of a heart attack and can prevent damage to the heart that may be permanent.

Another common form of heart disease is *congestive heart failure,* a chronic condition in which the heart cannot pump blood properly, causing tiredness and weakness, and fluid builds up inside body tissues. If the buildup is in the lungs, breathing becomes difficult. Fluid buildup can also result in swelling in the feet, legs, and abdomen. Uncontrolled blood glucose levels in people with diabetes may lead to small blood vessel (microvascular) disease, which contributes to loss of heart-muscle tone, resulting in congestive heart failure. People with diabetes have at least twice the risk of congestive heart failure as those without diabetes.

Staying heart-healthy

While having diabetes does increase your risk for heart disease, it doesn't make it inevitable. Work with your diabetes care team to learn all you can about the risks you have, the ongoing options for treatment, and the best action plan to keep you in good health. After all, it is truly a matter to take to heart! □

Dealing With Feelings

Tips 140–194 75

Relaxation Techniques for Stressful Times 79

Spiritual Self-Care and the Use of Prayer 83

Body Image 86
How You See Yourself

Overcoming Binge Eating Disorder 92

Making Positive Changes 97

Understanding Depression and Diabetes 101

How Stories Can Heal 106

Diabetes and Your Marriage 111
Making Things Work

Eight Tips for Managing Diabetes Distress 115

How to Ask For Help—And Get It 118

Getting a New Perspective on Your Diabetes 121

2

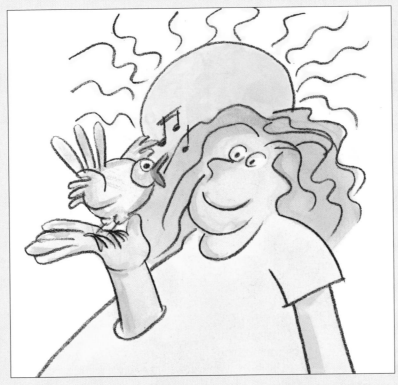

Dealing With Feelings Tips

140–194

140. If you hate your body, you cannot respect it or properly nurture it, and you may even punish or neglect it.

141. Try to separate the healthy behaviors you want to adopt from the attitudes that are just making you feel bad about yourself.

142. Having a stronger sense of self means learning to accept yourself the way you are now, warts and all.

143. When you catch yourself being judgmental about yourself or about someone else, stop and say, "I am not going to be judgmental or critical today."

144. Focus on your internal qualities and characteristics.

145. Each morning, make a written or mental gratitude list of all the things that you have, that you are, and that you are able to experience every day.

146. Make an effort to spend time with people who are supportive, affirming, and encouraging, not judgmental and critical.

147. Throw your fashion and celebrity magazines into the garbage.

148. Instead of viewing exercise as a chore, explore the way your body feels in motion.

149. Be a role model to others by acknowledging and taking them seriously for what they say, feel, and do rather than how

they look, and by curbing your own self-criticism.

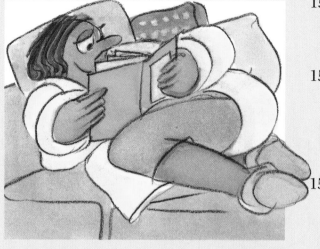

150. In addition to taking care of your diabetes, nurture your body regularly with pleasurable activities such as curling up on the couch with a good book, taking a nap, indulging in a wonderful-smelling body lotion or fragrance, or buying a new outfit that feels great and looks flattering to your figure the way it is now.

151. Diabetes can sometimes feel overwhelming because of the unending demands of self-management.

152. Many clinicians consider a person's levels of distress and depression to be as important to his or her care as measures of blood glucose, cholesterol, blood pressure, and weight.

153. Diabetes distress should be part of the conversation that people with diabetes have with their health-care providers on a regular basis.

154. Seek out others who are understanding about diabetes and are willing to listen without necessarily providing solutions.

155. The greater the number of things changed in a management plan at one time, the greater the probability that none of them will be accomplished. The slower the pace of change, the greater the probability that a goal will be achieved and, even more important, sustained.

156. The primary goal of most aspects of diabetes management is sustained behavior, not just reaching a target in the short term.

157. Dealing with diabetes distress and symptoms of depression is as important to your diabetes care as any drug taken or any behavior routinely practiced.

158. People who develop complications often find that they are manageable, that options for treatment and relief abound, and that even the onset of previously dreaded complications does not detract from the ability to live a meaningful life.

159. Diabetes management is not just a bunch of tasks involving meal plans, blood glucose monitoring, exercise, and medicines; it is also a lifelong process of learning and self-reflection.

160. Clinical trials have demonstrated that good blood glucose control reduces the likelihood of serious diabetes complications and improves health in many ways.

161. Exploring your beliefs about diabetes and about your ability to manage it can spark a reassessment of what you believe to be true about your ability to exert control over the course of your diabetes.

162. Although diabetes management needs continuous attention, when it becomes our world, and when we think that others could never understand the difficulties inherent in our special world, we forget to enjoy our lives.

163. Don't judge yourself harshly when you make a mistake; just observe the effects on your blood glucose, mood, and energy level, and use this information as a learning experience.

164. Don't let distressing thoughts about diabetes interfere with your vision of the future.

165. Try seeing your body and your management tools as miraculous, and see how your mindset and energy level changes.

166. Diabetes has no power to change anything in life that really matters.

167. It is estimated that about 40% of obese people have binge eating disorder. If you do not pursue weight loss in a way that is

Dealing With Feelings

realistic and flexible, you may raise your chances of falling into a binge eating cycle.

168. Don't eat when you are not hungry, and stop eating when you are comfortably full.

169. Be mindful and fully present when you are eating.

170. Some people find it useful to write about how they are feeling.

171. If you have diabetes, stress can make it harder to control your blood glucose level. Stress is a natural part of life, but when it becomes chronic, it can wear you down, both mentally and physically.

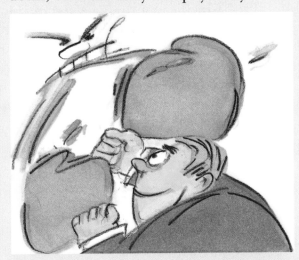

172. Even though life's problems can blindside you every once in a while, using relaxation techniques can help you to roll with the punches and adjust rather than letting stress knock you for a loop.

173. When looking for help, always consider the personality and abilities of the person you're asking, since inappropriate requests just lead to frustration for both of you. You are likely to get a better response if you target your requests for help appropriately.

174. When asking for assistance, decide in advance exactly what it is you will ask for. Make a list of all the forms of help that might be beneficial. Then narrow it down to the one or two most urgent items.

175. How you ask for help has a big influence on the response you get. Specify exactly what kind of help you need. And always give the other person a graceful way out.

176. For people with diabetes, having confidence in your ability to set and meet high standards means better health outcomes, a higher quality of life, and less reliance on the medical system.

177. Change is most successful when you work on things you want to accomplish, not on things you think you should do or things someone else tells you to do, even if that person is your doctor. You need to believe that the behavior change you are considering will actually do you some good if you're going to stick with it.

178. To make major changes more attainable, break your ultimate goal into manageable chunks.

179. Stay flexible and expect some ups and downs when trying to make changes in your life.

180. When you "relapse" into an unhealthy habit, don't give up. Ask yourself what went wrong, get some help if necessary, and try again.

181. Change usually takes longer than you think it should, and it often takes place when you're not looking for it.

182. Having the support of others can help ease the feelings of fear or frustration that often go along with having diabetes.

183. If your relationship is in trouble, admit it, talk about it, and recommit to nurturing the relationship.

184. Holistic principles that promote a more complete approach to wellness could enhance diabetes self-care efforts significantly.

185. For those comfortable with incorporating prayer into the fabric of their daily lives, the use of prayer may be yet another resource to enhance diabetes self-management and therefore, general wellness.

186. Remaining physically active should be an important health goal for people with diabetes and depression. The reduced physical activity and decreased attention

to self-care that accompany depression can worsen blood glucose control and increase risks for diabetic complications.

187. How you choose to find help for overcoming depression is not as important as just getting yourself to seek help if you feel you need it.

188. Much recent research suggests that low intake of omega-3 fatty acids may increase the possibility of depression, and that supplementing the diet with omega-3 fatty acids may help alleviate depression symptoms. Before supplementing with omega-3 fatty acids, talk to your physician or nutritionist about recommended doses and also about which supplement to use.

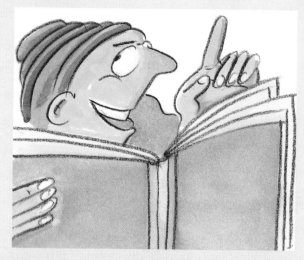

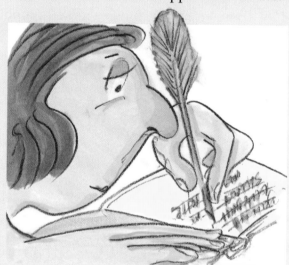

189. By telling your painful stories or writing them down, you can deal with the pain they cause, amplify the strength they give, and even change them for the better. If there is something you would like to tell others but can't for fear of embarrassment, writing about it can help resolve it in your mind.

190. Putting your experiences and feelings in the form of a story can help you deal with them in three important ways: Stories help you to make sense of your life, help you process trauma and loss, and allow you to communicate your experience to others.

191. Experiments have shown that writing or talking about painful memories and emotions can improve immune system.

192. Storytelling helps us make sense of our lives, which can give us a sense of control.

193. Don't use talking or writing as a substitute for action. If you can do something about a problem, do it.

194. Don't use writing as a way of complaining. Use it to discover how you feel and why. Just venting or complaining can sometimes make you feel worse.

RELAXATION TECHNIQUES FOR STRESSFUL TIMES

by Linda Wasmer Andrews

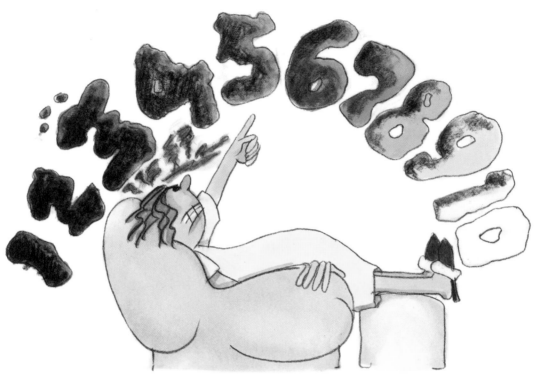

Stress is a natural part of life, but when it becomes chronic, it can wear you down, both mentally and physically. If you have diabetes, stress can make it harder to control your blood glucose level. It also may increase the odds of developing certain complications, such as heart and blood vessel disease and infections made worse by a weakened immune system. In addition, it may distract you so much that you forget to take good care of yourself and to follow your self-care regimen. Yet here's the catch: Diabetes itself can be a very stressful experience, as you're forced to adjust to having a chronic disease and making all the lifestyle changes that go along with it. That's why learning to manage stress is so important.

Stress and strain

To get a handle on stress, it helps to know a bit about the underlying physiology. The so-called fight-or-flight response is the body's way of gearing up to fight or flee when it encounters danger. Heart rate, blood pressure, breathing rate, and muscle tension all increase—changes that would come in quite handy if you were being attacked or chased. Another hallmark of the stress response is the rapid mobilization of energy stores along with the inhibition of further storage. Glucose and the simplest forms of proteins and fats come pouring out of their storage sites to fuel whatever muscles might be needed immediately for fight or flight. At the same time, digestion is inhibited since there wouldn't be time to derive benefits from this slower process.

Most situations in modern life don't involve much wrestling or running, however. Unfortunately, the body can't distinguish between the threat of a predator in the wild and that of an overdraft notice from the bank, so it goes into the same state of high alert.

Over time, a prolonged stress response may contribute to a range of health problems, including anxiety, depression, headaches, backaches, digestive difficulties, high blood pressure, and lower resistance to infection. As far as diabetes goes, many people say they see a link between stress and their blood glucose levels. In people with Type 2 diabetes, stress often raises blood glucose level. In people with Type 1 diabetes, the effects can vary.

"Some people who have Type 1 diabetes say stress drives their blood glucose level up, while others say it drives the level down, and still others don't notice any impact one way or the other," says Mark Peyrot, Ph.D., a sociology professor at Loyola College in Baltimore who has researched the stress–glucose connection. "Within a given individual, though, the reaction to stress tends to be consistent." In other words, if you've reacted to stress in the past with a spike in blood glucose, chances are you'll react that way in the future, too.

The means by which stress may affect diabetes is still unclear. However, part of the fight-or-flight response involves breaking down stored forms of glucose into blood glucose to ready the body for quick action. It's easy to see how this could lead to high blood glucose in the short term. Stress also blocks the release of insulin in people whose bodies still make that hormone.

In the long term, if stress becomes a frequent problem, a person might start to confuse its symptoms with other physical cues. This is why people aiming for tight diabetes control are often advised to record life events along with their blood glucose measurements and insulin or medicine doses. The goal is to identify patterns that make it easier to distinguish the effects of stress from other feelings, such as hunger and lightheadedness before a meal. In addition, stress may affect how people with diabetes take care of themselves. Some people react to stress by eating too much, drinking large amounts of alcohol, or vegging out rather than exercising. This behavior, in turn, may lead to unwanted fluctuations in blood glucose.

Turning off stress

Luckily, the body has a built-in mechanism for turning off the fight-or-flight response. Known as the *relaxation response,* it reverses the physiological changes brought on by stress. Heart rate, blood pressure, breathing rate, glucose mobilization, and muscle tension all decrease. While the stress response usually occurs involuntarily, people can learn to call up the relaxation response at will. This is what relaxation techniques such as meditation and imagery exercises are intended to do. So learning such techniques should help improve diabetes control, right? Surprisingly, the answer to that question is a resounding maybe.

"I think the jury is still out about the effectiveness of relaxation techniques for this purpose," says James Lane, Ph.D., an associate research professor of psychiatry at Duke University. The results of published studies to date have been mixed, and many of these studies have been too small to draw definitive conclusions in any case. Lane thinks another explanation for the lackluster results may be the absence of a good selection process for those taking part in the studies. "You would expect that relaxation training would be more beneficial to people who report feeling anxious or who say their glucose control is related to stress," he says. Yet most researchers have disregarded these issues when picking study participants.

One study that backs up the view that relaxation may help some people more than others was led by Angele McGrady, Ph.D., a psychiatry professor at the Medical College of Ohio. Her small study included 18 people with Type 1 diabetes. Half were assigned to get relaxation training that involved the use of biofeedback, a form of therapy in which a person is taught to gain control of a physiological process with the aid of feedback from an instrument. In this case, people were hooked up to instruments that measured muscle tension and finger temperature. They then were taught to decrease the tension and increase the temperature, two signs of greater relaxation, by breathing deeply and listening to a relaxation tape. The other half of the participants got no such treatment. The researchers didn't find any difference in blood glucose levels between the two groups overall. However, they did find that people with high scores on tests of stress, depression, and anxiety were more likely to have smaller changes in blood glucose as a result of the relaxation training.

Taking it easy

The bottom line: Relaxation techniques may help with blood glucose control very little or a lot, depending on your psychological makeup and your body's sensitivity to stress. Whatever the case, however, they probably won't hurt, and they may leave you feeling less tense and more at peace. While you can certainly take a class in meditation or go to a therapist who teaches imagery exercises, you also can try such techniques on your own at home. McGrady offers this caveat, however: "If you have frequent, long-lasting feelings of anxiety or depression, you should seek professional help." Based on her study, you may not be able to focus on your relaxation practice until you get these problems under better control. What's more, while deep relaxation usually leads to feelings of enhanced well-being and calmness, occasionally it can bring up disturbing emotions, such as fears, sadness, or despair.

Following are some simple techniques for getting the best of stress. You may find that one method is more effective or feels more natural than another. The best technique for you is the one that works. For more detailed instruction, see the books listed in "Relaxation Resources," or ask your health-care provider to refer you to a good stress-reduction program in your area.

Take a deep breath

Deep, abdominal breathing plays a role in many relaxation techniques. Here's a simple breathing exercise to help you get started:
1. Sit or lie in a comfortable position, and close your eyes.
2. Place one hand on your belly just below your navel, and notice your breathing.
3. Feel your hand rise slightly with each breath in. Feel it fall with each breath out.
4. Focus on this rising and falling motion for several breaths.

Have you ever been told to count to 10 to calm down? It really works, at least if you combine the counting with deep breathing:
1. Follow the steps above until you get a comfortable breathing rhythm going.
2. Now, say "ten" to yourself as you breathe in. Then breathe out.
3. With the next breath, say "nine" as you breathe in. Then breathe out.
4. Repeat until you reach "zero."

Meditate on it

Perhaps the best-known means of calling up the relaxation response is by meditation. This practice has its roots in religious rituals, and many people still use it as a path to spiritual enlightenment. However, you don't need to have any religious or spiritual intentions to reap the benefits of the technique. All forms of meditation have two key components. One is a mental focusing device, such as a repeated word, sound, phrase, or prayer or a repetitive movement. The other is a passive disregard for other thoughts that may come up. If you temporarily lose your focus, don't worry about it, but simply return your mind to the repeated word or motion. To get started meditating, try following these basic steps:
1. Pick a focus word or phrase. Keep it short enough to easily coordinate with your breathing. Some examples: "peace," "shalom," "let go," "hail, Mary."
2. Find a quiet place where you aren't likely to be disturbed.
3. Sit or lie in a comfortable position, and close your eyes.

RELAXATION RESOURCES

The plasma glucose goals published by the For more information on relaxation techniques, consult the following resources:

BOOKS
RITUALS OF HEALING
Using Imagery for Health and Wellness
Jeanne Achterberg, Ph.D., Barbara Dossey, R.N., and Leslie Kolkmeier, R.N.
Bantam Books
New York, New York, 1994
This book includes sample scripts that illustrate how to use imagery to both elicit relaxation and help manage a number of medical conditions, including diabetes.

THE WELLNESS BOOK
The Comprehensive Guide to Maintaining Health and Treating Stress-Related Illness
Herbert Benson, M.D., and Eileen M. Stuart, R.N., C., M.S.
Fireside
New York, New York, 1993
Dr. Benson is the one who first coined the term "relaxation response." This book is a classic guide to using relaxation techniques to improve health.

FULL CATASTROPHE LIVING
Using the Wisdom of Your Body and Mind to Face Stress, Pain, and Illness
Jon Kabat-Zinn, Ph.D.
Delta Trade Paperbacks
New York, New York, 1990
Dr. Kabat-Zinn pioneered the use of mindfulness in a medical setting. He is founder of a highly regarded stress-reduction program at the University of Massachusetts Medical Center.

WEB SITE
Benson–Henry Institute for Mind Body Medicine
www.mbmi.org
This nonprofit institute, located at Massachusetts General Hospital in Boston, evolved from the work of Herbert Benson, M.D., and his colleagues at Harvard Medical School. Today, it's at the forefront of research on the medical use of relaxation techniques.

4. Try to relax your muscles, and start noticing your breathing.

5. Repeat your focus word or phrase to yourself as you breathe out.

6. Passively disregard any distracting thoughts that come up.

7. Continue for 10–20 minutes. Meditate once or twice every day, if possible.

Mind your mindfulness

One popular variation on the meditation theme is mindfulness. In this technique, you're asked to focus on moment-to-moment awareness without judging or reacting to the things you notice. You can use mindfulness to become more aware of your breathing, much as you might do in traditional meditation. However, you also can use it to become more fully aware of your experiences in everyday life. The goal is to slow down, focus on one thing, and give it your full attention. Here's a quick exercise in eating mindfully:

1. Have an apple (or your favorite kind of fresh fruit) on hand.

2. Sit in a comfortable position. Relax with some deep, abdominal breathing.

3. Focus on what is happening in the here and now, and let go of other thoughts.

4. Now, focus your attention on the apple. Notice its appearance, feel, and smell.

5. Then, take a bite, and notice the flavor as if you had never tasted an apple before.

6. Note without judging any other thoughts that may come up. Then passively return your mind to focus on the apple.

7. Enjoy the feelings that arise as you savor the experience of eating an apple.

Imagine stresslessness

With mindfulness, you focus intently on the actual sensations you're experiencing. Imagery exercises are similar, except that you focus on imagined sights, sounds, smells, and tastes. This lets you harness the incredible power of imagination to help reduce stress and deepen relaxation. Often, the most potent images are ones you create for yourself. However, there are also a number of books and audiotapes on the market that guide you through the process of conjuring up soothing or healing images. Here is an example of the kind of script you might invent or follow:

1. Sit in a comfortable position. Relax with some deep, abdominal breathing.

2. Focus on the imaginary scenario: *Imagine that your body is made of very strong, clear crystal. Notice how beautifully the facets shine in the light. Now, with each breath in, see your body fill with colored mist in a soothing shade. Watch as the mist flows slowly from your head, to your chest and abdomen, to your arms and legs, and finally to your hands and feet. As the mist gradually fills your body, you are imbued with peace and well-being. With each breath out, watch as the mist flows in the reverse order, from your hands and feet to your head. As the mist leaves your body, it carries away any stress and fatigue, leaving you feeling relaxed and rejuvenated.*

Learning to cope

Stress can give you the intensity and energy to finish a project by a deadline, but chronic stress can affect your blood glucose control and your overall health. Even though life's problems can blindside you every once in a while, using relaxation techniques can help you to roll with the punches and adjust rather than letting stress knock you for a loop. □

SPIRITUAL SELF-CARE AND THE USE OF PRAYER

by Jacquelin Deatcher, A.P.R.N., B.C., C.D.E.

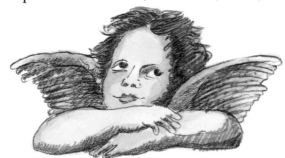

Diabetes self-management has evolved over the past few decades from relatively simple instructions to "avoid sugar" and take one's medicines on time to a much more comprehensive system that includes exercise, stress reduction, and meal plans as well as medicines. Current diabetes self-management guidelines, such as those of the American Diabetes Association, reflect a more holistic style that addresses the needs of the whole person rather than isolated parts. Holistic principles that promote a more complete approach to wellness could enhance diabetes self-care efforts significantly.

Holistic medicine is not a new concept. Socrates knew that it was important to treat the body as a whole when he wrote, "For the part can never be well unless the whole is well." An old Indian saying states that the body is like a house with four rooms: a physical, a mental, an emotional, and a spiritual room. To be a whole person, one must spend at least a little bit of time in each of these four rooms every day. For example, food and rest satisfy our physical needs; learning about the world and using what we learn enriches our minds; and validating and coping with our feelings meets our emotional needs. Our spiritual needs must also be addressed.

Spirituality can be defined as experiencing the presence of a power or force and experiencing a closeness to that presence. Spirituality may mean being involved with organized religion, taking time to contemplate one's place in the ultimate order of things, or focusing on the things that give life meaning, such as one's family or social group. No matter what one's personal motivation for seeking it, spirituality can be seen as part of the journey toward becoming whole.

Diabetes care is coming to address the four areas of needs in one's life. Insulin and diabetes medicines help the body. Diabetes educators teach people about blood glucose monitoring, meal plans, and exercise. Ideally, the health-care team also teaches people to manage stress or to recognize warning signs of depression to maintain emotional health. Recently, organized medicine has begun to address the spiritual aspect of self-care as well. Addressing each of these areas of our lives helps us to move closer to a holistic form of diabetes self-management.

Holistic health care seeks in part to enhance the body's natural healing ability. Much attention has been focused on developing sophisticated drugs and learning healthy life choices, but enhancing the body's natural healing ability hasn't been as rigorously studied.

Recent research in the field of mind/body medicine, or psychoneuroimmunology, though, has shown that the mind can and does have a profound effect on the body. Techniques such as the Relaxation Response and other forms of meditation, guided imagery, positive outlook, humor, hope, and even one's beliefs can all affect medical outcomes.

Perhaps it was the growing acceptance of involving the mind in the health process that made it easier for mainstream scientists to begin to take a serious look at spirituality and prayer. Prayer can be defined as communication with God, the creator of life, the collective unconscious, or one's higher self. Some studies have suggested that prayer can have an effect on both individuals who pray for themselves as well as on those who are prayed for by others (even without their knowledge). For example, in a study of patients in a car-

THE PRAYER WHEEL

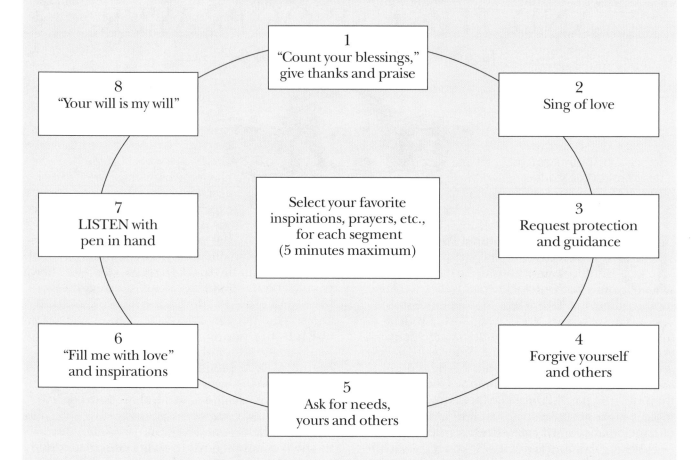

1
"Count your blessings,"
give thanks and praise

2
Sing of love

3
Request protection
and guidance

4
Forgive yourself
and others

5
Ask for needs,
yours and others

6
"Fill me with love"
and inspirations

7
LISTEN with
pen in hand

8
"Your will is my will"

Select your favorite
inspirations, prayers, etc.,
for each segment
(5 minutes maximum)

The prayer wheel was developed by Dr. John Rossiter-Thornton as a self-help tool that can be used by anyone, no matter what his background or beliefs. The wheel consists of eight components, and although five minutes are recommended for each, you can shorten or remove segments according to your preference. Dr. Rossiter-Thornton recommends that even if you shorten some of the steps you should keep a full five minutes for the "listen" segment. Proceeding clockwise from the top of the wheel, the steps of the prayer wheel as recommended by Dr. Rossiter-Thornton are as follows:

1. "Count your blessings" and give thanks and praise. Reflect on the things for which you are thankful.

2. Sing of love. Choose and sing a favorite love song.

3. Request protection and guidance. Ask for protection and guidance for you and your loved ones.

4. Forgive yourself and others.

5. Ask for needs, yours and others'. Record and date your requests for anything you or your loved ones need.

6. "Fill me with love" and inspirations. Think about the things that make you feel hope, love, and inspiration.

7. LISTEN with pen (and paper) in hand. The most important step, listening involves sitting quietly while being receptive to any thoughts, images, feelings, words, or ideas. Write down whatever comes to mind.

8. "Your will is my will." Put yourself in the hands of your higher power and trust that it has your best interests at heart.

Dealing With Feelings

diac intensive care unit, those who were prayed for (unbeknownst to them) by a group of community volunteers had about 10% fewer complications than those who were not prayed for by the volunteers.

Research at Duke University's Center for the Study of Religion/Spirituality and Health has looked at "intrinsic religiosity," which is defined as one's beliefs rather than participation in organized religious activities. Those with higher levels of intrinsic religiosity had better survival rates after severe illness, less depression in older age, less disability and mortality when faced with chronic disease, and possibly stronger immune systems. These and other studies raised interesting questions about the effect of prayer on both medical outcomes and general wellness.

One particular method of using prayer was developed by Dr. John F. Rossiter-Thornton, a psychiatrist in private practice in Toronto, Canada. He developed a tool he called the prayer wheel (not to be confused with the revolving prayer wheels of Tibet) for use with his psychotherapy patients. (See illustration on page 84.) The wheel is based on several distinct components of prayer, including giving thanks, singing of love, requesting protection and guidance, asking forgiveness for oneself and others, asking for needs, asking for inspiration, and surrendering to divine will. The suggested use of the wheel takes 40 minutes to allow at least five minutes for each component, including a "listen" segment in which one is encouraged to be receptive to any thoughts, images, or impressions that come to mind and to record them in a notebook. Use of the prayer wheel produced intriguing results for Dr. Rossiter-Thornton's patients,

including decreased anxiety, improved outlook, and improved family relationships.

One very small, unpublished study has looked at the possibility of enhancing diabetes self-management with the use of the prayer wheel. Nine study participants with Type 2 diabetes used the prayer wheel for three months in addition to their usual self-care. Glycosylated hemoglobin (HbA_{1c}) values were measured both before and after this three-month period and compared with the HbA_{1c} values of a similar group of nine people with Type 2 diabetes who were not involved in the study. Even though most of the participants reported that they used portions of the prayer wheel rather than the whole thing and that they used the prayer wheel anywhere from most days to occasionally but not every day, seven experienced a drop in HbA_{1c} levels during the study period; this drop in HbA_{1c} averaged 0.9%. The other two participants experienced an average increase of 0.4%. In the control group, five people experienced an average drop of 0.5% in HbA_{1c}, and four people experienced an average increase in HbA_{1c} of 0.8%. It should be noted that this study was conducted from October to January, a time of the year when common holiday behaviors often result in an increase in HbA_{1c} values for many people. Although this study was very small, the results suggest that the use of prayer, when combined with other holistic approaches to diabetes self-management, may have beneficial effects on one's HbA_{1c}.

More research in the field of spirituality is necessary, of course. However, for those comfortable with incorporating prayer into the fabric of their daily lives, the use of prayer may be yet another resource to enhance diabetes self-management and therefore, general wellness. □

BODY IMAGE
How You See Yourself

by Lisa Himmelfarb, C.S.W., R.D., C.D.E.

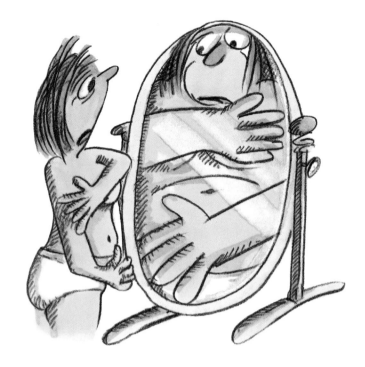

Joyce, a 42-year-old woman, sits on the couch across from me. She is a bright, creative, interesting, and successful attorney with a good sense of humor. Most people would describe her as attractive, although she is about 15 to 20 pounds overweight. Joyce, however, would use only one of these words to describe herself: overweight. Tearfully she says, "I loathe my body. If only I could get rid of these thunder thighs and my bulging stomach, my life would be so much better. I would be so much happier."

Because of her embarrassment about her weight and her fear of people "putting her under a microscope" and possibly rejecting her, Joyce rarely goes out socially. When she does go out for a work-related gathering or social event, she finds the experience painful. She becomes overly self-conscious and withdrawn and spends the majority of the time comparing her body to the bodies of other women in the room and wishing she were invisible. Joyce knows that she might not advance professionally if she doesn't get involved in more work engagements, but she still finds ways to skip these functions and to avoid social contact with her colleagues.

Shopping for clothes is another activity Joyce tries to stay away from. "I feel disgusted and ashamed when I see myself in the mirror," she says, "I try to avoid mirrors at all costs. And forget about going to the gym. I won't get into workout gear and stand next to the skinnies." Withdrawing more and more into the safety of her home, Joyce often feels very lonely and fears that she will never be able to find "someone special."

Dane, a 35-year-old man, is a dynamic, intelligent, personable, and good-looking real estate broker, but he doesn't see himself that way. Instead, he is miserable about his receding hairline and short stature. (He's 5'5".) "No woman will ever want to date a bald guy," he says. "Besides, I'm shorter than most women I meet. I don't stand a chance."

Dane spends close to an hour in the mornings staring in the mirror and trying to comb his hair in a way that will "save him embarrassment." Always wearing a baseball cap to hide his hairline, Dane goes out to bars and parties alone; he avoids women and tries not to stand near men who are taller than he is. Lacking self-confidence, he has trouble competing for clients and getting deals, especially when he perceives his competitors as "better looking." He sometimes describes himself as "a loser in his profession."

Just about everyone can relate to Joyce and Dane, at least to some extent. Both have what's called poor body image, negative thoughts and beliefs about their bodies that erode their already low self-esteem and self-confidence. Poor body image reinforces in their minds an idea that they are not good enough the way they are. The "defects" in their appearance have become almost an obsession and seem more important to them than any other qualities they might have. As you can see, body hatred is robbing them of joy and preventing them from embracing and improving their quality of life.

What is body image?

Body image is the way we see ourselves, our perception of the way others see us, and our beliefs about our physical appearance. Our body image is often entirely different from the way we look to others, because what we think or believe about our bodies is not based on facts or truths but on our emotions (how we feel about ourselves) and our physical sensations (how we feel in our bodies). Regardless of their actual appearance, people with poor body image see themselves as ugly and can't believe that others appreciate, admire, or even envy their looks.

Positive or negative, everyone has an image of his body. This image is not fixed or one-dimensional but ever-changing. It can be influenced by mood and overall emotional well-being, physical state of health, environment, and most important, self-esteem, or sense of self-worth. Like high or low self-esteem, positive or negative body image leads a person to like or dislike himself and to be content with or ashamed of who he is.

Having a healthy body image means that you are generally satisfied with your body and body parts and that your feelings toward your body are positive, respectful, and caring most of the time. That's not to say that you never have a "bad hair day" or dislike the way you look in a particular outfit. These are pretty normal thoughts and feelings that everyone has from time to time.

Negative body image ranges from moderate dissatisfaction with your body to outright hatred. People who have negative body image can become preoccupied and eventually obsessed with the idea that their bodies are ugly or flawed. These people may even develop a distorted body image, in which they are unable to accurately judge the size of their body, and what they see in the mirror is grossly disproportionate or inaccurate compared to what others see.

Poor body image can be emotionally and physically devastating. If you hate your body, you cannot respect it or properly nurture it, and you may even punish or neglect it. Extreme body dissatisfaction or distorted body image can lead to anxiety, depression, and eating disorders. Once negative body image develops, it can take decades to reverse.

How does body image develop?

Body image is learned; it is not something we're born with. It is shaped by a combination of factors, including societal ideals, media images, and the attitudes of family and peers.

Parents and siblings usually serve as our first role models and begin to give us direct and indirect messages about the way we should think and feel about our bodies when we are still very young. Joyce's mother, who was depressed, had very low self-esteem and frequently complained about her own body weight, sending Joyce the message that a person's size and appearance are related to his or her happiness. When she grew older, Joyce remembers her mother making more direct comments about Joyce's looks, such as, "You're not going out in those pants, are you? They make you look huge!" Dane's father undermined his self-confidence and encouraged negative feelings about his body with comments like, "You are not going to make it with that scrawny body of yours."

Coaches of some sports (especially wrestling, gymnastics, and figure skating) can influence the way we see our bodies if they take the attitude that slimness, musculature, or maintenance of an unrealistic weight are key to athletic achievement.

Peers can also reinforce negative messages, particularly during adolescence, when teens are impressionable, highly sensitive to the comments of their peers, and self-conscious about their changing appearance as they go through puberty. Joyce painfully recalls how she was teased by kids at school, who called her "chunky." Dane remembers being taunted by the other high school boys about being short. These messages stayed with them into their adult lives and clearly contributed to their negative body image and low self-esteem.

In cases of child abuse (whether verbal, physical, or sexual) or neglect, people may come to hate and feel shame about the object of abuse, their bodies, or they may feel that they, and thus their bodies, are not worthy of love and care.

People who grow up surrounded by family and friends who have a healthy body image and who value and accept them for who they are are far less likely to feel body dissatisfaction or to have low self-esteem, as children or as adults.

Even with supportive family and friends, however, it's nearly impossible to escape the media, which typically revere and showcase unrealistic images of appearance, weight, and musculature. Take a look at any billboard, fashion magazine, or men's fitness magazine, and you'll see glamorous men and women whose body proportions make up much less than one percent of the population. (The gap between the ideal and the attainable is even wider today than it was 25 years ago: Then, the average model weighed 8% less than the average woman. Today's models weigh about 23% less than the average woman.) Even models can't measure up to our image of perfection without a team of makeup artists, airbrushing, and computer retouching.

TV shows, movies, and advertisements reinforce the idea that women should be thin and big-breasted and men should be tall, muscular, and strong, like "real men." These rigid ideals suggest that people who look this way find it easy to win approval, fit in, and be successful. While this is certainly untrue, it makes it harder for people who don't look like models to feel comfortable with their own bodies and confident about their self-worth.

The goal of advertising is not to make people

feel good about themselves; it is to sell products. To do this, advertisers prey on our anxieties, vulnerability, and shame. The message they convey is, "You are not OK the way you are and here is the product you need to fix it." Ads for hair replacement products, breast augmentation, liposuction and other types of cosmetic surgery, weight-loss pills, teeth whitening kits, and various creams, potions, and powders saturate us with the message that improving your looks will improve your life.

This media message has helped make body image dissatisfaction such a pervasive and insidious problem in our society that it is almost considered normal, especially among women. But men are catching up. A 1997 survey taken by *Psychology Today* (in follow-up to landmark surveys in 1972 and 1985) polled over 3,000 women and 500 men from around the world. The survey revealed that 56% of women and 43% of men were dissatisfied with their overall appearance. It may come as a surprise that men are also dissatisfied with their looks, since they tend to suffer silently, feeling that "real" men shouldn't care about such things. It is more socially acceptable for women to be dissatisfied with their bodies and to verbalize their dissatisfaction. Recent surveys show, however, that men are increasingly concerned about their appearance and vulnerable to body image disorders such as muscle dysmorphia, in which a highly muscular man sees himself as weak and tiny.

According to the *Psychology Today* survey, gaining weight generated the most negative feelings about their bodies for two-thirds of the women and one-third of the men. In fact, reaching their ideal weight was so important that 15% of the women and 11% of the men said that they would be willing to give up more than five years of their life in exchange for the ability to reach their goal weight. This level of body dissatisfaction feeds today's $35 million diet industry; approximately 84% of the women surveyed and 58% of the men had tried dieting to lose weight. Studies also show that the more people are preoccupied with their looks, the more vulnerable they are to developing a negative body image and its accompanying distress, including disordered eating, dieting, and exercising patterns and low self-esteem.

How can disliking our bodies hold us back?

Body image, self-esteem, self-confidence, and self-respect are intertwined. When one is unhealthy, the others tend to suffer as well. When we have good self-esteem (that is, we accept and feel satis-fied with who we are and have a strong sense of self), nothing in our environment—not a mirror, not a picture in a magazine, not even a negative comment—can make us feel truly badly about ourselves, although we may be hurt or disappointed. When our self-esteem is low, however, we are much more easily wounded and more likely to take out our disappointments or difficulties on ourselves or on our bodies.

Negative body image, in turn, can undermine our mental, social, and physical health and create a vicious cycle of dissatisfaction with ourselves and an inability to effect positive change in our life. People like Joyce and Dane, who think very poorly of their bodies and themselves, tend to develop anxieties or feel limited in their careers, relationships, and sexuality, even though they may be talented and successful. Studies show that when we feel down about something, we tend to dislike our bodies more. Berating our bodies makes our mood sink lower, which makes our feelings toward ourselves even more negative and critical. When we are hypercritical of ourselves and focused only on our shortcomings, our self-confidence plummets. We may feel unable or afraid to express ourselves freely for fear of sounding dumb or drawing attention to ourselves and our bodies. We may feel inadequate and inferior in social situations and consequently start to avoid them. Isolation may intensify our negative thoughts about ourselves (such as, "I don't deserve to be loved or respected") and exacerbate our dead-end feelings of worthlessness, incompetence, and defeat, making it more difficult to take positive action.

Poor body image doesn't always develop into an eating or anxiety disorder, but beating up on your body can hold you back more than you may realize. Here are some thoughts and behaviors that indicate it's time to reassess your relationship with your body:

■ Avoiding mirrors or spending excessive time in front of them.

■ Putting considerable time and/or money into covering up flaws.

■ Frequently comparing your body to other peoples' bodies or seeking reassurance about your looks from a friend or partner.

■ Avoiding social or recreational activities or family visits because you are afraid others will criticize your body or simply view it negatively.

■ Weighing yourself several times a day.

■ Frequently dieting or trying extreme weight-control measures, such as skipping meals or severely limiting food choices.

■ Feeling embarrassed to eat in front of others.

■ Postponing doctor appointments because you will be weighed.

■ Being unable to accept compliments about your looks.

■ Feeling your life would be significantly improved if your body flaws disappeared.

Diabetes and body image

People with diabetes are particularly vulnerable to developing poor body image. When you were diagnosed with diabetes, you may have felt that your body let you down. Today, measuring or regulating what you eat, taking medicines or insulin, monitoring blood glucose levels, and keeping up with proper foot care can seem like constant reminders that there is something "wrong" with your body. In addition, you may be under pressure to attain or maintain a healthy weight, which is often a difficult part of managing diabetes. People with Type 2 diabetes may struggle constantly with losing weight, while some people with Type 1 diabetes can find it a challenge to gain weight, particularly when blood glucose levels are running high. Not being able to control your weight may make you feel weak or flawed.

Your body image directly affects the amount of respect and care you give to your body. Viewing your body as a burden or a traitor makes it nearly impossible for you to practice respectful self-care. If you don't care about your body, you may see no reason to eat right, get adequate sleep, dress in a manner that makes you feel good, engage in physical activity, or comfort yourself with healthy, gratifying activities that relax you and bring you joy. Neglecting these actions can make diabetes control more difficult or can lead to depression, which is common in people with diabetes and further impedes diabetes self-management. Some people may neglect their self-care to the point of seriously endangering their health by skipping meals or reducing insulin doses to lose weight.

If you are struggling with diabetes care, managing your weight, and feeling positive about your body, it's important to get some help. It is often useful to try to separate the healthy behaviors you want to adopt from the attitudes that are just making you feel bad about yourself. With the help of an understanding health-care provider and perhaps a counselor or therapist, you can learn to focus on making your positive behaviors, such as eating nutritious meals, working in some daily physical activity, and monitoring your blood glucose level, the measure of success—not how your body looks, what it weighs, or what your blood glucose readings are. Improving your body image is critical to better diabetes self-management and to living a healthier, longer, and more satisfying life.

Improving your body image

Developing a healthier body image and having a stronger sense of self means learning to accept yourself the way you are now, warts and all. It means learning to appreciate both your strengths and your weaknesses and recognizing that there is no such thing as perfection, physical or otherwise. If you have lived with a poor body image and self-image for a long time, developing a healthier body image also means giving up long-held beliefs about yourself and the world—and that's not easy. You may have to give up the belief that you will like yourself more or be happier if you change the way you look.

Accepting yourself the way you are doesn't mean throwing in the towel and giving up on your blood glucose goals, fitness objectives, or weight-loss efforts. Learning to feel good about yourself as a person will allow you to think, feel, and act more positively toward your body and to view good food and lifestyle choices as fuel and care for your body, not as punishment for your weakness or imperfections.

The following steps can help you adopt a healthier mindset about yourself and build a gentler relationship with your body:

■ Stop picking your body apart. If you look in the mirror long enough, you are sure to find something you don't like. This kind of inspection doesn't change your appearance, but it dramatically harms your body image. When you look in the mirror, identify something you like about your body. Take time to appreciate all the ways your body and specific body parts have served you. For example, reflect on how far your legs have carried you and how many things your arms have lifted and carried for you.

■ Work on changing negative, or "bad body," thoughts. Your thoughts about your body are based on core beliefs about yourself that are shaped from your past, cultural and societal messages, and interactions with people. It will take time and practice to reverse those negative thoughts, but you can do it. First, identify your negative self-talk and why and when you criticize your-self. Try replacing these negative thoughts with more positive, affirming ones. When Joyce is lonely, for example, she often thinks, "No one will ever want to date me because I'm so fat." If she tries interrupting this thought pattern and replacing the negative thought with a positive one, such as, "People like to spend time with me because

FOR MORE INFORMATION

The following books and Web sites provide further information on body image, how it develops, and how to improve yours.

BOOKS

THE BODY IMAGE WORKBOOK
An 8-Step Program for Learning to Like Your Looks
Thomas F. Cash, Ph.D.
New Harbinger Publications, Inc.
Oakland, California 1997

BODYLOVE
Learning to Like Our Looks and Ourselves
A Practical Guide for Women
Rita Freedman, Ph.D.
Gürze Books
Carlsbad, California 2002

LOVE YOUR BODY
Change the Way You Feel About the Body You Have
Tami Brannon-Quan, M.S., and Lisa Licavoli, R.D.
Trafford Publishing
Victoria, British Columbia 2007

MOM, I FEEL FAT!
Becoming Your Daughter's Ally in Developing a Healthy Body Image
Sharon Hersh
Waterbrook Press
New York 2001

THE ADONIS COMPLEX
The Secret Crisis of Male Body Obsession
Harrison G. Pope, Jr., M.D., Katharine A. Phillips, M.D., and Roberto Olivardia, Ph.D.
Free Press
New York 2000

MAKING WEIGHT
Men's Conflicts with Food, Weight, Shape & Appearance
Arnold Andersen, M.D., Leigh Cohn, M.A.T., and Thomas Holbrook, M.D.
Gürze Books
Carlsbad, California 2001

WHAT'S REAL, WHAT'S IDEAL
Overcoming a Negative Body Image
Brangien Davis
Hazelden Information Education
Center City, Minnesota 1999

WHEN YOU EAT AT THE REFRIGERATOR, PULL UP A CHAIR
50 Ways to Feel Thin, Gorgeous, and Happy (When You Feel Anything But)
Geneen Roth
Hyperion
New York 1998

WEB SITES

BODYPOSITIVE.COM
www.BodyPositive.com
This Web site is devoted to the discussion and improvement of body image. It focuses on improving quality of life, not body size, by relearning feelings of hunger and satiety, exercising for pleasure, finding a supportive community, and ending body disparagement. Users can read others' testimonials and post their own comments.

ADIOSBARBIE.COM
www.adiosbarbie.com
This Web site discusses body image in the media and society. Feature articles include a brief history of the Barbie doll, a discussion of men's body image issues, and ways to feel better about your body.

EATING DISORDER REFERRAL AND INFORMATION CENTER
www.EDreferral.com
This site provides information about all forms of eating disorders and offers free referrals to eating disorder practitioners, treatment facilities, and support groups. It also describes body image and offers guidelines for developing a healthier attitude toward your body.

4WOMAN.GOV
www.4woman.gov/bodyimage
This government-sponsored Web site, run by the National Women's Health Information Center, offers information on body image, nutrition, exercise, diabetes, and eating disorders. Fact sheets and links to other reliable health information sources are provided.

I'm kind and interesting, and I have a good sense of humor," gradually she can change the way she feels about herself and gain the confidence to get out and meet new people.

Here's one affirmation that might help you: "To live a carefree life, I will treat my body with

Compassion
Acceptance
Respect
Encouragement
Forgiveness
Reverence
Empathy
Enthusiasm."

■ Practice being less critical. When you catch yourself being judgmental about yourself or about someone else, stop and say, "I am not going to be judgmental or critical today."

■ Focus on your internal qualities and characteristics. What qualities do you like about yourself, and what qualities do you want others to see in you? Are you creative, compassionate, intelligent, kind, funny? Identify your skills, gifts, and dreams. How would people who care about you describe you? If you don't know, ask them. Chances are, they see positive qualities in you that you don't acknowledge often enough. How have you made the world a different place?

■ Each morning, make a written or mental gratitude list of all the things that you have, that you are, and that you are able to experience every day. Life is too short to spend all your time focusing on your shortcomings and striving for unobtainable goals.

■ Make an effort to spend time with people who are supportive, affirming, and encouraging, not judgmental and critical. Tell your friends how they can support you, especially during stressful times or when you feel blue. You're not the only one who occasionally feels insecure—show them the same support and encouragement they give you.

■ Throw your fashion and celebrity magazines into the garbage. Their unrealistic images made perfect with airbrush and flattering camera work can undermine your confidence in your own inner and outer beauty. Stop comparing your body to other peoples' bodies.

■ In addition to taking care of your diabetes, nurture your body regularly with pleasurable activities such as curling up on the couch with a good book, taking a nap, indulging in a wonderful-smelling body lotion or fragrance, or buying a new outfit that feels great and looks flattering to your figure the way it is now. Don't wait until you lose weight to feel good about what you wear. Most important, set realistic health, weight, and fitness goals and take care of your diabetes so that your body will take care of you.

■ Step up your "feel-good" physical activity. Instead of viewing exercise as a chore, explore the way your body feels in motion. Walk outside, swim or water walk, ride a bike, take a yoga or dance class, take up gardening, or get outside and play with your children or dog. Being active and moving your body more will help you to feel better about your body and yourself. Exercise is also a natural mood-booster that gives you more energy to tackle negative thoughts and feelings.

■ Be a role model to others by acknowledging and taking them seriously for what they say, feel, and do rather than how they look, and by curbing your own self-criticism.

Living with a negative body image is no fun for anyone. The good news is that no one has to live with it, because it can be changed. Since we only get one body to live in, it's worth making it an enjoyable place to be. □

OVERCOMING BINGE EATING DISORDER

by Lisa Himmelfarb, C.S.W., R.D., C.D.E.

Alice steals into the kitchen, her kingdom of solace. Her husband and two teenage sons have finally gone to bed. Alice has had a long day at the office; she had to deal with many demands from her clients, and her critical boss was on the warpath. Arriving home late, exhausted and hungry, she had to feed her husband and sons as well as herself.

Alice felt she did well on her diet today since she barely had time to eat. The one problem she had was that her blood sugar plummeted after she skipped lunch, so she ate a protein bar to bring it back up. For dinner, she ate her usual roasted chicken with vegetables while her family enjoyed a pizza.

Now that the day is almost over, Alice feels depleted, deprived, fatigued, and anxious. Her safe haven beckons her. Moving on what feels like automatic pilot, she starts eating out of a "healthy" box of cereal. Just one bowl, she thinks. Well, maybe one more. And one more.

After the third or fourth bowl of cereal, Alice thinks, "Why can't I stop? I'm not even hungry." Then, "I have no control. Why do I even bother?"

At that, she finishes off a bag of pretzels and moves on to a "forbidden" bag of cookies. After a couple of hours of eating, she staggers up the stairs in a shame- and guilt-ridden stupor. Careful not to wake up her husband, she stares at her body in the mirror in disgust and swears, "Tomorrow I'll get back on my diet."

Daniel dreads leaving his office on Friday in anticipation of an empty apartment and weekend of solitude. On his way home, he stops at several stores to arm himself with the reliable and predictable companion he has come to know so well: food. A pizza, beers, chips and dip, ice cream, and some steaks are all part of his repertoire. When friends call him later that evening to go out to a bar, Daniel declines the offer. He has already begun eating, already feels bad about himself, and doesn't think he can stop the binge cycle to go out; he takes a rain check. During his weekend of eating out of control and feeling miserable and disgusted with himself, he refuses another invitation from his friends to go to a football game on Sunday.

Like Alice and Daniel, you or someone you care about may be struggling with binge eating disor-

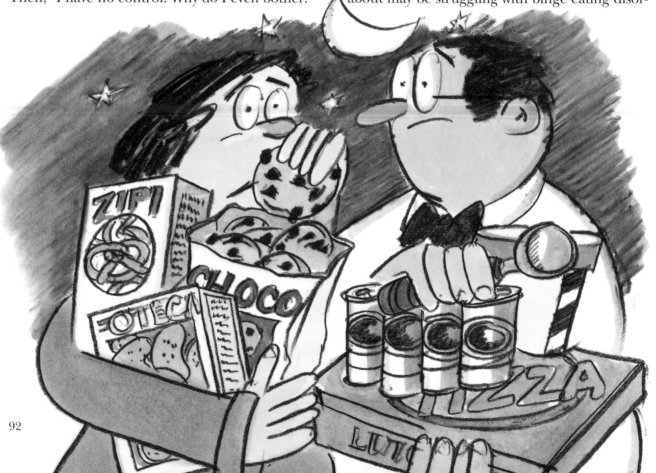

der. In fact, there are millions of people who do. Binge eating disorder affects both men and women, as well as people of all ages and ethnic backgrounds. If you have this disorder, what you probably do not realize is that you are not horrible, disgusting, or powerless—all common self-perceptions of the problem. There are multiple factors that contribute to binge eating disorder. The good news is that treatment and support are available.

What is binge eating disorder?

Sometimes people confuse binge eating with overeating. Everyone can identify with overeating, particularly at times like Thanksgiving. But binge eating is not the same as overeating from time to time or even every day, for that matter.

Simply put, overeating is eating more food than you normally would. You might feel a little uncomfortable after eating too much, express some regret for having done so, or comment that you'll eat less at the next meal, but you probably give it little thought after that.

Binge eating, on the other hand, is when you experience an overwhelming urge to eat and consume a large quantity of food more quickly than usual and in a short period of time. The amount of food you consume is definitely more than most people would eat in that amount of time. You eat despite the absence of hunger or how full you feel; you may not stop eating until you feel very painfully full.

It is not uncommon for a person with binge eating disorder to eat normally or restrictively in front of other people and to binge in secret to avoid embarrassment about the amount of food he consumes. A person might wait until the end of the day to binge, or he might snack all day so as never to feel empty. A key distinction between overeating and binge eating is that while binge eating, you feel like wild horses could not get you to stop eating once you have started. You are insatiable. You often feel guilty, distressed, and depressed, have low energy, and are riddled with shame and self-reproach after binge eating. These bad feelings often lead you to binge again, so ultimately you feel powerless and hopeless about the vicious and self-defeating binge eating cycle.

When episodes of binge eating become frequent (at least two times a week) and persist for six months, it is called binge eating disorder. Frequently referred to as compulsive overeating, binge eating disorder was first recognized in 1959 (although it surely existed well before that) but was not introduced as a medical diagnosis until 1994. It is similar to bulimia except that people with binge eating disorder do not attempt to rid themselves of the food they consume during a binge by vomiting, using laxatives or diuretics (pills that increase urination), decreasing or omitting insulin doses, or exercising excessively.

Who gets this, and why?

An estimated 4 million Americans struggle with binge eating disorder. The number may even be higher, but many people are ashamed and try to hide the problem, so they don't talk about it or seek help. Though most people with binge eating disorder are obese and have a history of weight problems and fluctuations, people who are overweight or normal weight can also be affected. It is estimated that about 40% of obese people have binge eating disorder.

Nobody is completely sure what causes binge eating disorder; more research is needed in this area. It is known, however, that the causes are complex and that it is produced by a variety of causes. Environmental, social, biological, psychological, developmental, and conditioned, or learned, factors work together in varying degrees to contribute to the disorder.

Environmental/social. We learn at an early age, either from family members, friends, authority figures, and especially the media, that appearance and body size are very important. In Western society, people are often admired, praised, and rewarded for their thinness, weight loss, and appearance. As a result, many of us perceive appearance as more important than internal qualities such as intelligence, kindness, and creativity or than our inherent self-worth.

If you ask participants in a weight-loss program if their self-worth is attached to their weight, most of them will say yes. Consequently, many people are preoccupied with their weight, shape, and size and have a poor body image. This preoccupation has fueled the multibillion-dollar dieting industry and has caused many people to resort to rigid and unrealistic dieting measures such as severely restricting calories or completely eliminating many enjoyable foods.

Biological. Up to half of all people with binge eating disorder have been depressed at some time, but it remains unclear whether depression causes binge eating disorder or binge eating disorder causes depression—or both. Current research is looking at the effect of brain chemicals such as serotonin, which affects mood and some other compulsive behaviors, and metabolism (the way the body burns calories) and their possible effects on binge eating disorder. Some experts hypothe-size that the hypothalamus, the part of the brain that controls appetite, doesn't properly signal hunger or fullness cues.

People with diabetes are particularly vulnerable to binge eating disorder. When you have diabetes, particularly Type 2 diabetes, and are overweight or obese, diet and weight loss are crucial in manag-ing your blood glucose level. If you do not pursue weight loss in a way that is realistic and flexible, you may raise your chances of falling into a binge eating cycle. Naturally, this is counterproductive to your diabetes control, since excessive food intake, weight gain, and distress only worsen blood glu-cose control.

Research has also demonstrated that depression is twice as common in people who have diabetes as in those who don't, and there is significant evi-dence that blood glucose control is poorer among those who are depressed.

Biological/psychological. When a person engages in strict "dieting," he can experience physiological and psychological hungers simultaneously. Going too long without eating—say, more than five hours—can cause you to become too hungry and make you want to take in a large amount of food when you finally do eat. If you "diet" all day, by the end of the day, if your body didn't get enough food, or "fuel," it seeks to make up for what it did-n't get during the day. The body's response to food deprivation is partly why a person can feel insatiable during a binge episode.

From a psychological perspective, if you are told you can't eat certain foods, you tend to be preoc-cupied with or crave those foods. When you finally succumb to the temptation of those "forbidden" foods, you are likely to adopt the attitude that you better eat all you can now that you've given in. If you do not enjoy the foods included in your diet or meal plan, you may never feel satisfied, no mat-ter how much of those foods you consume. And when you feel deprived, your desire for other, more satisfying foods is compelling.

To complicate matters, difficult emotions such as anger, anxiety, sadness, frustration, loneliness, and boredom may trigger a binge. You may use food as a way to cope with or alleviate these feel-ings. Some people, for example, use food to com-fort or nurture themselves, to numb their feelings, or to distract themselves from dealing with the source of these feelings. A person who feels sorry for himself because he has diabetes might look to food for comfort.

For others, feeling angry might trigger a binge. A person who hasn't learned to express anger in a productive way by acting assertively or confronting the person or situation that is making him angry is likely to become angry not only at the person or situation but also at himself for not being able to deal with them. His response may be to "eat over" those difficult feelings.

It's also common to use food to fill an empty void from loneliness or to feed psychological hunger from unmet childhood needs for atten-tion, affection, or love. A person might use food for reward or punishment or simply to calm his nerves. And some people even binge when they are happy.

Conditioned/learned/familial. How did you come to develop the type of relationship with food that you have? Many people can trace it back to their family of origin. In other words, the way you use food in your adult life may depend on how food was used in your family. Perhaps it was used for comfort or reward or was withheld for punish-ment. Maybe your mother gave you a cookie to soothe you when you scraped your knee. Or maybe you were given ice cream when you cleaned your plate at dinner or brought home top marks on a school assignment. Maybe you were not given ice cream when you said something to your little brother that you shouldn't have.

Food may have been used to handle stress or frustration or to avoid feeling at all. Alice remem-bers sitting with her father after an annoying and stressful day at the office; as he talked, they both dug into a bag of potato chips and dip. She recalls this as being the only quality time she had with her harsh and critical father. Daniel, on the other hand, barely ever saw his father, who worked long hours when he wasn't traveling, and his mother was depressed and always sleeping. Daniel ate con-tinuously to numb the pain of loneliness and per-ceived rejection and to satisfy his psychological hunger for attention and nurturing.

In most cases, parents do the best they can with what they know. Nonetheless, many people grow up without enough positive role modeling or effective and productive tools to identify, express, and manage difficult emotions. Some people are taught to suppress unhappy, unsettling, confusing, or even happy feelings. Having nowhere for these uncomfortable feelings to go, or as a way to deflate their happiness, they binge. Food provides instant gratification and is predictable and reli-able. But the physical and emotional effects of binge eating can be devastating.

Consequences. If left untreated, the major compli-cations of binge eating disorder are the diseases that accompany obesity, such as diabetes, high blood pressure, high cholesterol, heart disease, stroke, sleep apnea, respiratory problems, kidney disease, gallbladder disease, vascular diseases, and certain types of cancer. If a person already has diabetes, another possible result is difficulty controlling blood glucose level.

Treatment and support

There are some key points to remember when seeking treatment for binge eating disorder. There is no quick fix for the problem. Treatment is ongoing, and setbacks are part of the process. Because many factors contribute to the cause of binge eating disorder, and because each person is a unique and complex being, each person should be individually evaluated and have a plan tailored to his needs. Such a plan will often include any one or a combination of the following types of therapies. When you are looking for treatment providers, it is important that you work with people you trust and feel comfortable with. It's also important that they are willing to work with one another collaboratively. It is best to interview several people to find the best match for your needs.

Individual therapy. Psychotherapy is a good place to start, preferably with a psychologist, certified or licensed clinical social worker, or other professional counselor. Together you can explore, understand, and trace the origins of the intimate connection between food, thoughts, emotions, and your eating behaviors.

While many types of psychotherapy are used to treat binge eating disorder, research has shown that cognitive-behavioral therapy is the most successful in managing eating disorders. This type of therapy aims at targeting and changing counterproductive thoughts, feelings, and behaviors that lead to binge eating. It attempts to help you to learn alternative, healthier, and more effective coping methods to deal with difficult emotions and situations. Therapy should also address body image issues.

To find a therapist, try asking your endocrinologist, family physician, or nutrition specialist for a referral or use any of the resources listed on page 96.

Medication. During the course of your treatment, you and your therapist may decide that medication might be helpful to relieve depression and anxiety. Your therapist can refer you to a psychiatrist or psychopharmacologist for an evaluation.

Group therapy. This type of therapy can assist you in managing relationship issues more effectively. If you're interested in trying it, ask your therapist about groups in your area, or look to the resources listed on page 96.

Family therapy. Depending on your situation, you might see a family therapist with your family of origin or with a spouse and possibly children to work on problematic family dynamics.

Support groups. When used in combination with any of the other treatment options listed here, support groups can be helpful in breaking down isolation and alienation and provide you with valuable positive reinforcement and support.

Nutrition counseling. A registered dietitian (R.D.), preferably one who is a certified diabetes educator (C.D.E.), can help you develop an individualized, sensible, realistic, and flexible eating plan. Your therapist or diabetes care provider may be able to give you a referral to a dietitian. If not, check with The American Dietetic Association for an R.D. in your area.

Since attempting to follow a weight-loss diet can precipitate or exacerbate binge eating disorder, it should be discouraged for people who are at a normal weight. Even in people who are overweight, treating binge eating disorder and improving emotional well-being should be a priority over losing weight. For obese individuals, dieting should be approached in conjunction with one or more of the above therapies.

Useful strategies

While evaluating and pursuing treatment options, the following ideas may be useful to consider:

■ The single most important strategy and one that gives you control is to consume regular and balanced planned meals and snacks. To limit cravings, do not go more than three to four hours without eating, and avoid becoming too hungry.

■ Pay attention to internal cues. Learn to use true physiological hunger and fullness to regulate your eating. Don't eat when you are not hungry, and stop eating when you are comfortably full.

■ Make your environment work for you rather than against you. Don't keep foods that trigger bingeing in the house. However, don't completely deprive yourself of these foods either. When you are ready, reintroduce yourself to some of these foods in a more controlled setting. For example, if keeping a jar of peanut butter in the house causes you to consume the entire jar during one or two binges, make a point of ordering a peanut butter sandwich at a deli. If you can't keep a container of ice cream in the house, go out to an ice cream parlor on occasion and get a small cup of ice cream. This shows you how to incorporate normal foods into a healthy and flexible eating plan. You will likely discover that trigger foods become less alluring when you permit yourself to have them.

HELP FOR EATING DISORDERS

For more information about eating disorders and referrals to professionals who can help, contact the organizations listed here.

NATIONAL EATING DISORDERS ASSOCIATION
603 Stewart Street, Suite 803
Seattle, WA 98101
(800) 931-2237
www.nationaleatingdisorders.org
Toll-free line offers information and referrals to professionals and support groups.

ACADEMY FOR EATING DISORDERS
60 Revere Drive, Suite 500
Northbrook, IL 60062-1577
(847) 498-4274
www.aedweb.org
Web site contains links to numerous sources of information on eating disorders.

SOMETHING FISHY WEBSITE ON EATING DISORDERS
www.something-fishy.org
Provides news and information, chat support, and referrals to support groups and treatment centers worldwide.

THE AMERICAN DIETETIC ASSOCIATION
120 South Riverside Plaza, Suite 2000
Chicago, Illinois 60606-6995
(800) 877-1600
www.eatright.org
Provides general nutrition information, education materials, and referrals to a registered dietitian.

ANOREXIA NERVOSA AND RELATED EATING DISORDERS, INC.
www.anred.com
Web site includes information specifically on diabetes and eating disorders.

GURZE BOOKS
P.O. Box 2238
Carlsbad, CA 92018
(800) 756-7533
www.gurze.com
Sells books, audiotapes, videotapes, and other materials on eating disorders, body image, and related topics.

■ Be mindful and fully present when you are eating. In other words, give eating all your attention. Take in all of the sensory pleasures—the smell, taste, texture, etc. Not only does focusing on your food make it difficult to "escape," or disconnect from your emotions, it helps you to relax and slows down your eating. (Research shows that when you slow down and pay attention, you actually eat less.) Most important, slowing down and focusing helps you to feel more satisfied with the food.

■ If you have a powerful urge to binge, try to delay the urge as long as possible. Give yourself time to reflect on what you are feeling and may need in that moment. Ask yourself if you are feeling tired, lonely, anxious, bored, or frustrated. Try to think about what is going on in your life and how you might deal with it directly to feel better. Do you need to take a nap, take a walk, do a relaxation exercise, listen to soothing music, or talk to a trusted friend? Do you need to confront someone to tell them how you are feeling?

Some people find it useful to write about how they are feeling. A journal can be a powerful tool for self-expression and discovery. If you have too much unstructured time on your hands, plan ahead to meet with friends or to engage in interesting and satisfying activities. You might consider joining a club, taking up a hobby, or taking a class.

■ If, after considering your options, you decide to binge, state, "I choose to binge." This way you won't feel so powerless. Ultimately you—not the food—have control, even if it does not feel that way. At some point, you can say, "I choose not to binge." After a binge, spend less time beating yourself up and spend more energy examining the factors that triggered your binge and what can you do differently in the future to ward off a repetition. Be kinder and more forgiving of yourself. Repeat to yourself what you might tell a friend in a similar situation. This way, you don't fuel the vicious binge cycle.

With the right guidance and support, you do not have to be a slave to binge eating disorder, and you do not have to slay it alone. There is help available to you or those you care about. The sooner you seek help and the more you invest in your treatment and yourself, the better you will be able to ward off the complications of obesity and diabetes and live a healthier and more fulfilling and productive life. □

MAKING POSITIVE CHANGES

by David Spero, R.N.

"They don't understand," said Jessica. "My family, my friends, my doctor, they all want me to change everything—food, exercise, the way I cook…. But my life was hard enough before! I stick to my diet for a week, but then I slip up. I've started exercising a dozen times, but it doesn't last. Maybe I'm just not strong enough to change the way they want me to."

Sound familiar? Most people with diabetes can relate to Jessica's frustration. Like many major life challenges, learning to manage diabetes requires people to change their routines, their lifestyle, and their priorities. When there are so many changes to make—and all at the same time—it's easy to get overwhelmed. How can you possibly feel comfortable and confident with all those demands? How can you take charge of change?

Fortunately, there are some guidelines that can help you make successful changes with a minimum of suffering. Applying these guidelines has helped millions of people make changes they never thought possible, whether these changes related to diabetes care or to other areas of their lives. This article presents information and strategies to help you master the process of self-motivated behavior change.

Why change is hard

When someone is struggling to change old habits or start new ones, as Jessica was, they are often labeled "resistant to change," as if that were some kind of personality defect. But resistance to change is a normal attitude. In fact, our brains are wired to resist change. Every time you experience something new, you create a new neural pathway. Whenever that thought or action is repeated, the neurons involved receive more of certain chemical messengers called neurotransmitters, and the message is transmitted more efficiently. As the message is communicated, these neurons grow new connections to link up with even more nerve cells, making the message that much more powerful. This is why habits are so hard to break: Every time you do them or think them, they get stronger.

The good news is that you can "rewire" your brain and create new pathways to override old, unwanted ones. But changing habits isn't like putting on a new pair of socks. It's more like trying to grow flowers in a pot already filled with other plants. The new seeds will need a lot of tending if they are going to take hold.

For example, say you want to stop watching TV after dinner, because you know you tend to snack all the way through prime time. If you hang around the living room and rely on your willpower to keep you away from the remote control, you will have already lost the battle—not because you're a weak person, but because your brain is "wired" by habit to push that "on" button. If, however, you get out of the house and take a walk after dinner, or go to the bowling alley, or go to another room to write in a journal, do housework, or read a book, you may not even think about the TV. If you repeat that activity most evenings, the new habit will gradually become stronger and take the place of the old one.

For many people, the idea of change is intimidating because they don't think it is possible or they don't think they can do it successfully. If you never had much control over your life before, or if you haven't been successful at making changes or achieving goals in the past, it will be very hard to believe that you can succeed at diabetes management. This is one reason why diabetes tends to hit harder among people with less money, less education, and less power; not only is the incidence of diabetes higher among these groups, but the rate of diabetic complications is higher as well.

Psychologist Albert Bandura at Stanford University developed the notion of "self-efficacy"—a fancy term for self-confidence—as a measurement of people's belief in themselves and in their ability to effect positive change in their life. Research shows that a higher level of self-efficacy leads to higher goals and more success in making desirable changes. For people with diabetes, having confidence in your ability to set and meet high standards means better health outcomes, a higher quality of life, and less reliance on the medical system. It also makes you feel better about yourself and about your life in general.

Getting ready to change

It is possible and worthwhile to raise your level of self-efficacy, but like many other skills, it takes guidance and practice. A Stanford University program called Chronic Disease Self-Management offers one model for successful goal setting and behavior change that is also used by various diabetes self-help groups throughout the United States. Many of the guidelines that follow are based on this model.

Decide what you want to change. Change is most successful when you work on things you *want* to accomplish, not on things you think you *should* do or things someone else tells you to do, even if that person is your doctor. If you really want something, you'll put your energy behind doing or getting it. Without that energy, it's much more of a chore to instill new habits. For example, in one diabetes self-management program, each participant had to make a weekly action plan to work on a particular behavior. One student planned for three weeks in a row to do more walking, but she never did it. Finally, the truth came out: "I don't really like to walk," she said, "I just thought I should." Substituting another form of exercise—stationary bicycling while watching videos—got her going.

Where you start is really up to you. Physicians and health educators nearly always focus on behavior changes involving diet, medicines, exercise, or blood glucose self-monitoring. If you would like to work on one of these areas but aren't sure what steps would be effective, ask your health-care provider for guidance or do some research on your own to make sure your proposed action is both safe and beneficial.

But maybe you aren't ready to make health- or diabetes-related changes. As important as these behaviors are, sometimes other life situations—such as job stress, relationship problems, lack of physical security, or emotional distress—get in the way and must be dealt with first.

Alice, a student in a diabetes class at a hospital in California, was urged to make a meal plan and start blood glucose self-monitoring, but she refused to do so. She insisted that she had to get her kitchen and dining room cleaned up first. Apparently, the house was quite a mess, because it took her the whole four weeks of the class to get those rooms cleaned. She never got around to making any diabetes-care plans.

One month later, all the students came back to have their glycosylated hemoglobin (HbA$_{1c}$) monitored, to see if the class had helped their diabetes control. (HbA$_{1c}$ is a measure of blood glucose control over several months.) The educators in charge of the class were shocked at the results: Alice's HbA$_{1c}$ had dropped more than anyone else's in the class. They never determined exactly what it was about cleaning the kitchen and dining room that helped Alice's diabetes control, but the improvement was sustained. Perhaps the success with getting her house in order gave her the confi-

dence to tackle diet and exercise changes. Or maybe eliminating the chaos in her kitchen reduced her stress, which helped lower her blood glucose levels. Whatever the reason, her story illustrates that improving your life in any way can sometimes have unexpected health benefits.

Reward your efforts. You need to believe that the behavior change you are considering will actually do you some good if you're going to stick with it. In his book *Diabetes Burnout*, psychologist and diabetes educator William Polonsky writes that we all make cost–benefit analyses about whether a particular action is worth the trouble. If the costs seem too high and the promised benefits don't seem worth it, we won't be motivated to do it. If you feel that nothing you can do will improve your health, and that diabetic complications are inevitable, why would you bother making difficult lifestyle changes?

In the case of diabetes care, it's well known that controlling one's blood glucose is possible and does prevent complications. (If you still need convincing on this point, talk with a friend who also has diabetes, read books and articles about diabetes, or ask your doctor to provide evidence that lifestyle changes can improve your diabetes control and quality of life.) Unfortunately, though, many of the costs of not controlling diabetes (such as complications) come on very gradually and appear only as possibilities in the distant future. On the other hand, the reward of, say, eating chocolate cake is immediate and certain. The present, short-term consequences of an action usually win out over the future or potential consequences, even when you know what behavior is ultimately better for you.

There are ways to increase the immediate benefits of healthy behaviors and make them more rewarding. In her book *The Physician Within*, Catherine Feste (who has had diabetes for over 50 years, since age 10) recommends giving yourself frequent rewards for small successes. A reward is something you enjoy—maybe a hot bath, a movie, or a massage—that doesn't undermine the healthy behavior you are trying to reinforce. (You probably wouldn't reward yourself for sticking to your meal plan for a week with a big bowl of ice cream.)

As the new behavior becomes more automatic, another source of reward is noticing how your body starts to feel when you begin taking better care of it. Most people feel more comfortable and energetic when their blood glucose level is in the normal range, but they're often too busy to notice the good feeling! So paying more attention may raise the perceived benefits of lifestyle change and help make the new behavior its own reward.

Dealing With Feelings

Make changes that are realistically attainable.
When people decide to adopt new habits, they tend to want to do too much too fast. They end up turning self-care into a form of self-abuse. They decide, "I will run on the treadmill an hour a day" or, "I will lose 100 pounds in three months, like that person in the TV ad." Good luck! You have a much better chance of success if you make changes that feel good as you go along, and set a realistic timetable for your progress.

To make major changes more attainable, break your ultimate goal into manageable chunks. It is far better to start with a less ambitious goal and achieve it than to shoot for some gigantic transformation and fall short. The first pattern leaves you feeling good about yourself and ready for more; the second makes you want to forget the whole thing. You want to go from success to success, even if the successes are small.

Write an action plan. Self-help and self-management programs are built on accumulating small successes. The chief tool they use is called an action plan, a contract you make with yourself to work on one very specific behavior change for a set time period. The plan should be behavior-specific—that is, it should focus on what you will do, not on what the results will be. (Results are often beyond your control, but you can control what you do.) A good action plan might be, "I will walk four times this week, for 30 minutes, after dinner, around the block, with my spouse." Note how specific this plan is. It's not just, "I will exercise more." It details what type of exercise you'll do and when, where, for how long, and with whom. The more specific your plan, the better your chances of carrying it out.

The action plan should also specify your "confidence level." On a scale of 1 to 10, rate how certain you are of completing the entire plan. A confidence rating of 10 means you're absolutely sure you'll carry through with the whole plan; a rating of 1 means, "I'm just kidding myself. There's no way I'll do this." Research shows that if your confidence level is 7 or higher, you'll probably complete the plan; if it's lower than 7, you probably won't.

If your confidence level is less than 7, you have two choices: You can make the plan easier (for example, "I will walk *three times* this week," instead of "six times"), or you can evaluate what might get in your way and decide how you will remove these barriers. For example, maybe you want to walk but know you are restricted by child-care or elder-care commitments in the afternoon and evening. Could you get someone to watch the kids for an hour so you can exercise? Or try walking first

MAKING AN ACTION PLAN

An action plan is a commitment to yourself to take one specific step toward your longer-term goals. An action plan can be made for anything you want to work on, be it learning to ask for help or finding more time to exercise. Generally, the more specific the plan, the better, as in, "I will look in the phone book to find a home health aide," or "I will walk for 30 minutes three times this week." There are many variations on action plans, but a successful plan should meet the following criteria:

■ The action is something *you* want to do.
■ It's something you can reasonably accomplish within the time frame specified.
■ It spells out as much detail as possible, such as when, where, for how long, and with whom you'll work toward your goal.

The form that follows may guide you in setting attainable behavior-change goals.

MY ACTION PLAN
This week I will _____
_____
_____
_____ .
(state activity or behavior)

I will do this ____ times, for _____ .
(length of time or amount of activity)

I will do this activity _____
_____
_____
_____ .
(when, where, with whom)

On a scale of 1 to 10, my confidence level that I will do this is _____ .

The following barriers might get in my way:
_____
_____
_____ .

Here are the ways I might overcome those barriers: _____
_____
_____
_____ .

thing in the morning, before your duties begin? Brainstorming with a friend, a diabetes educator, a support group, or a family member might make it easier to find solutions to potential obstacles.

You can develop an action plan for almost any area of life, from marital relations ("I will have two conversations with my spouse this week during which I listen without interrupting for at least five minutes") to eating control ("I will limit my cookie consumption to one a day, four days a week"). There is nothing magical about a week, either; daily or monthly action plans are OK, too. You can read more about action planning in my book, *The Art of Getting Well*, or in *Living a Healthy Life with Chronic Conditions* (see "Resources" on this page for more details).

Smoothing the way

As you start working on your new behavior, you may find that even the best-laid action plan doesn't prepare you for some of the internal and external hurdles that you may encounter. The following hints can help you get back on track when obstacles get in your way.

Stay flexible. If the lifestyle change you want to make involves exercising more, it's not really critical that you do exactly the exercise you described in your action plan 100% of the time. If there's a blizzard outside, you're probably not going to go for a walk, but that doesn't mean you have to skip your workout altogether. Think of other options (indoor calisthenics, a trip to the gym, vigorous housework) that meet the same goal of getting you moving.

Expect some ups and downs. Drug and alcohol abuse counselors have a saying, "Relapse is part of recovery." Good ones often tell their clients, "You will probably backslide at some point. When you do, come back to me." Otherwise, when clients hit the inevitable bump in the road, they will feel like failures, bad people for whom there is no hope or help. So they relapse into old habits, and it may be years before they quit again.

The same applies to all kinds of behavior change. Making a great leap from couch potato to fitness fanatic, improving your ability to speak up for yourself overnight, permanently adopting a healthful diet—these things do not happen often in real life. For most people, there are good and bad days, good weeks and bad weeks, or months, or even years. Coming back from the bad patches is part of the process of successful change. When you "relapse" into an unhealthy habit, don't give up. Ask yourself what went wrong, get some help if necessary, and try again.

RESOURCES

The following books, available in most bookstores, give more in-depth guidance on making lifestyle changes.

THE ART OF GETTING WELL
A Five-Step Plan for Maximizing Health When You Have a Chronic Illness
David Spero, R.N.
Hunter House
Alameda, California, 2002

LIVING A HEALTHY LIFE WITH CHRONIC CONDITIONS
Kate Lorig, R.N., Dr.P.H., Halsted Holman, M.D., David Sobel, M.D., Diana Laurent, M.P.H., Virginia Gonzales, M.P.H., and Marian Minor, R.P.T., Ph.D.
Bull Publishing
Boulder, Colorado, 2000

THE PHYSICIAN WITHIN
Catherine Feste
Henry Holt
New York, New York, 1993

DIABETES BURNOUT
William Polonsky
American Diabetes Association
Alexandria, Virginia, 1999

All kinds of changes and stresses can knock you off your program. Maybe you've been walking every day, and then you sprain an ankle. You've been practicing daily relaxation when a noisy neighbor moves in and ruins the peace and quiet. Or maybe your partner leaves you, the rent goes up, you get bad news on a blood test, or your child flunks out of college. Most people could fill pages with similar disasters that have thrown them for a loop at one point or another. Good news can also throw you off schedule: When you get a new job, a new love, or an exciting new cause or hobby, it's suddenly hard to find time or energy to work on your goal. The important thing is to get back on track as soon as possible, because each time you relapse and make a comeback, you recover your progress a little more quickly and easily.

Get help when you need it. Many people have gotten the idea somewhere that life should be hard. If things are too easy, they think they must be doing something wrong. But your body likes things to be easy. When you are struggling with

Dealing With Feelings

making changes in your behavior or in your life, the answer is usually not more willpower or harder work but more help. Emotional support or advice, professional financial help, or practical assistance with cooking, housework, or transportation, for instance, can enable you to overcome many barriers to change.

Put it in perspective. For change to be worth the trouble, life has to be worth living. If you don't have a reason to get out of bed in the morning, it really won't matter how healthy you are, will it? So look for ways to get more pleasure, more purpose, and more fun into your life. Some people say that being healthy means giving up everything you like. They have it completely backward. Give up the things you don't like (such as high blood glucose, stressful arguments, or overworking when your body needs to rest) and appreciate the heck

out of the things you do enjoy, whether it's that cookie a day, the time you spend with your grandkids, or the "good" tired you feel after exercise. **Try to be patient.** Change usually takes longer than you think it should, and it often takes place when you're not looking for it. You may work and work toward getting in shape, say, but nothing seems to happen for the longest time. Then one day, you notice that you are not getting tired nearly as fast as you used to. You're breathing easier and feeling better throughout the day, too. When did this happen? Probably, it happened when you stopped watching for it. When you give up the need for miracles, miraculous changes begin to happen. And in the field of self-motivated behavior change, miracles happen every day. If you keep these guidelines in mind, they can happen for you, too. □

UNDERSTANDING DEPRESSION AND DIABETES

by Alisa G. Woods, Ph.D.

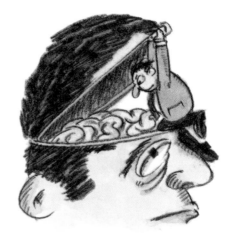

More than just a touch of "the blues," major depression is a serious illness that interferes with your daily life and affects your outlook, feelings, and physical health. The sadness and hopelessness that characterize depression lead a significant number of people with depression to commit suicide. But even those who don't kill themselves are often burdened by the feeling that life holds little enjoyment, pleasure, or meaning.

People with diabetes have special reason to be aware of depression, because their likelihood of developing it is double that of people who don't have diabetes. It is estimated that between 15% and 30% of people with diabetes also have depression at any given time. In addition, some studies have shown that being depressed in-creases the risk of developing diabetes, and that depression can worsen some diabetes-associated illnesses.

Diabetes plus depression

According to an article published in *The American Journal of Managed Care* by a group led by John D. Piette, Ph.D., Veterans Affairs Career Scientist and

Associate Professor of Medicine at the University of Michigan, depression affects people with diabetes in many different ways. For example, people with depression have reduced physical activity levels, which may contribute to poorer health. Dr. Piette believes this is of particular concern because "we know that being physically active helps both depression and diabetes." Remaining physically active should therefore be an important health goal for people with diabetes and depression.

People with both depression and diabetes may also be less likely to take the steps needed to manage their diabetes and care for their general health. They may fail to communicate effectively with their physicians about any of their health problems, including feeling depressed. This situation may be complicated by the fact that physicians may focus only on the problems associated with diabetes, making them miss the diagnosis of depression.

The reduced physical activity and decreased

attention to self-care that accompany depression can worsen blood glucose control and increase risks for diabetic complications. Depression also affects the immune and hormonal (endocrine) systems.

The immune–endocrine link

Clinical studies have shown that the system that controls the release of stress hormones does not function properly in people with depression, resulting in persistently high levels of stress hormones. Two parts of the brain that are important for controlling these stress hormones are called the hypothalamus and the pituitary gland. These two structures communicate with each other by releasing specific chemicals. One such chemical released by the hypothalamus is called corticotropin-releasing factor (CRF), which controls the release of adrenocorticotropin (ACTH) from the pituitary gland. ACTH, in turn, tells the adrenal glands (endocrine glands by the kidneys) to make the stress hormone cortisol. Cortisol helps mobilize the body by doing several things, including raising blood glucose levels to make energy available to overcome the stressful situation. In people with depression, this system may be impaired.

Studies suggest that the stress response system in people with depression does not shut down when a stressful situation ends. In some individuals with depression, abnormally high levels of cortisol have been measured, and there is also some evidence that they may have abnormally high levels of CRF as well. This is a problem because although cortisol is helpful for short-term responses to stress, prolonged high levels of cortisol may chronically elevate blood glucose, which damages organs, blood vessels, and nerves throughout the body. Cortisol also impairs the immune system and may cause or worsen insulin resistance, one of the major metabolic problems in Type 2 diabetes.

According to Larry Culpepper, M.D., M.P.H., Chairman of the Department of Family Medicine at Boston University School of Medicine, "Depression worsens diabetes at every step. It hastens its onset and is associated with more rapid development of diabetic complications." It should be noted that this statement applies to both Type 1 and Type 2 diabetes. Diabetic complications that may be worsened by depression include kidney failure, retinopathy (eye disease), and cardiovascular disease. In fact, depression is one of the best predictors for hospitalization in people with diabetes.

Identifying depression

So how do you know if you or someone you know is depressed? What distinguishes normal life disappointment and discouragement from a medical illness requiring treatment? Specific criteria for major depression are listed in the DSM-IV (Diagnostic and Statistical Manual of Mental Disorders, fourth edition), a tool used by physicians to identify and classify psychiatric illnesses such as depression. A major depressive episode is defined by the DSM-IV as "a period of at least two weeks during which there is either depressed mood or the loss of interest or pleasure in nearly all activities."

In addition to these two cardinal symptoms, people with depression also tend to have several of the following symptoms and signs: sleep problems (sleeping too much, being unable to get to sleep, or being unable to stay asleep), impaired concentration or memory, an increase or decrease in appetite and accompanying weight gain or weight loss, either restlessness and irritability or having everything seem in slow motion, a lack of energy, feelings of guilt or worthlessness, a dramatic decrease in sex drive, and negative thoughts of oneself and the future that may be tied to thoughts of death or suicide. Depression can also manifest itself physically in a number of ways, including backaches, diarrhea, constipation, headaches, excessive sweating, dry mouth, generalized itching, or blurry vision.

Health-care professionals are best qualified to evaluate whether someone is depressed, although they will often need you to speak up about your feelings or symptoms to clue them in to some of the warning signs. If you are concerned that you may have depression, Dr. Culpepper recommends that you talk about it with your primary-care physician and take a self-administered PHQ-9 (Patient Health Questionnaire for nine symptoms of depression). According to Dr. Culpepper, primary-care physicians "often focus on physical symptoms and causes rather than the psychological state of their patients, but if a patient calls attention to potential depressive symptoms, most primary-care physicians are equipped to respond appropriately." A score of 5 to 14 on a PHQ-9 should lead to a discussion about possible treatment for depression with one's health-care provider. A score of 15 or higher, according to the PHQ-9, "warrants treatment for depression, using [an] antidepressant, psychotherapy, or a combination of treatments." The PHQ-9 can be found on a number of Web sites or you may be given one by your physician. (See "Depression Resources" on page 104.)

If you are unwilling or unable to seek help from your family doctor, you can also get a referral to a therapist or psychiatrist for diagnosis or treatment from groups or individuals such as your health-maintenance organization, family or social service agencies, clergy, employee assistance programs, and local medical or psychiatric organizations. How you choose to find help for overcoming depression is not as important as just getting yourself to seek help if you feel you need it.

Current treatments

The good news is that there are currently many treatments available for depression. Although mental illnesses were once highly stigmatized as moral or mental weaknesses, seeking treatment for problems such as depression has become fairly well accepted. Health-care professionals beyond those traditionally involved in mental health care are more aware of the importance of diagnosing and treating depression. Current interventions include medicines, non-drug medical interventions, and psychotherapy. Your health-care provider can help you to decide on the intervention or combination of interventions to use.

Drugs. Available medicines are targeted at increasing levels of specific chemicals in the brain called neurotransmitters. Neurotransmitters allow cells of the nervous system to communicate. There is some evidence that depression may be linked to a deficit of specific neurotransmitters such as serotonin, dopamine, and norepinephrine. Numerous studies have shown that antidepressant medicines reduce symptoms of depression better than a placebo (sugar pill). (Interestingly, placebo itself seems to have an effect on alleviating depressive symptoms, and most trials of antidepressant drugs show a *placebo effect* [when a sham treatment causes an improvement simply because the person expects one to occur]. However, the mere presence of a placebo effect does not mean that antidepressants are ineffective.) Studies have also shown that people who have depression along with another illness, such as diabetes, respond just as well to antidepressants as people who only have depression.

The major types of antidepressants are the selective serotonin reuptake inhibitors (SSRIs), the selective serotonin norepinephrine inhibitor (SSNRIs), the tricyclic and tetracyclic antidepressants, and the monoamine oxidase inhibitors (MAOIs). These drugs are not miracle pills; it will take an average of four to eight weeks to see their full effects. During and after this adjustment time, you'll need to see your doctor regularly to assess your dose, gauge if you need to try a different medicine, and monitor side effects. In addition to those side effects experienced by all people who take an antidepressant, people with diabetes may need to adjust their insulin or diabetes medicine regimen while taking an antidepressant. SSRIs, SSNRIs and MAOIs can increase risks of hypoglycemia (low blood glucose), and some SSRIs have side effects that mimic hypoglycemia symptoms. Tricyclic and tetracyclic antidepressants can cause hyperglycemia (high blood glucose). Anyone who is taking multiple medications, including an antidepressant, should consult his physician regarding possible drug interactions. Any antidepressant that increases serotonin levels, for example, may cause a serious condition called serotonin syndrome if given with another medication that also increases serotonin. For this reason, SSRIs and MAOIs should not be given together. Antidepressants should also not be taken with dextromethorphan, commonly found in cough syrup, or with St John's wort, since this can also cause serotonin syndrome.

Psychotherapy. Psychotherapy ("talk therapy") is also effective for treating depression and can be administered alone or with antidepressant drugs. One form of psychotherapy that has been well studied for the treatment of depression is called cognitive-behavioral therapy, or CBT. CBT is a method for teaching an individual different ways of thinking in response to stressful situations. It is intended to replace habitual, negative thinking patterns with more realistic responses. CBT focuses more on present ways of thinking and behaving rather than exploring the origins of one's thought patterns and behavior. At least one study has shown that people who undergo CBT are less likely to have a recurrence of depression—at least in the short term—than people who only take antidepressants.

Patrick J. Lustman, Ph.D., of the Washington University School of Medicine in St. Louis, Missouri, with his colleagues, has shown that CBT is effective for treating depression specifically in people who have diabetes. In a study published in the *Annals of Internal Medicine* in 1998, Dr. Lustman and colleagues studied 51 people with Type 2 diabetes and major depression. After 10 weeks, more people (85%) who had received CBT were significantly relieved of depression symptoms when compared with a group that received no specific treatment for depression (27%). This effect persisted for up to six months following the end of treatment (70% of the CBT group were depression-free versus 33% of people in the group receiving no treatment for depression).

Although CBT is effective for treating depression, not all psychotherapists are trained in this specific method. You may have to ask around a bit to find one. Your health-care provider, your state's psychological or psychiatric association, or your local mental health clinic may be able to help.

DEPRESSION RESOURCES

There are a variety of depressive disorders such as major depression, dysthymia, bipolar disorder, seasonal affective disorder, and postpartum depression. Despite their various symptoms and causes, depression is treatable. The resources listed below can help you to learn more about depression and diabetes, treating depression, and preventing suicide.

DEPRESSION
AMERICAN DIABETES ASSOCIATION
www.diabetes.org
(800) DIABETES (342-2383)
The ADA has a Web page at www.diabetes.org/type-2-diabetes/depression.jsp that gives a brief overview of depression and diabetes. If you have symptoms of depression but your health-care provider is unable to refer you to a mental-health professional, visit the ADA Web site or call their national toll-free number to find your local ADA office, which might be able to refer you to a counselor in your area who has worked with people with diabetes.

DEPRESSION AND BIPOLAR SUPPORT ALLIANCE
www.dbsalliance.org
(800) 826-3632
THE DBSA is a not-for-profit organization that publishes a number of free publications about living with a mood disorder and preventing suicide. They also support a nationwide network of peer-led support groups.

THE HEALING POWER OF EXERCISE
Your Guide to Preventing and Treating Diabetes, Depression, Heart Disease, High Blood Pressure, and More

Linn Goldberg, M.D., and Diane L. Elliot, M.D.
John Wiley & Sons
New York, 2000

MACARTHUR INITIATIVE ON DEPRESSION & PRIMARY CARE
www.depression-primarycare.org
Choose "PHQ-9" from the drop-down menu to view or download a Patient Health Questionnaire that can help you and your physician assess your risk for depression. The questionnaire is also available in Spanish.

MAYO FOUNDATION FOR MEDICAL EDUCATION AND RESEARCH
www.mayoclinic.com
Search for "depression" to find overviews of the illness and information on spotting depression in yourself and others. Each page is linked to other pages you might find interesting such as coping with holidays and how exercise can help. The site also has a depression self-assessment quiz you can take that's similar to the PHQ-9 (Patient Health Questionnaire for depression).

NATIONAL INSTITUTE OF MENTAL HEALTH
www.nimh.nih.gov
(866) 615-NIMH (6464)
Click on "Publications." Then use the drop-down menu to select "Depression" (a particularly good booklet from 2000 is called "Depression") or "Depression and Other Illnesses" (which has a booklet called "Depression and Diabetes"). You can also call the toll-free number to obtain copies by mail. Materials are also often available in Spanish and easy-to-read formats.

(Some Web sites listed in "Depression Resources" above may also be helpful.)

Nutrition. Much recent research suggests that low intake of omega-3 fatty acids may increase the possibility of depression, and that supplementing the diet with omega-3 fatty acids may help alleviate depression symptoms. Essential fatty acids could help restore normal levels of neurotransmitters such as serotonin, or may increase levels of molecules that benefit the brain, such as brain-derived neurotrophic factor. Before supplementing with omega-3 fatty acids, talk to your physician or nutritionist about recommended doses and also about which supplement to use. It is important to use fish oil that is verified to be free of contaminants such as mercury, PCBs, and dioxins.

Relapse. Whether you and your health-care team select antidepressants, psychotherapy, nutrition, or a combination to treat your depression, it is important to know that the majority of people who have one episode of major depression are likely to have a recurrence. One small study of people with depression and diabetes suggests that the recurrence rate within five years of the first episode can be as high as about 90%.

There is some good news in that maintenance

COGNITIVE-BEHAVIORAL THERAPY
ACADEMY OF COGNITIVE THERAPY
www.academyofct.org
(610) 664-1273
This Web site has information on cognitive-behavioral therapy and a suggested reading list. You can also click on "Find a Certified Cognitive Therapist" to locate a therapist near you.

ASSOCIATION FOR ADVANCEMENT OF BEHAVIOR THERAPY
www.aabt.org
Click on "Find a Therapist" to find a database searchable by location and specialty. If you click on "Site Map" and then "General Public" you can also find information on topics such as finding and evaluating a therapist and what to expect from psychotherapy.

SUICIDE
NATIONAL HOPELINE NETWORK
www.hopeline.com
(800) SUICIDE (784-2433)
If you are actively considering suicide and have means available to you, call 911 or your local emergency services number (located in the front of your phone book) immediately. If you are depressed but are not considering hurting yourself, contact a member of your health-care team, clergy, a family member or friend, or a crisis hotline such as this one, because talking to others about your feelings can help to relieve your despair and help you get the treatment you need. This Web site is also a useful resource if you suspect someone close to you is depressed or considering suicide.

therapy (using antidepressants and/or psychotherapy for 6 to 12 months after the depression is first lifted) can help to reduce risks of recurrence. Because of the high risk of a relapse, it is important not to discontinue therapy as soon as the immediate symptoms resolve and to discuss an appropriate maintenance plan with your therapist or health-care provider. People who experience several episodes of depression may be advised to take long-term antidepressant therapy.

Other treatments. There are other treatments for depression that do not involve either medicines or psychotherapy (though they may be combined with these interventions). These treatments tend to be reserved for very severe and resistant cases of depression. Although it gained an unsavory reputation from books like *One Flew Over the Cuckoo's Nest*, electroconvulsive therapy is a safe and effective treatment for depression that has not responded to anything else. The reason it works is not completely understood, but it may once again be related to a stimulation of neurotransmitter production in the brain.

Transcranial magnetic stimulation (TMS) is used to stimulate the brain with special strong magnets that are placed on the patient's scalp. TMS is currently being investigated for use in depression and some studies have shown that it can improve symptoms of depression. In January of 2007, the FDA evaluated whether TMS should be approved to treat depression but there were mixed feelings regarding whether this device is really effective. Whether TMS will be approved by the FDA is still unknown and it is currently only used in research studies.

Electrical stimulation of the vagus nerve is a treatment that was approved for the treatment of depression in 2005. The vagus nerve is a major route of communication between organs of the body and the brain and is thought to be linked to a region of the brain involved in mood. Stimulating this nerve may help chronic depression sufferers who do not respond to other treatments. The treatment does not work for everyone, however, and the long-term effects are still unknown.

Treatments on the horizon

New medicines are being developed for the treatment of depression, but none are as close to having enough data to submit for review by the FDA. Some of these potential treatments are targeted at blocking hormones that are released during stress, such as drugs being explored as corticotropin-releasing factor (CRF) receptor antagonists. Other future treatments may be directed at inhibiting a molecule called substance P, which is involved in the perception of pain and may also play a role in depression. It remains to be seen whether these treatments will be effective and safe, and whether they will be made available.

The first step

It is important to identify and treat depression in anyone who has it. Dr. Piette is very optimistic that once depression is identified, most people will respond positively to therapy. According to Piette, "The positive spin is that if people do think that they have this, it is something that is eminently treatable and we do know what works." □

HOW STORIES CAN HEAL

by David Spero, R.N.

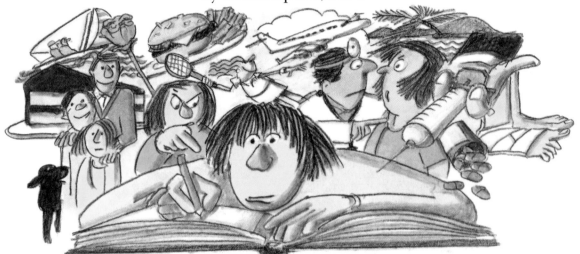

Lots of people struggle with diabetes self-care, but Mike didn't even try. In spite of his diabetes educators' best efforts, he wouldn't or couldn't pay any attention to food, blood glucose monitoring, exercise, or anything else related to his health. Mike was neither unintelligent nor uneducated, so what was the problem?

It turned out that Mike had a story he had never told. His beloved father had had diabetes and had gone from a foot infection to diabetic eye disease (retinopathy) to kidney damage and death within a single year. Mike had never talked about it. He rarely allowed himself to think about it, but the grief and terror he felt weighed him down, making his world seem empty and hopeless and making it impossible for him to take control of his health. When he finally told his story and dealt with his painful emotions, his depression lifted and he was able to start taking better care of himself.

Healers, from ancient shamans to modern psychoanalysts, have found storytelling among the most powerful forms of healing. We all have life stories, but we usually keep them to ourselves, if we are consciously aware of them at all. Some of our stories help us to keep going, while others cripple us. By telling them or writing them down, we can deal with the pain they cause, amplify the strength they give, and even change them for the better.

People can tell their stories in therapy, in groups, in interviews, or on their own. Psychiatrist Fred Busch says, "People come to therapy because they are living out somebody else's story, or [they are] afraid to see the story they're living out, or they cannot bear the story they've constructed.

The goal is to help people discover the stories they've been living, and in this way find the stories they choose to live."

Anyone with diabetes has a story that includes pain, loss, fear, and frustration—as well as joy, strength, and happiness. Putting your experiences and feelings in the form of a story can help you deal with them in three important ways: Stories help you to make sense of your life, help you process trauma and loss, and allow you to communicate your experience to others.

"Telling your story helps you understand where you have been and where you are going," says Teresa Campbell, whose book *Life Is an Adventure*, chronicles 25 years of travels with multiple sclerosis. "It helps you grieve your losses, celebrate your successes, acknowledge your fears, and move on."

Healing trauma

When pain, loss, or trauma goes ungrieved and untold, the result is often depression, which saps motivation and energy. Louise DeSalvo, Ph.D., author of *Writing as a Way of Healing*, says, "Depression is a story that has not yet been told."

Psychologist James Pennebaker of the University of Texas at Austin has studied the healing effects of storytelling for over 20 years. He found that writing about painful experiences for just 15 minutes a day for four days resulted in better health and a better mood for some college students. These students visited the doctor less often and reported less trouble getting used to college life. The beneficial effects were still in evidence six months later.

The students who benefited were those who

wrote about troubling memories and also about their feelings. Students who only described events or only vented feelings didn't benefit. It was writing a combination of descriptions of events and of related feelings that produced healing.

It didn't seem to matter whether students wrote in a journal or talked into a tape recorder. It didn't matter if anyone else heard it or read it. The important thing was to tell their stories for themselves. Participants said things like, "Although I have not talked with anyone about what I wrote, I was finally able to deal with it [and to] work through the pain instead of trying to block it out. Now it doesn't hurt to think about it."

Strengthening the immune system

Other experiments have shown that writing or talking about painful memories and emotions can improve immune system function. People's T-cells were more active; they responded better to vaccinations. Pennebaker believes these studies show that "inhibition"—holding back painful or shameful thoughts—takes energy. Inhibition becomes a powerful source of stress that slows the immune system and causes depression. When these inhibitions are released by talking or writing about traumatic events and their related emotions, the body starts to work much better.

When researchers looked at the brain waves of people who were telling their stories in this way, they found that writing or telling a coherent story used one side of the brain, while dealing with emotions used the other. So both sides of the brain are involved. Pennebaker believes that is an important reason why the storytelling method heals.

People who have been in accidents or experienced assaults or other traumatic events often talk about them over and over. Pennebaker says this seems to be the body's natural way of dealing with trauma. The problem comes when we are not allowed to talk about what happened (as often happens to sexually abused children, for example). If shame or fear keeps people from talking about their traumas, they often develop all kinds of physical and mental health problems.

Why is this relevant to diabetes? Like everyone else, most people with diabetes have painful memories that they may be reluctant to talk about and that may be affecting their health. Sometimes the memory of being diagnosed with diabetes itself is painful, or memories of insensitive treatment by health-care providers, family members, or others provoke feelings of anger or shame.

Cathy Feste, a diabetes educator who has had diabetes for over 50 years, writes about a young man who told her, "Anyone who has diabetes and doesn't admit that he's inferior is a liar!" She asked him how his diabetes had been introduced to him. He said, "I was 10 years old when I was diagnosed. My mother and doctor sat me down and told me I was sick. They said I couldn't go out for sports anymore or play with my friends the way I used to."

Most likely, this man's doctor thought he was doing the right thing for his young patient's health in warning him away from sports and activity, but his inaccurate information had the unfortunate side effect of making the boy feel bad about himself—for years if not decades. Had the boy been able to talk to other health-care providers or other people with diabetes who knew that sports were not off limits, he might not have developed a sense of inferiority. Talking or writing about his experiences as an adult can't change the past or make up for the years he felt inferior, but they can change the way he feels about himself now.

Telling your story

So talking or writing about your experiences with diabetes and other parts of your life can help you deal with them better. But what's the best way to do that, and what might stop you? In her book, Louise DeSalvo gives several suggestions.

■ Write or talk into a tape recorder for 20 minutes a day over a period of four days. Take days off between one four-day writing period and another. This way you won't feel overwhelmed.

■ Do it in a comfortable, safe, private place.

■ Write or talk about issues you're currently living with, things you're thinking or dreaming about a lot, or a trauma you've never disclosed or resolved.

■ Write about joys and pleasures too.

■ Include whatever positives you can find in the experience. What did you learn? Who helped you? What have you overcome?

■ Write or talk about both what happened and how you felt about it. Link events with feelings.

■ Writing will have benefits even if nobody else reads it. Keep your writing or tapes safe if you don't want others to read or hear them.

■ Going back to old memories may bring up sadness or anger or a confusing mix of feelings. People often report feeling troubled at first, but over time, you will feel more comfortable, clearer, and less stressed about those memories.

■ Because memories may provoke feelings of sadness or anger, it's a good idea to have someone available—such as a professional, a support group, or trusted friend or family member—you can talk with if you want some support in handling those feelings.

■ Storytelling is not therapy, but it can be just as powerful, and it can be complementary to therapy. You can do them together if you want.

Dr. Pennebaker says, "It is not necessary to write about the most traumatic experience of your life. It is more important to focus on the issues that you are currently living with. If there is something you would like to tell others but can't for fear of embarrassment, writing about it can help resolve it in your mind."

In dealing with issues and traumas about health, clinical social worker Bob Livingstone has clients keep journals, another way of writing your story. He asks them to think about some questions and pay attention to the feelings that come up.

■ How does my illness affect my personal relationships?

■ How has my illness changed my life? My outlook on life?

■ What fears do I have about my illness and how do I deal with them?

■ What was my experience of being diagnosed?

■ What have I learned about myself from dealing with my illness?

■ What gives me hope and inspiration during "down" times?

Livingstone says that many people benefit from thinking about these things while doing a physical activity or exercise. "Exercise releases endorphins," (our bodies' "feel-good" chemicals), he says. "The endorphins give you confidence and help you think about and deal with painful feelings." Thoughts and feelings can be written down after the activity or exercise.

Seeing the big picture

Without a story line, our lives tend to seem like a jumble of unconnected events. Things happen, we make choices, and we don't know why. Storytelling helps us make sense of our lives, which can give us a sense of control. However, many people discover in telling their story that they are really living other people's stories about who they are.

A man with Type 2 diabetes told Cathy Feste that he "couldn't exercise," even though his doctors had cleared him to do so. He meant that 35 years before, at age 17, a physical education teacher had called him a klutz and told him to get out of a game the class was playing. He had carried that story around ever since and had never rejoined the game.

But we can reclaim our stories and change them. A doctor in England told psychologist Lawrence LeShan that "her whole life had been a failure." She never wanted to be a doctor. She didn't really like patients and rarely read medical journals. She had moved to a small town to have a quieter practice, so she could devote more time to gardening, which she loved. She thought of herself as a bad doctor and a frustrated gardener.

In therapy with LeShan, though, she found a completely opposite way of seeing her story. Her parents had insisted she serve people with her intellect and had pushed her into medicine. By adopting a low-key medical practice, she was able to create the physical beauty of her lovely garden cottage. She now saw herself as having created a beautiful combination of her parent's values and wishes and her own. She was a success.

An African-American in Louisiana owned a small grocery store. He was extremely intelligent and had wanted to build a larger business, but childhood poverty and ongoing racism limited what he could do. Instead of feeling frustrated, he told his children, "I got as far as I could from where I started. Now you go and pursue your own dreams."

Ways to develop your story

Oral historian Nadine Wilmot collects people's stories in her job at University of California at Berkeley. She says the first task is helping people see that their stories are important. "People will say things like, 'I'm not important,' or 'Why do you want to talk to me?'" she says. "I have to let them know they are important, that their life is historically relevant, and they become quite excited about it once they begin talking."

Wilmot helps people remember by involving their senses. "We all have a canned story," she says. "You know, 'I was raised here, and it was this kind of town…' I focus on the sensory aspects, like what things smelled, tasted, and felt like, because the end result is richer if someone's engaged with their story in that way."

In my book, *The Art of Getting Well*, I suggest other ways to develop your story: "Think about where you came from, the times you've lived in, how they have influenced you, and you them. Remember the highs and lows, what you learned, whom you helped and who helped you."

Other questions you can think about include, What is the best thing that's ever happened to you? The worst? What's the best thing you have done so far? The worst? What are you proudest of? What has been the best period of your life? The worst? How did you get through that time?

It might be helpful to write or talk about how

diabetes fits into your life. In thinking about the role of diabetes in your life, you might want to consider philosophical questions such as, Where did your diabetes come from? What caused it? Is there something diabetes is trying to do for you? To teach you? To protect you from? Has diabetes given you any gifts? If your diabetes magically disappeared, how would you live differently?

Like archeologists, we sometimes need artifacts to help us build a story. In Kay Nelson's book *Writing Your Life Story: A Legacy to Your Family,* she provides lists of "memory joggers" to help us remember. She suggests looking through photo albums and old catalogs or magazines, listening to music or watching movies from different periods of your life, or going to historical museums. Nelson says remembering gets easier the more you work at it and the more cues you have.

Storytelling as communication

Most people are curious about their own family story. Telling your children and grandchildren about your life lets them understand you better and also tells them something about where they came from. Because they grew up or are growing up in a world very different from yours, they will probably enjoy hearing the details of a life they cannot even imagine. You may not be sharing painful traumas, but you will be building closer family ties. If you write down or tape-record your stories, you will also be creating a valuable memento to leave behind. The first person Nadine Wilmot ever interviewed was her grandmother, who has since died. "At the funeral," she says, "I felt so fortunate to be able to bring my uncle, father, and brother many CDs of her voice. That was a wonderful gift. She had a lovely voice."

Stories also help us communicate with doctors, other health professionals, and friends. Rather than tell your diabetes team, "I'm doing pretty good with my meal plan, but I'm having trouble exercising," or something vague like that, tell them a specific story about one event—maybe the day you planned to walk in the mall but wound up baby-sitting your niece's children instead. Hearing a story, including feelings, will give them a much better picture of what you're going through. It might also lead to your receiving some needed help.

Barriers to telling your story

Telling stories, especially painful ones, can be scary. You might not want to face memories that you have spent years repressing. But talking or writing about them can loosen their grip on you.

You may be embarrassed or ashamed and not

STORYTELLING RESOURCES

Here are some books and Web sites that can help you write your story.

WRITING AS A WAY OF HEALING
How Telling Our Stories Transforms Our Lives
Louise DeSalvo, Ph.D.
Beacon Press
Boston, 2000

OPENING UP
The Healing Power of Expressing Emotions
James W. Pennebaker, Ph.D.
Guilford Press
New York, 1997

WRITING YOUR LIFE STORY
A Legacy To Your Family
Kay Nelson
Westwinds Publications
Seattle, 1989

LIFE STORY WRITING NETWORK
www.lifestorywriting.net
A forum for writing about your life and sharing it with others.

These books can help you explore the effects of diabetes on your life:

THE ART OF GETTING WELL
Maximizing Health When You Have a Chronic Illness
David Spero, R.N.
Hunter House
Alameda, California, 2002

DIABETES BURNOUT
What to Do When You Can't Take It Anymore
William H. Polonsky, Ph.D., C.D.E.
American Diabetes Association
Alexandria, Virginia, 1999

To learn more about oral histories, visit these Web sites:

UC BERKELEY REGIONAL
ORAL HISTORY OFFICE
http://bancroft.berkeley.edu/ROHO

ABOUT.COM ORAL HISTORY PAGE
http://genealogy.about.com/od/oral_history/
This site is useful for those wanting to talk with family members.

want anyone else to know your story. If that's the case, you don't have to share what's uncomfortable. Telling the story to yourself and putting the events and feelings into clear, simple language can be healing even if no one else ever hears it. (But sharing with others can be powerful healing, too.)

If you feel you have nothing worth saying or that your life is so ordinary it isn't worth the effort of writing about, remember that every story has value. "Your mind is a storehouse," says Kay Nelson. "Its contents are precious. Your thoughts and memories seem ordinary to you because you've lived with them so long. But your story will be read by your descendents to whom life without the microchip will seem inconceivable!"

Some people believe they don't write well enough to tell their stories, even to themselves. But Louise DeSalvo says that anyone with a sixth-grade education is smart enough to get the emotional benefits of writing their story down. And if you can't write it down, you can tape-record it.

Some people may fear that creating a biography means they are getting ready to die. "Fear of mortality can come up when you start to look at and document your life story," says William Hazelwood, founder of Sojourna, a company that helps people tell their stories. "But we are going to die someday anyway. Why not take steps toward accepting, savoring, and celebrating life now? There is an old saying that funerals are for the living. So are personal legacies."

Technology of storytelling

What's the best way to record your story? And what do you do after you've recorded it? The answers depend on you. If you're telling about painful or traumatic events that you don't want anyone else to know about, you can keep a journal or talk into a tape recorder in private. You can always share them later if you want to.

A more interactive way to tell stories is by being interviewed. Perhaps a child or grandchild would like to record you talking on tape or even video-tape you talking about your life. The advantage of this method is that the interviewer will ask you about what is important to him, and you can also tell him what is important to you. You might also call the local college history department and see if anyone is doing oral histories.

Stories are more than words. You might want to illustrate your writing with photographs or, better yet, drawings. Sometimes art brings up feelings that words don't. But always write about the feelings too. That way you get both sides of your brain involved. If you're creating a life history for your descendants to read, Nelson's book has a lot of tips on creating a valuable and entertaining biography.

There are new ways to tell stories, too. Although we don't have research to document their health benefits yet, some people are using software like Microsoft PowerPoint and Apple's iPhoto to mix words and pictures. William Hazelwood of Sojourna says, "Unlike text-only formats, these programs allow easy revisions, visual attachments, and audio supplements."

Storytelling can be done in groups very effectively. Outfits like Sojourna often hold events where people can share and learn from others how to picture and tell their story. Local community colleges may have storytelling classes you can join. Support groups can be great venues for storytelling.

Although some biographies wind up getting published, don't feel you have to send your story to a magazine or book publisher. Some magazines want personal stories, while others (including this one) do not. You can easily show yours to the people who want to see it. Your story has value whether it is published or not.

No substitute for action

Dr. James Pennebaker and Louise DeSalvo give short lists of things not to do with stories.
■ Don't use talking or writing as a substitute for action. If you can do something about a problem, do it.
■ Don't use writing as a way of complaining. Use it to discover how you feel and why. Just venting or complaining can sometimes make you feel worse.
■ Concentrate on what happened and how you felt, not on why it happened or why you felt the way you did.

Although telling your stories might take some getting used to, especially if you have always been a quiet type, you may soon find that it enriches your life and even your conversation. You might find people becoming more interested in you and listening to you better when you talk in stories. You may grow in understanding and in your ability to deal with your life and your diabetes. Stories are powerful medicine. □

DIABETES AND YOUR MARRIAGE
Making Things Work

by Paula M. Trief, Ph.D.

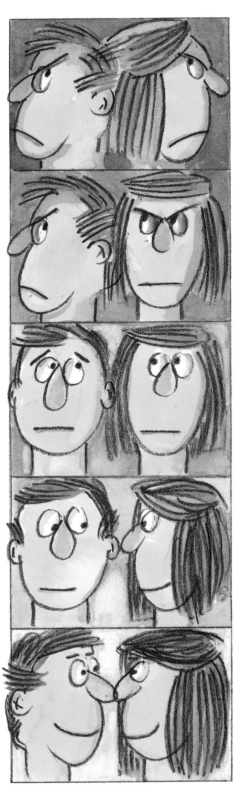

I t's hard to have a chronic illness like diabetes. You have to watch your weight, make healthy food choices, exercise, take insulin or oral medicines in many cases, and see several health-care providers on a regular basis. But there's more to it than that: You must carry out these tasks while also being worried that you may develop complications such as eye or kidney problems or while feeling depressed or overwhelmed.

Having the support of others can help ease the feelings of fear or frustration that often go along with having diabetes. Research has clearly shown that people who have social support tend to do better managing their diabetes. Social support can mean different things to different people. You may feel supported when a family member offers to take you to a doctor visit. You may feel supported when a friend listens and lets you cry about how frustrated you feel. Or you may feel supported when your sister walks with you each morning so that you can stick with your exercise program.

When people with diabetes feel they have people who care about them, people they can talk to about their deepest feelings, they are more likely to stick to their self-care regimen, to have better blood glucose control, and to feel positive about their ability to cope with diabetes.

When you are married (and 85% of adults are married at some point) or in a committed relationship, the most important source of support is usually your spouse or partner. However, the marital relationship can also be the greatest source of conflict and stress. This article explores how a couple's relationship may affect diabetes, how diabetes may affect the relationship, and how couples can work together to have both a healthy relationship and good diabetes control.

One affects the other

The quality of your relationship with your intimate partner can affect your general health and your diabetes control. Studies that have looked at the effect of marital stress on health have shown that your immune system, heart, and blood glucose control can all be negatively affected if you have a high degree of conflict and stress in your interactions with your partner. Your partner's involvement in your daily diabetes care can also make a lot of difference. It can make a positive difference if, for example, your partner prepares nutritious meals, keeps track of your medicines for you, or exercises with you.

As for diabetes affecting the relationship, a partner can experience many of the same negative feelings as the person with diabetes. He may feel scared about what the future holds. Will his partner develop complications? Will she get sicker? Will she continue to be able to do the things they have enjoyed doing together? These are common fears that partners have. A partner may be angry, especially if the diabetes has been linked to being overweight, or depressed about the extra medical bills. While fear and sadness are common feelings, different couples deal with these feelings differently, and how they cope can result in either greater conflict or more closeness.

A tale of two couples

The Smiths and the Joneses illustrate two different models for coping with diabetes as a couple. Both couples have been married for 20 years, both have two teenaged children, in both couples both partners work, and in both couples it is the husband who has had diabetes for 10 years. But their relationships are very different.

Mr. Smith hates the fact that he has diabetes and doesn't do much to take care of himself. He does inject insulin two times per day the way his doctor instructed him to, but he doesn't monitor his blood glucose level, he eats whatever he wants, and he regularly skips his medical appointments. He's had some vision and foot numbness problems. Mrs. Smith is very worried about her husband and frequently reminds him (Mr. Smith would call it "nagging") to monitor, take his blood pressure medicines, and watch what he eats. Mrs. Smith does the food preparation for the family, and she tries to limit the fat and sugar in their diet, but Mr. Smith gets mad if she says anything about his reaching for a second helping or getting ice cream when they are out. She responds by telling him he should feel grateful that she is trying to help. They fight about his diabetes a lot. With all of the tension, they have both decided that it's better to avoid the topic of diabetes altogether, so they try not to talk about it.

Mr. Jones has a different attitude about his diabetes. He also hates having it, but he's determined to "lick it" by "being the best darn diabetic I can be." He regularly meets with his health-care team. He is careful about what he eats, and he has asked Mrs. Jones to join him in following his diabetes meal plan. At first, she cooked special foods for him, but now the whole family follows the same meal plan as Mr. Jones. The Joneses try to take a walk together after dinner. Mrs. Jones is also worried about her husband, but she trusts that he is doing the best he can, and if he slips once in a while, she doesn't say anything. They talk about his diabetes when one of them wants to, but they try not to focus on it too much.

You can readily see that for the Smiths, diabetes is a big problem, and how they cope with it causes stress and conflict in their marriage. Mrs. Smith is trying to be supportive, but she is offering "directive support." This means that she takes responsibility for tasks that are really her husband's, and she often tells him what to do, feel, or choose.

In one study of adults with Type 1 diabetes, psychologist Edwin Fisher, Ph.D., and colleagues found that directive support causes more negative moods and is probably counterproductive. Partners who provide this type of support run the risk of joining the "diabetes police," a term coined by psychologist William Polonsky, Ph.D., C.D.E. The diabetes police are always watching to see if you eat the right things, check your blood glucose at the right times, and have the right blood glucose numbers. While they are usually doing this to protect you, it can be annoying and, by making you feel like a diabetes criminal, breeds anger, resentment, and shame. The way they are coping with diabetes leads to greater distance and will probably affect other aspects of their relationships.

In contrast, for the Joneses, diabetes is also a problem, but one they have both accepted as a challenge. They collaborate on how to deal with it. Mrs. Jones is providing "nondirective support." She assists her husband and cooperates with his requests, but the responsibility for his behavior lies with him; she has not taken it on. She tries to be actively involved in his self-care regimen, and she also recognizes that it's good for her and the whole family. Their nightly walks and talks contribute to more closeness and intimacy, so that they are ready to deal with the next problem that develops and work it out together.

In these examples, the husbands' attitudes play a big role in how the diabetes affects the relationship. But it's also true that the partner's attitude is very important. Even though Mr. Jones takes responsibility for caring for his diabetes, the Jones's relationship could still be marked by strife and tension if Mrs. Jones resisted making the changes that he requested or chose to simply ignore her husband's diabetes.

What is support?

To better understand what people with diabetes and their partners need as they cope with diabetes, my colleagues (Drs. Ruth Weinstock, Jonathan Sandberg, and Roger Greenberg) and I interviewed 42 people with diabetes and partners and asked them what is helpful and not helpful in their interactions with each other.

We found that help with diet is most important. Some partners help with grocery shopping and meal preparation.

One woman with diabetes said: "My husband likes to cook a lot of meat. I ask him not to fry my portion, and he is fine with that. He sautés it or broils it instead. He is very accommodating of my dietary needs."

Others focused on being sensitive to the need to time meals, especially if the partner injects insulin.

One partner said: "I've learned that he needs to eat within 30 minutes after the insulin, now that he is on that. So I am sure to let him know when I'll be serving supper so he can time his injection correctly."

Sometimes conflict develops, even with a supportive spouse.

One wife said: "I try to buy healthy foods. Unfortunately, my husband goes and buys other stuff that he likes to eat. I try to teach my kids how to eat healthy, how to live healthy. But my husband tells me not to tell him what to eat because he is going to eat what he wants."

Next most important is emotional support—not what your partner does for you but how it makes you feel.

One person with diabetes said: "She is very cooperative. She thinks of me. I can't ask for more than that."

One partner said: "Talking nicely and asking him how he feels instead of telling him helps him feel better."

Another person with diabetes said: "[I value] that discussion, that back and forth to try and figure out something that doesn't make sense right away, and sometimes it still doesn't make sense at the end. But sometimes there is a possible explanation, or we'll discover a pattern. It is helpful having a sounding board."

Finally, even though you want to avoid becoming a member of the diabetes police, our group said that it's helpful if a partner reminds the person with diabetes about things like when it's time to check blood glucose levels or take medicines or to pack a snack.

One person with diabetes said: "I am really active. I ski and bike, and I am out alone a lot. My partner is always asking me whether I have candy with me and whether I have my cell phone."

But crossing over to "nagging" or "bugging" or constant "critical" reminding was the least helpful behavior. It's often difficult for partners to find the line between helpful reminding and unhelpful nagging.

One partner who has struggled with this said: "[I have found that] nagging and being scared and nervous hasn't been helpful. I think [it's more helpful] if I am calm about things. If I see signs that suggest that he needs to check his blood sugar, I try to say something to him nicely. That basically helps and still makes him feel like a person, too."

Dealing with low blood glucose

Low blood glucose (hypoglycemia) can develop when people who use insulin have injected too much insulin, have eaten too little food, or have exercised without extra food. Some oral medicines can also cause hypoglycemia under similar circumstances. These include the sulfonylureas, which include glyburide (brand names DiaβBeta, Glynase, and Micronase), glipizide (Glucotrol and Glucotrol XL), and glimepiride (Amaryl) and the drugs repaglinide (Prandin) and nateglinide (Starlix).

Hypoglycemia can cause shakiness, weakness, nervousness, headache, hunger, mental confusion, and blurred vision. If blood glucose levels get very low, a person can have convulsions or become unconscious. A partner who notices such signs and symptoms may need to act fast by giving the person food or a beverage that contains carbohydrate. However, if the person with diabetes has become confused and is not thinking clearly, he may resist the help. If the person with diabetes has lost consciousness and can no longer safely swallow foods or liquids, the partner will need to inject glucagon, which makes the liver release stored glucose into the bloodstream. In some cases a partner might also need to call emergency services.

Hypoglycemia is upsetting, both for people with diabetes and their partners. Both get scared, both get frustrated, and both can get angry, at each other and at the diabetes.

One partner's comments captured the mix of emotions that can accompany a hypoglycemic episode, when he said, "I get very concerned about her having a low sugar and I become very annoyed at the fact that it is going to go down or is down. We had an incident this morning. I woke up, went in the shower and came out, and I generally check her blood sugar before I come down and have breakfast. Well, she is laying there in a cold sweat and she has a 36 blood sugar. I get aggravated because I am on a tight schedule [and now] I've got to feed her something."

A person with diabetes remarked, "Sometimes I get angry because of something that has happened. But sometimes it is a direct function of my sugar getting too low and affecting my mood and my thought processes. On at least one occasion, I more or less came to my senses to find myself sitting at the kitchen table and my wife sitting on the couch at the other end of the house crying because of something I did. I still don't know exactly what happened."

Another person with diabetes said, "If I developed hypoglycemia while we were out because the meal was late or for some other reason, he would get very angry and say, 'This is why I don't take you out anyplace.' Then I would cry and cry and cry."

Ways to collaborate

Having diabetes puts unique strains on a relationship, but it can also bring you closer together if you learn how to work together. Here are some ways to do that.

Get educated. It helps if both partners know what diabetes is, what must be done to manage it, and what to expect in the future. Your health-care team can provide the information, but in some cases, the person with diabetes may have to encourage his partner to join in the learning. If this is true in your case, ask your partner to come to a medical visit with you. Ask your partner what questions he has, and decide together how to get the answers. In addition to presenting general information about diabetes, educate your partner about your own specific self-care plan. If you set achievable and realistic goals and share them with your partner, he may be able to help you work toward achieving them.

Communicate. Talk about what you both need from each other. Talk about what is helping and not helping. Try not to be critical of each other but to approach this conversation with an open, nondefensive attitude.

Listen. Ask your partner how he feels about the changes you are making, then listen to the response. Don't interrupt, don't argue, don't try to convince him that he's wrong; just listen, not just to the words, but also to the feelings that are being shared.

Set shared goals. If you work together, you will probably get closer. So set goals for your diabetes management, like walking together after dinner, and talk about how to achieve them. Also, set goals for your relationship, like improving com-

munication, and talk about how to achieve that, like setting time aside to talk.

If you and your partner are not working toward the same goals, you will get frustrated and angry. If, for example, you are doing your best to prepare nutritious meals, but your partner who has diabetes eats a lot of junk food and then gets angry when you criticize, you know what I mean. A frank discussion about what each of you sees as the problem, what goals you have, and what you are each willing to do to work toward those goals is essential. **Make room for negative emotions.** Dealing with diabetes can lead to depression, anger, guilt, and fear, for both the person with diabetes and his partner. Sometimes, people get persistently angry or depressed, causing fights and emotional outbursts. These feelings become barriers in your relationship.

While it helps to be positive, recognizing negative emotions is part of the coping process. By accepting and experiencing these emotions, you can come to terms with the emotional impact of diabetes. And by sharing these feelings with your partner, you will decrease conflict and build intimacy in your relationship.

Get support from others. Even though your partner may be your main source of support, allow yourself to turn to other family members and friends, too. Doing so decreases the stress on your partner and provides an opportunity for other people in your life to feel involved and important and to experience the gift of giving.

Commit to nurturing the relationship. If your relationship is in trouble, admit it, talk about it, and recommit to nurturing the relationship. You can set aside time to take a daily walk and talk, go out on a weekly "date," find ways to be thoughtful of each other (such as offering flowers or doing your partner's chores), kiss good night, and make an effort to express physical closeness.

There is no standard for a healthy, satisfying relationship, and there are no limits on ways to develop and maintain one. Think about what happens in your relationship, and come up with creative ways to make things better. If you need some help, see a couples therapist. Often, a few sessions with an impartial observer can help you clarify the issues and develop a strategy to address them.

If you and your partner think of diabetes as a challenge that can either help or hurt your relation-ship—and choose to focus on what you have, not what you don't have—you can be grateful that there is someone in your life to walk with you on this road that includes diabetes toward a healthier and happier place. □

EIGHT TIPS FOR MANAGING DIABETES DISTRESS

by Lawrence Fisher, Ph.D.

Many people experience considerable distress about having diabetes and the amount of hands-on management that diabetes requires. This often includes frustration with the ongoing obligations of diet, physical activity, blood glucose monitoring, and taking medicines. Other equally important but less frequently acknowledged stresses can center around fears about the future, concerns about complications, difficulties dealing with caring but potentially intrusive friends and family members, and keeping up with all of the new drugs, treatment options, and related recommendations from the diabetes community. It is no wonder that as a group, people with diabetes report relatively high levels of personal distress, fatigue, frustration, anger, burnout, and feelings of poor mood and depression. Diabetes can feel overwhelming because of the unending demands of self-management.

The distress associated with diabetes and its management can have an effect on diabetes itself. For example, several studies have shown that people with diabetes who report more depressive symptoms have poorer management of their diet, physical activity, oral diabetes drug usage, and blood glucose monitoring, report more family conflict around diabetes, have more contact with the health-care system, and have higher levels of both diabetes complications and death from any cause over time than people with diabetes who do not have elevated levels of depressive symptoms.

The reasons for these associations are not completely clear, but two mechanisms have been proposed. First, research has indicated that distress and symptoms of depression are linked to the production of *cortisol*, a hormone produced by the adrenal glands. Among other actions, cortisol has been shown to reduce insulin sensitivity and to affect cardiovascular functioning. Second, stress and depression interfere with diabetes management behavior. It can be very hard to keep up with a complicated diabetes routine when you are having intense feelings of tension, distress, sadness, and frustration. So distress and depression can have both biological and behavioral effects on diabetes management. In fact, many clinicians consider a person's levels of distress and depression to

be as important to his or her care as measures of blood glucose, cholesterol, blood pressure, and weight.

In light of the considerable impact of distress on diabetes management—and on a person's well-being in general—what can be done in response to feeling burned out, overwhelmed, and blue? The good news is that diabetes distress can be managed and reduced if a few important tips are kept in mind. Not every tip will work for every person, because people with diabetes have different personal styles, life contexts, and preferences. But the ideas underlying these tips are applicable to most people with diabetes.

1. Feelings of being overwhelmed and burned out are to be expected. Almost everyone who has diabetes feels frustrated and distressed from time to time, and some more than others. Diabetes *is* burdensome, and it is normal to react to this burden. Some people feel particularly depressed and frightened when a new development occurs, such as a new eye or kidney problem. They may blame themselves, other family members, or their health-care practitioners, or they may simply feel that they should give up ("What's the use anyway?"). Others are more likely to feel burned out because of the unending demands of diabetes management. Having these feelings for more than a week or two signals that these feelings need to be attended to, just as other aspects of health and well-being need to be attended to on a regular basis. Disregarding or ignoring one's feelings often makes matters worse, while paying attention to the intensity and type of feelings experienced often provides a clue for what to do next.

2. Consult your health-care provider. Diabetes distress should be part of the conversation that people with diabetes have with their health-care providers on a regular basis. Admittedly, however, many people feel awkward bringing up issues about distress and feelings of discouragement, particularly when office visits are short and a large amount of material must be covered during any one visit. Furthermore, practitioners often make suggestions for care that overload people by asking them to do too many things too quickly, not explaining things clearly, or proposing a management plan that is not practical and realistic given each person's unique life context. One can leave a practitioner's office far more distressed than when one arrived.

While many health-care providers fail to initiate discussions about the feelings a person is having, most know that even the best diabetes plans will not work if the person is distressed, depressed, or burned out, and most will attend to these issues if a person brings them up directly. Sometimes a short course of antidepressant drugs can be helpful; sometimes reworking the management plan or coming up with alternative coping behaviors can address the problem; or sometimes a referral to a behavioral specialist is in order. In many cases, a simple airing of the problem relieves much of the tension and distress and helps put things back into perspective.

3. Talk to family members, friends, or others with diabetes. Put your feelings into words and express yourself. Talking about how diabetes feels is not necessarily whining or complaining; it is sharing what is going on internally in ways that inform others and in ways that force you to articulate your concerns verbally. Talking it out can help a person gain perspective, identify specific aspects of self-management that have become problematic, and make plans to address each aspect of the problem in a focused way. Keeping feelings inside and unexpressed often forces them into an internal box, where they fester and build upon one another. When this occurs, the risk of expression at the wrong time, at the wrong target, or with the wrong intensity increases dramatically.

Seek out others who are understanding about diabetes and are willing to listen without necessarily providing solutions. Telling the tale is often more helpful than finding the supposed solution.

4. Do one thing at a time. When distressed, many people with diabetes attempt to tackle all of their problems head-on or to alter their entire management plan in the hopes of making diabetes more tolerable. They double their physical activity regimen, sharply reduce calories with a new diet, or perhaps purchase a new blood glucose meter as a cue to monitor more frequently. The greater the number of things changed in a management plan at one time, though, the greater the probability that none of them will be accomplished. The lack of accomplishment then increases feelings of frustration and failure, and the process escalates to another level. To deal with diabetes distress effectively, create a list of priorities for change, and address each separately, one at a time.

5. Pace yourself. This tip follows directly from #4.

The slower the pace of change, the greater the probability that a goal will be achieved and, even more important, sustained. For example, people who drastically increase their physical activity may do very well for a week or two, even with sore muscles. But the probability is low that they will be able to sustain the program over time. Fatigue will increase, other lifestyle factors will compete for time, and motivation to continue will suffer. The primary goal of most aspects of diabetes management is sustained behavior, not just reaching a target in the short term. A slow pace of change enables the new behaviors to become more easily incorporated into a person's general lifestyle, and the new behaviors become self-reinforcing because many small goals are achieved sequentially over time. Furthermore, a slow pace enables each individual to experiment with alternatives in ways that make the most sense, and barriers to success are less overwhelming and can be dealt with more slowly and consistently.

6. Behavior change works best when not done alone. Diabetes distress often occurs when diet and physical activity goals are not achieved. In fact, of all the behavioral tasks associated with diabetes management, people with diabetes report that they experience the most distress about these two components of their management plan. A number of studies, however, have shown that for most people, behavior change works best when others are involved. People tend to reinforce each other, and joint actions are usually sustained far longer than actions taken by individuals alone. A related study showed that a weight-reduction program worked best for marital partners when both spouses sought to lose weight together. Studies of smoking cessation have shown similar results.

Some ways to involve others in your diabetes management routine include soliciting members of your household to help remind you to take medicines or monitor blood glucose levels (as long as these individuals are helpful and not critical); walking with friends or family members at a set time each day; and joining a physical activity program at a nearby neighborhood center, school, or gym. By engaging with others, the probability increases that a person's behavioral goals will be achieved and sustained, and distress about this portion of the management plan will be reduced.

7. Focus on behavioral goals. No person with diabetes can directly control his weight or blood glucose level. A person can consume fewer calories, take blood-glucose-lowering drugs, and expend energy through physical activity, but these are indirect behaviors, not direct methods of weight or blood glucose control. Many people with diabetes become very frustrated with how difficult it is to lose weight, for example, and their frustration increases when difficult diets are adhered to over time with relatively few pounds shed.

The reason is that many factors play a role in weight loss, just as many factors play a role in reducing blood glucose levels. Body size, age, sex, ethnicity, and medicines taken for blood glucose control all influence weight and blood glucose levels. Setting a goal of losing 25 pounds, therefore, is far more frustrating and difficult to achieve than setting a goal of staying on a 2,000-calorie-a-day diet. A person cannot directly control his weight, but he can control the number of calories consumed.

This is an important distinction that can help reduce frustration and distress: Focus on goals that can be directly controlled with behavior. A person with diabetes can control the number of calories he consumes, the amount of physical energy he expends, how regularly he takes his medicines, and how frequently he monitors his blood glucose. Completing all of these tasks regularly as part of an overall management plan *will* affect his diabetes control if his plan is designed properly. A focus on behavioral goals, then, rather than goals that are less directly controllable, helps people with diabetes stay focused on things that they can do and the goals that they can achieve and sustain. If a person's behavioral goals have been achieved but his HbA_{1c}, cholesterol, or blood pressure levels remain high, it is time to review his management plan with a health-care provider.

8. Take responsibility for your diabetes. Even though health-care providers play a crucial role in managing diabetes, fundamentally, management is up to the person who has it. This fact can be either overwhelming or empowering, acknowledging full well that it is a tough job in either case. It can be empowering by motivating people with diabetes to be proactive in gathering new information, devising experiments to test how different behaviors affect their blood glucose levels and other important measures, and addressing dia-

betes management difficulties both on their own and with their health-care providers. Being proactive may involve using a health library, the American Diabetes Association Web site (www.diabetes.org) and other Internet resources, and others in the diabetes community so that information about alternatives and strategies for care can be gathered. It may also involve raising concerns with practitioners and seeking out educators, nurses, physicians, and other health-care providers who specialize in diabetes. Studies clearly show that people who are engaged in their care, who take responsibility for their diabetes, and who are often one step ahead of their health-care providers do much better over time than people with diabetes who remain passive and uninvolved in their care. They are less frustrated, more inquisitive, and more upbeat about having diabetes than those who simply "go along" with what they are told. Holding back and feeling afraid to ask questions or pursue problems independently increases the probability of struggling alone and feeling overwhelmed and overburdened, since far fewer of the tools needed for success will have been obtained.

Putting it all together

As time passes, life changes, diabetes changes, drugs change, and management requirements change as well. Caring well for diabetes requires persistence, motivation, knowledge, and collaboration with family members, friends, and a team of health-care professionals. But keeping on top of the seemingly endless series of personal tasks associated with diabetes can often lead to frustration, fatigue, distress, and symptoms of depression, all of which can have negative effects on diabetes management, outcomes, and general well-being.

It is important to pay attention to these feelings, to use them as signals to take action, and to address them with your health-care providers. Dealing with diabetes distress and symptoms of depression is as important to your diabetes care as any drug taken or any behavior routinely practiced. Awareness of these issues is an inherent part of good diabetes self-management. □

HOW TO ASK FOR HELP — AND GET IT

by Linda Wasmer Andrews

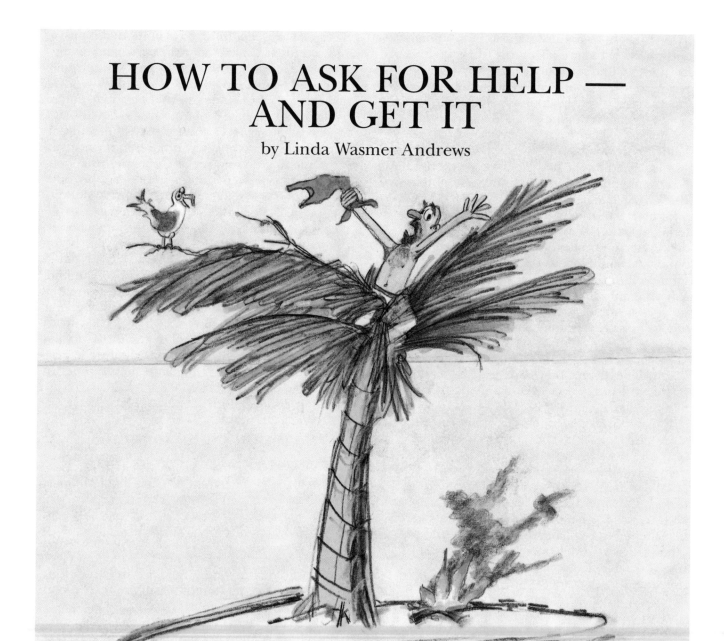

Everyone can use a helping hand now and then, and people with diabetes are no exception. The condition itself ensures that there will be ample opportunity to request help, whether it's asking your spouse to leave the doughnuts at work, your exercise partner to help you stay motivated, or your friend to remind you to take your medicine when you're out together. Unfortunately, asking for assistance doesn't come naturally for many of us. But like any other skill, it can be learned and honed with practice.

Truly mastering this skill may take some effort and patience, though. We live in a culture that prizes self-reliance, where *not* asking for help is often seen as a badge of independence and maturity. As a result, many people feel guilt and shame when they lean on others, as if they have somehow failed a central test of adulthood. Some are embarrassed about revealing a vulnerable side. Others are worried that they'll be a nuisance or, worse yet, a burden to family, friends, and coworkers.

Yet, used appropriately, asking for help doesn't indicate failure or weakness. To the contrary, it often shows that you understand how to manage your diabetes and are taking the necessary steps to do it well. There are times when asking for help is the most independent thing you can do, because it allows you to stay healthier, more active, and more self-sufficient in the long run.

Getting by with a little help

Study after study has shown that getting the right type of help in the right amount can promote better diabetes management. Among other things, research has found an association between greater family support and better blood glucose control, improved adherence to a treatment plan, increased weight loss, and reduced stress levels. On the other hand, what's intended as support can sometimes feel like nagging or smothering to the person on the receiving end. One study of people with chronic diseases, including 204 people with diabetes, found that misplaced "help" with chores and diabetes-related tasks was associated with more, not less, depression in the diabetes group.

In another study, 40 people with diabetes and 32 spouses participated in detailed interviews in which they were asked about helpful support. Transcripts of the interviews were then analyzed. When asked to describe what partners did to help, both groups most frequently mentioned something involving dietary control: grocery shopping, meal preparation, a shared diet plan, changes in the timing of meals, and so forth. Other forms of helpful help included general morale boosting and reminders to check blood glucose levels, take medicines, and pack extra snacks. In contrast, when spouses nagged, criticized, communicated poorly, or undermined healthy eating habits, their behavior was decidedly unhelpful.

Keep in mind, though, that support is in the eye of the beholder. For one person, reminders from a spouse to check blood glucose levels might be much appreciated. For another, the same reminders might be extremely aggravating. Your family and friends aren't mind readers. They may be walking a fine line, trying to offer welcome assistance without being overly intrusive. When you spell out what you need clearly and precisely, you actually make life easier for everyone.

Who, what, when, where

You are likely to get a better response if you target your requests for help appropriately. Your spouse may be the logical person to pick up a prescription at the pharmacy or remind you about a new diabetes drug schedule, but a friend with diabetes might be better equipped to provide useful tips when it comes to adapting recipes. When looking for help, always consider the personality and abilities of the person you're asking, since inappropriate requests just lead to frustration for both of you.

Decide in advance exactly what it is you will ask for. Make a list of all the forms of help that might be beneficial. Then narrow it down to the one or two most urgent items. If possible, give those items a shot on your own before asking for a hand. You may surprise yourself and discover that you don't need help after all. But even if it turns out that you do need assistance, you may feel better about asking once you've done everything in your power to help yourself.

Choose your time and place carefully. The middle of an argument is definitely not the optimal time to ask for help. Nor is the end of a long, tiring day, when the other person may already be feeling overwhelmed by life's demands. Instead, pick a moment when both of you are rested and relaxed enough to discuss your request calmly. In addition, make sure you have privacy. You'll only engender resentment if you put the other person on the spot in a public situation.

Asking for it

How you ask for help has a big influence on the response you get. It's obvious that a polite request will get a more positive reaction than a rude demand. A simple "please" can go a long way. But beyond that, there are more subtle factors that may affect how likely you are to get your desired outcome. These tips can help you master the art of asking for help effectively.

State your request calmly. Don't whine, wheedle, cry, yell, threaten, or try to make someone feel guilty. If you're feeling angry or hurt, wait until you have calmed down to present your request. Otherwise, the person you're asking for help is likely to feel manipulated or trapped, and you're almost guaranteed to get a negative response, ranging from outright refusal to grudging agreement.

Specify exactly what kind of help you need. Take the guesswork out of the situation. The more information you provide, the easier it is for the other person to comply, and the more likely you are to get what you really want. Instead of dropping vague hints, such as "I could sure use some help with my diet," spell it out: "Honey, you know I have a hard time resisting chocolate chip cookies. Instead of bringing home a whole box, could you buy just the number you plan to eat right away? That way, we won't have extra cookies around to tempt me."

Counter vague offers with specific suggestions. You've heard it a hundred times: "Let me know if there's anything I can do." Next time, take the offer seriously. Be prepared with a specific idea for how that person can help. If you don't need anything at the moment, ask if you can have a rain check. Most people sincerely want to help, but simply don't know where to start. They'll be grateful for well-focused suggestions that point them in the right direction.

Make it clear that "no" is an option. Always give the other person a graceful way out. Then don't be hurt if someone takes it—you may not be aware of all the factors in that person's life that could make it hard to honor your request right now. Those who do decide to help will appreciate feeling that they had a choice in the matter. They're less likely to react as if you're imposing on them, and you, in turn, are less apt to feel that you're being a burden.

Expand your support network. Avoid overwhelming any one person with too many requests. Asking four people for two favors each is likely to be much better received than asking one person for eight. If several family members, friends, and neighbors have agreed to help out in various ways, make a list so you can keep track of who offered to do what and when. With an organized list in hand, you're less likely to keep going back to the same person over and over, and you're better able to time your requests to the other person's convenience.

Ask someone to be on emergency standby. In fact, you may want to ask several people, such as your spouse or closest friend as well as other family members, friends, or coworkers with whom you spend time regularly. Make sure they can recognize the signs of severe hypoglycemia (low blood glucose) and know what to do if the situation arises. This is no small favor, since it might involve giving you a glucagon injection or forcing you to accept help when you're confused and irritable. Be sure to provide the information each person needs to feel comfortable with the responsibility.

Plan ahead for other upcoming needs. When you can foresee that your needs will be increasing soon—for example, if you have surgery scheduled—line up your support team in advance. Your doctor should be able to give you an idea of what kind of help you'll need and for how long. If possible, have both a Plan A and a Plan B ready. For example: "My daughter will stay with me for a few days after surgery. When she can't be here, my friend has offered to help."

Guard against becoming overly dependent. While many people find it very difficult to ask for help,

others find it far too easy. Watch out for sneaky ulterior motives. Do you really need your spouse to prepare your insulin injections and plan all your meals, or do you just like keeping your spouse close by your side? It's natural to enjoy a loved one's attention and concern, but asking for unnecessary help isn't the best way to get it. By doing so, you're taking advantage of your loved one's kind intentions, and you're depriving yourself of the chance to learn diabetes self-management skills that can serve you well for a lifetime.

Be sensitive to financial concerns. Your retired neighbor may be happy to drive you to doctor appointments, and your daughter may be glad to stock up on the organic foods you like whenever you visit. But the cost of gas or groceries can be a real hardship for someone with a limited income. Don't wait for the other person to ask, since it can be awkward to bring up money issues. Instead, volunteer to buy a tank of gas or a few bags of groceries.

Find thoughtful ways to say thank you. The words are important, of course, but actions speak even louder. Look for personal ways to let family and friends know how much you appreciate their help. Homemade gifts from your kitchen, garden, or woodworking shop are always welcome. So are gifts of time and attention. Rent the person's favorite movie, invite him or her for a walk, or share a hobby that the person has shown an interest in learning about.

Be there to help your helpers. We all need a friendly boost from time to time. Lending a hand when your helper needs support not only makes you feel good, but also helps keep the relationship in balance. If your spouse has been your biggest cheerleader while you struggled to lose weight, return the favor when your spouse decides to quit smoking. If your friend is going through a rough patch at work, be a sympathetic listener while she talks about the problem. Both parties gain when you take turns filling the roles of giver and receiver.

Volunteer a hand to others. Another way to relieve any sense of unpaid obligation you might feel is by giving back to your community. Numerous studies have found an association between volunteering and mental health. In addition, a recent study from Stanford University involving nearly 7,500 older Americans found that frequent volunteers were significantly less likely than nonvolunteers to die during the eight-year study period. By generously sharing your time and knowledge, you just might end up helping yourself to a longer life. □

GETTING A NEW PERSPECTIVE ON YOUR DIABETES
Confronting Fears and Building Motivation

by Susan Shaw, C.Ht.

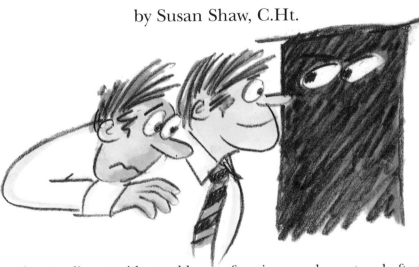

I magine that you're standing outside an old movie theater with a towering, lighted marquee. In huge, red letters, the marquee reads, "Your Future With Diabetes." If you bought a ticket, went inside, and waited quietly in the dark while the curtains parted, what kinds of images would appear on the screen?

What is the rest of your life with diabetes going to be like? What changes are likely to happen to your body? How might other parts of your life change? How long will your life be?

If you feel a great deal of anxiety about the answers to these questions, you're not alone. Studies show that 73% of people with diabetes are concerned about developing serious complications, and almost half worry that these complications will render them helpless. For the most part, these fears are unwarranted. Although complications can and do occur, total helplessness usually does not. People who develop complications often find that they are manageable, that options for treatment and relief abound, and that even the onset of previously dreaded complications does not detract from the ability to live a meaningful life. But when you don't know that your fears are excessive and irrational, they can detract from your quality of life and destroy your motivation to perform diabetes self-care routines.

Diabetes management is not just a bunch of tasks involving meal plans, blood glucose monitoring, exercise, and medicines; it is also a lifelong process of learning and self-reflection. Con-fronting our deepest and often false beliefs about ourselves and our diabetes, and learning to change beliefs based in fear to form a more positive outlook can improve motivation to perform self-care.

Building self-efficacy

Clinical trials have demonstrated that good blood glucose control reduces the likelihood of serious diabetes complications and improves health in many ways. Unfortunately, subsequent studies have found that the majority of people do not maintain the current recommended level of blood glucose control, nor do they meet current blood pressure and lipid (cholesterol and triglycerides) goals. But according to a 2004 study on psychological barriers in the *European Journal of Endocrinology*, "Nearly all the barriers to effective self-management of diabetes lie in individual's personal and social worlds."

Health-care professionals are now recognizing that to empower people to reach their health-related goals, their social, psychological, emotional, and even spiritual issues must be addressed, in addition to medical issues. The need to promote self-efficacy is becoming clearer. But what exactly is self-efficacy? More than just self-confidence, it involves an individual's personal beliefs about his ability to reach goals and exert influence over events that affect the course and quality of his life. Albert Bandura, a Stanford University professor who pioneered the theory of self-efficacy, writes in the *Encyclopedia of Human Behavior,* "Self-efficacy beliefs determine how people feel, think, motivate themselves and behave."

People with a strong sense of efficacy see new tasks as challenging and strive to master them. They set challenging goals and sustain their efforts in the face of failure. According to Bandura, people with a strong sense of efficacy also experience reduced stress and are less vulnerable to depression.

People with low confidence in their abilities, on the other hand, strive to avoid difficult tasks and view them as threatening. They tend to dwell on personal inadequacies and obstacles and to focus on the worst possible outcome. People with a low sense of efficacy give up quickly, are slow to recover from failure, and are easy prey for burnout, stress, and depression.

"Self-belief does not necessarily ensure success, but self-disbelief assuredly spawns failure," Bandura says. "Unless people believe they can produce desired effects and forestall undesired ones by their actions, they have little incentive to act, or to persevere in the face of difficulties."

Diabetes is widely recognized as one of the most difficult chronic conditions to manage. A typical day with diabetes presents challenge after challenge: making food choices, counting carbohydrate grams, taking injections or medicines, checking blood glucose levels, and writing everything down to monitor blood glucose trends. The demand for self-efficacy is intense and never ending. Doctors know they can't write "self-efficacy" on their prescription pads, but they are becoming aware that this characteristic can and should be strengthened.

Exploring your beliefs

Exploring your beliefs about diabetes and about your ability to manage it can spark a reassessment of what you believe to be true about your ability to exert control over the course of your diabetes. Of all the beliefs people with diabetes can have, none are more disabling than those based on fear. Fears can have little basis in fact and can cause us to lose belief in our ability to control our diabetes. And unfortunately, a culture of what Andrew Weil, M.D., calls "medical pessimism," the established practice of predicting negative outcomes, as well as the widespread use of fear as an attempt to motivate others, allows fear to thrive in the lives of people with diabetes.

Many of us have experienced the power of what Weil calls a "medical hex." When I was nine, for example, a nurse shook her finger at me and proclaimed that if I didn't do what I was supposed to

do, I would go blind. "And it will happen just like that!" she said, snapping her fingers. Her hex was effective; as a teenager, I panicked whenever my vision seemed blurry and worried that my sight would disappear all at once. Many years later, I did develop retinopathy, but I also became better educated and discovered that retinopathy is treatable and that abrupt and total blindness is highly unlikely, especially with regular eye exams. With more accurate information, the hex was undone.

A woman at one of my workshops seemed proud of her efforts to motivate her husband. "My husband's brother died of the worst possible complications of diabetes," she reported, "So I throw that in my husband's face every day!" Although this type of scolding might be well intentioned, a German study found that "fear of complications can lead to patients dealing as little as possible with their diabetes, largely neglecting self-management." In other words, well-meaning relatives and health-care providers who take this approach can actually drive people with diabetes, especially those with a poor sense of efficacy, further into denial and inaction.

One often overlooked reason for fear and burnout in people diabetes is that diabetes care providers can suffer from both themselves. They may fear that their patients will suffer from complications for which they will feel partly responsible. In response to those difficult feelings, they may redouble their attempts to "help" patients, often by using gloomy predictions as motivators.

In addition to being based on misguided warnings from health-care providers, beliefs about diabetes can be founded on outdated information, old wives' tales, negative talk around the dinner table, or colorful family legends about distant relatives with diabetes. It's important to examine these beliefs, decide what aspects are factual, and discard the rest. I suggest that you proceed slowly through the following list of common beliefs, taking a moment to reflect on each one, and noticing what thoughts, feelings, and images come up.

I will die early. Sit with this thought for a moment and see how you feel about it. Many of us were told this when we were diagnosed, and recent television commercials inform parents of overweight children that Type 2 diabetes will significantly shorten their children's lives. Providers often feel compelled to report the statistics on early death to their patients with diabetes, even though many of them will defy these statistics. This information can cause people with diabetes to experience panic, despair, and immobility. I was startled by the number of young people I met at my workshops who believed they would die by age 45 or who thought they shouldn't have children because they wouldn't live long enough to raise them.

I am bad. "I'm a diabetic, but I'm bad," one woman announced. "I don't do what I am supposed to do." Countless others have approached me to report how "bad" their relatives with diabetes are. We often think negatively about ourselves and see only our errors instead of the multitude of self-care tasks that we perform correctly. We may tend to magnify every transgression (such as eating an extra snack) and can even be burdened with guilt over a sense that we caused diabetes in the first place, or could have or should have prevented its onset.

I must be perfect. Although the pursuit of perfection may seem worthy on the surface, perfectionism is a self-defeating attempt to escape what we fear by setting goals that are likely to be unattainable. In the end, perfectionism kills motivation. In diabetes management, where some miscalculations and unexpected blood glucose swings are unavoidable, trying to achieve perfection in our habits and our blood glucose numbers will leave us burned out and disappointed.

I am special, but flawed. Some of us allow our diabetes to be the most prominent and distinguishing characteristic of our life and feel that diabetes makes us "special." But this sense of being special can isolate us from others and from the ordinary activities and fun of living. Some of us make the management of our diabetes our greatest focus or our biggest achievement. Although diabetes management needs continuous attention, when it becomes our world, and when we think that others could never understand the difficulties inherent in our special world, we forget to enjoy our lives.

I have to change my lifestyle NOW! You just got an e-mail saying that your cousin went on kidney dialysis, and a jolt of fear hit you like a lightning bolt. "I'm going to control my blood sugars starting right now!" you promise yourself. But the motivation that comes from panic wears thin only hours later, in the face of the reality that making a major lifestyle change takes many small efforts over a very long period of time. When change doesn't occur immediately, the belief that we are "bad" and incapable of change is reinforced. In this way, urgency can be a motivation killer.

Complications are coming; they will be sudden and unmanageable. When we think of complications, our minds often conjure up the worst. We fear that if complications occur in the future, they will be overwhelming and take away all quality of life, and that we will have no ability to cope,

adjust, or adapt. With this view of complications, hope goes out the window.

Gaining insight and new awareness

Fortunately, new beliefs can arrive in one "Aha!" instant or in a series of many instants. Education or an honest discussion might be all it takes to start turning fear-based beliefs into motivating ones.

One workshop participant said, "I don't worry about dying early; I'm just afraid of the pain."

"What pain?" I asked.

"I don't know exactly," she responded, "I just always thought there would be pain at the end."

"Well, there can be pain if you get neuropathy, but not everyone will, and even if you do, there are drugs that can help you manage pain," I said. "There are also new non-drug treatments that can help control neuropathy pain." She looked perplexed for a moment and then her face broke into a grin. "Really!" she exclaimed. She later told me that her life with diabetes had turned around that day. This is a perfect example of how intelligent people can inadvertently develop dysfunctional beliefs based on hearsay.

As a hypnotherapist, I've worked with hundreds of people using hypnosis, a state of relaxation similar to meditation, to unravel dysfunctional beliefs and discover the positive power within each person. The insights that arise when the body is relaxed, brain waves are slowed, and the mind is anxiety-free can be spectacular.

One man fiddled with his insulin pump and blood glucose monitoring paraphernalia with great anxiety, worried that his body was on the brink of disaster. But in a hypnotic trance, he discovered a new way to perceive his physical being.

"This is a good body!" he said when he opened his eyes, surprised. "It's strong, it's flexible, it's active; it does a lot of things, and it does them really well!" People with diabetes can tend to focus on what may go wrong in the future and forget to appreciate that in the present, we're mostly fit and healthy.

Here are two simple exercises that can help you examine your own beliefs and discover new ones.

Exercise #1. Get a piece of paper and write the beginnings of these sentences three times each. Leave room on the page so that you can complete the sentence with a word or a phrase. Then imagine that your diabetes is speaking to you and completing the sentences. Write down whatever words pop into your mind.

A word of caution: This can be a disturbing

experience, since deep down, you may fear that diabetes is destroying you. But stick with it; the information the process uncovers is worth revealing. If you are startled by what comes up, discuss your experience with a trusted friend or therapist. Completing each sentence three times will allow you to penetrate deeper into your belief system.

I am _____ .

I feel _____ .

I need _____ .

I believe _____ .

I want _____ .

I will _____ .

I secretly _____ .

When you're done writing, read what's on the paper and consider it. Go through each belief and ask yourself:
- Is this true? Partly true? Totally false?
- Is this belief based on fact? If not, where did this belief come from?
- Which beliefs can be rejected or modified?
- What could I believe that would show confidence in my ability to manage diabetes?

Exercise #2. Find a place where you can recline comfortably and be undisturbed for 25 minutes. Close your eyes and take five deep, slow breaths. Count backward from 21 to 0 as you imagine yourself walking down a staircase. Notice your body relaxing. At the bottom of the staircase, someone wise and loving who knows you well awaits. Your wise guide will take you to three different places to show you something about hope. Take plenty of time, notice that your inner world is colorful—like being in a dream except while awake—and allow your journey to unfold.

Some new beliefs to consider

Now that we know that fear-based beliefs undermine motivation, let's look at some beliefs that enhance a sense of efficacy and your motivation to do the best possible job of self-care.

It's OK to make mistakes. Mistakes are part of learning. Don't judge yourself harshly when you make a mistake; just observe the effects on your blood glucose, mood, and energy level, and use this information as a learning experience.

I have plenty of time. Pressure and panic don't mix well with the careful attention that diabetes management demands. If feeling like you need to make changes right now has you panicked, focus on your breathing and your body, and notice that for the most part, things are OK. You do have time. Be willing to slow down and invest whatever

amount of time is needed. In the words of Steven Edelman, a physician with diabetes, "It's never too late to do something to improve your diabetes."

I can shape my future. Don't let distressing thoughts about diabetes interfere with your vision of the future. Will Cross imagined himself on the summit of Mount Everest, and new insulins and insulin delivery systems allowed it to happen. All of us have personal summits to reach. Create a vision of a healthy, rewarding future in your mind, and be willing to utilize all available management tools, as well as the new ones that are certain to come, to make your desired future happen.

I have unique and special talents. Don't let diabetes be the thing that makes you special. Develop your abilities and talents, be proud of them, and let diabetes be only a small part of who you are.

My body and the tools I have to manage my diabetes are miracles. The first insulin injections in the 1920's pulled people back from the brink of coma and death and allowed them to live for many years in relatively good health. These events were celebrated as miracles. Today, medical pessimism and a culture of negativity have overshadowed reality. Instead of being grateful for medicines and management tools that most of the developing world still goes without, we see them as burdensome chores. Insulin is *still* a miracle. Our bodies are miracles; they are surviving and thriving. Try seeing your body and your management tools as miraculous, and see how your mindset and energy level changes.

I am a survivor. At events like the Avon Walk for Breast Cancer, cancer survivors join hands and walk with their arms overhead in a victory parade. They celebrate the fact that they are alive and refuse to feel shamed or stigmatized by a disease. People with diabetes, and especially those living with complications, deserve to do the same. Stop feeling shame over having diabetes and celebrate the fact that you are surviving in spite of it.

Diabetes cannot diminish my ability to love or be loved. This simple truth puts diabetes into perspective. Diabetes has no power to change anything in life that really matters.

It is worth it

Being diagnosed with diabetes can be a frightening experience, but developing the right attitude can go a long way in helping you manage this condition. So the next time you are faced with a diabetes chore you resist, take a moment and say to yourself, "I can do this, this will work, my body is a miracle, and taking care of it is worth it." □

Blood Glucose Control

Tips 195–257 127

HbA$_{1c}$ 132
What It is and Why It Matters

Blood Glucose Monitoring 137
What Do the Numbers Tell You?

The Myth of Brittle Diabetes 141

Strike the Spike 146
After-Meal Blood Glucose Highs

Take a Bite Out of Hypoglycemia 153
10 Proven Strategies for Cutting Down on
Low Blood Glucose

Continuous Glucose Monitoring 160
Getting Started

3

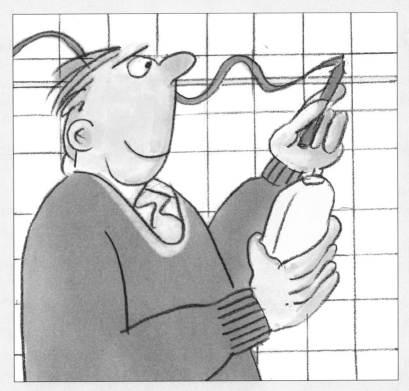

Blood Glucose Control Tips

195–257

195. The HbA$_{1c}$ test gives an indication of your blood glucose control over the previous 2–3 months and is an important part of your diabetes-care regimen.

196. Because the red blood cells in a blood sample used for an HbA$_{1c}$ test are a mixture of cells of different ages, the test gives a "weighted" average of recent blood glucose levels.

197. Even if you haven't met your HbA$_{1c}$ goal yet, you might be pleased to know that just about any decrease in blood glucose levels can help.

198. Exactly how often your HbA$_{1c}$ level should be checked depends on your degree of blood glucose control and your physician's judgment. Because everyone's health situation is unique, you need to work with your health-care team to set a HbA$_{1c}$ goal that will work best for you.

199. Current American Diabetes Association recommendations are to first get low-density lipoprotein (LDL) cholesterol (the "bad" cholesterol) levels below 100 milligrams per deciliter.

200. Every health insurance and managed-care company has its own policies, so you'll need to check your plan for specifics on whether it will cover the cost of an HbA$_{1c}$ test.

201. Continuous monitoring systems must be periodically calibrated with conventional blood glucose meters using fingerstick blood samples for accurate readings.

202. People using a continuous glucose monitor are advised to do a conventional blood glucose check before making any changes in their diabetes care regimen.

203. Remember to keep an eye on glucose trends, not just individual glucose numbers. Focus on prevention and catching potential problems early.

204. Speak to your health-care provider if your attempts at improved diabetes control aren't having the effects you intended.

205. Research presented in 2004 suggests that a person's HbA_{1c} correlates closely to his average blood glucose levels during the three hours after—not before—eating.

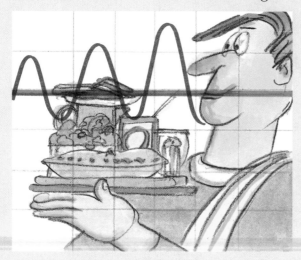

206. Even though after-meal high blood glucose levels are temporary (often resembling a spike when plotted on a graph), frequent between-meal rises can cause your HbA_{1c} to go up.

207. Perhaps the most practical measure for detecting after-meal blood glucose spikes is to check your blood glucose level about one hour after completing a meal or snack using a blood glucose meter.

208. When checking your blood glucose level after meals or snacks, you should use a blood sample from a finger rather than an alternate site sample.

209. Check your blood glucose before and after breakfast, lunch, and dinner several times to determine whether postprandial spikes are a problem at a specific meal.

210. Substituting foods with a lower glycemic index for foods with a higher glycemic index in your diet will help to reduce your after-meal blood glucose spikes.

211. Look at your after-meal blood glucose levels from time to time, and determine whether a problem exists. If it does, take the necessary steps to achieve better after-meal control.

212. Both your premeal blood glucose level and the glycemic index of the foods you are planning to eat should be taken into consideration when deciding when to take a mealtime insulin dose.

213. For a person with diabetes, detailed written records can reveal blood glucose patterns and, more important, what is contributing to those patterns.

214. A good set of records should include blood glucose values, insulin and/or oral medicine doses, the amount of carbohydrate eaten at meals and snacks (with notes about high-fat or extra-large meals), and physical activities.

215. The onset, duration, and peak action times of NPH and Regular insulin vary depending on where the injection is given.

216. If you use NPH or Regular and you want to rotate your injection site, use the same body part for each time of day for greater overall consistency.

217. Make sure to rotate your insulin injections within each site, giving each shot at least a finger's width away from the previous shot.

218. Check the expiration date on your insulin before using it, and never use an open vial for more than a month.

219. Matching what you eat to how much insulin is available (whether injected or secreted from the pancreas) is the crux of diabetes management.

220. Some people who use insulin can achieve tighter blood glucose control by adjusting their insulin doses based on the amount of carbohydrate they consume at a meal or how active they plan to be.

221. To avoid low or high blood glucose around mealtimes, be sure you know how much time to allow between taking the drug or insulin you use and eating.

222. To keep blood glucose levels more stable, count the grams of carbohydrate in your meals and snacks and try to keep the total at each meal or snack consistent from day to day.

223. If you know that you will be eating more than usual, you may need to increase your insulin or fast-acting oral medicine dose prior to eating.

224. When you have symptoms of low blood glucose, use your meter to confirm them, then limit yourself to consuming 15–30 grams of carbohydrate to treat the low.

225. Using preportioned glucose tablets or gel to treat hypoglycemia instead of food or juice may help you control the amount of carbohydrate you consume.

226. Check your blood glucose more frequently following intense or extended exercise, and reduce your long-acting insulin dose or consume an extra snack after the activity if necessary.

227. Check your blood glucose before and during high-intensity exercise, and check for ketones if it goes above 300 mg/dl.

228. Try to exercise at about the same time of day on a consistent basis.

229. Learning some simple meditation techniques or other relaxation methods can help you cope with everyday stresses.

230. If a difficult situation can be anticipated (for example, a funeral or an exam), and you know how your body typically responds to stress, you may be able to prepare for it by increasing your basal insulin or oral medicine dose, or by engaging in more exercise.

231. Unless otherwise directed, don't skip insulin or oral medicines when you're sick, even if you're eating less than usual.

232. Communicate with your (or your child's) health-care team frequently during your child's growth years; insulin adjustments may need to be made on a monthly basis.

233. If you notice a regular pattern of high blood glucose around the time of your period, talk to your doctor about making a monthly adjustment to your insulin or oral medicine regimen.

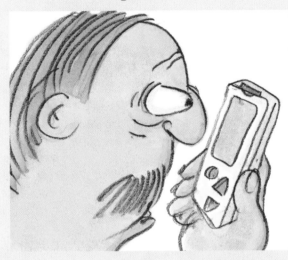

234. Check your blood glucose level before meals whenever possible. If you decide to check after meals as well, expect the readings to be higher than they usually are before eating.

235. Always check the expiration date before starting a new vial or box of strips. Keep your strips sealed in their packaging and away from extreme temperatures.

236. If your blood glucose levels are rising despite your best efforts to control them, speak to your physician about adding, increasing, or changing your dose of diabetes medicines.

237. If you have trouble falling or staying asleep, try cutting down on caffeine, avoiding naps during the day, and getting regular exercise early in the day.

238. If caffeine appears to affect your blood glucose level, either keep your caffeine intake modest (but consistent), or work on cutting it out of your diet completely.

239. When traveling, allow your body a day to adjust to time zone changes, but try to get back to your usual meal and sleep schedule on the first full day at your destination.

240. Ask your health-care provider what guidelines you should use to evaluate your blood glucose readings before and after meals.

241. Remember that the goal for blood glucose monitoring is to be within a target range, not to get a specific number each time.

242. When analyzing your blood glucose readings, it helps to recognize the difference between an isolated reading and a pattern of readings; one isolated reading is far less noteworthy than a pattern.

243. Be sure to consider the variety of factors that can influence your blood glucose levels when trying to determine the causes of a single reading. These include food, medicines, exercise, stress, and infection, and normal hormonal variation in the body.

244. If you must use a limited number of test strips because of their cost, try to use them in a way that lets you see a pattern in your blood glucose readings.

245. It may be helpful to record your blood glucose readings in a logbook along with comments about what might have influenced it.

246. If you are confused about what your blood glucose readings mean or about what could have caused a reading, go over them with a diabetes educator or with your health-care provider.

247. Since the brain's ability to detect hypoglycemia (low blood glucose) is reduced with each episode of it, don't assume you'll know if it happens again based on how you felt the last time it happened.

248. All types of insulin and many oral medicines for diabetes can cause hypoglycemia. If you're not sure whether this risk applies to a medicine you take, find out from your health-care provider or another reliable source.

249. If you are aiming for tight diabetes control with insulin or another medicine that creates the risk of hypoglycemia, accept that an occasional low will occur and have a plan for when it does. This is usually better than keeping blood glucose higher than recommended to avoid hypoglycemia.

250. Following any episode of severe hypoglycemia (one that results in seizure, loss of consciousness, or unresponsiveness), greater attention to blood glucose control and possibly a change in therapy are in order.

251. To avoid hypoglycemia, try to have no more than 10% of your blood glucose readings before meals or at bedtime below 70 mg/dl (80 mg/dl for very young children).

252. For people with Type 2 diabetes, multiple episodes of hypoglycemia are usually a sign that insulin and/or oral medicines should be reduced.

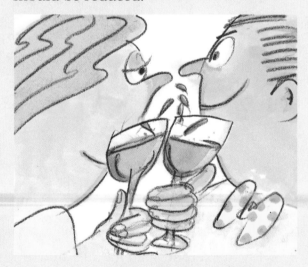

253. Beware of the effect of alcohol; it may cause blood glucose to drop several hours after it is consumed, even as it raises blood glucose at first if the drink is carbohydrate-rich. Adjust medicine and/or carbohydrate intake based on this effect.

254. Work with your doctor to determine an ideal premeal blood glucose level, and aim for this level when making mealtime dosing decisions for insulin or other medicines. A target below 100 mg/dl may

result in a greater frequency of low blood glucose, especially for those who use insulin.

255. Be careful when taking extra insulin to "cover" for high blood glucose. Take into account any insulin that is still active from your previous dose, as well as any variability in the effect of the "correction" insulin based on the time of day or other factors.

256. Since carbohydrate has the most profound effect on blood glucose levels, monitor your carbohydrate intake and use this information to calculate your insulin and/or oral medicine doses.

257. Take low blood glucose seriously; any single low reading presents more of a threat to your well-being than a single high reading.

H-B-A-1-C
(WHAT IT IS AND WHY IT MATTERS)

by Mark Nakamoto

You've pulled out your logbook and are taking off your jacket to bare your upper arm for the blood pressure cuff, when the nurse walks in and asks you to hold out a finger. "Does it matter that I had breakfast this morning?" you ask, trying to remember if you were supposed to fast before coming in, as she pricks your finger and collects a blood sample. "No, it doesn't," she says. "There; all done. The doctor will be in shortly to discuss your result." And, indeed, several minutes later, your doctor walks in and says with a smile, "Looks like things are coming together for you. You're at 6.8%."

For some people, the doctor's words would be enough for them to realize that the fingerstick in the imaginary scenario above was for a glycosylated hemoglobin (HbA_{1c}) test. The HbA_{1c} test gives an indication of your blood glucose control over the previous 2–3 months and is an important part of your diabetes-care regimen. This article discusses what the test is, why it's important, and how it's used to help better blood glucose control.

The ABC's

Figuring out how the HbA_{1c} test can help with your blood glucose control starts with understanding a bit about the test and what it measures.
Hemoglobin. Hemoglobin is a molecule found in great quantities in each of the body's red blood cells. As red blood cells travel through the circulatory system, the hemoglobin molecules join with oxygen from the lungs for delivery to the peripheral tissues, where they exchange it for some of the carbon dioxide destined for release to the lungs. The hemoglobin molecule is made up of two pairs of protein chains (two alpha chains and two beta chains) and four *heme* groups (iron-containing structures that act as the site of oxygen attachment and give red blood cells their color). Adults usually have a variety of types of hemoglobin, each with slightly different properties. The type of particular interest to people with diabetes is called HbA_{1c}.

Besides carrying oxygen, hemoglobin molecules were discovered to have a secondary property that could be used to monitor blood glucose levels, namely the ability to join with glucose. Unlike cells that have insulin-controlled gating mechanisms to regulate how much glucose enters

cells (such as muscle and liver cells), red blood cells allow glucose from the blood to freely enter and leave. The concentration of glucose inside a red blood cell is therefore the same as its concentration in the blood. The level of glucose in the blood affects how much glucose is available to bind to hemoglobin.

Once bound to hemoglobin, the sugar molecules mostly remain attached for the life of the red blood cell, which averages about 120 days. Your blood cells don't all die at the same time: New blood cells are constantly being created, and younger cells outnumber older cells. Because the red blood cells in a blood sample used for an HbA_{1c} test are a mixture of cells of different ages, the test gives a "weighted" average of recent blood glucose levels. This average is heavily influenced by more recent blood glucose levels because of the greater number of younger red blood cells; blood glucose levels from the past three months determine most of an HbA_{1c} test's result. In fact, blood glucose levels in the 30 days before the test determine roughly half of the HbA_{1c} test's result. Therefore, the HbA_{1c} test is often said to give an indication of blood glucose levels for the previous 2–3 months.

HbA_{1c} test results are given as a percentage that indicates the percentage of your HbA_{1c} molecules that are linked to glucose molecules. A chart like the one on page 133 can help you to figure out what your average blood glucose levels were that caused your HbA_{1c} result.
What's in a name? If you look through both the scientific literature and the information produced specifically for people who have diabetes, you will probably see a variety of terms to describe the HbA_{1c} test, such as glycosylated hemoglobin, glycated hemoglobin, and glycohemoglobin, and abbreviations such as GHb and A1C. For the purposes of the average person with diabetes and his health-care team, these terms are all basically referring to the same thing.

When a molecule is said to be glycosylated, it means it has been linked to a *glycosyl* group (a derivative of a glucose molecule). Glycosylation can either be aided by helper molecules called enzymes or occur chemically without the enzymes. The nonenzymatic form of glycosylation is called glycation. When being precise in their writings for scientific journals, biochemists tend to call the form of hemoglobin examined in the HbA_{1c} test a "glycated hemoglobin," because the process by which glucose links itself to hemoglobin is nonenzymatic. "Glyco-" is a prefix that usually refers to a sugar, so a glycohemoglobin is a hemoglobin with some sort of sugar attached. GHb is used as a catch-all shorthand for glycosylated and glycated hemoglobin and glycohemoglobin.

To reduce the confusion that all these different-sounding terms could cause, in August 2001, the American Association of Clinical Endocrinologists and the American College of Endocrinology recommended that health-care providers use the shorthand term "A1C" when speaking with people with diabetes, a change that the American Diabetes Association (ADA), the National Glycohemoglobin Standardization Program (NGSP), and the National Diabetes Education Program (NDEP) came to endorse. Researchers were encouraged to continue to use the term "glycated hemoglobin" in scientific papers aimed at their peers.

Setting a standard

In the past, a physician's previous personal experience with a certain illness or the opinion solicited from a specialist at the local medical center used to be considered the basis for good medical care. Over the years, however, physicians came to desire more research-based, statistical data to support long-standing medical practices and to ensure that people were given the best medical care possible. The tail end of the 20th century saw the increasing use of controlled clinical trials to compare the effectiveness and safety of various drugs and therapies. To test theories on whether high blood glucose levels were responsible for some of the complications of diabetes and if complications could be reduced or reversed by lowering blood glucose levels, a number of trials involving volunteers with diabetes were conducted.

Type 1 diabetes. The longest and largest well-conducted study of controlling high blood glucose in people with Type 1 diabetes was the Diabetes Control and Complications Trial (DCCT). Between 1983 and 1993, the DCCT enrolled and studied over 1400 people with Type 1 diabetes, assigning them to receive either a conventional therapy (one or two daily injections of insulin and either urine testing for glucose several times per day or blood glucose monitoring once per day) or a more intensive regimen intended to achieve near-normal levels of blood glucose. The intensive regimen consisted of monitoring blood glucose levels

BLOOD GLUCOSE CORRELATIONS

If your lab is using methods certified by the National Glycohemoglobin Standardization Program, you can convert your glycosylated hemoglobin (HbA_{1c}) result into your average plasma glucose levels over the past 2–3 months. (Laboratories and most blood glucose meters give plasma glucose levels; however, we included whole blood glucose values here as well for people with older meters.)

HbA_{1c} (%)	PLASMA GLUCOSE LEVEL (milligrams/deciliter)	WHOLE BLOOD GLUCOSE LEVEL (milligrams/deciliter)
6	135	121
7	170	152
8	205	183
9	240	214
10	275	246
11	310	277
12	345	308

four times daily and either the use of an insulin pump or three or four daily injections of insulin. The HbA_{1c} test was used to assess the level of blood glucose control achieved by each group and to compare the groups. After an average of 6.5 years of follow-up, people in the intensive-treatment group attained an average HbA_{1c} of 7.3%, while the average HbA_{1c} in the conventional-therapy group was 9.1%.

These differences in HbA_{1c} results translated into significant differences in risks for diabetes complications such as nephropathy (kidney disease), retinopathy (eye disease), and neuropathy (damage to and malfunctioning of nerves, especially those of the legs and feet). When the kidneys are functioning normally, they do not allow proteins from the blood to be filtered out in the urine. Kidneys damaged by diseases such as diabetic nephropathy can allow a blood protein called albumin to pass into the urine. Intensive control of blood glucose reduced the development of *macroalbuminuria* (large amounts of albumin in the urine) by 56%. Every 10% decrease in HbA_{1c} (say, from 11% to 9.9%) led to a 25% decrease in risk for developing signs of nephropathy.

Those participants in the intensive-therapy group who entered the study with no signs of retinopathy and very low to no protein in the urine had a 76% reduction in progression to retinopathy compared with those in the conventional treatment group. Even people with mild to moderate retinopathy and *microalbuminuria* (very small quantities of albumin in the urine) benefited from intensive therapy, seeing a 54% reduction in retinopathy progression. Even if you haven't met your HbA_{1c} goal yet, you might be pleased to know that just about any decrease in blood glucose levels can help. The study found that every decrease of 10% of one's HbA_{1c} was linked to a 39% decrease in risk of retinopathy.

Diabetic neuropathy was reduced by 60% in the intensive-treatment group compared with the conventional treatment group.

Type 2 diabetes. The DCCT's findings about the link between HbA_{1c} levels and risks for complications in people with Type 1 diabetes were complemented by similar findings in another large study—this one of people with Type 2 diabetes—called the United Kingdom Prospective Diabetes Study (UKPDS). The UKPDS studied over 4500 people with Type 2 diabetes, assigning them to receive either a diet-based treatment regimen or a more intensive regimen utilizing a sulfonylurea (a class of diabetes pills that stimulate the pancreas to produce more insulin), metformin, or insulin. Those people treated with diet achieved average HbA_{1c} levels of 7.9%, while those on the more intensive regimen attained an average HbA_{1c} of 7.0%. The study found that there was a direct relationship between HbA_{1c} levels and risks for some diabetes complications; people with lower blood glucose levels had lower risks of *microvascular* (small blood vessel) complications such as retinopathy, neuropathy, and nephropathy.

For every percentage point decrease in HbA_{1c} (say, from 11% to 10%), there was a corresponding 37% decrease in microvascular complications and a 21% decrease in deaths related to diabetes.

"DCCT-comparable." When HbA_{1c} tests were first introduced, different laboratories used different methods to compute HbA_{1c} levels. The multitude of methods lead to different results being reported—a result above, say, 8%, which would indicate high blood glucose levels in a DCCT participant, might represent normal blood glucose levels at some laboratories. People who switched physicians or physicians who changed the laboratory to which they sent their samples had to be careful about interpreting HbA_{1c} results.

To reduce confusion and to make HbA_{1c} results readily comparable with the results of the DCCT, the National Glycohemoglobin Standardization Program (NGSP) was begun to certify labs and their testing methods. Most HbA_{1c} tests done by laboratories in the United States today are performed using methods certified by the NGSP as being standardized to DCCT results.

Current recommendations

The ADA recommends routine checking of HbA_{1c} levels. Exactly how often yours should be checked depends on your degree of blood glucose control and your physician's judgment. Because the HbA_{1c} test is an indicator of blood glucose control over the previous 2–3 months, people who are having trouble meeting their goals or people whose medicine, diet, or exercise regimens have changed may be helped by having HbA_{1c} assessments every three months. Many experts recommend having the HbA_{1c} test at least twice a year for people who are meeting their blood glucose control goals.

In some cases, your physician may decide to order more frequent HbA_{1c} tests. Very large changes in your average blood glucose level can be reflected in your HbA_{1c} in about two weeks, so a person who's been newly diagnosed may have HbA_{1c} tests every few weeks while his initial therapy is adjusted. Pregnant women with diabetes may also have their HbA_{1c} monitored every month or every two months to help them achieve the tight blood glucose control recommended to prevent health problems for the fetus. (See "The Fructosamine Test" on page 135 for more information on a related test sometimes recommended for pregnant women for gauging long-term blood glucose control.)

Your personal target. Currently, the ADA recommends that most people with diabetes work with their health-care team to achieve HbA_{1c} results below 7%. Other groups, including the American College of Endocrinology, the American Association of Clinical Endocrinologists, the European Association for the Study of Diabetes, and the International Diabetes Federation, advocate a target of 6.5%.

Even the carefully monitored people in the DCCT's intensive-treatment group had to work hard to achieve that group's average 7.3% HbA_{1c} result. Because everyone's health situation is unique, you need to work with your health-care team to set a HbA_{1c} goal that will work best for you.

The big picture. Some people—and even their physicians—focus so much on controlling blood glucose levels that they forget that diabetes is more than just abnormal blood glucose. It's important to remember that heart disease is the number one killer of people with diabetes, yet the large studies only found modest relationships between blood glucose levels and cardiovascular disease. High blood pressure and cholesterol abnormalities, two major risk factors for cardiovascular disease, are also problems for people with diabetes.

The UKPDS researchers understood that people with Type 2 diabetes also tend to have or develop high blood pressure, so they used a subset of volunteers from the blood glucose study to study the effects of tighter blood pressure control. Their results along with those from a number of other large studies have shown that tight control of blood pressure reduces the risk of strokes, microvascular complications (such as nephropathy and retinopathy), and diabetes-related deaths in people with diabetes. The ADA currently recommends that people with diabetes aim for a blood pressure below 130/80 mm Hg.

People with Type 2 diabetes also tend to have decreased blood levels of high-density lipoprotein (HDL) cholesterol (the so-called "good" cholesterol) and high blood levels of triglycerides (fat). Current ADA recommendations are to first get low-density lipoprotein (LDL) cholesterol (the "bad" cholesterol) levels below 100 milligrams per deciliter. After that has been achieved, HDL cholesterol levels should be raised above 40 milligrams per deciliter in men (or above 50 milligrams per deciliter in women) and triglyceride levels should be lowered below 150 milligrams per deciliter.

To remind people that controlling cholesterol and blood pressure are also important components of diabetes care, national health groups recently began a concerted effort to get the word out with nationwide campaigns and catchy slogans involving the letters "ABC" (for A1C, blood pressure, and cholesterol). The American College of Cardiology and the ADA collaborated to create a resource for physicians and people with diabetes called "Make the Link! Diabetes, Heart Disease, and Stroke" (www.diabetes.org/MaketheLink), which contains health information and an interactive, visual program explaining the link between diabetes and heart disease. You can also call to order publications such as the Diabetes Outcomes Wallet Card at http://store.diabetes.org. The National Diabetes Education Program (NDEP) started a campaign called "Be Smart About Your Heart: Control the ABCs of Diabetes" (www.ndep. nih.gov/campaigns/BeSmart/BeSmart_overview. htm); the Web site contains basic information as

THE FRUCTOSAMINE TEST

Hemoglobin is not the only blood component that can be *glycated* (linked to a glucose molecule). Blood proteins such as albumin can also be glycated. One test to measure the glycation level of proteins in the blood is called the fructosamine test. Blood proteins have a shorter life span than red blood cells, so the fructosamine test gives an overview of just the 1–2 weeks before the test.

Studies have not yet shown that fructosamine levels can be linked to risks for long-term diabetes complications, so a fructosamine test is not a substitute for an HbA_{1c} test. There is also some controversy over how to calibrate the test properly.

The manufacturer of the first combined home blood glucose and fructosamine meter recalled the product in 2002 because of problems obtaining accurate readings, but laboratories can still perform the test if a physician deems it necessary. Some doctors prescribe this test for pregnant women to aid in tight control or for people who have health conditions that interfere with obtaining accurate HbA_{1c} results.

well as links to statistics and publications. You can also call the NDEP at (800) 860-8747 or visit http://ndep.nih.gov/diabetes/pubs/catalog.htm to order printed copies of brochures such as "Be Smart About Your Heart" (http://ndep.nih.gov/ diabetes/pubs/BeSmart_Article.pdf).

Everyday HbA_{1c}

Although another fingerstick and another blood test may seem redundant to people who monitor their blood glucose levels three or more times per day, self-monitoring of blood glucose and HbA_{1c} tests actually work together and don't just rehash the same information.

Use in therapy. Using a home blood glucose meter allows people with diabetes to fine-tune their diabetes regimen and detect low blood glucose levels (hypoglycemia). Blood glucose monitoring several times a day gives people the opportunity to adjust insulin doses before meals and to know if a snack is needed before or after exercising.

The HbA_{1c} test can corroborate the daily blood glucose measurements you take or they can signal the need for a closer look at your therapy. A logbook full of blood glucose results that are in your target range and an HbA_{1c} of 6.5% can leave you and your physician confident that your treatment is going well. However, if you only check your fasting blood glucose once a day and usually find it around 120 mg/dl yet your HbA_{1c} is above 8%, you can be sure your blood glucose is much higher than 120 mg/dl at other times of the day. You will need to work with your health-care team to figure out when and why your highs are occurring. You may be encouraged to check your blood glucose levels more frequently as you and your team review your meal plan, physical activity levels, and medicines. Even people who monitor several times a day with few to no high results may be surprised to find they have a high HbA_{1c}. In such cases, a little detective work might uncover a simple lab or meter error or the need to make changes in your meal plan, the timing of your blood glucose checks, or your blood glucose meter technique.

Who pays? Every health insurance and managed-care company has its own policies, so you'll need to check your plan for specifics. However, most companies and Medicare cover the costs of HbA_{1c} tests.

Most variations tend to occur in the number of tests covered per year and who runs the tests. Some plans allow quarterly tests while others cover 10 or more per year. Several devices have been approved by the U.S. Food and Drug Administration for giving HbA_{1c} results right in a doctor's office (called *point-of-service testing*) or even at home. (Most home tests involve taking a blood sample at home and mailing the sample to a lab for analysis, although at least one of these products can give results at home in a few minutes.) Although some physicians use the office-based test and like that they can give people feedback about their results at the time of an office visit, some insurers do not cover these tests and may require physicians to send your blood sample to an approved laboratory. In such cases, a physician may have you make another appointment to go over the results or may call you when results come in. Coverage of home HbA_{1c} tests is variable, and although such tests can be as accurate as any other lab test, they should not be used as a substitute for a regular visit with your physician.

Risks. For people with diabetes, especially those who use insulin, the main risk in trying to achieve tight control is low blood glucose levels (hypoglycemia). In the DCCT, people in the intensive-control group had three times the risk of hypoglycemia as people in the conventional-treatment group. Severe hypoglycemia can result in altered consciousness, coma, or convulsions; impaired neuropsychological or intellectual function in children; or strokes or heart attacks in older adults.

For some people, the risk of severe hypoglycemia may necessitate higher target blood glucose levels. For others, hypoglycemia is a risk that can be managed by being more aware of when lows can occur, by learning how to treat them effectively, and by reversing any *hypoglycemia unawareness* (the inability to sense the physical and mental side effects of low blood glucose) by setting temporary, higher blood glucose targets.

HbA_{1c} error. Several medical conditions can affect the HbA_{1c} test result, including anemia, sickle cell disease (and sickle cell trait), and chronic kidney disease. Simple lab error is a possibility, too. Because HbA_{1c} results are based on hemoglobin levels, anything that affects hemoglobin or the life of red blood cells can affect the HbA_{1c} result. Shortened life spans of red blood cells, such as can happen in people with most forms of anemia or when recovering from blood loss, can falsely lower one's HbA_{1c} result because the red blood cells have less time to interact and bind with glucose molecules. Iron-deficiency anemia and some forms of genetic abnormalities of hemoglobin may falsely elevate HbA_{1c} results. High levels of vitamins C and E in the blood may interfere with glycation—falsely lowering results.

In some cases, the testing method may contribute to skewed HbA_{1c} results. Alcoholism, the taking of large quantities of aspirin, chronic use of opiate-containing drugs, high levels of blood triglycerides, uremia (high blood levels of nitrogen-containing wastes such as urea—usually caused by kidney failure), high blood levels of vitamin C, and high levels of bilirubin (a product of hemoglobin destruction) in the blood can falsely elevate HbA_{1c} results, depending on a laboratory's testing method. If your HbA_{1c} test results don't seem to match your blood glucose monitoring results, talk to your doctor about why this might be the case.

HbA_{1c} and you

The HbA_{1c} test is another tool that you and your health-care team can use to tighten your blood glucose control and reduce your risk for diabetic complications. Work with your team to determine the best, lowest HbA_{1c} goal for you. □

BLOOD GLUCOSE MONITORING
What Do the Numbers Tell You?

by Virginia Peragallo-Dittko, A.P.R.N., M.A., B.C.-A.D.M., C.D.E.

"I must admit that I stopped checking my blood sugar," Dave said. "I used to stick myself and write the numbers in a book, but I had no idea what they meant. I'd eat the same thing and get different numbers. Finally, I just gave up."

Sound familiar? Many people dutifully check their blood glucose levels but have no idea what the numbers mean. Part of the problem is that blood glucose levels constantly fluctuate and are influenced by many factors. The other part of the problem is that no two people are alike. A blood glucose reading of 158 mg/dl in two different people might have two different explanations.

Most people know that their bodies need glucose to fuel their activities and that certain foods or large quantities of almost any food will raise blood glucose. That's the easy part. But just as cars require a complicated system of fuel pumps, ignition timing, batteries, pistons, and a zillion other things to convert gasoline into motion, our bodies rely on an intricate system to convert glucose into energy.

Back to basics

Insulin is a hormone secreted by the pancreas that helps regulate the way the body uses glucose. Its main job is to allow glucose in the blood to enter cells of the body where it can be used for energy. In people who don't have diabetes, the pancreas changes how much insulin it releases depending on blood glucose levels. Eating a chocolate bar? The pancreas releases more insulin. Sleeping? The pancreas releases less insulin until the wee hours of the morning when the hormones secreted in the early morning naturally increase insulin resistance, so the pancreas needs to release a little more.

Insulin also controls how much glucose is produced and released from the liver. Glucose is stored in the liver in a form called glycogen. When blood glucose levels drop, the liver turns glycogen into glucose and sends glucose to the bloodstream. When there is enough glucose in the bloodstream, the pancreas signals the liver to stop sending glucose into the bloodstream. This system of signals and feedback loops keeps the delicate coordination of insulin release and blood glucose in balance.

In Type 1 diabetes, the coordination of insulin release and blood glucose is completely out of balance because the pancreas stops making insulin. Injected insulin is used to replace what is missing and supply insulin's signals again.

With Type 2 diabetes, the pancreas makes insulin but not enough to keep up with the body's demand. Studies have shown that Type 2 diabetes is progressive, meaning that the beta cells of the pancreas make less insulin over time. In addition, the cells of the body are unable to take glucose out of the bloodstream when needed because they resist the insulin that you need to allow glucose to enter cells. On top of that, the liver continues to send a lot of glucose into the bloodstream even when it isn't needed because the signals telling the liver to shut off aren't working. So there are three problems facing those with Type 2 diabetes: not enough insulin, insulin resistance, and a liver that won't stop releasing glucose into the bloodstream.

What's normal?

Before any blood glucose reading has meaning, you need to know what you're aiming for. Target goals for blood glucose set by the American Diabetes Association (ADA) are 90–130 mg/dl before a meal and less than 180 mg/dl two hours after the start of a meal. The American Association of Clinical Endocrinologists (AACE) has defined stricter blood glucose target goals of less than 110 mg/dl before a meal and less than 140 mg/dl two hours after the start of a meal. Ask your health-care provider whether you should use the ADA or the AACE targets as your goal. Both guidelines are based on evidence showing the blood glucose readings that are needed to prevent the complications of diabetes.

The words you use to describe blood glucose monitoring may affect how you feel about it. For example, it might help to call it a blood glucose check, not a test, because the word "test" implies pass or fail. It might also help to refer to blood glucose readings as either in or out of target range rather than "good" or "bad."

It's also good to remember that your blood glucose goal is to aim for a target *range*, not an exact number each time. Before-meal blood glucose readings of 101 mg/dl, 114 mg/dl, 126 mg/dl, and 97 mg/dl may look like they are up and down, but they're all within the target range defined by the ADA.

BLOOD GLUCOSE METER AVERAGES: DON'T BE FOOLED

Most blood glucose meters store a certain number of readings in their memory, along with the date and time of each reading. Most also report either a 14-day or 30-day average of readings. An average is calculated by adding up all the numbers in a set and dividing the sum by the number of numbers in the set. For example, if you checked your blood glucose level 25 times in 14 days, your meter would tally all of your readings and divide the sum by 25 to get your 14-day average.

Blood glucose averages can be useful, but they can also be misleading. Compare the before-dinner blood glucose readings of two different people over four days:

Rhoda's blood glucose before dinner:
    Monday 158 mg/dl
    Tuesday 178 mg/dl
    Wednesday 174 mg/dl
    Thursday 161 mg/dl

Raul's blood glucose before dinner:
    Monday 82 mg/dl
    Tuesday 302 mg/dl
    Wednesday 200 mg/dl
    Thursday 87 mg/dl

Both Rhoda's and Raul's four-day average is 168 mg/dl, but there is a big difference in the patterns. Raul's average gives no indication of the wide fluctuations in his blood glucose readings. By relying on the average, he'd miss the opportunity to correct the highs and lows.

Luckily Raul keeps a logbook, which reveals that he exercises before dinner on Monday and Thursday, so he'll probably require a change in his medicine dose on exercise days. On Tuesday he had a very stressful business meeting over lunch in a restaurant. That explains the reading of 302 mg/dl.

Many people don't check their blood glucose level if they suspect that the result will be high, so the average doesn't tell them anything meaningful. Others only check before meals, then say, "How could my HbA_{1c} be 8.8% when my average blood glucose is 148 mg/dl?" Your HbA_{1c} (an indication of your average blood glucose over the previous 2–3 months) could be elevated because your after-meal readings are out of range. The average only reflects the blood glucose checks you did before meals.

An average can be useful if it helps to give you the big picture. A change in your average from 130 mg/dl in the summer to 170 mg/dl in the winter might reflect a decrease in exercise during the winter months. An average that slowly climbs or falls over time can alert you to look for changes in your blood glucose patterns.

When you begin to analyze your blood glucose readings, it is helpful to recognize the difference between an isolated reading and a pattern of readings. Say you check your blood glucose before lunch one day, and you get a reading of 246 mg/dl. You know that the reading is out of range, but so what? To make sense of that reading, you would need to know your pattern of blood glucose readings before lunch. If you checked three days in a row before lunch and recorded readings of 118 mg/dl, 110 mg/dl, and 113 mg/dl, you'd see that the reading of 246 mg/dl doesn't fit your usual pattern before lunch and therefore isn't noteworthy.

Knowing your pattern gives you a background for comparison. Isolated readings can still be helpful, especially when your blood glucose is low. But an isolated reading is meaningless without knowing the story behind it. And the story includes the factors that affect blood glucose level, including food, medicines, exercise, stress, and infection.

How often should I check?

Most people check their blood glucose level once a day, first thing in the morning. It's a common time to check because it's easy: You get up, check your blood glucose, take your medicines, and eat breakfast. Then you're done with your diabetes for the day and don't have to think about it anymore.

The problem with this routine is that it only tells you about your blood glucose pattern before breakfast. You don't learn what is happening after meals or later in the day. To find meaningful patterns at other times of the day, you have to check at other times of day.

One option for finding more patterns is to check your blood glucose four times per day three days per week. Checking before breakfast, two hours after breakfast, before dinner, and two hours after dinner three times per week for a few weeks will help you identify your patterns throughout the day.

Try to make blood glucose monitoring a useful tool by checking your blood glucose at times that serve you. Blood glucose monitoring should help you make a decision, give you feedback about a decision, and help you learn about your usual patterns.

You also need to consider the cost of the test strips. For those who do not take insulin, Medicare pays for one strip per day, so you want to put those strips to good use. Instead of just checking before breakfast every morning, you might decide to check before and after breakfast on Monday, before and after lunch on Wednesday, and before and after dinner on Saturday. If you take insulin, Medicare and most health insurance plans will pay for the number of strips written by your health-care provider on the prescription.

There are many ways to keep track of your blood glucose readings so that you can evaluate the patterns. You can use a logbook in which you write down the readings along with any comments (such as what you had for lunch or how stressed you were feeling). Depending on what meter you use, you may be able to use computer software that displays the contents of your meter memory in graphic forms. Or you could use a meter with an electronic logbook, such as the OneTouch UltraSmart, Accu-Chek Complete, or FreeStyle Tracker.

Here are some common patterns and probable explanations that will help you make sense of your numbers:

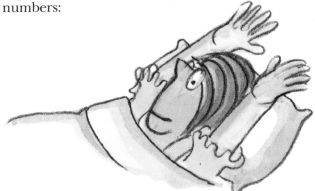

My blood glucose is always higher in the morning when I get up and is lower during the day.

■ Your liver might be sending a lot of glucose into the bloodstream because the signals telling it to shut off aren't working. The drug metformin may be prescribed, because its main action is to signal the liver to shut off.

■ Your dinner or bedtime snack choices might be raising your blood glucose the next morning. Try changing your food choices and portions to learn more about their effect on your blood glucose levels.

■ Your body may be unable to handle the effect of the hormones secreted at dawn that work against insulin. This early-morning release of hormones is called the dawn phenomenon. High blood glucose that results from it can be managed with oral medicines or insulin.

■ Your insulin or oral medicine dose may need to be adjusted.

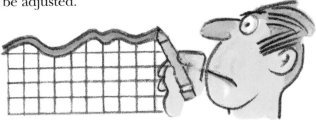

My blood glucose is high all day.

■ If you have Type 2 diabetes, your cells may be resisting your insulin. Exercise, weight loss, and certain medicines will help to make your body more sensitive to insulin and lower your blood glucose.

■ If you have Type 2 diabetes, your pancreas may not be making enough insulin to meet your needs, and you may require oral medicines or insulin.

■ If you have Type 1 diabetes, you may need an increase in your basal insulin doses. Basal insulin is the amount of insulin your body needs in the background all day long. Insulin glargine (brand name Lantus) or NPH can provide basal insulin. An insulin pump is also programmed to deliver basal insulin.

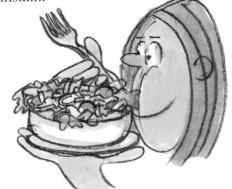

My blood glucose is within range before I eat but high two hours later.

■ It is helpful to understand how the secretion of insulin changes in Type 2 diabetes. The pancreas secretes insulin in response to a meal in two phases. In the first 10 minutes after glucose enters the bloodstream, there is an early burst of insulin release called *first-phase* insulin secretion. This is followed by the *second-phase* insulin secretion, a sustained release of insulin that lasts for several hours. One of the early changes in Type 2 diabetes is the loss of first-phase insulin secretion following a meal. This means that not enough insulin enters the bloodstream as quickly as it is needed, resulting in high blood glucose after meals.

Certain medicines taken at mealtimes can help. Nateglinide (Starlix) and repaglinide (Prandin) stimulate the pancreas to release more insulin when blood glucose levels are higher, while acarbose (Precose) and miglitol (Glyset) slow the rate at which certain carbohydrates are absorbed from the small intestine.

The rapid-acting insulin analogs lispro (Humalog) and aspart (NovoLog) also work effectively to lower blood glucose after meals. Regular insulin peaks too slowly to completely lower blood glucose following meals although some people find Regular insulin is the best choice for them.

■ What you eat makes a difference, too. Your blood glucose reading taken two hours after you start to eat should be about 30 mg/dl higher than before you eat. After-meal readings can tell you about the impact of food on your blood glucose levels. If your blood glucose reading was 111 mg/dl before eating two cups of pasta and 322 mg/dl two hours later, you've learned that two cups of pasta is too much for you. However, a reading of 157 mg/dl two hours after eating *one* cup of pasta tells you how much pasta you can eat to keep your after-meal readings within the target range.

Many people are shocked by how high their readings are after meals. Ralph was convinced that his large restaurant meals every night didn't really raise his blood glucose levels because his fasting readings weren't elevated. But when he actually checked two hours after dinner and got readings over 400 mg/dl, he decided to make some changes.

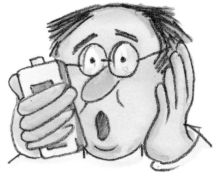

My blood glucose is usually no higher than 130 mg/dl, but for the past two days every reading is over 200 mg/dl.

■ A sudden change in your blood glucose pattern is usually due to infection. The stress hormones released when you are sick tend to raise blood glucose levels. Infection is a physical stress, and when stress occurs, the body reacts by secreting more epinephrine, cortisol, and glucagon. These hormones cause extra glucose to be released from the liver to give the body added energy to cope. Most times, your blood glucose levels will rise even before you get symptoms of an infection.

Two heads are better than one

Dave stopped checking his blood glucose levels because the numbers didn't mean anything, but some people stop checking simply because the numbers upset them. It's especially hard when you've been following all the rules, eating right, exercising, and taking your medicines and the numbers are still high.

Learning what the numbers mean and evaluating the patterns are tools that can help you cope. It's also helpful to remember that there are blood glucose readings that defy explanation. Sometimes we just don't know why a reading is out of range. That's why it is wise to team up with a diabetes educator or your health-care provider who can offer guidance and a fresh perspective. What do the numbers tell you? The answer lies in knowing your targets, patterns, and who to call when you have a question. □

THE MYTH OF BRITTLE DIABETES

by Gary Scheiner, M.S., C.D.E.

The Loch Ness Monster. The Abominable Snowman. The World Series Champion Chicago Cubs. All myths of epic proportions. Well, here's another: brittle diabetes. What is brittle diabetes? To be honest, it's a term health-care providers made up when there were no easy answers to why blood sugar levels were sometimes unexpectedly high or low. If you were ever "diagnosed" as brittle, it initially may have been a relief to have an explanation for those yo-yo blood sugar levels—kind of like finding something in your shoe that was making your foot sore. How nice it must have been to fall back on that "brittle diabetes" answer for everything:

"Yes, honey, my blood sugar is high now, probably because my diabetes is so brittle. What's that? Why was it low at the same time yesterday? Same thing: I'm just brittle."

While brittle diabetes can be a convenient excuse for anything that doesn't make perfect sense, assuming that you are "just brittle" can keep you from looking for the *real* causes of—and solutions to—your diabetes control problems. Diabetes management is far from an exact science, but there usually is a logical explanation for the variations in your blood sugar readings. If you look hard enough, you can almost always find them, and finding those explanations is the first and most important step toward a solution.

The value of records

A complete set of data can reveal the answers to many of life's problems. That's how a smart businessperson determines the best places to invest money. It's where detectives turn for clues to solving a crime. It's even how weather forecasters can predict (with amazing 50% accuracy) whether or not it will rain tomorrow.

For a person with diabetes, detailed written records can reveal blood glucose patterns and, more important, what is contributing to those patterns. A good set of records should include blood glucose values, insulin and/or oral medicine doses, the amount of carbohydrate eaten at meals and snacks (with notes about high-fat or extra-large meals), and physical activities, including both formal exercise and daily activities such as shopping, yard work, and extended walking. By organizing

the records so that you can view several days on a page, it is easier to look for trends and patterns.

Sometimes, written records reveal not-so-obvious answers to common blood glucose control problems. For example, one woman's records showed that her blood glucose level would rise the week before her menstrual period, then drop immediately after her period started. A devotee of horror movies found that he would have very high readings following scare flicks, and that they would be even higher if he ate buttery popcorn during the movie. A young boy found he experienced high blood sugar while participating in competitive sports, followed by hypoglycemia the next morning. All of these people had been told by their physicians that their diabetes was—you guessed it—brittle.

Sources of variability

So, you say you want some answers. If there is no such thing as brittle diabetes, what is causing your blood sugar to be high one day and low the next or to vary from meal to meal? The fact is, there is an almost unlimited number of possibilities, ranging from chemical to physical to metaphysical. Below are some of the more common causes of inconsistent blood sugar levels and steps you can take to iron out some of the wrinkles in your diabetes control.

Insulin

Each type of insulin has a different activity profile. That is to say, the onset of action (the time it takes to start working), duration of action, and peak action (when it is working the hardest) are different for each type. Ideally, the activity profiles of the insulins you use are matched to your meal and activity patterns so that your blood glucose level stays fairly stable. However, there are variables besides activity profile that can affect how well your insulin regimen works. Here are just a few.

Injection site. The onset, duration, and peak action times of NPH and Regular insulin vary depending on where the injection is given. These types of insulin are absorbed most rapidly from the abdomen and slowest from the buttocks. Insulin analogs, including lispro (brand name Humalog), aspart (NovoLog), glulisine (Apidra), detemir

(Levemir), and glargine (Lantus), are absorbed at the same rate regardless of injection site.

If you use NPH or Regular and you want to rotate your injection site, use the same body part for each time of day for greater overall consistency. For example, inject in your abdomen in the morning, thigh in the evening, and buttocks at bedtime. You also need to make sure to rotate your injections within each site, giving each shot at least a finger width away from the previous shot. Repeated injections in the same spot can create a hard lump of fat under the skin, which can slow insulin absorption.

Insulin type. Make sure you are taking the proper type of insulin at each injection. Sounds obvious, but most insulin bottles look alike, and mix-ups can cause serious problems. The appearance of the insulin may help you distinguish quickly between bottles: NPH insulin has a cloudy look, while all others are clear. However, don't hesitate to label vials with tape and a big marker. People with visual impairment may benefit from the Accu-Chek Voicemate meter (made by Roche Diagnostics), which reads aloud the type of insulin you have selected.

Incorrect dose. Imprecise or inconsistent insulin doses will give inconsistent blood glucose control. If you have difficulty reading the syringe, use a magnifier such as the BD Magni-Guide (made by Becton, Dickinson) or consider switching to an insulin pen, which allows you to dial up to the correct dose. Be sure to eliminate any large air bubbles from the syringe by tapping the syringe and redrawing the dose, if necessary. Air in the syringe reduces the amount of insulin you receive.

Insulin strength. In some cases, elevated blood sugar levels can be attributed to insulin that has gone bad or lost its potency. Check the expiration date on your insulin before using it, and never use an open vial for more than a month. (Discard whatever insulin remains at the end of the month and start a new vial.) Store the vial you are using currently at room temperature, and store extra insulin in the refrigerator. Do not expose your insulin to extreme heat or cold or direct sunlight.

Mixing improperly. If you mix two insulins in the same syringe, but you draw them up in the wrong order, the fast-acting insulin can become contaminated, and its onset may be delayed. Always draw the clear (fast-acting) insulin into the syringe before the cloudy (longer-acting) insulin. (Note, though, that the long-acting insulin analog glargine, which is also clear, should never be mixed with another insulin.)

In addition, if a cloudy insulin is not mixed evenly before you draw it up, you may not get the insulin at full strength. Roll the longer-acting insulin bottle or pen between your hands 5–10 times to ensure an even mixture. Never use insulin that appears "clumped" or has crystals in it.

Pump problems. Insulin in a pump and tubing can lose its potency over time; its effectiveness deteriorates the longer you use your infusion set. Change your infusion set every 2–3 days, and change the insulin cartridge at least once a week. Also, check for kinks in the tubing and for leaks between the pump and tubing.

Food

Matching what you eat to how much insulin is available (whether injected or secreted from the pancreas) is the crux of diabetes management. Some people who use insulin can achieve tighter blood sugar control by adjusting their insulin doses based on the amount of carbohydrate they consume at a meal or how active they plan to be. The same concept may help people who take oral medicines at meals, particularly fast-acting repaglinide (brand name Prandin) or nateglinide (Starlix). If interested, ask your diabetes team for help with this. In addition, keeping records of what you eat can help you detect some common food-related causes of unusual or unexpected blood glucose readings and fine-tune your treatment regimen.

Meal-to-medicine timing. Once you've injected your mealtime insulin or taken certain oral medicines, delaying meals or snacks too long can cause low blood sugar. Oral medicines that can cause hypoglycemia on their own are those that stimulate insulin secretion from the pancreas. These include repaglinide, nateglinide, or any of the sulfonylureas (chlorpropamide [Diabinese]; glipizide [Glucotrol, Glucotrol XL]; glyburide [DiaBeta, Glynase PresTab, Micronase]; glimepiride [Amaryl]; tolazamide [Tolinase]; and tolbutamide [Orinase]).

On the other hand, if you inject your insulin too soon before eating or too long after eating, you can experience high blood sugar before your insulin starts working.

To avoid low or high blood glucose around mealtimes, be sure you know how much time to allow between taking the drug or insulin you use and eating.

Varying carbohydrate intake. Gram for gram, all types of carbohydrate (except for fiber) raise blood sugar fairly quickly and about the same amount. So if your carbohydrate intake varies from day to day, your blood glucose levels will, too.

To keep blood sugar levels more stable, count the grams of carbohydrate in your meals and snacks and try to keep the total at each meal or snack consistent from day to day. Read food labels and serving sizes, measure your portions carefully, and get a good nutrition book detailing the nutrients in the types of foods you typically consume. Changes in carbohydrate intake will require changes to your insulin dose or possibly to the amount of exercise you do.

Fat or fiber. Fat and fiber can slow down the digestion of carbohydrate. Even if they contain the same number of carbohydrate grams, meals that contain mostly low-fiber carbohydrate will lead to a quicker rise in blood sugar than those that are higher in fat or fiber. High-fat meals may lead to a blood sugar rise several hours later.

To prevent this late blood glucose rise, try exercising a few hours after a high-fat meal, increasing the basal rate on your pump, or taking some extra Regular or NPH insulin (but not rapid-acting insulin) with the meal. Be sure, though, to get your doctor's OK before making these kinds of adjustments on your own.

Gastropathy. Another factor that can affect digestion rate is gastropathy, a form of diabetic neuropathy (nerve disease) in which the stomach empties much more slowly than usual. As a result, your blood sugar level might rise several hours after eating rather than right after the meal, or you may have low blood glucose after eating if your insulin or medicine begins working before the food is absorbed.

If you experience this sort of blood glucose pattern or any other symptoms of gastropathy, including nausea, diarrhea, constipation, bloating, vomiting, or stomach cramps, see your doctor. Gastropathy can be treated with drugs that help promote digestion, but it is also helpful to eat frequent, small meals rather than a few large meals each day, and to minimize the fat and fiber content of your meals. Insulin or diabetes pills may need to be taken after meals rather than before.

Extra-large meals. Meals eaten at restaurants or at friends' or family members' houses and take-out foods tend to contain more fat and carbohydrate than meals you prepare at home. Portions are usually larger, too.

If you know that you will be eating more than usual, you may need to increase your insulin or fast-acting oral medicine dose prior to eating. If you don't already know how to do this, ask your health-care provider for help.

Overtreatment of low blood sugar. Every gram of carbohydrate you ingest is converted to glucose and enters your bloodstream at some point. Overtreating hypoglycemia is a common mistake that can result in very high readings within a few hours of the low.

When you have symptoms of low blood sugar, use your meter to con-firm them, then limit yourself to consuming 15–30 grams of carbohydrate to treat the low. Be patient. Give your blood sugar level 15–30 minutes to come up before monitoring again. Keep yourself occupied and out of the kitchen while waiting. Using preportioned glucose tablets or gel instead of food or juice may help you control the amount of carbohydrate you consume to treat hypoglycemia.

Physical activity

Physical activity has all sorts of benefits, but sometimes its effects on blood glucose can be baffling. Glucose is almost always burned as fuel during exercise, and exercise also makes insulin work more efficiently. For these reasons, exercise can lead to low blood sugar, and some people need to consume extra carbohydrate prior to activity or cut back on insulin on days they exercise. Your diabetes-care team can help you adjust your treatment regimen to your regular exercise habits. However, there are several problematic situations to watch out for.

Delayed-onset hypoglycemia. Long, intense bouts of exercise can continue to lower blood sugar for up to 24 hours after the workout, as the body replenishes depleted glucose stores in the muscles with glucose from the blood.

Check your blood sugar more frequently following intense or extended exercise, and reduce your long-acting insulin dose or consume an extra snack after the activity if necessary.

High-intensity exercise. Competitive or high-intensity activities (such as weight lifting, sprinting, or basketball) usually cause the body to produce adrenaline, which makes blood sugar levels rise. If you don't have much insulin in your system before the activity, ketones can develop, especially in people with Type 1 diabetes. Check your blood sugar before and during high-intensity exercise and check for ketones if it goes above 300 mg/dl. You may need *extra* insulin prior to these types of activities.

Exercise time. Because physical activity can have both an immediate and a lasting effect on blood sugar levels, varying the time of day you work out can affect insulin sensitivity and create inconsistencies in blood sugar patterns from day to day. Try to exercise at about the same time of day on a consistent basis.

Unaccounted-for activities. Be aware that even if it doesn't seem like exercise, anything that has you using your muscles in a repetitive manner will tend to bring your blood sugar down. This includes occupational and recreational activities like taking the grandkids to the zoo, planting petunias, raking leaves, or even having sex. In many cases, extra exercise is a good thing, but if you are prone to hypoglycemia, you may need to reduce your long-acting insulin dose to account for prolonged or unusual physical activities, or have a snack to prevent low blood sugar.

Hormones

If food, exercise, and insulin or medicine doses are factors you control, hormones produced by the body are the wild cards, raising or lowering blood glucose levels in response to stress, sickness, or other internal stimuli you may not even be aware of. If you're doing everything right but your blood glucose levels are still erratic, hormones could be to blame.

Stress. Short-term emotional stress (say, getting stuck in traffic or having an argument) can cause an immediate and sharp rise in levels of stress hormones. These hormones increase heart rate, blood pressure, and, yes, blood sugar level. Chronic stress (such as marital difficulties or an overly demanding job) can have the same effect on a long-term basis. To make matters worse, stress can also distract you from taking good care of your body and your diabetes.

Learning some simple meditation techniques or other relaxation methods can help you cope with everyday stresses. If a difficult situation can be anticipated (for example, a funeral or an exam), and you know how your body typically responds to stress, you may be able to prepare for it by increasing your basal insulin or oral medicine dose, or by engaging in more exercise (this may help you relax, too). If you are under long-term stress, you may also want to work with a licensed psychologist to resolve the underlying causes.

Illness or infection. Any type of infection in the body—from a common sinus infection to a major foot ulcer—will increase the production of stress hormones, causing the body to release extra glucose to fight off the infection.

Check your feet daily for cuts or bruises (and report any that don't heal quickly to your doctor), and work with your doctor or diabetes educator to develop a sick-day plan for adjusting your insulin or oral medicine regimen during an illness. Unless otherwise directed, don't skip insulin or oral medicines when you're sick, even if you're eating less than usual. Even people who normally don't use insulin may need it to control blood sugar during an illness.

Growth. During a person's growth years, up to age 20 or so, insulin needs steadily increase due to growth hormone and sex hormone production and changes in body size. Erratic hormone production can also trigger wild swings in blood glucose level.

Communicate with your (or your child's) health-care team frequently during these years; insulin adjustments may need to be made on a monthly basis.

Menstruation. Throughout the menstrual cycle, the body produces hormones (mainly estrogen and progesterone) that can affect blood sugar level. Production of these hormones increases right before menstruation, and many women find that their blood sugar levels are higher than usual during this time, returning to normal or lower-than-normal levels immediately after menstruation begins. For some women, the stress or carbohydrate cravings that often go along with the premenstrual period can also result in blood glucose fluctuations.

If you notice a regular pattern of high blood sugar around the time of your period, talk to your doctor about making a monthly adjustment to your insulin or oral medicine regimen.

Nighttime hormone production. A common cause of high blood glucose in the morning (especially in Type 2 diabetes) is the dawn phenomenon, which is caused by the nighttime production of hormones that cause the liver to increase glucose production. Ordinarily, this effect is balanced with increased insulin secretion, but in people with diabetes who either do not produce insulin or whose bodies do not respond well to it, high blood glucose can result.

Another possible reason for high readings in the morning is a *drop* in blood sugar level in the middle of the night. This can stimulate the production of stress hormones that prompt the release of glucose from the liver and inhibit insulin's action. This rebound effect can cause high blood sugar several hours later—when you wake up in the morning.

To make sure your blood sugar level is not dropping during the night, check your blood sugar at bedtime, at 3 AM, and upon waking in the morning for a few nights. If your blood sugar is dropping at around 3 AM, you may need to take less insulin or medicine at bedtime. If your blood sugar is high during the middle of the night, the dawn phenomenon is in effect, and you may need to increase your bedtime dose.

Monitoring miscues

When your diabetes seems out of whack, monitoring your blood glucose more frequently can help you figure out why. But if your monitoring technique is incorrect, inaccurate results could be adding to the confusion.

Monitoring timing. Blood glucose readings taken soon after meals tend to be elevated; readings taken before meals are typically closer to normal.

Check your blood sugar level before meals whenever possible. If you decide to check after meals as well, expect the readings to be higher than they usually are before eating.

Insufficient blood sample. If not enough blood is applied to the test area of the test strip, the reading may be artificially low. However, most meters display an error message if the blood sample is inadequate, and many test strips now "draw in" the blood, making it easier to get enough.

Obtain the blood sample and apply it to the strip according to the meter manufacturer's instructions. If a strip is not fully dosed and the reading seems low, ignore the result and start over with a new strip and a fresh blood sample.

Improper coding. Most meters require a code number or code chip or strip to be entered with each new vial or box of strips you use. If the meter is not coded to match that specific batch of strips, the readings will not be accurate.

Code your meter with every new box or vial of strips, according to the manufacturer's instructions.

Outdated or spoiled test strips. Using outdated test strips may produce false readings. Test strips may also give false results if they have been exposed to heat or humidity.

Always check the expiration date before starting a new vial or box of strips. Keep your strips sealed in their packaging and away from extreme temperatures. (The proper storage temperature range is listed on the package.) Do not leave test strips in your car!

Disease progression

Even if you've become an expert at self-care, diabetes control can get harder the longer you live with it. As your body changes, it may take continued adjustments to therapy and lifestyle to keep on top of blood sugar control.

Beta cell loss. Over time, Type 2 diabetes becomes progressively more difficult to manage as the pancreas loses the ability to produce sufficient amounts of insulin.

If your blood sugar levels are rising despite your best efforts to control them, speak to your physician about adding, increasing, or changing your dose of diabetes medicines. Some people with Type 2 diabetes start insulin therapy when oral medicines alone are no longer effective.

After the "honeymoon." Soon after diagnosis and the initiation of treatment, many people with Type 1 diabetes resume some insulin production. This results in blood glucose levels that are stable and near normal for a while, with less (or even no) injected insulin. Gradually, though, the pancreas loses this ability to produce insulin, blood sugar levels become higher and more erratic, and more injected insulin is needed to control them. Work closely with your health-care team to adjust insulin doses as your honeymoon period comes to an end.

Weight gain. Many people tend to gain weight with changes in job or lifestyle or just as a natural part of getting older. Even modest weight gain—especially around the middle—can increase insulin resistance and cause blood sugar to rise.

The good news is that losing just a few pounds can reduce insulin resistance, and exercise can greatly improve insulin sensitivity even when it doesn't lead to weight loss. If weight gain is a problem (whatever your age), try to increase your activity level and work with a dietitian to modify your food intake.

Other stuff

You probably think you've heard enough already, but there are a few more sources of blood glucose fluctuations worth mentioning.

Irregular sleep patterns. People with diabetes are especially prone to sleep-disordered breathing, which can reduce sleep quality. Difficulty sleeping and sleep deprivation can alter normal production of hormones that help regulate metabolism and appetite. Lack of sleep may affect your mood, eating habits, and exercise patterns, and it can impair your sensitivity to insulin.

If you have trouble falling or staying asleep, try cutting down on caffeine, avoiding naps during the day, and getting regular exercise early in the day. Try to get out of bed (at a reasonable hour) and go to bed at about the same time daily. If necessary, discuss sleep-inducing medication with your doctor.

Caffeine. A natural stimulant, caffeine (found in coffee, black tea, cola, and chocolate) can cause a temporary rise in blood sugar level. If caffeine appears to affect your blood sugar level, either keep your caffeine intake modest (but consistent), or work on cutting it out of your diet completely.

Alcohol. Alcoholic beverages that contain significant carbohydrate (such as regular beer, sweet wine or wine coolers, or mixed drinks) tend to raise blood sugar in the short term. However, alcohol can lower blood sugar several hours later by suppressing the liver's natural release of stored glucose. Drinking on an empty stomach or after exercise can result in hypoglycemia, which may be more difficult to recognize, since its symptoms can mimic those of tipsiness. Speak with your health-care team for individual guidelines on alcohol use.

If you take a long-acting insulin or a sulfonyl-urea that will be active for several hours after you drink, you may need to reduce the dose or eat a snack to prevent the blood sugar drop that can occur after drinking.

Steroidal medicines. Steroidal anti-inflammatory drugs such as cortisone and prednisone are commonly used to treat asthma, arthritis, emphysema, and muscle and joint disorders. These drugs create insulin resistance and raise blood sugar levels, sometimes dramatically.

When taking a steroidal medicine, monitor your blood sugar frequently. If you see a rise in your blood sugar levels, ask your doctor about temporarily increasing your insulin or diabetes medicine dose.

Travel. Traveling—especially when it involves changing time zones—can disrupt your sleep, meal, exercise, and insulin or medicine patterns. A health-care provider can help you come up with a temporary insulin or medicine schedule based on the direction and duration of your trip. Monitor your blood glucose frequently during the trip and have snacks on hand in case of delayed meals. Allow your body a day to adjust to time zone changes, but try to get back to your usual meal and sleep schedule on the first full day at your destination.

What you can expect

Everyone with diabetes has out-of-range blood sugar readings at times. By keeping detailed records and eliminating the possible causes one by one, you should be able to pinpoint the source of most of your unusual readings, and more important, do something about it, particularly when you see a pattern of highs or lows. Don't hesitate to ask your health-care provider for help in this process, and don't expect perfection. Despite your best efforts, there will still be some blood sugar readings that just don't make any sense. Does it mean you're brittle? Hardly. It just makes you human. □

STRIKE THE SPIKE
Controlling After-Meal Blood Glucose Highs
by Gary Scheiner, M.S., C.D.E.

Today's the big day! After months of working hard to achieve tight blood glucose control and actually succeeding most of the time, you're about to get the result of your latest glycosylated hemoglobin (HbA$_{1c}$) test, the blood test that gives you an indication of your overall blood glucose control over the previous 2–3 months.

"It's just got to be lower than last time," you think as you wait in your doctor's exam room.

"I've been good. Really good. My average on my meter is lower than it's been in years. He's going to be impressed for sure. No lectures about the risks associated with a high A$_{1c}$ this time! I'll be out of here in 10 minutes, easy."

In walks your doctor, with the results of your latest lab work in hand. Thirty minutes later, after a series of careful examinations and a lengthy lecture on the need to get your HbA$_{1c}$ down, you walk out shaking your head.

"I don't get it. How can my A_{1c} still be so high? My mealtime readings are almost always where they should be. It just doesn't make sense. Maybe the lab made a mistake. Maybe my blood is different from everyone else's."

Or maybe you've been the victim of postprandial hyperglycemia.

Post-what?

Postprandial hyperglycemia refers to high blood glucose levels that occur soon after eating meals or snacks. For anyone with diabetes, it is normal for blood glucose to rise somewhat after eating. But if your after-meal rises are dramatic and occur consistently, they can result in higher HbA_{1c} test results than your premeal blood glucose readings would otherwise indicate, and the higher your HbA_{1c}, the higher your risk of serious diabetes complications.

The HbA_{1c} reflects an average of all blood glucose levels at all times of day—before eating, after eating, during the night, etc.—over 2–3 months. (To see how HbA_{1c} levels compare to average blood glucose levels, see the table on this page.) However, research presented in 2004 suggests that a person's HbA_{1c} correlates closely to his average blood glucose levels during the three hours after—not before—eating. So even though after-meal high blood glucose levels are temporary (often resembling a spike when plotted on a graph), frequent between-meal rises can cause your HbA_{1c} to go up.

Research on the effects of postprandial hyperglycemia has shown an increase in the risk of death from heart disease in those with Type 2 diabetes and earlier onset of kidney disease in those with Type 1. But postprandial hyperglycemia can have more immediate effects as well. Just as a big turkey dinner can turn the peppiest person into a slumbering slug, a rapid rise in blood glucose levels after meals has been shown to affect the ability to concentrate, stay alert, and perform athletically and intellectually.

How high is too high?

In most cases, blood glucose levels peak about an hour after finishing a meal or snack. Ideally, the blood glucose level at the peak should be below 180 mg/dl, or less than 80 mg/dl higher than it was before the meal. With children, after-meal peaks can be a bit more liberal. Teenagers should try to keep peaks below 200 mg/dl, school-age children below 225 mg/dl, and preschoolers and toddlers below 250 mg/dl.

In practice, these ideals may not be achieved by

BLOOD GLUCOSE AND HbA$_{1c}$ CORRELATIONS

If your lab is using methods certified by the National Glycohemoglobin Standardization Program, you can convert your glycosylated hemoglobin (HbA_{1c}) result into your average plasma glucose levels over the past 2–3 months. (Laboratories and most blood glucose meters give plasma glucose levels; however, we included whole blood glucose values here as well for people with older meters.)

HbA_{1c} (%)	PLASMA GLUCOSE LEVEL (milligrams/deciliter)	WHOLE BLOOD GLUCOSE LEVEL (milligrams/deciliter)
6	135	121
7	170	152
8	205	183
9	240	214
10	275	246
11	310	277
12	345	308

POSTPRANDIAL BLOOD GLUCOSE GOALS

Ideally, your plasma glucose level about an hour after finishing a meal or snack should be in the range specified here and less than 80 mg/dl higher than it was before the meal or snack. Goals are somewhat more liberal for children than for adults.

AGE	POSTPRANDIAL GOAL
Adult (older than 18)	less than 180 mg/dl
Teen (12–18)	less than 200 mg/dl
School age (6–11)	less than 225 mg/dl
Preschool (up to age 5)	less than 250 mg/dl

many. Research conducted at Yale University on children with Type 1 diabetes indicated that after-meal blood glucose peaks are generally much

HOW BOLUS TIMING AFFECTS AFTER-MEAL SPIKES

When Gary took his mealtime insulin boluses as he sat down to eat, the result was after-meal spikes as shown in Graph 1. When he took boluses 15 minutes before meals and snacks, the spikes flattened out, as shown in Graph 2.

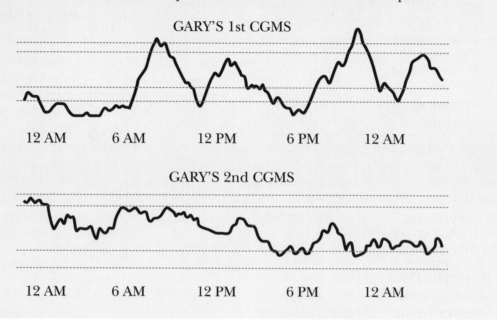

higher than the recommended levels. After breakfast, the average peak blood glucose level was 293 mg/dl; after lunch it was 291 mg/dl; after dinner, 280 mg/dl. In fact, nearly half (46%) of meals were followed by a blood glucose peak of over 300 mg/dl!

Detecting the spikes

A number of good options exist for measuring after-meal blood glucose spikes. Perhaps the most practical is to check your blood glucose level about one hour after completing a meal or snack using a blood glucose meter. When checking your blood glucose level after meals or snacks, you should use a blood sample from a finger rather than an alternate site sample. Because of the way blood circulates in the body, samples from the fingers may show changes in blood glucose level sooner than samples from other sites. Check before and after breakfast, lunch, and dinner several times to determine whether postprandial spikes are a problem at a specific meal. It is more common to see significant spikes after breakfast than at other meals, but it is worth checking after each meal just to make sure.

When interpreting your results, take your pre-meal readings into account since you are interested in not just your after-meal reading but also in how much your blood glucose level increased because of your food intake. For example, a post-meal blood glucose reading of 240 mg/dl following a premeal reading of 210 mg/dl shows just a 30-point rise, whereas a 240 mg/dl following a 110 mg/dl shows a 130-point rise. Having a mildly low blood glucose value (around 65 mg/dl, for example) before a meal can result in a temporary "rebound" to a higher-than-usual level after the meal and may not reflect a true postprandial spike.

A more detailed analysis of after-meal blood glucose can be obtained through use of a continuous glucose monitor (such as the Abbott FreeStyle Navigator, MedTronic Guardian RT, Dexcom STS, and MiniMed Paradign REAL-Time combined monitor/insulin pump). A continuous monitor measures glucose levels in interstitial fluid by way of a tiny sensor inserted just below the skin. Each of the monitors currently on the market displays a glucose reading every five minutes and graphs the previous 9 or 24 hours (depending on the model), from which included software can analyze trends so that you and your

BOLUS TIMING IN RELATION TO MEALS

Both your premeal blood glucose level and the glycemic index of the foods you are planning to eat should be taken into consideration when deciding when to take a mealtime insulin dose. The timing shown here assumes you use lispro (Humalog) or aspart (NovoLog) to "cover" meals. If you use Regular, by itself or in a premixed preparation, back up the timing by 20–30 minutes.

	FOR HIGH-GI FOODS	FOR MODERATE-GI FOODS	FOR LOW-GI FOODS
Blood glucose above target range	30–40 minutes before eating	15–20 minutes before eating	0–5 minutes before eating
Blood glucose within target range	15–20 minutes before eating	0–5 minutes before eating	10–15 minutes after eating
Blood glucose below target range	0–5 minutes before eating	15–20 minutes after eating	30–40 minutes after eating

health-care team can see exactly how much your blood glucose levels are rising after meals and snacks. (See sample printouts on page 148).

Spike control

Reducing after-meal spikes does not always mean taking more insulin or oral medicine at mealtimes. In fact, if your premeal readings are already close to normal, increasing your dose of insulin or oral medicine would result in *low* blood glucose before the next meal. Remember, the idea is to reduce the between-meal peak, but not necessarily lower the blood glucose level before the next meal.

To accomplish this feat, a number of strategies can be used, including the following:

Get moving. Physical activity after eating has a multitude of benefits. If insulin was taken with the meal or snack, the enhanced blood flow to the skin surface caused by physical activity is likely to make the insulin get absorbed quicker so that it can act quicker. This means that the insulin will do a better job of keeping the blood glucose from rising too high right after eating. In addition, muscle activity diverts blood flow away from the intestines, resulting in slower absorption of glucose and other simple sugars into the bloodstream. The sugars that do enter the bloodstream are likely to be "consumed" by the working muscles.

How much activity is required to experience these benefits? Not much. Ten or 15 minutes (or more) of mild activity will get the job done. The key is to avoid sitting for extended periods after eating. Instead of reading, watching TV, or working on the computer, go for a walk, shoot some

hoops, or throw a few darts. In the course of your usual day, try to schedule your active tasks (housework, yardwork, chores, errands, walking pets) for after meals. Make an attempt to schedule your exercise sessions for after meals to take advantage of their blood-glucose-lowering effect. (Individuals with heart disease or other circulatory complications should consult their physician before attempting to exercise after eating.) When you go out for a meal, resist the urge to sit and talk for hours or head straight for a movie. Instead, get up and go out dancing, bowling, or skating.

Think lower GI. The glycemic index of a food refers to the speed with which the food raises blood glucose level. While all carbohydrates (except for fiber) convert into glucose eventually, some do so much faster than others.

Many starchy foods, including many types of bread, cereals, potatoes, and rice have a high glycemic index; they digest easily and convert into glucose quickly. Some starchy foods, including pasta, beans, and peas, have a lower glycemic index because the starches contained in them do not digest as easily. Similarly, some sweet foods have a high glycemic index while others do not. Table sugar (sucrose), for example, has a moderate glycemic index. Foods that contain fiber or fat tend to have lower glycemic index values than foods that do not. Foods in solid form tend to have a lower GI than similar foods in liquid or "sauce" form, and cold foods tend to digest more slowly than hot foods.

A number of books contain extensive information about the glycemic index, including Dr. Jen-

GLYCEMIC INDEX OF COMMON FOODS

The glycemic index of a food is a measure of how quickly it raises blood glucose after eating. The higher the number, the faster it raises blood glucose.

BREAD/CRACKERS	
Bagel	72
Crispbread	81
Croissant	67
French baguette	95
Graham crackers	74
Kaiser roll	73
Pita bread	57
Pumpernickel	51
Rye, dark	76
Saltines	74
Sourdough bread	52
Stoned Wheat Thins	67
White bread	71
Whole wheat bread, high-fiber	68

CAKES/COOKIES/MUFFINS	
Banana bread	47
Blueberry muffin	59
Chocolate cake	38
Corn muffin	102
Cupcake with icing	73
Doughnut	76
Oat bran muffin	60
Oatmeal cookie	55
Pound cake	54
Shortbread cookie	64

CANDY	
Chocolate bar	49
Jelly beans	80
LifeSavers	70
M&M, peanut	33
Skittles	69
Snickers bar	40
Twix bar	43

CEREALS/ BREAKFAST FOODS	
All-Bran	42
Bran Chex	58
Cheerios	74
Cornflakes	83
Cream of Wheat	70
Grape-Nuts	67
Oatmeal	49
Pancakes	67
Pop-Tarts	70
Raisin Bran	73
Rice Krispies	82
Shredded Wheat	69
Special K	66
Total	76
Waffles	76

COMBINATION FOODS	
Chicken nuggets	46
Fish fingers	38
Macaroni and cheese	64
Pizza (cheese)	60
Sausages	28
Stuffing	74
Taco shells	68

DAIRY	
Chocolate milk	34
Ice cream	62
Milk, skim	32
Milk, whole	27
Pudding	43
Yogurt, low-fat	33

FRUITS & JUICES	
Apple	38
Apple juice	41
Banana	55
Cantaloupe	65

nie Brand-Miller's *Glucose Revolution* series, which is readily available in bookstores. For a list of the glycemic index values of many common foods, see the list above. (Higher numbers mean faster conversion to glucose). Substituting foods with a lower glycemic index for foods with a higher glycemic index in your diet will help to reduce your after-meal blood glucose spikes.

Medicate wisely. Whether you take insulin or oral medicines to control your blood glucose levels, the right program can make or break your ability to control those after-meal spikes. In general, insulin and medicines that work slowly over a prolonged period do a poorer job of controlling after-meal spikes than those that work quickly and for a short period.

For insulin to control after-meal spikes, the insulin's "peak" action must match the peak blood glucose level after eating. If you take a morning injection of NPH to "cover" the food you eat in the middle of the day, your postprandial blood glucose is likely to be very high after lunch and after any late-morning or afternoon snacks. That's because the peak for these insulins is less pronounced than that of the rapid-acting insulins and it is spread over several hours. To remedy this, consider taking a dose of a rapid-acting insulin analog such as lispro (brand name Humalog), glulisine (Apidra), or aspart (NovoLog) before each meal and snack, with an intermediate insulin at nighttime only.

Even Regular insulin, with a peak taking place 2–3 hours after injection, rarely works as well at controlling after-meal blood glucose levels as does lispro or aspart, both of which peak about an hour after injection.

Your choice of oral medicine can also affect your after-meal control. Sulfonylureas (glyburide,

Cherries	22	Macaroni	45	**SPORTS BARS/DRINKS**	
Cranberry juice	68	Spaghetti	41	Gatorade	78
Fruit cocktail	55	Spaghetti, whole wheat	37	PowerBar	58
Grapefruit	25	Tortellini	50	**SUGARS & SPREADS**	
Grapefruit juice	48	**RICE**		Glucose tablets	102
Grapes	46	Brown rice	55	High-fructose corn syrup (found in most regular sodas)	62
Orange	44	Instant rice	87	Honey	58
Orange juice	52	Long grain rice	56	Pancake syrup	66
Peach	42	Risotto	69	Strawberry jam	51
Pear	37	**SNACK FOODS**		Table sugar (sucrose)	64
Plum	39	Corn chips	74	**VEGETABLES**	
Raisins	64	Granola bars	61	Carrots, boiled	49
Watermelon	72	Nutri-Grain bars	66	Carrots, raw	16
LEGUMES		Peanuts	15	Corn	46
Baked beans	48	Popcorn	55	French fries	75
Black beans	30	Potato chips	54	Potato, baked	85
Black-eyed peas	42	Pretzels	81	Potato, boiled	88
Chickpeas	33	Rice cakes	77	Potato, instant	83
Lentils	25	**SOUPS**		Potato, mashed	91
Pinto beans	45	Black bean	64	Sweet potato	44
Red kidney beans	19	Lentil	44	Tomato	38
PASTA		Minestrone	39		
Couscous	65	Split pea	60		
Fettuccini	32	Tomato	38		

glipizide, glimepiride), which are generally taken once or twice a day, stimulate the pancreas to secrete a little extra insulin throughout the day, without regard to meal timing. Because these medicines fail to concentrate the insulin secretion at times when it is needed most, after-meal blood glucose levels can run very high. However, the drugs repaglinide and nateglinide, which also stimulate the pancreas to secrete more insulin, are much faster- and shorter-acting. When taken at mealtimes, these drugs stimulate the pancreas to secrete extra insulin for a concentrated period of time, thus producing better after-meal control.

Another class of diabetes medicines called alpha-glucosidase inhibitors improve after-meal control by partially blocking the transport of some carbohydrates across the intestines and into the bloodstream. However, these drugs can sometimes cause temporary gas, bloating, and gastrointestinal upset. You might recall that physical activity after meals will also slow the movement of carbohydrates into the bloodstream, but without the side effects!

Back up your bolus. In the real world, the fourth dimension (time) is of the essence. The timing of your mealtime insulin doses (often called boluses) can significantly affect how high your blood glucose level rises after meals. Boluses given too late to match the digestion of most carbohydrates can result in significantly high blood glucose soon after eating. However, a properly timed bolus can result in excellent after-meal control.

The advice presented here assumes that you are using either lispro or aspart for your mealtime boluses. If you use Regular insulin, either by itself or premixed with NPH, take all the advice given below and back everything up by 20–30 minutes. It is also assumed that you do not have a condition

HOW THE GLYCEMIC INDEX
AFFECTS BLOOD GLUCOSE LEVEL

Carbohydrates that break down quickly, and therefore have a high glycemic index value, cause a fast and high blood-glucose rise after meals. Carbohydrates that break down slowly and have a low glycemic index value release glucose into the bloodstream more gradually.

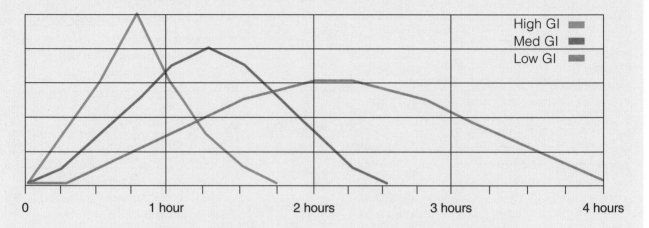

MAKING LOWER GLYCEMIC INDEX
FOOD CHOICES

Substituting foods with a lower glycemic index for those with a higher glycemic index may help keep your after-meal blood glucose levels closer to target range. Here are some ideas for food substitutions.

MEAL	HIGH-GI CHOICES	LOWER-GI CHOICES
Breakfast	Typical cold cereal, bagel, toast, waffle, pancake, corn muffin	High-fiber cereal, oatmeal, yogurt yogurt, whole fruit, milk, bran muffin
Lunch	Sandwich made with white or whole wheat bread, French fries, tortillas, canned pasta	Chili, pumpernickel bread, corn, carrots, salad vegetables
Dinner	Rice, rolls, white potato, canned vegetables	Sweet potato, pasta, beans, fresh or steamed vegetables
Snacks	Pretzels, chips, crackers, cake, doughnut	Popcorn, fruit, chocolate, ice cream, nuts

that impairs your digestion, such as gastroparesis (a nerve disorder that slows emptying of the stomach) or gastritis (nausea and upset stomach). These conditions can significantly delay the rate at which carbohydrates raise blood glucose level, and they usually require that boluses be administered after food has been consumed.

Foods with a high glycemic index (greater than 70), such as cold cereals, bread, potatoes, rice, and snack chips, tend to raise blood glucose the fastest,

with a significant peak occurring in 30–60 minutes. For these types of foods, it is best to bolus 15–20 minutes prior to eating. This will allow the insulin peak to coincide as closely as possible with the blood glucose peak. And that, of course, will produce the best possible after-meal control. Bolusing for high-GI foods as you are eating them will cause an after-meal spike, because the insulin action will lag behind the blood glucose rise by almost half an hour.

Foods with a moderate glycemic index (approximately 45–70) digest a bit slower, resulting in a slightly less pronounced blood glucose peak approximately 60–90 minutes after eating. Examples include ice cream, orange juice, cake, and carrots. It is best to bolus immediately prior to eating foods with a moderate GI. This will allow the insulin peak to closely match carbohydrate digestion and result in the best possible after-meal control.

Foods with a low glycemic index (below 45) tend to cause a slow, gradual blood glucose rise. The blood glucose peak is usually modest and may take several hours to appear. Examples of foods with a low glycemic index include pasta, milk, yogurt, and kidney beans. For these types of foods, a few bolus options are available. One option is to bolus 10–15 minutes after finishing your main course. This usually gives the food enough of a head start before the insulin kicks in. A second option is to split the bolus into two or three parts and to take each about an hour apart, starting at the mealtime. A third option is to take Regular insulin with the meal, rather than a rapid-acting insulin analog. One other option, available to users of insulin pumps, is to extend the bolus delivery over an hour or two.

Another variable to consider when determining the timing of your mealtime bolus is your premeal blood glucose level. To avoid an after-meal drop or spike in your blood glucose level, it is best to give the bolus earlier when your blood glucose is elevated and later when it is below your target. The chart on page 149 combines the glycemic index and premeal blood glucose level to determine optimal bolus timing.

Does earlier bolusing make a difference? Check out the results of my own CGMS reports on page 148. The first was taken six months ago, when I was bolusing just as I would sit down to eat. Notice the after-meal spikes. The second was taken more recently, with boluses taken 15 minutes before each of my meals and snacks. Notice the lack of after-meal peaks!

Mull, measure, and manage

Postprandial blood glucose spikes are a force to be reckoned with. The acute and chronic problems caused by after-meal highs can be significant. Start by looking at your after-meal blood glucose levels from time to time, and determine whether a problem exists. If it does, take the necessary steps to achieve better after-meal control. Get some activity after eating. Make wiser food choices. And make sure your oral medicine or insulin program is working in your favor.

With better after-meal control, perhaps your next HbA_{1c} will be right where you want, expect, and *deserve* it to be! □

TAKE A BITE OUT OF HYPOGLYCEMIA

10 PROVEN STRATEGIES FOR CUTTING DOWN ON LOW BLOOD GLUCOSE

by Gary Scheiner, M.S., C.D.E.

Is it really possible to have too much of a good thing? Take my own "good things" list as an example. I really enjoy eating popcorn at the movies, lying on the beach, and taking my kids to ballgames. Good things, yes, but only in moderation. If left unchecked, I might become broke, obese, and badly sunburned.

For millions of people with diabetes, insulin and oral medicines that stimulate the pancreas to release more of its own insulin are good things. Without them, blood glucose levels would become wildly out of control. But when taken in too great a quantity, they can produce the opposite extreme: low blood glucose, or hypoglycemia.

Physicians usually advise people to avoid blood glucose levels below 60 or 70 mg/dl (it varies depending on which book you read and where your health-care provider studied). At this low level, many of the body's key organs, especially the brain and nervous system, become deprived of the fuel they need to function properly.

Greatest limiting factor

Hypoglycemia presents a serious threat to a person's physical, intellectual, and emotional well-being. It has been called the "greatest limiting factor" in diabetes management. Were it not for the risk of hypoglycemia, a person with diabetes could simply load up on insulin or pancreas-stimulating medicines to keep his blood glucose level from ever rising too high. Unfortunately, hypoglycemia does exist, and it creates a number of problems.

First and foremost is the risk to one's personal safety. The brain is one of the first organs to be affected by low blood glucose. When the brain receives inadequate fuel, confusion and poor decision-making often result. This can easily lead to life-threatening accidents, loss of consciousness, coma, and possibly even death if left untreated for too long.

Personal performance is another area affected by hypoglycemia. The ability to perform in sports, school, work, and social situations is affected negatively by low blood glucose. In many ways, having low blood glucose is similar to being drunk: It affects our movements, our thoughts, and virtually everything we say and do.

The brain's ability to detect low blood glucose is an important protective mechanism. However, this mechanism is blunted by repeated bouts of hypoglycemia. With each low, the brain becomes less and less sensitive to the lows—perhaps not recognizing them at all. Without the brain's reaction to the low, a person with diabetes may remain completely oblivious to the problem. This condition, known as *hypoglycemia unawareness,* puts a person at risk for severe hypoglycemia (leading to loss of consciousness, etc.) due to the lack of an "early warning" system.

In extreme cases, hypoglycemia can even cause permanent brain damage. With every episode of hypoglycemia, some brain cells die. Considering that you start with billions of brain cells, losing a few here and there is not likely to make any significant difference. However, repeated bouts of severe or prolonged hypoglycemia have the potential to create noticeable cognitive deficits.

In many instances, low blood glucose also causes anxiety or embarrassment. Some people with diabetes worry about the impression left on others by a hypoglycemic episode. Does it make me look sick? Different? Like I'm not "in control"? The fear of experiencing hypoglycemia in a social setting leads many people toward the opposite

extreme: maintaining high blood glucose levels around the clock.

Because of the need to eat extra food to treat low blood glucose, weight gain can also become an issue. Hypoglycemia can produce a werewolf-size appetite, resulting in the consumption of excessive calories for several hours. If low blood glucose occurs frequently or is consistently overtreated, weight gain will likely result.

Additionally, did you know that low blood glucose can produce significant highs? A rebound, as this is called, is the body's natural hormonal response to the low. Once hypoglycemia is detected by the brain, adrenaline starts to flow into the bloodstream along with other blood-glucose-raising *counterregulatory* hormones such as cortisol and glucagon. Collectively, these hormones stimulate the liver to release stored glucose, which can cause blood glucose to stay high for many hours following a bout of hypoglycemia.

What should I aim for?

With the current state of medical technology, it is usually not realistic to achieve tight blood glucose control without any episodes of hypoglycemia. This holds true for everyone with Type 1 diabetes and many people with Type 2 diabetes who use insulin or pancreas-stimulating oral medicines. All types of insulin as well as the following oral medicines can cause hypoglycemia:

- Chlorpropamide (Diabinese)
- Glimepiride (Amaryl)
- Glipizide (Glucotrol)
- Glyburide (DiaBeta, Glynase, Micronase)
- Glyburide and metformin (Glucovance)
- Nateglinide (Starlix)
- Repaglinide (Prandin)
- Tolazamide (Tolinase)
- Tolbutamide (Orinase)

So what is realistic? For starters, accept that an occasional low can occur. It is reasonable to experience mild low blood glucose a couple of times each week—lows that you can detect and treat without outside assistance. It is never acceptable to experience a severe episode of hypoglycemia (a low that causes a loss of consciousness, seizure, or unresponsiveness). Following any low that requires emergency medical assistance, additional self-management education and greater attention to control is always in order. A change in therapy may also be necessary.

If you check your blood glucose at each mealtime and bedtime, try to have no more than 10% of your readings below 70 mg/dl (or 80 mg/dl for very young children) at each test time. For example, let's say you collect your readings for an entire month (31 days) and find the following:

Before breakfast: 3 lows (10%)
Before lunch: 2 lows (6%)
Before dinner: 0 lows (0%)
Bedtime: 5 lows (16%)

The conclusion would be that there are too many lows at bedtime. A reduction in the dinner-time insulin (or oral medicine) may be in order. The number of lows at breakfast, lunch, and dinner appears to be acceptable.

For people with Type 2 diabetes, multiple episodes of hypoglycemia are a sign that insulin and/or oral medicines should be reduced. This, in turn, will help with any weight-loss efforts. In addition, people with existing heart disease should try to avoid hypoglycemia entirely. If you have heart disease, let your doctor know if you experience any lows.

Prevention strategies

Part of avoiding low blood glucose involves—how shall I put this?—just dumb luck. That's why it is usually considered acceptable to have lows up to 10% of the time. But the majority of hypoglycemia avoidance is well within your control. My top 10 strategies for preventing lows are as follows:

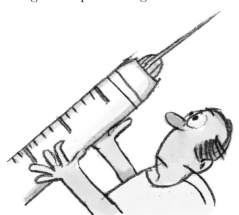

1. Match your insulin or medicine program to your needs.
The "peaks and valleys" in your insulin should coincide with the peaks and valleys in your blood glucose levels. This usually means utilizing a basal–bolus insulin approach—having a long-acting, or basal, insulin working at a low level throughout the day and night, and rapid-acting, or bolus, insulin at each meal or snack. Most adults experience a *dawn phenomenon*, in which more basal insulin is needed during the early morning hours, and less in the middle of the day. Daytime doses of intermediate-acting insulin, such as NPH, peak in the middle of the day or too early at night and

increase the risk for hypoglycemia at these times.

Mealtime insulin should match your typical blood glucose rise caused by dietary carbohydrate. Most starchy and sugary foods cause a rapid blood glucose rise, with a peak occurring about an hour after eating. Rapid-acting insulin analogs do a nice job of covering the rapid blood glucose rise and then dissipating before they can cause hypoglycemia later on. Regular insulin tends to peak too late and last too long, increasing the risk of hypoglycemia several hours after eating.

For those taking pancreas-stimulating oral medicines, be aware that some—glimepiride, glipizide, glyburide, chlorpropamide, tolazamide, and tolbutamide—work constantly (whether you are eating or not), while others—nateglinide and repaglinide—work for a short time (just after eating). Obviously, nateglinide and repaglinide are less likely to cause between-meal lows.

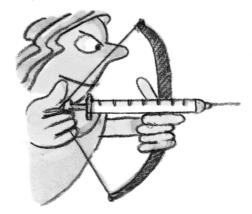

2. Set an appropriate target.
Work with your doctor to determine an ideal pre-meal blood glucose level. This is the level that you aim for when making your mealtime dosing decisions. For most people with diabetes who take insulin, this is usually 100, 120, or 140 mg/dl. A target below 100 mg/dl does not leave much margin for error and may result in a greater frequency of low blood glucose. For those with Type 2 diabetes who use oral medicines, targets of 80, 100, or 120 mg/dl are common.

3. Take a look at your schedule.
Are you eating at the times your insulin or medicine is working its hardest? For those using an insulin pump, this is not generally an issue as long as the basal rates are set properly. For those using a long-acting basal insulin, there may be a tendency for the blood glucose to drop gradually during the daytime, so it will be necessary to eat at regular intervals. For those using daytime NPH, meal timing is a major issue: This insulin begins to work hard approximately four hours after injec-

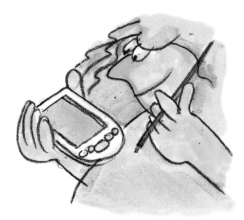

tion, so carbohydrates must be consumed in specific amounts at specific times. For those taking sulfonylureas (glimepiride, glipizide, glyburide, chlorpropamide, tolazamide, and tolbutamide), it is not a good idea to skip or delay meals since the medicine is stimulating extra insulin production throughout the day and night.

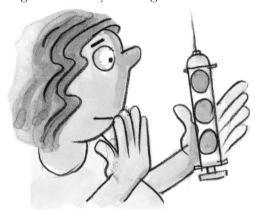

4. Use caution when "covering" high blood glucose.

Each unit of insulin will cause the blood glucose to drop by a certain amount, but the amount may vary by time of day. For many people, each unit lowers the blood glucose more at nighttime than during the day. Make sure your "correction" doses take this into account.

Also, be certain to account for "unused" insulin (the amount that is still active from the previous dose). With rapid-acting insulin analogs, it usually takes about 3–5 hours for the insulin's activity to fade completely. Regular insulin takes about 5–6 hours. A blood glucose reading taken 2 hours after a meal can be misleading since the insulin still packs a good deal of punch and the blood glucose should continue to drop. (See "Accounting for Unused Insulin" on this page for guidelines on how to take still-active insulin into account.)

For those who take daytime intermediate-acting insulin, it can be difficult and dangerous to cor-

ACCOUNTING FOR UNUSED INSULIN

Rapid-acting insulin continues to lower blood glucose levels for 3–5 hours after it is injected. It is important to account for the activity of previous injections or boluses when deciding how much to give in a correction dose to lower high blood glucose after a meal. In most cases, a person in whom rapid-acting insulin analogs last about 4 hours can expect the insulin's activity to decline as follows:

TIME SINCE INSULIN WAS GIVEN	INSULIN "USED UP"	INSULIN REMAINING
½ hour	10%	90%
1 hour	30%	70%
1½ hours	50%	50%
2 hours	70%	30%
2½ hours	80%	20%
3 hours	90%	10%
3½ hours	95%	5%
4 hours	100%	0%

For example, if you gave yourself 5 units for a 4 PM snack then checked your blood glucose at 6 PM, you'd still have 30% of your insulin remaining. 5 units × 30% = 1.5 units. This amount should be deducted from any dose that you are about to give yourself.

Although insulin does not truly stop working in a linear fashion, for the sake of simplicity, some people in whom rapid-acting insulin remains active for 4 hours choose to assume that one-fourth of their insulin is "used up" each hour.

TIME SINCE INSULIN WAS GIVEN	INSULIN "USED UP"	INSULIN REMAINING
1 hour	25%	75%
2 hours	50%	50%
3 hours	75%	25%
4 hours	100%	0%

If you find that rapid-acting insulin lasts shorter or longer than 4 hours for you, you would need to adjust these tables to fit your situation. For example, a person who finds that rapid-acting insulin lasts 3 hours could assume that 33% is used up per hour.

rect for high blood glucose until the intermediate-acting insulin has worn off. NPH insulin does not always get absorbed or act in a predictable manner. In general, to avoid hypoglycemia, it is best to wait at least 10 hours after taking NPH before correcting for high readings.

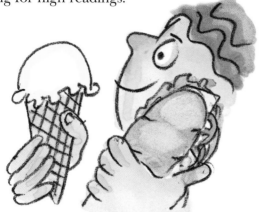

5. Adjust doses based on carbohydrate intake.

Of everything you eat, carbohydrate has the most profound influence on blood glucose levels. Virtually all forms of carbohydrate convert into blood glucose fairly rapidly. If your carbohydrate intake varies, your insulin and medicine doses should vary as well.

Carbohydrate also acts differently throughout the day. Most people need different doses of insulin or oral medicine to cover their carbohydrate at different meals. This is caused by varying levels of stress, insulin sensitivity, and physical activity throughout the day.

And if you're going to go to the trouble of matching your doses to your carbohydrate intake, be sure that your carbohydrate counts are reasonably accurate. Look up the exact carbohydrate count for foods you are unfamiliar with. (An excellent resource for looking up carbohydrate counts is *The Doctor's Pocket Calorie, Fat and Carb Counter,* which is available through your local bookstore or online.) Measure your portions. And don't forget to deduct all of the ebifr grams and half of the sugar alcohols from the total carbohydrate count; fiber is a carbohydrate that is not digested, and sugar alcohols only raise the blood glucose about half as much as an equivalent amount of ordinary carbohydrate.

6. Extend or delay your mealtime insulin when necessary.

Not all foods are digested at the same rate, so in some instances you will need to prolong your insulin's action to prevent hypoglycemia after eating. For example, foods with a low glycemic index

value (such as pasta, beans, and dairy products) usually take several hours to digest. With these kinds of foods, it might take 2–4 hours to see a significant blood glucose rise. (The glycemic index is a system of rating carbohydrate-containing foods based on how quickly they are absorbed; a food with a high glycemic index raises blood glucose levels faster than foods with a lower glycemic index.) If you were to take your full dose of rapid-acting insulin with your meal, the insulin would peak long before the blood glucose rises, resulting in hypoglycemia. To add insult to injury, your blood glucose may rise significantly several hours later once the mealtime insulin stops working and the food finally kicks in.

It is advisable to extend or delay your insulin when consuming food for a prolonged time, such as at a holiday meal or when eating a bucket of popcorn at the movies. Very large food portions also take a long time to digest. Think of your stomach as an hourglass and the food as sand trickling through. A very large portion of food, especially with a high fat content, might take several hours to pour through the stomach and into the intestines where it can be absorbed into the bloodstream, while a small portion will pour through relatively quickly.

In addition, a person who has gastroparesis (a nerve condition that causes the stomach to empty more slowly than usual) would also benefit from extending or delaying his mealtime insulin.

Extending or delaying insulin delivery can be accomplished in a number of ways. People who use mealtime rapid-acting insulin can take it 15–30 minutes *after* eating instead of before or during the meal. The dose could also be split into two injections—taking 50% with the meal and taking the other 50% an hour or two later. Alternatively, Regular insulin can be used instead of rapid-acting insulin when a slow-digesting meal is consumed.

For those who use an insulin pump, there are several options for prolonging or delaying the action of the mealtime bolus. Almost all pumps allow the bolus to be delivered over an hour or more (using the Square Wave or Extended boluses feature). Some allow a portion of the bolus, such as 33%, to be delivered immediately while delivering the remainder over the next couple of hours (Dual Wave or Combination boluses).

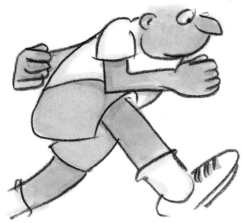

7. Adjust for physical activity.

With the exception of short bursts of high-intensity exercise, physical activity of almost any kind will lower blood glucose levels by accelerating the uptake of glucose by muscle cells. Note the term *physical activity* and not *exercise*. Physical activity includes exercises such as jogging, sports participation, and almost any form of physical conditioning. It also includes occupational activities and chores such as cleaning, shopping, yardwork, and home or auto repair. Recreational activities such as golf, gardening—and yes, even sex—count, too.

Work with your health-care provider to develop a plan to reduce your insulin or oral medicine when physical activity is anticipated. There is no way to tell exactly how much the activity will lower your blood glucose, so you might start out by reducing your dose by 33% when activity is planned within 90 minutes of the meal. For more intense activity, a 50% (or greater) reduction can be made; for less intense activity, a 20% or 25% reduction may be sufficient.

For activity that will take place before or between meals, it makes more sense to check your blood glucose and have a snack before you exercise. Again, the size of the snack depends on many variables, including your body size, the nature of the activity, and the timing and amount of your last dose of insulin or oral medicine. As a general rule, people who weigh 100 pounds will need approximately 15–25 grams of carbohydrate per hour of activity to keep their blood glucose steady. Those who weigh 150 pounds will need 20–30 grams; 200 pounds: 25–35 grams; 250 pounds: 30–40 grams, and so on.

Don't forget that physical activity that is very intense and prolonged can produce a blood glucose drop several hours later. This is called "delayed-onset hypoglycemia." Many people find that their blood glucose drops during the night following heavy daytime exercise, or in the morning following heavy exercise the night before.

Check your blood glucose more often than usual for up to 24 hours following heavy exercise. If you detect a pattern of delayed-onset hypoglycemia, you can prevent it by consuming extra carbohydrate or by lowering your insulin or oral medicine at the appropriate time. For example, to prevent the late-morning drops following nighttime exercise, try lowering your insulin dose at breakfast by 33%.

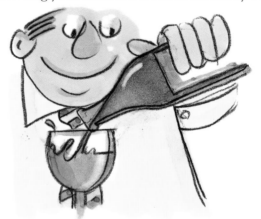

8. Be aware of alcohol's effects.

While many alcoholic drinks contain carbohydrate that raises blood glucose levels fairly quickly, the alcohol itself has a tendency to make blood glucose drop several hours later. This is because alcohol inhibits the liver's secretion of glucose into the bloodstream. When the liver is releasing less glucose than usual, the blood glucose level may drop.

After drinking alcohol, it is recommended that you reduce your insulin or diabetes medicine dose or consume extra carbohydrate. People who use insulin pumps can lower their basal insulin by 40% to 50% for approximately two hours for every drink consumed. Those who take NPH at night can lower their dose by a similar percentage after drinking. If you choose to eat to offset alcohol's blood-glucose-lowering effects, choose a food that will take time to affect blood glucose levels such as ice cream, peanut butter, or yogurt. Fifteen to thirty grams of carbohydrate at bedtime should serve as a good starting point.

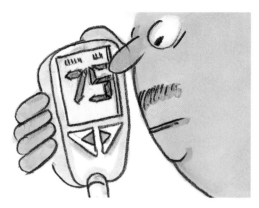

9. Check often.

Managing blood glucose is a lot like driving a car. If you pay attention and keep your hands on the wheel, you're not likely to veer off the road. Close your eyes or let go of the wheel for too long and you'll probably wind up in a ditch. Likewise, the more often you check your blood glucose, the less likely you are to suffer from extreme highs and lows. Checking before breakfast, lunch, dinner, and bedtime on a consistent basis, whether or not you take insulin or medicine at those times, will allow you to catch potential problems before they become too serious. A blood glucose level of 75 mg/dl at lunchtime should alert you to the need to either reduce your insulin or medicine or have some extra carbohydrate. Without knowing this, you could easily wind up hypoglycemic in the afternoon.

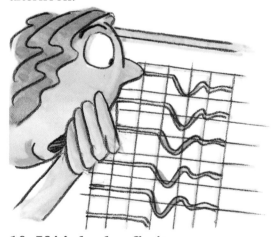

10. If it's broke, fix it.

Take a good look at your blood glucose monitoring logbook every couple of weeks. If you see too many lows at a particular time of day, do something about it! Don't keep doing the same things over and over, expecting different results. Perhaps you need to reduce or change your medicine. Maybe your insulin-to-carbohydrate ratio at a particular meal needs to be adjusted. Or maybe you just need to eat more carbohydrate when you are active.

As the saying goes, the one constant in life is change. The same goes for your diabetes self-care. What worked yesterday may not work today, so don't hesitate to make changes if you see a pattern of low readings. A single low could be caused by just about anything, but a pattern of lows indicates a problem with your current program.

Strategize to minimize

Living with diabetes can be a real pain in the rear sometimes (no pun intended). And nothing makes diabetes more disruptive in daily life than low blood glucose. Take the lows seriously. They present a greater threat to your well-being than any single high reading. While it may not be possible to eliminate the lows entirely, the 10 strategies listed here should allow you to lessen their frequency and severity.

It may not be possible or practical to implement all 10 strategies at once, so take them one at a time. Try focusing on one each week, and then add another the next week. If in 10 weeks you're not completely satisfied, simply return this issue along with a completed blood glucose logbook for a full refund. Or better yet, give me a call or send an e-mail. Maybe we can figure it out together. □

CONTINUOUS GLUCOSE MONITORING
Getting Started

by Linda Mackowiak, M.S., R.N., C.D.E.

Even with regular blood glucose monitoring, one of the big unknowns in diabetes self-management is what happens to glucose levels between blood glucose checks. In recent years, however, the development of continuous glucose monitors that check glucose levels in the fluid just under the skin have started to change all that. The newest continuous glucose monitors measure glucose levels continually around the clock and display results every few minutes.

The first continuous glucose monitoring systems simply collected data, which had to be uploaded to a computer for analysis. When the numbers were plotted on a graph, it became possible to see, for example, whether glucose levels were rising after meals or getting too low overnight.

The newer systems display glucose readings on a screen, so the user can see, in real time, what his glucose level is and whether it is rising or falling. The newer systems can also be programmed to sound an alarm when the user's glucose reaches high or low levels. Some systems are able to display graphs showing glucose levels over a certain number of hours on the display screen. And the data collected by all the systems can still be uploaded to a computer for graphing and analysis, if desired.

For all the information they provide, however, continuous monitoring devices do not replace regular blood glucose monitoring. Continuous monitoring systems must be periodically calibrated with conventional blood glucose meters using fingerstick blood samples for accurate readings. In addition, users are advised to do a conventional blood glucose check before making any changes in their diabetes care regimen.

How glucose sensors work

The glucose sensors used in continuous glucose monitors are small electrodes that the user places under the skin using an introducer needle and a spring insertion device that is similar to a lancing device or insulin pump infusion set inserter. Once the sensor is inserted, the introducer needle is removed, and only the sensor remains under the skin, held in place with an adhesive patch. The sensor must be changed every few days, according

to the manufacturer's recommendation. Inserting a glucose sensor should not be painful, and wearing a sensor should be comfortable.

The sensor produces a very small electrical current based on the amount of glucose in the body fluid (called interstitial fluid) around the sensor. When the glucose level rises, the current rises. When the glucose level goes down, the current goes down.

The sensors presently on the market need a number of hours to settle in to the body before they can start giving accurate glucose information. When the sensor is ready, the user calibrates the device by doing a fingerstick blood glucose reading and inputting the reading into the device (different systems have different methods for inputting information). The continuous monitoring device uses the reading to determine what the measured electrical current means in terms of glucose concentration. Additional calibrations are performed while wearing the sensor, according to the manufacturer's recommendations.

To get the most accurate readings from a continuous glucose monitor, it is important to calibrate carefully and correctly. You must use your best blood glucose monitoring technique, including checking on clean, dry fingers, using strips that have been stored properly, and coding and using your meter correctly. Remember: The sensor glucose information you get is only as accurate as the quality of the calibration you do.

Even with the best calibration possible, there can sometimes be differences in the level of glucose in your blood and the level of glucose in your interstitial fluid because of the way the body uses glucose. A noticeable difference is particularly likely if the glucose level in your blood is changing rapidly, which can occur just after eating or taking insulin or during exercise, but there can be differences at other times, too. It is best not to calibrate your continuous monitoring device when your blood glucose level is likely to be changing rapidly. Some people find the best time to calibrate is just before a meal.

With time and experience, you will learn when the difference between the sensor readings and your blood glucose monitoring readings is normal and when there may be a technical problem that needs addressing, such as a sensor that needs changing. If you're concerned about the accuracy of your readings, however, speak to your health-care provider, or call your monitor's manufacturer for help.

Getting started

It may take some time to get the most from continuous glucose monitoring. Start by learning as much as you can about the technical aspects of your new device, such as how to insert the sensor properly, how to calibrate the device with finger-stick blood glucose readings, how to set the alarms, how to put the alarms on vibrate mode, and how to transfer your monitoring data to a computer. Once you are up to speed on operating the system, you can work on learning to analyze and respond to the information you're getting from it.

Don't be surprised if you have an emotional response to seeing all of the glucose changes you experience over the course of a day. For some people, all this new information can be confusing or even frightening. If you're feeling overwhelmed, try not to tune out, but instead take the challenge to see how you can use this technology to help your diabetes care. Although there is a lot of information, you will quickly learn how to focus on the important trends and worry less about each individual number.

Keep in mind that even though you are using a continuous monitor, there are still times you should use your blood glucose meter. For example, you should still check your blood glucose level with your meter if you have symptoms of low blood glucose (hypoglycemia) and before making any diabetes care changes, including taking a "correction" dose of insulin for high blood glucose. (Also remember to consider how much insulin is already active in your system before you take more.) You should also check your blood glucose level before driving or doing anything that could be dangerous if you had low blood glucose.

Responding to your readings

Continuous glucose monitoring can offer information that can be of use immediately, over the intermediate term, and over the longer term.

Immediate information. Your blood glucose meter gives you point-in-time blood glucose levels, so you know where your blood glucose is, but not necessarily where it's going. Your continuous monitor, on the other hand, reports glucose levels every few minutes, so you can see not only where it is but

also which direction it's headed. With this added information, you may decide to respond differently to the same number, depending on whether your glucose is rising or falling. Being able to see trends in your glucose levels may enable you to take preventive action—by eating a snack, for example—before your glucose reaches a level considered problematic.

As you use this new technology, you may discover that you don't always know how to respond to the glucose trends you're seeing. Should you take more insulin? Less insulin? Delay your meal? Do something different before eating a similar meal in the future?

If you're not sure how to use the information you're collecting, speak to your health-care provider.

Intermediate term. If you develop a problem requiring immediate care, such as an episode of hypoglycemia, your monitoring data may be able to help you determine when the problem started and what may have caused it. Your data can also help you evaluate how well your response to the problem worked. Did your treatment raise your blood glucose level fast enough? Did it raise it too much? Best of all, your data may give you some ideas on preventing the same problem from happening again.

Longer term. Looking at the glucose information collected over-night, over some portion of the day, or over the course of several days can help you to see the big picture. Depending on which device you're using, you may need to upload your data to a computer to make a graph showing glucose ups and downs, or you may be able to display graphs covering certain time periods on the monitor itself.

You may notice that some days look much different from others. Why is that? You may discover that exercise, school, work, or dining out can have a big effect on your glucose pattern for the day.

What usually happens after eating? Does it vary depending on the time of day, foods eaten, or timing of your premeal insulin dose?

When does hypoglycemia happen? Do you ever get delayed hypoglycemia after exercising?

If you use an insulin pump, does the length of time between infusion set changes appear to have any effect on your glucose pattern?

It may help to keep detailed written records of your daily routine, food intake, exercise, and stress level for a few days to look at alongside a graph of your glucose levels. Bring your records along with your continuous glucose monitoring information to your next appointment with your diabetes care provider. Together you can evaluate how well your

DEVICES ON THE MARKET

All of the continuous glucose monitoring systems currently on the market measure glucose levels continuously and display glucose levels on a screen every five minutes. However, all must be calibrated with conventional blood glucose meter readings several times a day. They are approved for use in adults age 18 and older and require a prescription for purchase.

Product: Freestyle Navigator Glucose Monitoring System
Manufacturer: Abbott Diabetes Care
(888) 522-5226
www.abbottdiabetescare.com
The FreeStyle Navigator system is composed of three parts: a sensor, a transmitter, and a receiver. The sensor, worn for up to five days and then replaced, is placed just under the skin and is attached to a plastic sensor mount with adhesive to adhere to the skin, like a patch. The transmitter snaps into the sensor mount and sends glucose information wirelessly to the pager-sized receiver. The system discreetly measures glucose levels once per minute; provides high/low glucose alarms based on customizable levels; and delivers early-warning alarms that indicate if glucose levels are likely to be too high or too low 10, 20, or 30 minutes in advance. The system also stores up to 60 days worth of glucose information that can be analyzed by the user or a health-care professional.

Product: DexCom Seven Continuous Glucose Monitoring System
Manufacturer: DexCom, Inc.
(877) 339-2664
www.dexcom.com
The DexCom Seven System consists of a tiny wire-like sensor that is inserted by the user just under the skin. The sensor continuously measures glucose levels, which are transmitted wirelessly to the Seven Receiver. With the push of a button, the handheld receiver provides real-time glucose measurements and trends, as well as providing alerts to warn of high and low glucose levels. The system can display graphs covering 1 hour, 3 hours, and 9 hours.

According to the manufacturer, interpretation of the Seven System results should be based on the trends and patterns seen with several sequential sensor readings over time.

Product: MiniMed Paradigm REAL-Time Insulin Pump and Continuous Glucose Monitoring System
Manufacturer: Medtronic Mini-Med
(800) MINIMED (646-4633)
www.minimed.com/products/insulin pumps
The MiniMed Paradigm REAL-Time System combines a MiniMed Paradigm insulin pump with a continuous glucose monitoring system that can transmit data to the pump. The glucose sensor, which is a tiny electrode that is inserted just below the skin, sends updated readings every five minutes via a transmitter to the insulin pump, which displays the reading and can additionally show graphs of glucose trends from the previous 3-hour and 24-hour periods. An alarm sounds when glucose levels have risen above or dropped below thresholds programmed into the pump by the user.

The system cannot automatically adjust the amount of insulin being delivered by the pump.

Two MiniMed pumps can be used with this system: the MiniMed Paradigm 522 insulin pump, which holds up to 176 units of insulin, and the MiniMed Paradigm 722 insulin pump, which holds up to 300 units of insulin.

Product: Guardian REAL-Time Continuous Glucose Monitoring System
Manufacturer: Medtronic Mini-Med
(800) MINIMED (646-4633)
www.minimed.com/products/guardian
The Guardian REAL-Time Continuous Glucose Monitoring System displays glucose values on a monitor every five minutes and has alarms to alert the user to high or low levels. It cannot display graphs showing glucose trends, however. The data collected by the system, which can record up to 288 glucose readings per day, must be transferred and analyzed on a computer via a docking station and software.

diabetes regimen is keeping your blood glucose levels in target range and what changes you might make for improvement.

A word on alarms

Finding the right alarm settings may take some time. You want the alarms to alert you to situations that require action, but you don't want the alarms to overwhelm you or interrupt your day or your sleep too often. The best setting for an alarm may not always be the actual glucose value at which you wish to take action. You may have to move the settings up or down and reassess until you find the best setting. Also, different times of day (or night) and different situations, such as work or recreational activities, may require different settings. Expect to have to change your settings occasionally; you may even choose to silence the alarms in some circumstances.

Setting the low alarm. The higher you set your low glucose alarm, the more low alarms you are likely to get. In fact, if you set your low alarm fairly high, you may get alarms when your blood glucose level is simply at the low end of normal. One reason this may happen is that the rise in interstitial fluid glucose level lags behind the rise in blood glucose level after meals. While some people may find "low normal" alerts helpful, others may consider them a nuisance. You can avoid such alerts by setting your low glucose alarm lower, but if you do, you may not always get enough warning for real lows.

If you have *hypoglycemia unawareness,* meaning you do not sense the early signs of hypoglycemia, you may decide to set your low alarm on the high side to help you to prevent episodes of hypoglycemia and keep your blood glucose level in a safe range.

Setting the high alarm. The high glucose alarm on your continuous monitor can be useful in a number of situations. For one thing, it can alert you to a missed insulin dose or a problem with insulin delivery from a pump. (In both cases, the likely result is glucose that is higher than normal.) It can also be useful to evaluate the effect of food choices on your glucose level or, for those who use rapid-acting insulin, the amount and timing of premeal insulin doses.

As mentioned earlier, however, because the rise in interstitial glucose level lags behind the rise in blood glucose level just after eating, if you put the high alarm setting too high, you may not get an early warning that your glucose level is out of range. On the other hand, if you set the alarm too low, it may go off every time you eat.

Some health-care providers may suggest that you turn off the high and low glucose alarms for the first few days of using a continuous monitor (or that you set the low alarm very low and the high alarm very high), so that you can get used to wearing the device and to getting a lot more information about your glucose level than you are used to. If you decide not to use the alarms at first, keep in mind that you do not have the protection of this safety net.

Skin and tape issues

If you experience irritation or redness under the tape holding your sensor in place, or if the tape isn't sticking well, talk to your health-care provider about it, and call the monitor manufacturer as well to report any problems. There are other tapes and skin wipes that you can try that may keep your sensor secure without bothering your skin. (The products used to hold glucose sensors in place are the same as those used to hold insulin pump infusion sets in place.) Don't ignore the problem; it can make the difference between being willing to use continuous glucose monitoring and not being willing to use it.

Staying grounded

With all of the new glucose information you'll be getting from a continuous glucose monitor, it's easy to feel overwhelmed, but try to keep things in perspective.

Aim for improvement, not perfection, and don't try to fix everything at once. If you're not sure what to do first, try learning about and preventing some lows. Some people find that their overall diabetes control improves when they do this. Work with your health-care provider to make small changes, reassess, and make some more small changes. In many cases, cumulative small changes can make a big difference.

Remember to keep an eye on glucose trends, not just individual glucose numbers. Focus on prevention and catching potential problems early.

If your blood glucose control improves as a result of using a continuous monitor, you may find you are gaining weight. This can happen as your body becomes able to store glucose it was previously losing in urine. You will need to rebalance your food, exercise, and insulin to stop the weight gain and stay at a healthy weight. Talk to your health-care provider about how to do this safely.

Whatever you do, try not to get discouraged. Speak to your health-care provider if your attempts at improved diabetes control aren't having the effects you intended. □

Insulin and Injection Devices

Tips 258–302 167

Understanding Insulin 171

Rapid-Acting Insulin 177
Timing It Just Right

Getting Down to Basals 182

Insulin Therapy for Type 2 Diabetes 187

Insulin Delivery Devices 191

4

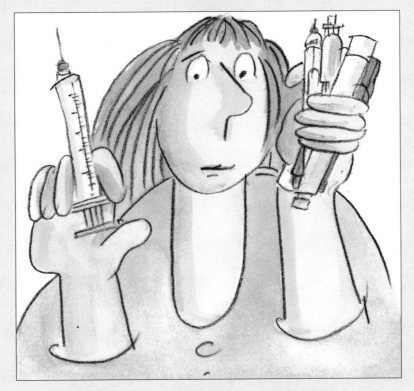

Insulin and Injection Devices Tips

258–302

258. Know the timing of your insulin's onset, peak, and duration so that you can coordinate it with meals and exercise. Use your own experience to find out how an insulin affects you personally.

259. If you take rapid-acting insulin with meals, try taking it 15 minutes before eating, with your first bite, and 15 minutes after starting to eat, on different occasions, to determine which timing is best for you to control your postmeal blood glucose spike. Check your blood glucose level one, two, and three hours after your meal to gauge the effect.

260. When taking insulin, pay attention to the thickness of fat under the skin at the injection site, timing of exercise, and temperature, all of which can affect how insulin is absorbed. Injection site does not seem to affect the action of rapid-acting insulin, as it does for slower-acting insulins.

261. Try to "stay ahead" of your blood glucose with your insulin doses; it's easier to control blood glucose by preventing

large spikes than by reducing already high levels.

262. If your blood glucose is high before a meal, calculate a dose of rapid-acting insulin to cover the high, then wait until that insulin begins to lower your blood glucose before eating. If you can't delay a meal, check your blood glucose an hour before you eat and take a corrective dose then.

263. If your blood glucose is low before a meal, wait until you have eaten for 15 minutes before taking your insulin.

264. If you don't know how much carbohydrate is in a meal, consider splitting your rapid-acting insulin dose. Take enough insulin at the beginning of the meal to cover the amount of carbohydrate you know you will eat, then take more insulin as soon as you know the meal's total carbohydrate content.

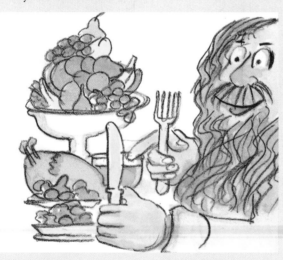

265. If you plan to eat a long, drawn-out meal, consider taking half of your mealtime insulin at the beginning of the meal and the other half an hour or two later.

266. Take rapid-acting insulin with any amount of carbohydrate over 10 grams, including snacks.

267. Remember that rapid-acting insulin can lower blood glucose for as long as five hours. If you plan on taking another dose within five hours of your last one, reduce it somewhat to lower the risk of hypoglycemia.

268. Getting the correct amount of basal insulin is essential to prevent both high and low blood glucose.

269. Taking NPH insulin at bedtime may reduce or eliminate the blood glucose spike that many people experience during the predawn hours. Timing the insulin to peak when blood glucose spikes can, however, be difficult.

270. Insulin pump therapy offers the greatest flexibility in matching the body's basal insulin needs.

271. With an ideal basal insulin regimen, blood glucose should change no more than 30 mg/dl during sleep.

272. Talk with a member of your diabetes team if you feel that your insulin delivery device is not working for you or that you may not be using it correctly.

273. If you keep syringes prefilled with insulin in your refrigerator, discuss with your health-care provider how long they can be safely stored.

274. Insulin leakage at the injection site or worsening blood glucose control may indicate that a syringe with a longer needle is needed.

275. For people who have trouble injecting insulin or who are afraid of needles, various injection aid devices exist. Before purchasing an injection aid, make sure that it is compatible with the type of syringe you use.

276. It is important to prime an insulin pen to make sure that insulin is flowing properly and that there is no air in the cartridge or needle.

277. When delivering a dose with an insulin pen, hold the needle in place with the dose knob pressed down for five seconds to make sure that no insulin leaks out of the skin.

278. Insulin pen needles should be used only once; they should be removed and discarded after an injection.

279. Never store an insulin pen with a needle (new or used) attached, as this may allow insulin to leak out or air to leak in.

280. Do not store an insulin pen in the refrigerator; once a cartridge is placed in the pen, it should be stored at room temperature to prevent condensation in the insulin container.

281. Insulin pens hold the advantages of accurate dosing and easy use over syringes.

282. An insulin pump can offer more flexibility in food choices and the timing of meals and activities, but it also requires a strong commitment to self-management of diabetes.

283. Always place used lancets, syringes, and other sharp devices in a hard, firmly closed container that is clearly marked as "used sharps" before disposing of them if you have no containers created for this purpose. Specific guidelines for disposal vary by state.

284. When traveling, keep your diabetes supplies with you; never place insulin or other liquid supplies in checked baggage. Make sure that prescription information accompanies the supplies.

285. If you have Type 2 diabetes and your HbA_{1c} level is rising despite consistent diabetes control, you may need to begin insulin therapy.

286. If you are apprehensive about beginning insulin therapy or about any aspect of your diabetes management, share your concerns with a member of your health-care team; they may be able to help once they know what is worrying you.

287. If you feel that you have "failed" your diabetes management because you need to start insulin therapy, reassure yourself that it is your pancreas that is failing; this is part of the regular progression of Type 2 diabetes.

288. In some cases of Type 2 diabetes, if the function of the pancreas has not deteriorated, it may be possible to reduce or eliminate insulin use through weight loss, diet, and exercise.

289. In most cases, it is important for a basal insulin to be taken at the same time of day, every day, at the prescribed intervals.

290. Never mix two types of insulin unless this is approved by your health-care provider.

291. Insulin stored at room temperature beyond the recommended period of time should be discarded; its effectiveness may be severely compromised.

292. If you suspect you may have hypoglycemia (low blood glucose), check your blood glucose level immediately.

293. To treat low blood glucose, eat or drink 15 grams of fast-acting carbohydrate, wait 15 minutes for it to be absorbed, and check your blood glucose level again. If it has not increased, consume 15 more grams of carbohydrate and check again.

294. Good choices for treating low blood glucose include 4 ounces of orange juice, 6 ounces of ginger ale, 6 saltine crackers, 3 BD glucose tablets, or 4 Dex4 tablets.

295. Always report episodes of low blood glucose to your health-care provider.

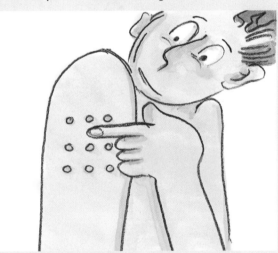

296. If you use insulin, change the site of injection each time you take it by at least a finger's width. This prevents the skin in the area from becoming thick, hard, or pitted.

297. Weight loss, healthy eating habits, regular exercise, and taking prescribed drugs can, for some people with Type 2 diabetes, prolong the life of pancreatic beta cells and delay the need to take insulin.

298. Your diabetes care team can help you determine your insulin-to-carbohydrate ratio, or how much insulin you need to

take for a certain amount of carbohydrate, by looking at your food records and records of your premeal and postmeal blood glucose levels.

299. In women with Type 2 diabetes who are pregnant, insulin is usually the drug of choice to manage blood glucose levels even if an oral medicine was used before the pregnancy. If a pregnancy is planned, it is usually best to switch to insulin therapy even before becoming pregnant.

300. If your diabetes plan requires mixing different types of insulin and you struggle to do this, ask your health-care provider about premixed insulin options.

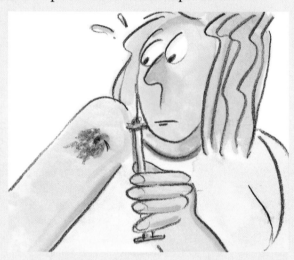

301. It is possible to have an allergic reaction to injected insulin; contact your doctor if you experience swelling, itching, or redness at the injection site. It will be important to determine the exact cause of the reaction.

302. If you experience shortness of breath, wheezing, a fast heart rate, clamminess, or a full-body-rash after injecting insulin, get immediate medical attention as this may indicate a severe, systemic allergic reaction.

UNDERSTANDING INSULIN

by Laura Hieronymus, M.S.Ed., A.P.R.N., B.C.-A.D.M., C.D.E.,
and Patti Geil, M.S., R.D., C.D.E.

In any discussion of diabetes, the word insulin is almost certain to come up. That's because a lack of insulin or trouble responding to insulin (a condition called insulin resistance) or both is what is responsible for the high blood glucose levels that characterize diabetes.

Thanks to years of medical research, however, *endogenous* insulin (that produced by the pancreas) can be replaced or supplemented by *exogenous* insulin (insulin produced in a laboratory). For people with Type 1 diabetes, injecting insulin (or infusing it with an insulin pump) is necessary for survival: Before the discovery of insulin in 1921, the life expectancy for a person diagnosed with what was then known as juvenile diabetes was less than a year. For some people with Type 2 diabetes, using insulin may be the best—or only—way to keep blood glucose levels in the recommended range, and maintaining blood glucose control is one of the most important things you can do to lower your risk of developing potentially devastating complications.

But even if you never have to take insulin to control your diabetes, it is important to understand what insulin is and what it does in the body. That's because your lifestyle choices affect the health of your insulin-producing beta cells. Making an effort to lose excess weight, eat healthfully, exercise regularly, and take any prescribed drugs as instructed can prolong the life of your beta cells, so they continue to make the insulin you need.

The role of insulin

Insulin is a hormone that is released by the beta cells of the pancreas, a glandular organ located in the abdomen, in response to a rise in the level of glucose in the blood. Blood glucose levels rise when a person consumes carbohydrate-containing food or drinks, as well as during periods of physical and sometimes mental stress. Insulin prevents a further increase in the blood glucose level and causes it to fall gradually by enabling the glucose to enter the body's cells, where it is burned for energy or stored as glycogen or fat for later use. While many hormones raise blood glucose levels, only insulin lowers them.

The body needs a small amount of insulin at all times to keep blood glucose levels controlled between meals and overnight. In a person who does not have diabetes (or who does have diabetes but whose pancreas still produces insulin), the pancreas constantly secretes this small amount of so-called background, or *basal,* insulin. A person whose pancreas does not produce insulin (or does not produce enough) can compensate by injecting an intermediate- or long-acting insulin or by using an insulin pump that is programmed to continuously deliver small pulses of short- or rapid-acting insulin.

At mealtimes, blood glucose levels rise as carbohydrates are broken down to glucose and other simple sugars and enter the bloodstream. A healthy pancreas responds by releasing a burst of insulin in two phases, the first occurring almost as soon as food is eaten and lasting about 15 minutes, and the second occurring more gradually over the next 1½–3 hours. In a person who doesn't have diabetes, the amount of insulin released matches the rise in blood glucose. In people with Type 2 diabetes, a diminished first-phase insulin response is often the first sign of pancreatic insufficiency.

People who use insulin can match the pancreas's action by injecting a dose of short- or rapid-acting insulin before the meal or by taking a *bolus* dose with an insulin pump. Since the goal is to match the premeal insulin dose to the expected rise in blood glucose following the meal, and since the amount of carbohydrate in the meal predicts the rise in blood glucose, the current practice is to match the premeal insulin dose to the amount of carbohydrate in the meal. This requires knowing your insulin-to-carbohydrate ratio—or how much insulin you need to "cover" a certain number of grams of carbohydrate. Your diabetes care team can help you determine your insulin-to-carbohydrate ratio by looking at your food records and your blood glucose monitoring records for before-meal and after-meal blood glucose levels. They will also take your overall insulin requirements into consideration.

Types of diabetes

In Type 1 diabetes, an autoimmune process destroys the insulin-producing beta cells of the pancreas, leaving it unable to make insulin. People with Type 1 diabetes must therefore inject or infuse insulin for survival. While some people appear to have a genetic predisposition to develop Type 1 diabetes, exactly what sets off the autoimmune destruction of the beta cells is unknown.

In Type 2 diabetes, some degree of insulin resistance is typically present. Initially, the pancreas may release more insulin than normal to compensate for the insulin resistance, but eventually, the pancreas is believed to "burn out" from overproduction, and blood glucose levels rise. However, treatments other than insulin therapy are usually tried first for Type 2 diabetes. In most cases, insulin resistance can be improved with moderate weight loss, so treatment recommendations generally include lifestyle adjustments such as changes in diet and increased physical activity. Oral blood-glucose-lowering medicines are also often used in the treatment of Type 2 diabetes. (These oral medicines are not insulin.) If dietary changes, increased physical activity, and oral medicines are unable to keep blood glucose levels adequately controlled, insulin therapy may be added to the diabetes treatment regimen or substituted for the oral drugs.

Diabetes and pregnancy

In any pregnancy, the need for insulin dramatically increases around the 16th week of gestation. From then on, more and more insulin is necessary to maintain normal blood glucose levels as the pregnancy progresses.

In women with Type 1 diabetes who are pregnant, careful blood glucose monitoring to adjust insulin doses is necessary over the course of the pregnancy. In women with Type 2 diabetes, insulin is usually the drug of choice to manage blood glucose levels during pregnancy and also requires adjustments, as needed, throughout the pregnancy. Women with Type 2 diabetes who are taking oral blood-glucose-lowering medicines prior to pregnancy are urged to plan their pregnancy and, typically, to begin using insulin prior to conception. While a few studies have examined the use of oral diabetes drugs during pregnancy, many health-care providers feel they do not yet know enough about the effect of these medicines on the fetus to advocate their use at this time.

A temporary type of diabetes that complicates about 7% of all pregnancies among women not diagnosed with either Type 1 or Type 2 diabetes is called *gestational diabetes*. The high blood glucose levels that occur in gestational diabetes are usually first recognized around the 24th to 28th week of pregnancy. They are due to increased insulin resistance, which is generally caused by the pregnancy hormones as well as the weight gain that normally occurs in pregnancy. About 75% of women with gestational diabetes can maintain normal blood glucose levels by making lifestyle changes, such as following a meal plan and getting regular physical activity. However, if blood glucose levels remain too high, insulin is currently the drug of choice for treatment for gestational diabetes.

Synthetic insulin

Insulin that is used in diabetes treatment is not and never was extracted from human pancreases (although earlier forms of insulin were, in fact, extracted from pig and cow pancreases). Human insulin is manufactured using recombinant DNA technology (often called genetic engineering) in a laboratory; it is identical in structure to what a human pancreas produces. Insulin analogs, which are structurally different from human insulin, are also manufactured in labs using similar processes.

Although genetically engineered human insulin is identical to the natural product, insulin that is injected into the fatty tissue under the skin does not act the same as insulin secreted from the pancreas directly into the bloodstream. Injected insulin reaches the bloodstream more slowly, so there's a delay in when it starts lowering blood glucose levels. Because these differences make it difficult to control blood glucose levels with injected insulin, much research has gone into altering synthetic insulin so that it behaves more like the insulin that is secreted by a pancreas. The rapid-acting insulin analogs are one of the results of this research.

Insulin is now available in a variety of types that are categorized according to action time. These types include rapid-acting insulin, short-acting insulin, intermediate-acting insulin, and long-acting insulin. Insulin can also be purchased in mixtures of intermediate-acting and either rapid-acting or short-acting insulins. (For a list of the insulins currently approved for marketing in the United States, see page 173.)

Rapid-acting insulin. The rapid-acting insulin analogs currently available include insulin aspart (brand name NovoLog), insulin lispro (Humalog), and insulin glulisine (Apidra).

Rapid-acting insulin typically starts working in 5 to 15 minutes, is strongest (peaks) in 45 to 90 minutes, and diminishes in activity 3 to 5 hours after injection. Because it starts working so quickly, rapid-acting insulin is generally taken within 15 minutes of eating—either within the 15 minutes before a meal or as much as 15 minutes after starting to eat. Rapid-acting insulin comes close to mimicking the pancreas's first-phase insulin

TYPES OF INSULIN

TYPE OF INSULIN	BRAND NAME	ONSET OF ACTION	PEAK ACTION	DURATION OF ACTION	APPEAR-ANCE	CAN BE MIXED WITH
RAPID-ACTING (BOLUS/MEALTIME) INSULINS						
Insulin aspart	NovoLog	5–10 minutes	1–3 hours	3–5 hours	clear	NPH, but only on the advice of a doctor. If mixed, aspart should be drawn into the syringe first, and the mixture injected immediately
Insulin glulisine	Apidra	15 minutes	30 minutes to 1½ hours	3–5 hours	clear	NPH
Insulin lispro	Humalog	15 minutes	30 minutes to 1½ hours	4–5 hours	clear	NPH, but only on the advice of a doctor. If mixed, lispro should be drawn into the syringe first, and the mixture injected immediately.
SHORT-ACTING (BOLUS/MEALTIME) INSULIN						
Regular	Humulin R Novolin R	30 minutes to 1 hour	2–4 hours	5–7 hours	clear	NPH
INTERMEDIATE-ACTING (BASAL/BACKGROUND) INSULINS						
NPH	Humulin N Novolin N	1–2 hours	6–14 hours	24+ hours	cloudy	Regular
LONG-ACTING (BASAL/BACKGROUND) INSULINS						
Insulin detemir	Levemir	1½ hours	"peakless" action	up to 24 hours	clear	Do not mix with other insulins.
Insulin glargine	Lantus	1½ hours	"peakless" action	24 hours	clear	Do not mix with other insulins.
PREMIXED INSULINS						
Insulin aspart protamine suspension/ aspart	NovoLog Mix 70/30	10–20 minutes	1–3¾ hours	up to 24 hours	cloudy	Do not mix with other insulins.
Insulin lispro protamine suspension/ lispro	Humalog Mix 75/25	15–30 minutes	30 minutes to 2½ hours	14–24 hours	cloudy	Do not mix with other insulins.
NPH suspension/Regular	Humulin 50/50	30 minutes to 1 hour	2–5½ hours	14–24 hours	cloudy	Do not mix with other insulins.
NPH suspension/Regular	Humulin 70/30 Novolin 70/30	30–60 minutes	2–6 hours	14–24 hours	cloudy	Do not mix with other insulins.

The insulins and insulin mixtures listed in this table are currently approved for marketing in the United States. All are stable at room temperature for 28 days in the original vial. For insulin pens and similar delivery devices, see the package insert for the amount of time the pen or device may be stored at room temperature. All of the action times shown are estimates: The onset, peak, and duration of action may vary considerably from the times listed due to individual variations.

release in response to food. If timed correctly and accurately matched to the amount of carbohydrate in the meal, a dose of rapid-acting insulin before a meal can help keep blood glucose levels in target range after the meal.

All of the rapid-acting insulin preparations are approved for use in insulin pumps. In the case of pump therapy, rapid-acting insulin is used not just for bolus doses at mealtimes but also as basal insulin around the clock.

Short-acting insulin. Regular, or short-acting, human insulin usually starts working about 30 minutes after injection, is strongest (peaks) 2 to 4 hours after injection, and decreases in activity 5 to 7 hours after injection. People who use Regular insulin are typically advised to take it approximately 30 minutes before eating a meal so that the rise in the level of insulin in the bloodstream matches the rise in blood glucose level.

Intermediate-acting insulin. Intermediate-acting human insulins (Humulin N and Novolin N) generally start working in 1 to 3 hours. They peak in 6 to 14 hours, and their activity decreases 16 to 24 hours after injection. Intermediate-acting insulins are commonly prescribed once or twice daily, usually before breakfast and/or supper, to enhance overall blood glucose control. In some cases, intermediate-acting insulin may be recommended at bedtime to help control overnight and early morning blood glucose levels. In either situation, the insulin would be providing a basal-type effect.

Long-acting insulin. Long-acting insulins, sometimes called basal insulins, are typically given once daily and include the insulin analogs glargine (Lantus) and detemir (Levemir). Glargine and detemir, which stand apart from other longer-acting insulins by being clear rather than cloudy or milky in appearance, are considered to be "peakless" insulins. Their effects last for up to 24 hours. They should never be mixed with another type of insulin.

Premixed insulins. Premixed insulin preparations contain intermediate-acting insulin that is mixed with either rapid- or short-acting insulin in varying percentages. The advantage to using a premixed preparation is that you don't have to mix the insulins yourself when drawing up an injection or take two injections rather than one.

All of the insulin analogs require a prescription from a physician for purchase. Human insulin does not require a prescription for purchase in some states; however, a prescription is usually necessary for insurance coverage. Use of insulin therapy should always follow a physician's recommendation and prescription.

TREATING HYPOGLYCEMIA

Treating for hypoglycemia (low blood glucose) is usually recommended when a person's blood glucose level is 70 mg/dl or less. The "rule of 15" is commonly used as a guideline for treatment: After checking your blood glucose level with your meter and seeing that your level is under 70 mg/dl, consume 15 grams of carbohydrate, wait about 15 minutes, then recheck your blood glucose level. If your blood glucose is still low, consume another 15 grams of carbohydrate and recheck 15 minutes later. Since blood glucose levels may begin to drop again about 40–60 minutes after treatment, it is a good idea to recheck your blood glucose approximately one hour after treating a low.

Although the "rule of 15" is an accepted method for treating hypoglycemia, it should not replace the advice of your diabetes care team.

The following items contain 15 grams of carbohydrate:

- 3–4 glucose tablets
- 1 dose of glucose gel (in most cases, 1 small tube is one dose)
- ½ cup of orange juice or regular soda (not sugar-free)
- 1 tablespoon of honey or syrup
- 1 tablespoon of sugar or 5 small sugar cubes
- 6–8 LifeSavers
- 8 ounces of skim (nonfat) milk

Challenges of insulin therapy

Insulin may be a lifesaver for people with Type 1 diabetes and may offer the best chance of achieving optimal blood glucose control for many with Type 2, but it can be a challenge to use. The body's need for insulin is based on many things—including body weight, stage of growth, food intake, physical activity, use of certain drugs, and physical or mental stress—all of which can change from day to day.

When there is too much insulin in the bloodstream relative to the body's needs, *hypoglycemia*, or low blood glucose, results. Hypoglycemia can occur as the result of skipping or delaying a meal, taking more insulin than is necessary to control blood glucose levels, engaging in unusual or more frequent physical activity than normal, and consuming alcohol. People who use insulin should be aware of the signs and symptoms of hypoglycemia, as well as how to treat it. (See "Treating Hypoglycemia" on page 174.)

Many people gain weight when they start insulin therapy, usually because their bodies are now absorbing glucose that was previously exiting the body in the urine. For people who had lost a lot of weight because of their diabetes, the weight gain may be welcome, but for many, it is not. To slow any weight gain and maintain a healthy weight, it's necessary to consume only as many calories as your body needs, given your level of physical activity. A registered dietitian can help you determine what and how much to eat to maintain a healthy weight and optimal blood glucose control. It's also worth noting that weight loss (through burning more calories than are consumed) can lower insulin needs, while weight gain can increase it.

It's possible to have an allergic reaction to insulin. Symptoms of a local reaction at the injection site include slight swelling, itching, and redness. Local reactions can occur as the result of preservatives used in the insulin (not the insulin itself), the material used in the needle, products used to cleanse your skin prior to injection, or using an injection technique that injures the skin. Determining the cause is important. Let your diabetes care team know if any of these symptoms occur. Symptoms of a more serious, systemic allergic reaction include shortness of breath or wheezing, fast heart rate, clamminess, and a rash that occurs all over your body. If any of these occur, notify your physician immediately.

Skin changes due to repeated insulin injections, such as slight pitting or areas of thickened skin, are rare but possible. If you notice that your skin is changing in the area you inject insulin, consult your diabetes care team. A change in injection technique or needle size may solve this problem.

When insulin doses are inadequate relative to the body's needs, high blood glucose results. Common causes of high blood glucose include not taking enough insulin for the amount of food eaten and physical stress such as an illness or infection. Very high blood glucose can lead to serious consequences such as diabetic ketoacidosis or hyperosmolar hyperglycemic state, both of which usually require hospitalization. Chronically elevated blood glucose, even when it doesn't cause an acute crisis, can damage the blood vessels and nerves in the body over time. Your diabetes care team can help you learn to keep your blood glucose in target

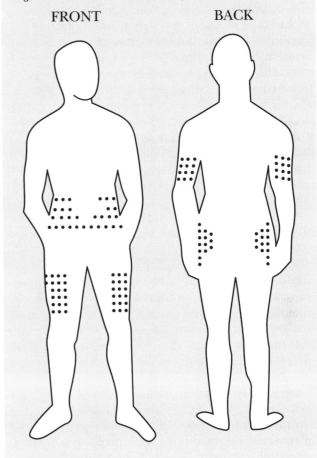

INSULIN INJECTION SITES

Self-administered insulin is injected or infused into the fatty tissue just under the skin. The body areas used most commonly for insulin injections are the abdomen, buttocks, and thighs. The backs of the upper arms may be used as well. To avoid skin problems, inject at least a finger's width away from your last injection. To avoid absorption problems, don't inject near moles, scars, or your navel.

FRONT   BACK

range and develop a plan for responding to high blood glucose if it occurs.

Insulin delivery

While alternative delivery methods continue to be researched, currently the only way to take insulin outside a medical setting in the United States is to inject it into the fatty tissue just below the skin. There are a few device options for doing this. The body areas used most commonly for insulin injections or to insert an insulin pump infusion set are the abdomen, buttocks, and thighs. (see "Insulin Injection Sites" on page 175).

Insulin vial and syringe. The traditional way of taking insulin, using a syringe to draw insulin from a vial and inject it, is widely used in the United States. Technique is important when administering insulin with a syringe and is best learned with guidance from a health-care provider. Insulin syringes come in a variety of sizes to accommodate larger or smaller doses. Different lengths and gauges of needles are available, too. Your diabetes care team can help determine the right size syringe and needle for you.

Insulin pens and dosing devices. Insulin pens are usually the size of a large fountain pen, with other dosing devices about the size of a cell phone. Some are reusable, and some are disposable. Reusable insulin pens and devices use cartridges of insulin that are replaced as they are emptied. Disposable pens and devices are prefilled with insulin and discarded when empty. However, there is a limited time an insulin pen or device can be stored at room temperature. Check package inserts for specifics, and discard any cartridge or disposable pen or device that has been kept at room temperature longer than specified by the manufacturer.

The general procedure for injecting insulin with a pen or dosing device is as follows: A disposable pen needle is attached, the dose is dialed in, the needle is inserted into the skin, and a button on the pen is pressed to deliver the insulin. However, because the steps for using a pen are somewhat different from those for using a syringe, and because each device may work a little differently, it's important to read the manufacturer's package insert for specific instructions for each pen or dosing device.

Insulin pump. Insulin pumps are small, computerized, mechanical devices about the size of a pager. Insulin pumps deliver insulin by pumping rapid- or short-acting insulin through plastic tubing to a small catheter or needle that is inserted into the fat layer under the skin and taped in place. Pumps are generally programmed to deliver a steady, small dose insulin (basal insulin), and the user delivers larger amounts of insulin (bolus doses) based on the amount of carbohydrate in meals and snacks. To learn more, consultation with a physician and a diabetes educator with expertise in insulin pump therapy is recommended.

Insulin jet injectors. Jet injectors send a fine spray of insulin through the skin using a high-pressure air mechanism instead of a needle. If used incorrectly, injectors can be painful, injure the skin, and result in inaccurate dosing, so education and training on use of the injector device is important.

When insulin is prescribed, it is important that the method of delivery be individualized. Expense and insurance coverage may influence your choice, as may issues such as convenience and level of manual dexterity. Work with your diabetes care team to choose and learn to use the best method for you.

How am I doing?

Blood glucose self-monitoring lets you know how well your treatment is working. Your diabetes care team can help you decide when and how often to monitor and also how to interpret your monitoring results. Most insulin users should check their blood glucose level at least three times daily. Checking both before meals and after meals (one to two hours after eating) can be useful for fine-tuning bolus, or premeal, doses. Checking first thing in the morning, before meals, at bedtime, and in the middle of the night can assist with determining basal insulin needs. Any changes in insulin dosing should be made cautiously and with the direction of your diabetes care team.

Powerful medicine

While no one necessarily enjoys injecting insulin or inserting a pump catheter, for many people with diabetes, insulin is the most effective therapy for maintaining blood glucose control, along with healthy lifestyle behaviors such as meal planning and getting regular physical activity. This is important to remember, because the devastating complications that are associated with diabetes result largely from high blood glucose levels—and can be prevented by keeping blood glucose levels close to the normal range.

If you have questions about your insulin therapy or whether it might be a good time for you to start using insulin, speak to your diabetes care team. The more you understand your diabetes treatment, the more you are able to benefit from it. □

RAPID-ACTING INSULIN
TIMING IT JUST RIGHT

by Hope Warshaw, M.M.Sc., R.D., B.C.-A.D.M., C.D.E.

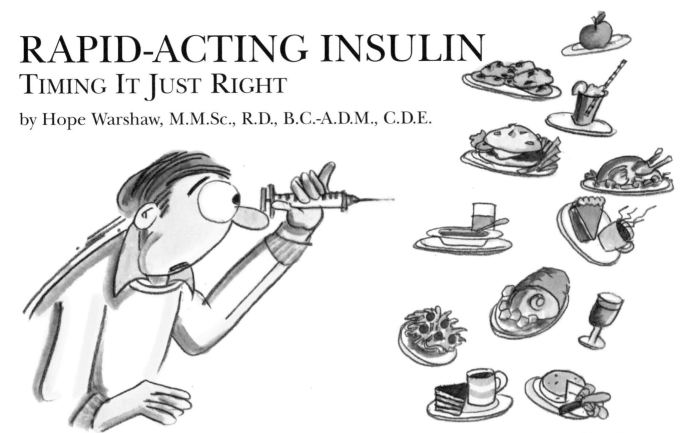

E ven when you think you're doing everything right with your diabetes care regimen, it can sometimes seem like your blood glucose levels are hard to control. One potential source of difficulty that you may not have thought of is how you time your injections or boluses of rapid-acting insulin with respect to meals.

Since the first rapid-acting insulin, insulin lispro (brand name Humalog), came on the market in 1996, most diabetes experts have recommended taking it within 15 minutes of starting a meal (any time between 15 minutes before starting to eat to 15 minutes after starting to eat). This advice is based on the belief that rapid-acting insulin is absorbed quickly and begins lowering blood glucose quickly. However, several years of experience and observation suggest that this advice may not be ideal for everyone who uses rapid-acting insulin. As a result, the advice on when to take it needs updating.

Insulin basics

The goal of insulin therapy is to match the way that insulin is normally secreted in people without diabetes. The illustration on page 178, "Normal Insulin Release for Food," gives a graphic representation of how a healthy pancreas releases insulin.

Basal insulin. Small amounts of insulin are released by the pancreas 24 hours a day. On aver-

age, adults secrete about one unit of insulin per hour regardless of food intake.

Bolus insulin. In response to food, larger amounts of insulin are secreted and released in two-phase boluses. The first phase starts within minutes of the first bite of food and lasts about 15 minutes. The second phase of insulin release is more gradual and occurs over the next hour and a half to three hours. The amount of insulin that is released matches the rise in blood glucose from the food that is eaten.

In people with normal insulin secretion, insulin production and release is a finely tuned feedback system that maintains blood glucose between about 70 mg/dl and 140 mg/dl at all times, no matter what or when a person eats or when he engages in physical activity. During illness, when insulin needs may rise, the pancreas just produces more.

People whose pancreas does not secrete insulin normally often must inject insulin or infuse it with an insulin pump. People who have Type 1 diabetes, in which the pancreas secretes no insulin or virtually no insulin, must inject or infuse insulin. But learning when to take insulin and how much to take is challenging, because injected or infused insulin does not act exactly like insulin released from the pancreas. The first step to figuring out when to take insulin and how much to take is understanding an insulin's action curve.

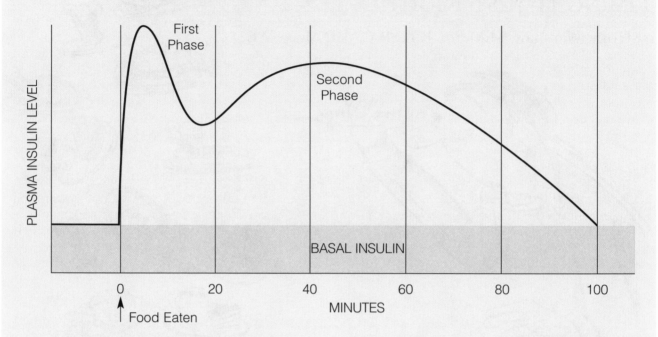

NORMAL INSULIN RELEASE FOR FOOD

(chart axes: PLASMA INSULIN LEVEL (vertical); MINUTES (horizontal) with marks at 0, 20, 40, 60, 80, 100; labels: First Phase, Second Phase, BASAL INSULIN, Food Eaten)

This diagram shows how the body normally releases insulin. The pancreas constantly secretes a background (basal) level of insulin. When a person eats, the pancreas releases a surge (bolus) of insulin in two phases to take care of the blood glucose rise caused by the food. (Reprinted with permission from *Using Insulin,* by J. Walsh, R. Roberts, C. Varma, and T. Bailey. Copyright © 2003, Diabetes Services, Inc.)

Insulin action

An insulin's action curve has the following three phases:

■ Onset: when the insulin starts to lower blood glucose

■ Peak: when insulin has its greatest effect on blood glucose

■ Duration: how long the insulin continues to have some blood-glucose-lowering effect

Rapid-acting insulin is often called mealtime insulin because its action curve most closely resembles the body's normal release of insulin at mealtimes. (However, most people who use an insulin pump use rapid-acting insulin as a basal insulin as well, infusing small amounts 24 hours a day.) The three rapid-acting insulins currently approved by the U.S. Food and Drug Administration—lispro, aspart (NovoLog), and glulisine (Apidra)—have similar action curves, with an onset occurring in 5–15 minutes, a peak in 45–90 minutes, and an overall duration of about 3–4 hours.

However, Howard Wolpert, M.D., editor of the book *Smart Pumping* and Senior Physician and Director of the Insulin Pump Program at Joslin Diabetes Center, cautions against blind-faith acceptance of insulin action curves or standard advice about when insulin works, noting that insulin can show "a lot of variability…between individuals and even within the same person from day to day." The time ranges given for an insulin to reach its peak action are averages, so they may not fit everyone or every situation. You may find through blood glucose monitoring and experience that rapid-acting insulin typically reaches peak effectiveness within 45–90 minutes or possibly sooner or later. This information can affect when you take your premeal doses.

Matching insulin and food

In addition to understanding an insulin's action curve, it's important to understand how the food you eat affects your blood glucose level so that you can match your insulin's action to the expected rise in blood glucose level following a meal. In general, people with normal stomach emptying can expect some glucose from the carbohydrate they've eaten to start raising their blood glucose level within minutes of starting to eat. Blood glucose level tends to peak about one to two hours after the start of a meal and gradually drops over the next three hours.

When to inject. If rapid-acting insulin always started working almost immediately and peaked one to two hours later, injecting it anytime within 15 minutes of starting to eat would work well. But newer observations suggest that rapid-acting insulin doesn't get absorbed and start working that quickly in all people. John Walsh, P.A., C.D.E., coauthor of the book *Using Insulin,* for example, believes the maximum blood-glucose-lowering effect of rapid-acting insulin may occur much closer to two hours after an injection rather than 45–90 minutes. If this is the case, the optimal time to take rapid-acting insulin is on the earlier end of the spectrum—about 10 to 15 minutes before eating—rather than with the first bite or 15 minutes after starting a meal. Walsh's belief is based on research suggesting that insulin's *pharmacodynamics* (when, how much, and how long insulin seems to be acting on cells, working to reduce blood glucose levels) may be different from its *pharmacokinetics* (when, how much, and how long insulin is detectable in the bloodstream). In other words, insulin may be measurable in the bloodstream before it begins actively lowering blood glucose.

Some other factors that may cause insulin action to differ from the action curve given in product literature or to vary from person to person include thickness of the subcutaneous fatty layer at an injection site, temperature, blood flow, exercise, and dose size. (The choice of injection site—abdomen, thigh, arm, buttock—does not seem to affect the absorption rate of rapid-acting insulin as it does for slower-acting insulins.) Injecting into areas that have more subcutaneous fat tends to slow insulin absorption. Widened blood vessels (caused by higher temperatures or exercise) allow insulin to be absorbed more quickly; constricted blood vessels (caused by colder temperatures or smoking) can cause slower absorption. Large doses of insulin may also be absorbed somewhat more slowly than smaller doses.

The importance of staying ahead. Fine-tuning the timing of your premeal boluses or injections is important, but it should not overshadow one of the basics of blood glucose control: counting the carbohydrates in a meal or snack and using enough insulin to cover the anticipated rise in blood glucose. (If you don't know how to count carbohydrates or to match your insulin dose to the amount of carbohydrate you plan to eat, speak to your health-care provider.) Many people find themselves in a reactive mode when it comes to dosing insulin, taking it in response to high blood glucose rather than using enough of it before a meal to cover the rise of blood glucose in the hours after a meal or snack. Experts agree that it's much harder to bring high blood glucose back down than to control blood glucose levels with sufficient insulin in the first place.

Variable impact of food

To achieve a good match between the amount of insulin you take and an anticipated rise in your blood glucose level, you need to know how much carbohydrate you intend to eat, because carbohydrate has the greatest effect on blood glucose level. Some experts also encourage people to take into account the type of carbohydrate consumed as well as the amount.

Walsh, Wolpert, and Gary Scheiner, a certified diabetes educator in private practice in Pennsylvania, agree that the glycemic index of the foods in a meal or snack as well as the fiber and fat content can dramatically affect how quickly or slowly blood glucose level rises. (The glycemic index ranks foods based on how quickly they raise a person's blood glucose.) "Using this knowledge is especially helpful at breakfast," adds Wolpert, because "some people are more insulin-resistant in the morning and therefore have more of a problem controlling blood glucose around the breakfast hours." For these reasons, both Wolpert and Scheiner suggest that people have foods with a lower glycemic index such as yogurt or a bowl of oatmeal with a piece of fruit for breakfast rather than foods with a higher glycemic index such as some cold cereals, pancakes, or muffins.

In general, foods and combinations of foods that have a low glycemic index and high fiber content will raise blood glucose more slowly. Meals and snacks that have a higher glycemic index and are lower in fiber will raise blood glucose more quickly. Meals and snacks that are high in fat content tend to cause a delayed rise in blood glucose.

The extent to which the glycemic index or fat content of a meal speeds or slows the rise in blood glucose following a meal varies from person to person. If you find that certain meals affect your postmeal blood glucose levels in a predictable fashion, you may be able to fine-tune the timing of your premeal injections or boluses accordingly.

Practical tips

Meticulously timing your rapid-acting insulin dose and carefully calculating your dose according to the carbohydrate you will eat is usually best for blood glucose control, but it may not always be possible. There are times when you know exactly when and how much you will eat and times when you don't. For example, if you are trying out a new restaurant, eating at a friend's home, or not feeling well, you may not know exactly when or what you will be eating, which can make it difficult to know how much insulin you'll need and when to take it. In addition, if your blood glucose level is low before a meal, you may have to give the food, not the insulin, a head start. The following practical tips may help you adjust for the realities of daily life:

High blood glucose before a meal. If your blood glucose is high before a meal, use your *insulin sensitivity factor* (how much your blood glucose level falls in response to one unit of insulin) to calculate a dose of rapid-acting insulin to cover the high, then wait until that insulin begins to lower your blood glucose before you eat. This method is easier and more convenient for insulin pump users. (For people who are willing to take an extra injection but who don't want the hassle of carrying a vial of insulin and syringes, an insulin pen may also add some convenience.)

Claudia Shwide-Slavin, a dietitian and certified diabetes educator in private practice in New York City, advises the following: "If your blood glucose level is between 140 mg/dl and 180 mg/dl, take the rapid-acting insulin and wait half an hour before eating. If it's between 180 mg/dl and 200 mg/dl, wait 45 minutes. If it's higher than 200 mg/dl, wait at least an hour." She also notes, however, "I have seen it take two hours after an injection for blood glucose levels to budge." If a person is hungry or must eat at a specific time, Shwide-Slavin recommends limiting the amount of carbohydrate at the meal by eating mainly protein and nonstarchy vegetables.

Another suggestion from Shwide-Slavin if you can't delay a meal is to "check your blood glucose an hour before you think you will eat. If it is high, take a correction dose so that your blood glucose will be on the downswing by the time you eat."

Low blood glucose before a meal. If your blood glucose is low before a meal (below about 80 mg/dl), "Wait to take your insulin," says Shwide-Slavin. "Let the food have 15 minutes to raise your blood glucose before taking your insulin."

Low glycemic index foods. On a related note, Wolpert advises, "If your blood glucose is less than 100 mg/dl before a meal and you plan to have a meal with a low glycemic index, wait until you start to eat to take your rapid-acting insulin."

Uncertain carbohydrate intake. If you don't know how much carbohydrate you will eat at a meal, consider splitting your rapid-acting insulin dose. Take enough insulin before the meal to cover the amount of carbohydrate you are sure you will eat. Then as the meal goes on and you know how much more carbohydrate you will eat, take more insulin to cover that amount. This method is easiest if you are on an insulin pump.

Large meals. Splitting your rapid-acting insulin dose can also work well for meals that are larger than normal. It has been shown that large meals can delay the rise of blood glucose regardless of the nutrient composition of the meal.

Drawn-out meals. Pump users who are planning to have a meal that is eaten over time, such as a cocktail party or Thanksgiving dinner or a meal that is higher in fat or lower in glycemic index and high in fiber, may want to consider using one of the optional bolus delivery tools on their insulin pump. Most insulin pumps allow you to deliver a bolus over time rather than all at once or to deliver some of the bolus immediately and the rest over the next few hours. People who inject insulin could take half their bolus at the start of a meal and the other half an hour or two later.

Snacks. Regardless of whether the carbohydrate you eat is part of a meal or snack, it has the potential to raise your blood glucose level. Alison Evert, R.D., C.D.E., a diabetes educator at Joslin Diabetes Center at Swedish Hospital in Seattle, advises people to "take rapid-acting insulin with any amount of carbohydrate over 10 grams." Although it is common to think that a few grams won't make a big difference, the reality is that 10 grams of carbohydrate can raise many peoples' blood glucose 30 or more points.

Unused bolus insulin

While the duration of action of rapid-acting insulin is usually given as 3–4 hours, some diabetes experts believe it may continue to lower blood glucose level for as long as 5 hours. Walsh believes that a good rule of thumb is to assume that about 20% of a dose of rapid-acting insulin is used each hour after it is given. In his book *Using Insulin* and on his Web site http://diabetesnet.com/diabetes_control_tips/ bolus_on_board.php, he provides a table that shows insulin activity at 1, 2, 3, 4, and 5 hours after bolus doses of insulin from 1 to 10 units.

This information becomes important if you give bolus doses of rapid-acting insulin less than four to five hours apart. When two doses of rapid-acting insulin overlap, their effects overlap, too, and the result can be hypoglycemia. Therefore, when you're considering the size of a bolus dose of insulin, it is critical that you factor in what Walsh calls "the unused insulin" or "bolus [insulin] on board." This is the amount of "active" rapid-acting insulin left from a previous injection or bolus dose from a pump that continues to lower your blood glucose.

To illustrate this idea, consider the following example. Before lunch, you take a bolus of rapid-acting insulin. Three hours later you decide to have a snack with 30 grams of carbohydrate. You check your blood glucose and find that it's high at 195 mg/dl. Assuming your insulin sensitivity factor is 45 mg/dl, you calculate you'll need two units of insulin to bring your blood glucose level down to your premeal target of 100 mg/dl and another two units to cover the snack you're about to eat (assuming an insulin-to-carbohydrate ratio of 1:15). You take the insulin, and several hours later, your blood glucose has dropped to 55 mg/dl. Why? Because you didn't factor in the hour or so of action left on the bolus you took at lunch.

To prevent hypoglycemia from unused insulin, get in the habit of thinking about when you took your last bolus dose and how much (if any) action is still left before taking another bolus to "correct" high blood glucose.

The latest generation of insulin pumps, which some people call "smart pumps," has a built-in feature that keeps track of how much of a previous bolus dose is still active. If the user attempts to administer a bolus dose while a previous bolus is still active, the pump will suggest subtracting the amount of insulin still "on board" from the requested amount.

How are you doing?

Measuring and observing your postmeal (postprandial) blood glucose values will help you to determine how well you are timing your rapid-acting insulin and figuring your doses. Walsh suggests that "much of the postprandial high blood glucose values observed are because people aren't giving rapid-acting insulin long enough before a meal to act in tandem with their food. Most foods affect the blood glucose within two hours, while most of the effect of rapid-acting insulin is seen over five hours."

The American Diabetes Association advises that postprandial blood glucose shouldn't exceed 180 mg/dl (plasma value) at two hours after the start of a meal. Other associations and experts believe

INSULIN RESOURCES

To learn more about how to fine-tune your insulin regimen, take a look at some of the following resources.

BOOKS
SMART PUMPING
A Practical Approach to the Insulin Pump
Howard A. Wolpert, Editor
McGraw-Hill
New York, 2002

THINK LIKE A PANCREAS
A Practical Guide to Managing Diabetes
with Insulin
Gary Scheiner
Marlowe & Company
New York, 2004

USING INSULIN
Everything You Need to Know for Success
with Insulin
*John Walsh, Ruth Roberts, Chandrasekhar Varma,
Timothy Bailey*
Torrey Pines Press
Torrey Pines, California, 2003

INTERNET
DIABETES MALL
www.diabetesnet.com
Web site selling diabetes products founded by John Walsh and Ruth Roberts. The site also has helpful information on diabetes and tips for managing your blood glucose.

INTEGRATED DIABETES SERVICES
www.integrateddiabetes.com
Gary Scheiner's Web site has premade charts for logging your insulin, carbohydrate intake, and blood glucose readings that you can download and print for free (Click on "Log Sheets"). There is also some helpful information on insulin pumps.

the two-hour postmeal goal should be less than 140 mg/dl.

Occasionally checking your blood glucose after a meal at hours one, two, and three can help you determine when your blood glucose level peaks and starts to come down again. According to Scheiner, "Research shows that it is common for people to have elevated blood glucose levels after meals." One key to controlling these highs is better timing of rapid-acting insulin.

Because responses to insulin and carbohydrate can vary (because of, say, activity level or meal composition), some people find it helpful to record their experiences for future reference in a notebook, computer file, or logbook. Chart the foods you eat and the amounts, the amount of insulin you take to cover the food, your blood glucose levels before and after you eat, when you exercise and how vigorously, and any lessons you learn. Although perfect control is impossible, your personal database can help you obtain a better understanding of your blood glucose readings and how to fine-tune your diabetes control.

The right time

Delivering rapid-acting insulin at the proper time can help you to achieve optimal blood glucose control. It's not easy, but by learning when it's best for you to take your insulin and putting a few tips into practice, you can increase your chances of hitting your blood glucose targets more regularly. □

GETTING DOWN TO BASALS

by Gary Scheiner, M.S., C.D.E.

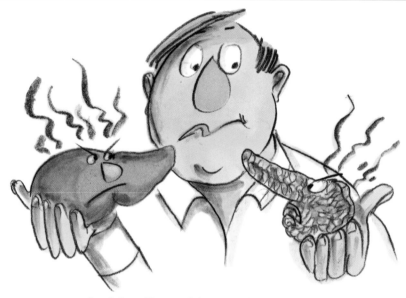

To borrow a phrase from the late, great Rodney Dangerfield, "Basal insulin gets no respect." Very few people know how to spell it correctly (basil? bazal? I mean, really!), and even fewer know what the heck it's for. That's a shame, because basal insulin (no "z") is the foundation upon which insulin therapy is built.

Unlike its more famous little brother *bolus,* which is the rapid-acting insulin given to cover those delicious carbohydrates in our diet, basal's job is much more mundane: to match the liver's secretion of glucose into the bloodstream (and to prevent the liver from oversecreting glucose). Everyone's liver does it, and a healthy pancreas responds by secreting a small amount of insulin into the bloodstream every few minutes.

How would we manage without basal insulin? Not so well. Because the liver is secreting glucose into the bloodstream continuously, a complete lack of insulin, even for just an hour or two, would result in a sharp rise in blood glucose level. Basal insulin also makes sure that the body's cells are nourished with a steady supply of glucose to burn for energy. Without basal insulin, many of the body's cells would starve for fuel. Some cells would resort to burning only fat for energy, and that leads to production of acidic waste products called ketones. The combination of dehydration (caused by high blood glucose) and heavy ketone production (from excessive fat metabolism) leads to a life-threatening condition known as diabetic ketoacidosis (DKA).

Suffice it to say that basal insulin is necessary for maintaining blood glucose control, not to mention survival. So where does one find basal insulin? How much is needed? And when should it be taken?

Basal options

Each person's basal insulin requirement is unique. It's affected by factors such as body size, activity level, stage of growth, hormone levels, and the amount (if any) of internal insulin production from one's own pancreas.

During a person's growth years (up to age 21), basal insulin requirements tend to be heightened throughout the night. This is due to the production of hormones (growth hormone and cortisol) that stimulate the liver to release extra glucose

BASAL INSULIN ACTION

This graph illustrates the approximate level of basal insulin activity
using various types of insulin programs.

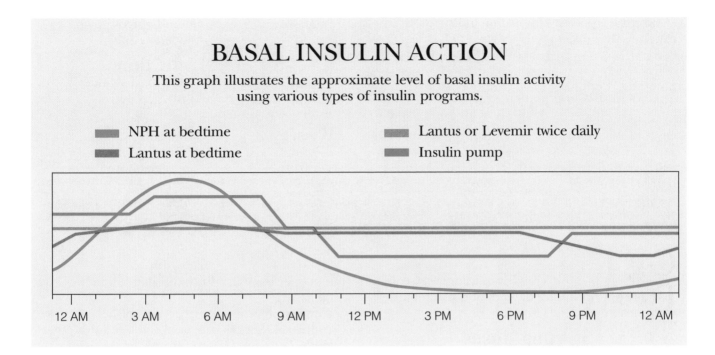

into the bloodstream. After the growth years, production of these hormones is reduced and limited primarily to the predawn hours. The dawn effect, or dawn phenomenon, as this is called, results in an increased secretion of glucose by the liver in the early morning. As a result, basal insulin requirements in most adults tend to peak during the early morning hours.

To match these requirements, basal insulin can be supplied in a variety of ways. Intermediate-acting insulin (NPH) taken once daily will usually provide basal insulin around the clock, albeit at much higher levels 4–8 hours after injection and at much lower levels 16–24 hours after injection. Insulin glargine (brand name Lantus) taken once daily offers a relatively peakless insulin presence for approximately 24 hours, although the insulin level may wane a few hours earlier in some people. Insulin detemir (brand name Levemir) provides approximately 16–24 hours of insulin activity with a mild peak near the midway point. Taken twice daily, detemir produces a relatively flat basal insulin level throughout the day and night. Insulin pumps deliver basal insulin in the form of tiny pulses of rapid-acting insulin every few minutes. With a pump, the basal insulin level can be adjusted and fine-tuned to closely match the liver's ebb and flow in glucose secretion.

The chart on this page illustrates the approximate level of insulin in the bloodstream using various types of basal insulin programs.

Basal option 1: NPH at bedtime. The advantage of this program is the peak that occurs during the

predawn hours—for those who need it. The disadvantages include the unpredictability of the peak and the potential for a blood glucose rise in the daytime and evening as the insulin action falls to very low levels at these times.

Basal option 2: Glargine once daily or detemir twice daily. The main advantage here is the relatively unwavering flow of basal insulin and consistent absorption pattern that is unaffected by exercise and skin temperature. The disadvantages include the potential for blood glucose rises during the night (due to the lack of a predawn peak) and the potential for blood glucose drops in the afternoon and evening (if meals are delayed), if the basal insulin level exceeds the liver's production of glucose. In some people, glargine begins to wear off in less than 24 hours, resulting in a blood glucose rise prior to the next injection.

Basal option 3: Insulin pump therapy. Pump therapy offers the greatest degree of flexibility in terms of matching basal insulin to the body's needs. Because small pulses of rapid-acting insulin analogs—lispro (Humalog), aspart (Novolog), or glulisine (Apidra)—are used to deliver basal insulin, the "basal rate" can be adjusted hourly, if needed, to match the liver's normal, 24-hour pattern. Pumps also permit temporary changes to basal insulin rates to accommodate short-term changes in basal insulin needs (for situations such as illness, high or low activity levels, stress, and menstrual cycles).

Perhaps the greatest drawback to pump therapy is the risk of ketoacidosis. Any mechanical prob-

TYPICAL BASAL REQUIREMENTS

In people whose pancreases produce virtually no insulin, such as those with Type 1 diabetes, basal insulin requirements vary fairly predictably according to age, size, and physical activity level. Here are some typical basal insulin requirements.

	50-POUND CHILD	120-POUND ADOLESCENT	150-POUND ADULT	150-POUND OLDER ADULT
MOSTLY INACTIVE	6–14 units/day	21–50 units/day	17–40 units/day	14–34 units/day
MODERATELY ACTIVE	5–12 units/day	17–40 units/day	14–34 units/day	10–27 units/day
VERY ACTIVE	4–10 units/day	13–32 units/day	10–27 units/day	7–20 units/day

lem resulting in stoppage of insulin delivery can cause a severe insulin deficiency and production of ketones in just a few hours.

Starting doses

Once you have selected a strategy for supplying basal insulin, the next step is to determine the proper dose. Ideally, this should be done in cooperation with a physician who is experienced at setting and adjusting insulin doses.

In most cases, the daily dose of basal insulin is not very different from the total daily dose of bolus insulin. The daily basal insulin requirement generally depends on a person's body weight and sensitivity to insulin, which is affected greatly by physical activity and hormone levels. For those with Type 2 diabetes, the daily basal insulin requirement can vary considerably: Some people who still produce their own insulin may require only a few units daily, while people who are obese and highly insulin resistant may require hundreds of units daily.

For people who produce virtually no insulin on their own (including those with Type 1 diabetes), insulin requirements are somewhat more predictable. The chart above provides typical ranges for daily basal insulin needs.

Fine-tuning basal insulin

In the absence of food and exercise, basal insulin should hold the blood glucose level fairly steady. That's because, as mentioned earlier, the level of basal insulin should come as close as possible to matching the liver's secretion of glucose throughout the day and night.

It is a good idea to fine-tune your basal insulin before settling on specific bolus doses to use at mealtimes. When high or low blood glucose appears, it is difficult to know what to adjust unless

the proper basal insulin levels have already been established.

For people who take injections of NPH, glargine, or detemir, the goal is to set a dose that maintains a steady blood glucose level during sleeping hours and does not produce significant hypoglycemia or hyperglycemia during the day. Ideally, your blood glucose level should change no more than 30 mg/dl while you're sleeping, assuming that no food is eaten and no heavy exercise is performed before going to sleep. A consistent rise or drop of more than 30 mg/dl overnight indicates a need to change your basal insulin dose.

To determine whether your overnight basal insulin dose is set correctly, try the following:
1. Have a fairly healthy dinner that does not contain a great deal of fat. Avoid restaurant or take-out food before this test. High-fat food will cause a prolonged blood glucose rise and will contaminate the test results. Take your usual doses of dinner-time and nighttime insulin.
2. If you normally exercise in the evening, go ahead and do so, but keep the intensity and duration modest. Very heavy exercise may cause blood glucose to drop several hours later, which would also contaminate the test.
3. At least three hours after dinner, perform a bedtime blood glucose check. As long as your blood glucose level is above 80 mg/dl and below 250 mg/dl, do not eat any food or take any rapid-acting insulin. If your blood glucose level is below 80 mg/dl, have a snack and try the test another night. If it's above 250 mg/dl, give a correction dose of insulin and try again another night.
4. If your blood glucose level was above 80 mg/dl and below 250 mg/dl and you have decided to go ahead with the basal insulin test, check your blood glucose again in the middle of the night (or the middle of your sleep time) and again when you

INSULIN PUMP BASAL RATE TESTING SCHEDULE

You can test whether your insulin pump basal rates are set correctly by not eating and not taking any bolus doses for a controlled period of time. Starting with the overnight period, test, adjust your rate, and retest until your blood glucose level changes by no more than 30 mg/dl between bedtime and when you wake up. When one rate is set, move on to the next time period.

TEST TIME PERIOD	EAT AND BOLUS NO LATER THAN	CHECK BLOOD GLUCOSE AT	OK TO EAT AND BOLUS AGAIN AFTER
OVERNIGHT	7 PM (Eat dinner, then skip evening snacks.)	11 PM, 1 AM, 3 AM, 5 AM, 7 AM	7 AM
MORNING	3 AM (Have a bedtime snack, then skip breakfast and morning snack.)	7 AM, 9 AM, 11 AM, 12 noon	12 noon
AFTERNOON	8 AM (Eat breakfast, then skip morning snack, lunch, and afternoon snacks.)	12 noon, 2 PM, 4 PM, 6 PM	6 PM
EVENING	2 PM (Eat late lunch, then skip afternoon snack. Have dinner near bedtime.)	6 PM, 8 PM, 10 PM, 11 PM	11 PM

first wake up the next day. The middle-of-the-night reading is needed to rule out the Somogyi phenomenon, in which low blood glucose causes "rebound" high blood glucose.

If your blood glucose remains within 30 mg/dl from bedtime to wake-up time, your basal dose is probably OK. If it rises more than 30 mg/dl, increase your basal insulin dose by 10% and repeat the test. If it drops by more than 30 mg/dl, decrease your basal insulin by 10% and repeat the test. Continue adjusting and repeating the test until your blood glucose holds reasonably steady through the night.

For example, if your bedtime reading was 185 mg/dl and your wake-up reading was 122 mg/dl, your basal insulin dose is too high, because your blood glucose dropped by 63 mg/dl while you slept. Had your bedtime blood glucose level been closer to normal, you would have experienced hypoglycemia during the night. Reduce your basal insulin dose by 10%, and run the test again the following night. Had your blood glucose risen from 87 mg/dl to 160 mg/dl—a rise of 73 mg/dl—an increase in your basal insulin dose would be in order. If your bedtime reading was 95 mg/dl and you woke up at 87 mg/dl, your basal insulin dose would not need to be adjusted because your blood glucose level changed by only 8 mg/dl.

Fine-tuning pump basal rates

Appropriate basal rates must be established to obtain quality blood glucose control and enjoy the flexible lifestyle afforded by an insulin pump. Remember: The right basal rate is one that keeps your blood glucose at a fairly constant level when you have not eaten or taken a bolus dose for several hours and are not exercising.

To test your basal insulin settings, you will need to wait approximately four hours after your last bolus and meal or snack. This will give the carbohydrates in your food time to finish digesting and the bolus dose time to finish working. The meal (or snack) eaten before the test should be fairly low in fat (no restaurant or take-out food) so that you don't have a delayed blood glucose rise. You must stay connected to the pump continuously during the test and go about your normal, daily activities. However, heavy exercise should be avoided during the fasting phase of the test. Testing should not be performed during an illness or onset of menses, following hypoglycemia, or if your blood glucose level is greater than 250 mg/dl at the beginning of the test.

Here's what to do:

■ Check your blood glucose level about four hours after your last bolus of lispro, aspart, or glulisine.

- If your blood glucose is above 250 mg/dl, bolus for the high blood glucose and cancel the test.
- If your blood glucose is below 80 mg/dl, eat to bring your blood glucose level up, and cancel the test.
- If your blood glucose level is neither too high nor too low, proceed with the test.

I prefer to test and fine-tune the nighttime basal rates first. Once the overnight rate is set properly, move on to the morning segment, then the afternoon, and finally, the evening segment.

Basal testing should be set up around the framework of your usual mealtimes and sleep patterns. The schedule above can be used as a guide for performing a complete set of basal tests.

If your blood glucose drops by more than 30 mg/dl during the test period, the basal rate is probably too high. If it rises by more than 30 mg/dl, the rate may be too low. The basal rate should be changed in increments of 0.05 to 0.2 units per hour, depending on your usual settings and the magnitude of the rise or drop that took place. The next day, retest to see whether the adjustment produces a steadier blood glucose level. Continue to adjust and retest until steady blood glucose levels are attained.

Note: Basal rates are usually changed one hour prior to an observed rise or fall in the blood glucose, since the rapid-acting insulin infused by the pump takes about an hour to peak. For example, if your blood glucose rises between 3 AM and 7 AM, you would increase the basal rate between 2 AM and 6 AM.

The Somogyi phenomenon

What about those pain-in-the-neck blood glucose readings you took during the night? Nobody likes getting up in the middle of the night to prick their finger, so those extra tests had better be worth it! Believe me, they are.

In many people, blood glucose can drop during the night to levels below 70 mg/dl without the person knowing it. The drop causes the body to secrete hormones that raise the blood glucose level by morning. This occurrence, known in the medical community as the Somogyi phenomenon (after its discoverer), can interfere with basal dosing decisions if it goes undetected.

As shown on the graph on this page, Larry, Moe, and Curly all started and finished the night with the same blood glucose levels, indicating a rise during the night. Without knowing their blood glucose level in the middle of the night, our first instinct would be to increase the basal insulin for all three. But that wouldn't solve the problem for all three.

OVERNIGHT BLOOD GLUCOSE PATTERNS

People can have high blood glucose in the morning for several different reasons, as illustrated in this graph. Larry's blood glucose rise is steady throughout the night, while Moe's occurs during the predawn hours, and Curly experiences a low, which is followed by a "rebound" effect.

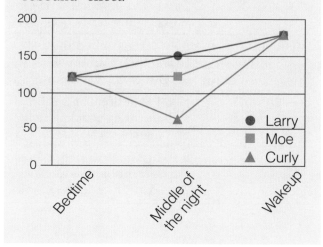

Larry, as it turns out, is experiencing a steady rise throughout the night. An increase in his basal insulin is in order.

Moe also experienced a rise, but primarily during the pre-dawn hours. Adding a few units of intermediate-acting insulin (NPH) at bedtime (if he takes injections) or raising his basal rate in the early morning (if he uses a pump) would likely work best for Moe.

Curly, on the other hand, experienced the Somogyi phenomenon. He dropped low in the middle of the night and rebounded to a higher level by morning. Increasing his basal insulin would make the problem worse, not better. A *reduction* in his basal dose by 10%, or possibly adding a bedtime snack, would make the most sense.

Giving basal a little respect

Having the right basal insulin program and setting the right doses is important for anyone who uses insulin. Taking too much basal insulin, or taking it at the wrong times, can result in frequent (and perhaps severe) hypoglycemia, not to mention weight gain. Taking too little basal insulin will produce high blood glucose and make it very difficult to set appropriate mealtime bolus doses. However, a properly set basal insulin level will allow you a great deal of flexibility in your schedule and should allow you to go to sleep confident about where you'll be when you wake up.

Fine-tuning basal insulin can be complex, so don't hesitate to ask a member of your health-care team for help with this task. An endocrinologist, certified diabetes educator, nurse practitioner, or insulin pump specialist can usually help you put your basal insulin on the right track. □

INSULIN THERAPY FOR TYPE 2 DIABETES

by Virginia Peragallo-Dittko, R.N., B.C.-A.D.M., M.A., C.D.E.

Al just couldn't believe what he was hearing. "Insulin for me? But I exercise almost every day. I eat so much less than I used to, and I never skip my pills. What more can I do? Why has my diabetes gotten worse?"

Every number in Al's blood glucose log is over 200 mg/dl and his glycosylated hemoglobin reading (HbA$_{1c}$ or A1C, a measure of long-term blood glucose control) has slowly increased from 7.2% to over 10%. (The American Diabetes Association recommends aiming for an HbA$_{1c}$ less than 7%.) You can empathize with his frustration; he's trying to do his part to keep his blood glucose within range, but his HbA$_{1c}$ keeps increasing. Why have his blood glucose readings gotten higher?

To understand the answer to this question, it helps to first understand why our bodies need insulin. Insulin is a hormone secreted by the beta cells of the pancreas that helps regulate the way the body uses one of its main sources of fuel, glucose. Its main job is to allow glucose in the blood to enter the cells of the body, where the glucose can be used for energy. Insulin also controls the rate at which glucose is produced and secreted by the liver. Glucose is stored in the liver in the form of *glycogen*. When a person's blood glucose level drops, the liver converts glycogen to glucose and releases this glucose into the bloodstream. When there is enough glucose in the bloodstream, insulin secreted by the pancreas signals the liver to shut down glucose production. In people who do not have diabetes, the pancreas continually measures blood glucose levels and responds by secreting just the right amount of insulin—whether it is during the night, before meals, or during periods of stress. However, in people with Type 2 diabetes, there is a flaw in the system.

The two main problems behind Type 2 diabetes are insulin resistance and inadequate insulin secretion because of a defect in the beta cells.

When a person has insulin resistance, the cells of his body are unable to take as much glucose from the bloodstream as they should, even when there's a lot of insulin in the bloodstream. That is, the cells resist the insulin. On top of that, the liver may continue to secrete a lot of glucose into the bloodstream even when it isn't needed. So insulin resistance can lead to higher blood glucose levels, especially following meals, and this causes the pancreas to secrete more insulin to compensate. At first, this may keep blood glucose levels within the normal range, but eventually the overworked beta cells produce less and less insulin.

So what happened to Al? His beta cells no longer secrete enough insulin for his needs. He could exercise like a professional athlete, follow a restricted diet, and follow every guideline for self-management, and his blood sugar levels would remain high simply because his pancreas cannot make enough insulin.

It's not his fault...

Al is upset because he has tried hard to keep his blood glucose level within his target range, and he feels as though he has failed. But the truth is that Al didn't fail; his pancreas did. In fact, his efforts at exercise and healthy eating probably created an environment that prolonged the life of his beta cells. Research confirms that the nature of Type 2 diabetes involves the progressive loss of beta-cell function. Taking the burden of producing lots of insulin off the beta cells by treating insulin resistance through weight loss, healthy eating, exercise, and certain medicines is clearly effective. In fact, the research devoted to the delay and prevention of Type 2 diabetes has shown the importance of preserving beta-cell function as well as reducing insulin resistance.

For years, people worried that one group of pills used to treat diabetes, the sulfonylureas, might be contributing to the decline of the beta cells. These pills, namely glyburide (DiaBeta, Glynase, Micronase), glipizide (Glucotrol, Glucotrol XL), and glimepiride (Amaryl), work by stimulating the pancreas to secrete more insulin. But research has proved that it is the beta-cell defect and progressive nature of Type 2 diabetes, not overstimulation by these pills, that leads to the decline in insulin production by the pancreas. Some people have a robust pancreas that continues to produce insulin when stimulated by these pills, and they never require injections of insulin. But if your pancreas no longer makes insulin, these pills will not help you.

There's a lot you can do to manage your diabetes. You can make healthy food choices, eat reasonable portions, exercise, lose weight, take your prescribed medicines, manage stress, and visit your health-care team regularly. In combination, these self-management practices can keep your blood glucose level (and blood pressure and cholesterol levels) within target range for a long time. But there are two things that you cannot control: your genes and the beta-cell defect of Type 2 diabetes. The need to make the transition to insulin therapy is not your fault.

Psychological resistance to insulin

Insulin resistance is one of the metabolic hallmarks of Type 2 diabetes, but psychological resistance to insulin is a horse of a different color. When faced with the need to take injections of insulin, many people resist. They plead, bargain, or never return to the health-care provider's office. But much of this aversion is caused by fear over misperceptions, because insulin is a highly effective treatment, one that some diabetes experts would one day like to see started sooner rather than later.

Fear of needles. This is one of the most common reasons people avoid insulin therapy and one of the easiest to surmount. Syringe and pen needles are so small and fine that you barely feel them, but don't take my word for it. Your diabetes educator or the nurse in your doctor's office can show you the tiny needle and help you to do an injection on yourself. Most people are immediately relieved by the ease of injection and absence of discomfort.

If you can't bring yourself to insert a needle in your skin, there are gadgets that will do it for you. These devices are designed so that you don't have to see the needle. With the BD Inject-Ease Automatic Injector and Medicool InstaJect, you just press a button and the needle is inserted under your skin. The Owen Mumford Autoject 2 not only inserts the needle but injects the insulin as well. There are devices to hide needles too, such as the NeedleAid device, which can be used with a syringe or insulin pen, and the PenMate, which conceals the needle on the NovoPen Junior and NovoPen 3. Jet injectors, including Medi-Jector Vision, AdvantaJet, GentleJet, and Vitajet 3 are needle-free. They force a stream of insulin through your skin with pressure, not a needle.

Having a negative experience or association with insulin. When some people are confronted with the need to inject insulin, they immediately think of someone they know who had a bad experience. One woman associated insulin with causing her aunt's blindness, because soon after her aunt started insulin therapy, she lost her vision. In reality, years of untreated diabetes was responsible for her aunt's loss of vision, not insulin. The most effective strategy for dealing with these negative experiences or associations is to share them with your health-care team. By learning what is worrying you, they can help you.

Feeling defeated. Some people report a sense of failure when they learn of their need for insulin therapy. They feel that they didn't take care of themselves, often because of a few pieces of cake they "shouldn't" have eaten or because of those times they were "too lazy" to exercise. Family members may reinforce these feelings because they don't understand that Type 2 diabetes is progressive, and they blame the person with diabetes for self-neglect.

If you feel defeated, remember that perfection is not the goal of diabetes self-management. Even if you chose not to make healthy food choices or to exercise in the past, insulin therapy is not a punishment. But it can be an opportunity to reevaluate your choices and get involved in managing your health. Once you know the facts about Type 2 diabetes, you'll see that you didn't fail; your pancreas did.

Insulin therapy as threat. For years, your doctor threatened you with insulin therapy if you didn't stop overeating. Unfortunately, this practice continues. Some well-intentioned health-care providers use insulin injections as a threat to motivate people. However, this only serves to send the message that insulin injections are something to be avoided, not that insulin is one of many effective treatments for diabetes. Health-care providers need to learn other methods for helping people who struggle with managing their diabetes.

Insulin inconvenience. It's true; it is easier to take pills. However, newer insulin delivery devices minimize the inconvenience of taking injections, and insulin regimens can be tailored to your needs and your routines to make it easier.

Permanent or temporary?

In the treatment of Type 2 diabetes, insulin therapy may be prescribed for a variety of reasons and may be permanent or temporary. For example, some people require short-term, or temporary, insulin therapy when they take certain drugs such as steroids to treat other medical conditions. Because steroids such as prednisone can cause extremely elevated blood glucose levels, insulin may be used to lower blood glucose levels during steroid use. Generally, when the steroids are discontinued, the person no longer requires insulin therapy.

Infection or long periods of untreated diabetes may cause a condition called *glucotoxicity*. When someone is glucotoxic, elevated blood glucose levels interfere with the body's ability to lower blood glucose. Short-term insulin therapy is used to lower blood glucose levels, eliminating the glucotoxicity and restoring the body's normal glucose regulation.

Effective treatments for insulin resistance include weight loss, exercise, and insulin-sensitizing medicines such as pioglitazone (Actos), rosiglitazone (Avandia), and metformin (Glucophage). But some people may also require large doses of injected insulin, at least initially, to get past the barrier of insulin resistance and keep their blood glucose within range. Once these people have lost weight and begun exercising, they may be able to discontinue insulin therapy—as long as their pancreas continues to produce insulin. But people who have both insulin resistance and a pancreas that cannot secrete enough insulin require permanent insulin replacement.

Insulin replacement strategies

Just as there are different reasons to use insulin therapy, there are different formulations of insulin that are prescribed based on what your body needs. To get past the barrier of insulin resistance or to combat glucotoxicity, long- or intermediate-acting formulations of insulin may be prescribed. The insulin analog glargine (Lantus) is a type of long-acting insulin that is typically injected at bedtime and usually effective for up to 24 hours. Other long-acting insulins include insulin analog detemir (Levemir) and NPH insulin. These insulins are effective for less than 24 hours. They are generally injected once or twice per day.

When both insulin resistance and inadequate secretion of insulin by the pancreas are the prob-

lem, two different insulin formulations are needed: one long-acting *basal* insulin and one short-acting *bolus* insulin. The basal insulin supplies the low-level, background insulin needed by the body at all times; the short-acting bolus insulin supplies the insulin your body needs at mealtimes to handle the glucose from food. So-called "mealtime" insulins include Regular and the rapid-acting insulin analogs lispro (Humalog), aspart (NovoLog), and (Apidra).

Some people who need both long-acting basal and short-acting bolus insulins use premixed insulins such as Humulin 50/50, Humulin 70/30, Novolin 70/30, Humalog Mix 75/25, Humalog Mix 50/50 or NovoLog Mix 70/30. A dose of 50 units of Humulin or Novolin 70/30 provides a combined basal insulin (NPH) dose of 35 units and a bolus insulin (Regular) dose of 15 units. Other people mix their own long-acting and short-acting insulins or take each separately.

Practical concerns

If you are considering insulin therapy or if your health-care team is recommending insulin therapy, you're probably wondering about the day-to-day mechanics of using insulin. Although this is not an exhaustive list, it may help you to get an overview of the subject.

Timing of injections. Taking your injections around the same time of day is important because insulin formulations release insulin into your system over a period of time, and although some basal insulins maintain a rather constant level of insulin in your bloodstream, other increase, peak, and decrease. If you inject your NPH insulin at 6 PM one night and 11 PM another night, you will see potentially wide variations in your blood glucose levels.

The rapid-acting insulins aspart, glulisine and lispro can start to lower your blood glucose within five minutes of an injection, so they should be taken just before or after meals. If you wait too long to eat after injecting aspart or lispro, your blood glucose level could drop too low.

Mixing insulins. Insulin glargine (Lantus) and insulin detemir (Levemir) cannot be mixed in the same syringe with any other insulin. NPH insulin can be mixed with Regular, insulin aspart, glulisine, or lispro.

Insulin delivery systems. Insulin is injected into a fatty part of the body so that the blood supply that feeds fat can absorb the insulin for use in the body. A syringe filled with insulin from a vial is the traditional method of delivering insulin. Pen-shaped devices called insulin pens, which are either prefilled with insulin or loaded with a cartridge of insulin, are also used. Devices prefilled with insulin called insulin dosers, which have a large display or dial for easier measurement of insulin doses, are also available.

The insulin delivery system that you choose to use can be based on your preferences, cost of the system and reimbursement, manual dexterity, visual acuity, and your unique lifestyle issues.

Storage. All insulin vials or pens not in use should be stored in the refrigerator. Most opened vials of insulin can be stored at room temperature for up to 28 days (insulin detemir is 42 days), after which they should be discarded. Prefilled insulin pens, insulin dosers, and insulin cartridges have very specific room temperature storage guidelines of 10, 14, or 28 days depending on the type of insulin. Insulin stored beyond the room temperature storage guideline may be significantly less effective if used.

Checking blood glucose levels. There is no exact formula for deciding on an insulin dose, but one of the key factors used in regulating insulin doses is your blood glucose level. Blood glucose monitoring becomes an indispensable tool when you make the transition to insulin therapy. How often you need to check your blood glucose depends at least in part on the type of insulin prescribed. Plan to check more frequently when you first begin insulin therapy so that adjustments to your regimen can be made.

Side effects

The most common side effect of insulin therapy is hypoglycemia, or low blood sugar. Hypoglycemia is also a side effect of the sulfonylureas, the pills that stimulate the pancreas to secrete more insulin. Most episodes of hypoglycemia can be traced back to one of the following: taking too much insulin or oral medicine, skipping or delaying a meal, exercising strenuously without having a snack or carbohydrate drink, and drinking alcohol. Common signs and symptoms of hypoglycemia include sudden weakness, shaking, sweating, headache, hunger, palpitations, confusion, blurred vision, and irritability.

If you suspect you have hypoglycemia, check your blood glucose level with your meter to confirm it. To treat low blood sugar, eat or drink 15 grams of carbohydrate, wait 15 minutes for the carbohydrate to be absorbed, and check your blood glucose level again. If it has not increased in 15 minutes, eat or drink another 15 grams of carbohydrate and check again in 15 minutes. Some common foods containing 15 grams of carbohy-

drate include 4 ounces of orange juice, 6 ounces of ginger ale, 3 BD glucose tablets, 4 Dex4 tablets, and 6 saltine crackers.

Some people put up with frequent hypoglycemia because they can manage it well. But frequent hypoglycemia is a sign that something is wrong, and it can even be dangerous. When untreated or unrecognized, hypoglycemia can lead to seizures and loss of consciousness. Report episodes of hypoglycemia to your health-care provider.

Other than hypoglycemia, serious reactions to human insulin are rare. However, injecting insulin into the same spot over and over can cause the area to become thick and hard (a condition called lipohypertrophy) or pitted and dented (a condition called lipoatrophy). When tissues become damaged in these ways, insulin injected into these sites may not be absorbed consistently, causing your blood glucose levels to fluctuate. Lipohypertrophy and lipoatrophy can be avoided by changing the site of injection within an injection area such as the abdomen each time you inject. For each shot, pick a new site a finger's width away from your last injection.

Frequently asked questions

People who are starting insulin therapy naturally have questions. I've listed and answered some of them below.

Does insulin make you gain weight?
In addition to allowing glucose in the blood to enter the cells of the body, insulin also helps the body store fat. If you don't have enough insulin, you lose weight, and if you have too much insulin, you gain weight.

If you routinely take more insulin (or sulfonlyureas) than your body needs, you will gain weight. This could happen, say, if you kept your blood glucose in the 60–70 mg/dl range and endured frequent bouts of hypoglycemia. If your blood glucose levels fall too low frequently, contact your health-care provider and talk about lowering your insulin dose.

Some people view insulin therapy as a license to eat whatever they want because they can just take more insulin to keep their blood sugar level in range. If you frequently overeat and inject extra insulin, however, you will gain weight.

If your pancreas is not secreting enough insulin and your blood glucose is elevated, your cells will use fat for energy, and you will lose weight. Once insulin therapy is initiated and your body burns glucose instead of fat, you will gain the weight back. This is a positive sign that your body is working properly again.

What is an insulin pump?

Another option for delivery of insulin, an insulin pump is a beeper-size device that contains a cartridge filled with short-acting insulin analog. Most pumps are connected to small, flexible tubing, and the tip of the tubing is inserted into the fatty tissue under the skin. One pump model does not require tubing as the insulin is contained in a pod that is worn on your skin. Insulin pumps release small amounts of insulin into the body every few minutes. When food is eaten, the pump can deliver a larger quantity of insulin right away. With a pump, you get closer to receiving the right amount of insulin at the right time: large amounts when you eat and small amounts between meals. The rate of insulin delivery can also be adjusted for exercise, periods of stress or illness, and other activities or occurrences that might affect blood glucose level. Insulin pumps are used most commonly by people with Type 1 diabetes, but people with Type 2 diabetes who require insulin therapy can be candidates for insulin pump therapy. Even Medicare provides reimbursement to people who meet certain criteria.

What does it mean if I have to keep taking more insulin?

Taking more insulin does not mean that you are getting sicker. Health-care providers use a formula to decide your starting dose, but they always begin with a small dose because the formula only serves as a guideline. When beginning insulin therapy, you would expect to slowly increase the dose of insulin based on your blood glucose monitoring results. The dose of insulin that works for you depends on factors such as the amount of insulin your pancreas still makes, how resistant you are to insulin, your activity level, other medicines you take that raise blood glucose, and how much you eat.

You can make a smoother transition to insulin therapy when you have help. Seek the counsel of a certified diabetes educator with whom you can share your concerns and feelings about insulin therapy. Starting insulin is a big step, but the payoff—better blood glucose control—is worth the effort. □

INSULIN DELIVERY DEVICES

by Stacy Griffin, Pharm.D., and Laura Hieronymus,
M.S.Ed., A.P.R.N., B.C.-A.D.M., C.D.E.

Change does not necessarily assure progress, but progress implacably requires change. Education is essential to change, for education creates both new wants and the ability to satisfy them.
—Henry Steele Commager

Insulin is a necessary part of the treatment plan for all people with Type 1 diabetes and many with Type 2. Insulin helps get glucose from the bloodstream into the muscle and fat cells to be used for fuel. It cannot be taken as a pill or a swallowed liquid, because it would be broken down by the digestive system before it reached the bloodstream, where insulin does its work. Instead, insulin is injected or infused into the fatty tissue under the skin or absorbed through the lungs when aerosolized and inhaled through the mouth.

There are a number of devices that can be used to deliver insulin, including syringes, insulin pens, jet injectors, insulin pumps, and an inhaler. No single device or type of device works well for everyone. The decision of which to use may be based on a person's insulin regimen, ability to manipulate or operate a particular device, visual ability, insurance coverage or ability to afford a particular device and related supplies, occupation, and daily schedule or leisure-time activities. Discussing your needs and preferences with your diabetes care team is the best way to pick the device that will work well for you and get the training you need to use it correctly.

Syringes

The most common method of insulin delivery in the United States is by syringe. Medical syringes are relatively small, are disposable, and have fine needles with special coatings that make injecting as easy and painless as possible. To take insulin with a syringe, the user first pulls back on the plunger to draw in air equal to the amount of insulin to be drawn, inserts the syringe needle into a vial of insulin, pushes the air into the vial, pulls back on the plunger until the correct dose is drawn into the syringe barrel, then inserts the nee-

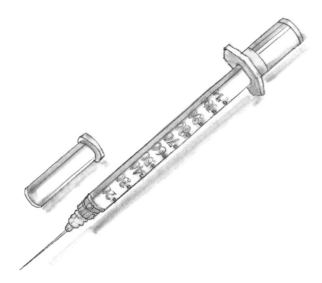

dle through the skin and presses down on the plunger until the barrel is emptied.

People who have difficulty drawing up insulin doses on their own may be able to have a caregiver draw up doses in advance and store the filled syringes in the refrigerator with the needles pointing upward until needed. (Placing the needles in a small cup will keep them upright.) If you use this option, be sure to discuss with your diabetes care team how far in advance syringes can be filled.

Syringes come in a variety of sizes, with different barrel sizes, different needle gauges (thicknesses), and different needle lengths. The higher the gauge, the finer (thinner) the needle. Your diabetes care team will help choose the appropriate syringe for you based on the sizes of your insulin doses and your personal preference for needle gauge and length. While some people may prefer a shorter needle, insulin leakage at the injection site or worsening blood glucose control are signs that a longer needle may be necessary to deliver the insulin properly.

Reusing syringes is not recommended due to potential complications such as more painful injections as the needle dulls with use, infection, or tissue damage. The best practice is to use a new syringe for each injection.

If you travel outside of the United States, it is important to be aware that insulin is manufactured in different strengths; however, U-100 (100 units of insulin per milliliter [ml] of fluid) is the most common strength. The syringes for administering insulin are specifically designed for each different strength. Therefore, a U-100 syringe should normally only be used with U-100 insulin. All insulin syringes in the United States are designed for use with U-100 insulin.

While most insulin sold in the United States is U-100, people who are severely insulin resistant may use U-500 (500 units of insulin per ml). However, no U-500 syringes are manufactured, so people who are prescribed U-500 insulin must work with their diabetes care team to learn how to draw up the correct dose in a U-100 syringe.

Injection aids. Various types of injection aids can make injecting with a syringe easier in some situations. Injection aids that hide the syringe needle can be helpful for people with needle phobia. Those that guide or insert the needle into the skin or that insert the needle and inject the insulin can be useful for children who give their own injections, people who have difficulty seeing, or people who have unsteady hands, pain or numbness in their hands, or difficulty manipulating syringes for some other reason. Vial stabilizers and syringe magnifiers may be helpful in drawing up accurate doses of insulin. Brightly colored vial sleeves and caps can help with identifying different types of insulin if more than one type is used.

Before purchasing any kind of injection aid, make sure it is compatible with the type and brand of syringes you use.

Insulin pens

Insulin pens look similar to oversized ink pens, making them a potentially convenient and discreet way of carrying insulin. To use an insulin pen, the pen cap is removed and a pen needle is attached. The pen is then "primed" by dialing in a very small dose (exactly how much depends on the particular pen) and expelling the insulin into the air. Priming is done to ensure that insulin is flowing through the pen properly and that there is no air in the cartridge or needle.

After priming is completed, the actual dose of insulin to be administered is dialed in using a dial or dose knob. The needle is inserted into the skin,

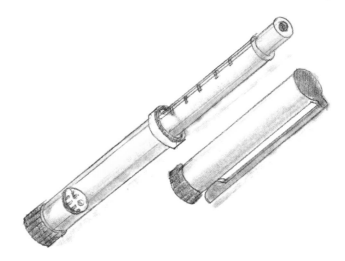

and the dose is delivered by pressing on the dose knob until it is fully depressed. It is important to hold the pen in place and to continue pressing the dose knob while counting slowly to five before removing the needle from your skin to ensure that no insulin leaks out. Pen needles are intended for one use only and should be removed and discarded after an injection.

Insulin pens should never be stored with the needle still attached because doing so may allow insulin to leak out or air bubbles to form in the insulin cartridge. Between uses, the pen's cap should be put on to protect the insulin cartridge. In-use pens or pen cartridges should not be stored in the refrigerator because of the possibility that condensation will form in the insulin container. (As soon as an insulin cartridge is placed in a pen, it is considered "in-use" and should no longer be stored in the refrigerator, even if the pen is not actually used for an injection for several days.)

Most pens hold 300 units (3 ml) of insulin and deliver doses in one-unit increments, with up to 60 to 80 units per dose. The NovoPen Junior and the HumaPen Luxura HD deliver insulin in half-unit increments. One of the biggest advantages of insulin pens is accurate dosing. Ease of use is another advantage of pens over syringes because they require less manual dexterity and coordination, and they may be easier to use for people with low vision.

Like syringes, pen needles also come in a variety of needle gauges and lengths. However, pen needles may be slightly thinner and in some cases shorter than syringe needles, so injections may be more comfortable.

Some pens are disposable, while others use replaceable cartridges of insulin that are inserted into the pen.

Prefilled pens. Prefilled, plastic, disposable insulin pens have a self-contained insulin cartridge. Several different types of insulin are sold in prefilled pens. Once you have used all of the insulin in the cartridge (or the insulin has reached its in-use expiration date), you dispose of the entire pen.

While most insulin pens look like writing pens, one exception is the InnoLet, a disposable device that looks more like a kitchen timer with a big round dial. The big dial with large, easy-to-read numbers makes the InnoLet easier to use for some people with visual difficulties or dexterity problems. In addition, the relatively large size of the device also may make it easier to hold securely against the skin while administering insulin doses, particularly for people with arthritis, tremors, or shaky hands. The InnoLet holds 300 units of insulin.

Durable pens. Insulin pens that use replaceable cartridges of insulin are also available. Most reusable pens are made of metal but otherwise have about the same features as disposable pens and a comparable cost. One exception is the HumaPen Memoir, which was approved for use in April 2007. It has some additional features, including a memory of the 16 most recent doses delivered (including priming doses) and the time they were administered, as well as a five-second timer to help the user hold the pen in place long enough after injecting.

Jet injectors

Another option that has been available for several years is insulin jet injectors. Jet injectors use a mechanism to produce high-pressure air to deliver a fine spray of insulin through the skin. Once the appropriate dose of insulin has been loaded into the injector, it is placed against the skin and the trigger, or button, is pushed. The high pressure causes the insulin to vaporize and penetrate the skin so that it reaches the subcutaneous tissue.

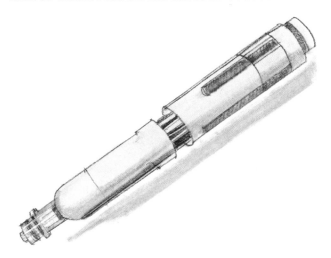

Some bruising may occur from injections using a jet injector, but bruising can be minimized by adjusting the pressure (setting) of the spray. The pressure may have to be adjusted differently for different injection sites.

It is extremely important to follow the manufacturer's guidelines on the care and cleaning of the device to maintain sterility. Jet injectors are generally not recommended for people who take blood thinners, are undergoing dialysis, or have hemophilia.

If you are interested in using a jet injector, work with your diabetes care team to learn the proper technique. In addition, check with your insurer to determine whether the cost of the device is covered.

External insulin pump

Insulin pumps are becoming more popular as the technology improves and additional features are added. Some pumps are now available that work in conjunction with continuous glucose monitors that can alert the user to high or low blood glucose levels if programmed to do so.

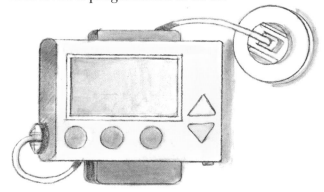

Insulin pumps have traditionally been used primarily by people with Type 1 diabetes, but they are becoming a treatment of choice for many with Type 2 diabetes, as well. Most insulin pumps are small devices about the size of a pager. (The exception is the OmniPod, which is even smaller and is attached directly to the skin, with no tubing necessary.) The pump itself can be clipped onto the waistband of your pants or skirt or placed in a pocket. A length of plastic tubing connects the insulin reservoir within the pump to the infusion set, which is taped onto the skin and contains a small catheter (often called a cannula), through which insulin enters the body. The catheter is commonly inserted into the abdomen or buttocks and needs to be changed every 48 hours.

The pump user programs the insulin pump to deliver insulin at a slow, continuous (basal) rate as well as in supplemental (bolus) doses before meals and to correct for high blood glucose. Basal and bolus dosing most closely resembles how the pancreas releases insulin in a person without diabetes.

Using an insulin pump requires commitment and frequent blood glucose monitoring. According to the American Diabetes Association, people who demonstrate the following characteristics are more likely to do well with pump therapy:
■ Strongly motivated to improve glucose control
■ Willing to work with their diabetes care team
■ Willing to assume substantial responsibility for their day-to-day care
■ Able to understand and demonstrate use of the insulin pump

■ Willing and able to frequently perform self-monitoring of blood glucose
■ Knowledgeable about using their blood glucose monitoring data to make dose adjustments

Many people are willing to put in the work necessary to use an insulin pump because it gives them more flexibility with respect to food choices and the timing of meals and activities, while helping to achieve tighter control of their blood glucose.

Disposal of needles

Most states require that used needles and other "sharps" (such as lancets) be disposed of in a way that reduces the risk of accidental needle sticks. Once you've used a needle or lancet, place it in a puncture-resistant container such as a liquid detergent bottle or a sharps container purchased at your local pharmacy. (When traveling, carry a small container with you.)

Some communities offer a sharps disposal program that allows you to drop off your sharps at particular locations such as hospitals or pharmacies. If your area does not have such a program, discard your puncture-resistant sharps containers by placing the lid securely onto the container, taping it shut, and marking it "USED SHARPS." Place the container in the trash, not in a recycling container. Other options for disposing of sharps include sharps mail-back programs and home needle destruction devices.

Your diabetes care team can help you learn the guidelines that are specific to your state. Another place to find information on relevant state laws and regulations is the Center for Disease Control and Prevention Web site www.cdc.gov/needledisposal.

Traveling with diabetes supplies

When traveling, keep your diabetes supplies with you. Never place insulin or other liquid medicines in checked baggage, where they could be exposed to freezing or very hot temperatures. The Transportation Security Administration currently allows the following items on commercial airplanes once they have been screened at the security checkpoint in the airport:
■ Insulin and insulin-loaded dispensing products (vials of insulin, jet injectors, pens, infusers, and preloaded syringes) that are clearly identified with a prescription label containing a name that matches the passenger's name on his ticket
■ Other liquid prescription medicines such as Symlin, Byetta, or a glucagon emergency kit that are clearly identified with a prescription label containing a name that matches the passenger's name on his ticket

INSULIN DELIVERY DEVICE COMPARISON

DEVICE	ADVANTAGES	DISADVANTAGES
Syringe	Costs less than other devices. Syringes are available in range of sizes. Caregiver can draw up doses in advance.	More difficult to manipulate than other devices, particularly for people with low vision or numbness, stiffness, or tremors in the hands.
Prefilled pen	Accurate dosing. Convenient, discreet, and easy to use.	May have to give two shots if dose size exceeds maximum allowed at one time. Not covered by all insurance plans.
Durable (refillable) pen	Accurate dosing. Convenient, discreet, and easy to use. At least one pen offers a memory function to track recent doses.	May have to give two shots if dose size exceeds maximum allowed at one time. Not covered by all insurance plans. Must choose compatible cartridges.
Jet injector	Convenient and discreet. No needles.	Can be costly. May cause bruising. Device requires regular cleaning. Not covered by all insurance plans.
Insulin pump	More lifestyle flexibility. Most similar to how a healthy pancreas releases insulin. Medicare covers for Types 1 and 2 diabetes, if eligible. Some pumps work with continuous glucose monitor.	Pump and supplies can be expensive. Not covered by all insurance plans. More complex treatment regimen.

■ An unlimited number of unused syringes, when accompanied by insulin or other injectable medicine
■ Clearly labeled nonprescription liquid medicines, such as Regular insulin, which in some states does not require a doctor's prescription to dispense
■ Blood glucose meters, test strips, continuous glucose monitors, lancets, and other monitoring supplies
■ Insulin pump and insulin pump supplies
■ An unlimited number of used syringes when transported in a sharps disposal container or other similar hard-surface container

In general, liquids, gels, and aerosols (such as toothpaste and shampoo) must be in three-ounce or smaller containers and must be placed in a single quart-size, zip-top plastic bag to be brought aboard an airplane. However, there are no limits on the amounts of prescription or over-the-counter medicines that come in a liquid, gel, or aerosol form that may be brought onto an airplane. These items should be packed separately from the items in the quart-size plastic bag.

Cost considerations

Always check with your insurance company to determine whether and which insulin injection devices and supplies are covered by your plan and what out-of-pocket costs are involved. If you do not have insurance coverage (or do not have prescription coverage), many pharmaceutical manufacturers offer patient assistance programs, which offer free or low-cost drugs and supplies to individuals who are unable to pay for their medicine. For more information, look on a specific company's Web site or the Web sites www.rxassist.org or www.needymeds.com, or contact the Partnership for Prescription Assistance either online, at www.pparx.org, or by telephone, at (888) 477-2669.

Making your choice

The basic purpose of all insulin delivery devices is the same: to deliver the desired dose of insulin into the body to keep blood glucose levels under control. The device you choose should be one that's easy for you to use and to afford. But picking one insulin delivery device now doesn't mean you can't switch to another—or to a combination of devices—in the future. If your needs, lifestyle, or fortunes change, you may decide that a different device might work better for you in your new situation.

To learn more about your insulin delivery device options, speak to the members of your diabetes care team, look at the Web sites or call the companies that manufacture such devices, and look for articles and product reviews in magazines such as this one or on reliable Web sites about diabetes. Work closely with your diabetes care team to make sure you know how to use the device you choose effectively so that you can take the best care of yourself possible. □

Drugs and Dietary Supplements

Tips 303–365 199

Vitamins in Food and Supplements. 204

Minerals in Food and Supplements. 211

Antioxidants. 219
Should You Supplement?

Amylin 224
Insulin's Partner

Exenatide 227
From the Gila Monster to You

Oral Medicine for Type 2 Diabetes 230

Blood Pressure Drugs 236
What Are the Options?

5

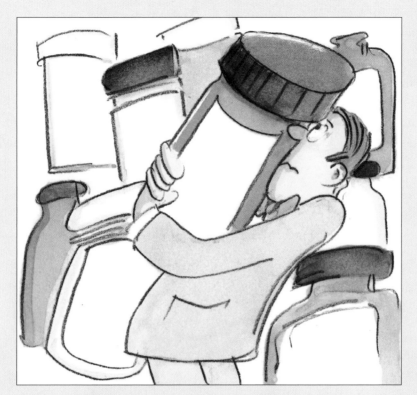

Drugs and Dietary Supplements Tips

303–365

303. Exenatide (brand name Byetta) may provide better blood glucose control for people with Type 2 diabetes when oral medicine is inadequate.

304. People who take both a sulfonylurea drug and exenatide should watch out for low blood glucose, a risk of this drug combination.

305. Exenatide may reduce appetite and cause weight loss in addition to its main purpose of stimulating insulin secretion in response to high blood glucose.

306. Pramlintide (brand name Symlin) can smooth postmeal blood glucose spikes in people with both Type 1 and Type 2 diabetes by delaying the entry of glucose into the bloodstream: It suppresses the appetite, slows stomach emptying, and inhibits the release of glucose by the liver.

307. Evidence is mounting that high postmeal blood glucose levels, in particular, contribute to a higher incidence of kidney, eye, nerve, heart, and blood vessel complications.

308. Pramlintide may reduce oxidative stress, a process driven by excess glucose in the bloodstream that may be responsible for many diabetic complications.

309. Pramlintide may increase the risk of low blood glucose, and insulin doses must be modified to account for pramlintide's glucose-lowering effects.

310. If you and your doctor decide to supplement your oral diabetes medicine with a new one, you may be able to take a single combination pill of both drugs.

311. Alpha-glucosidase inhibitors may be a good drug choice to control postmeal elevations in blood glucose; these drugs inhibit the breakdown absorption of carbohydrates from the digestive system.

312. If alpha-glucosidase inhibitors are taken with another drug that carries a risk of low blood glucose, many carbohydrate sources will no longer be effective at raising blood glucose levels quickly because of the effect of the drug; sources of pure glucose are recommended.

313. Metformin may be useful in treating insulin resistance that can occur during puberty in adolescents with Type 1 diabetes, in addition to the drug's normal use for Type 2 diabetes. This is, however, not an FDA-approved use of the drug.

314. If you are supposed to take an oral diabetes drug with a meal, do not take it any other time without first checking with your health-care provider. Some types of medicine increase insulin secretion and could result in low blood glucose if taken without a meal.

315. Vitamins C and E, carotenoids such as beta-carotene, and other nutrients from plants play an important antioxidant role in the body. Oxidative damage has been linked to heart disease, nervous system disorders, cancer, arthritis, kidney disease, multiple sclerosis, bowel diseases, eye disorders, and diabetes.

316. Vitamin C may protect against damage to DNA within cells throughout the body.

317. Good sources of vitamin C include guava, red and green bell peppers, kiwifruit, and oranges.

318. Vitamin E can prevent oxidative degradation of cell membranes and fatty nerve tissue.

319. Good sources of vitamin E include wheat germ and wheat germ oil, sunflower seeds and sunflower oil, almonds, safflower oil, and hazelnuts.

320. Some studies have shown increased oxidative damage and decreased antioxidant activity in people with diabetes, suggesting that an increased intake of antioxidants may be helpful.

321. Research indicates that adequate vitamin E intake may significantly reduce the risk of developing Type 2 diabetes. Vitamin E may also reduce the HbA_{1c} level of people with Type 2 diabetes and improve heart function.

322. Studies have shown that carotenoids (such as beta-carotene) may improve glucose metabolism by reducing insulin resistance and fasting blood glucose levels.

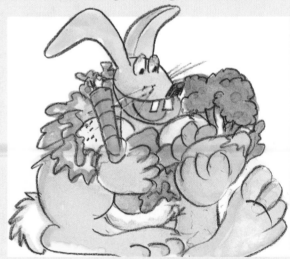

323. Good sources of beta-carotene include apricots, broccoli, cantaloupe, carrots, papaya, sweet potatoes, pumpkin and other winter squashes, and leafy green vegetables.

324. Consuming alpha-lipoic acid may improve blood glucose control and more generally reduce oxidative damage in people with Type 2 diabetes. It has

Drugs and Dietary Supplements

also been shown to reduce some symptoms of neuropathy and improve blood circulation.

325. Although a vitamin supplement is generally no match for a nutritious diet, it may offer benefits if a diet lacks essential nutrients.

326. Older people with a decreased appetite, reduced taste or smell, dental problems, or a decreased ability to absorb nutrients like zinc, vitamin D, calcium, vitamin B_{12} folate, or vitamin B_6, may need to use vitamin supplements to achieve adequate nutrition.

327. People who smoke generally need to consume a higher level of vitamin C.

328. Premenopausal women, teens, and pregnant women may benefit from iron and calcium supplements.

329. People who consume excess alcohol may have various increased nutrient requirements due to alcohol's interference with nutrient absorption.

330. Vegans (people who consume no meat, eggs, or dairy) may require zinc, calcium, vitamin D, and vitamin B_{12} supplements.

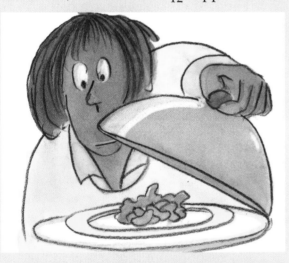

331. People whose daily diet contains less than 1200 calories may need nutritional supplements.

332. People who must avoid large categories of food because of allergies, or who have gastrointestinal disorders, may need various types of nutritional supplements.

333. Blood glucose control is essential to maintaining adequate levels of vitamins and minerals in the body. People with diabetes who have frequent high blood glucose may need nutritional supplements because of the loss of nutrients with glucose in the urine.

334. Some medicines that may reduce nutrient absorption include metformin and many diuretics. If you take either of these, ask your health-care provider about supplementation.

335. Some supplements may affect how certain medicines are absorbed, so be sure to tell your doctor about anything that you take.

336. If you take a nutritional supplement, you should know the established % Daily Value (%DV) or adequate intake (AI) of the nutrient or nutrients included, as well as the tolerable upper intake level (UL), to make sure that you are not oversupplementing.

337. Moderate doses of niacin may improve cholesterol and triglyceride levels without worsening blood glucose control, as high doses have been shown to do.

338. People who do not get regular sun exposure and who do not get enough vitamin D from fortified foods such as milk may want to consider a supplement; however, vitamin D supplements should only be taken with a doctor's supervision due to a higher chance of oversupplementation than with most nutrients.

339. Remember that more is not better when it comes to vitamins: Choose a multivitamin that supplies no more than 100% of the % Daily Value for each nutrient included.

340. Many people stand to benefit from stand-alone calcium supplements; most other essential nutrients can be found in a multivitamin.

341. Look for supplements with the U.S. Pharmacopeia (USP) symbol to ensure quality.

342. Always check the expiration date and follow storage guidelines of a supplement.

343. The most important nutrients to have in a supplement are vitamins, A, B_6, B_{12},

D, and E, thiamine, riboflavin, niacin, folic acid, zinc, magnesium, calcium, and iron.

344. To make dietary changes to include more vitamins and minerals in the diet, plan ahead—prepare fruits and vegetables ahead of time so that you can eat them right away when you're hungry.

345. Stock up on canned, frozen, or dried fruits and vegetables, in addition to fresh ones, so that they are always available with a smaller risk of spoilage.

346. Try adding canned beans, whole-grain pasta, nuts, canned or dried fruit, or frozen peas or corn to salads to increase the nutritional value.

347. Bring healthy, nonperishable foods to work to eat as snacks or as part of lunch.

348. In people with diabetes, having high blood pressure increases the risk of stroke, aneurysm (bulging of a blood vessel), heart attack, heart failure, narrowed arteries in the legs, eye damage, and kidney damage.

349. Have your blood pressure measured regularly; until damage occurs, hypertension generally has no symptoms. Numerous treatment options, including drug treatments, are available.

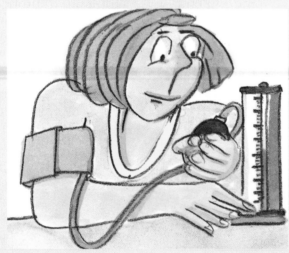

350. If you have been advised to take your blood pressure regularly, you may want to invest in a home blood pressure monitor. They start out under $30, and your insurance might cover part or all of it.

351. In people over the age of 50, systolic blood pressure (the top number) over 140 mm Hg has been found to be a greater risk factor for cardiovascular disease than diastolic blood pressure.

352. People with a systolic blood pressure of 120 to 139 mm Hg and a diastolic pressure of 80 to 89 mm Hg should consider themselves "prehypertensive" and make lifestyle changes to help prevent cardiovascular disease.

353. Some antihypertensive drugs could cause problems if stopped suddenly; never stop taking one without first consulting your doctor.

354. If you take a diuretic, in may be helpful to take it early in the day to reduce the chance of having to get up during the night to urinate.

355. Take your drugs at the same time every day. Try to link taking them with something else that you do regularly, like brushing your teeth. If your doctor told you to take your pills with food, try taking them at the same time as you have your meal every day.

356. The best way to achieve a diet with adequate vitamins and minerals is to emphasize fruits, vegetables, whole grains, fat-free or low-fat milk products, lean meat and poultry, beans, eggs, and nuts.

357. Adequate intake of the mineral chromium is necessary for normal blood glucose metabolism, as well as for metabolism of blood fats. Chromium has been shown in clinical trials to reduce the HbA_{1c} levels of people with Type 2 diabetes.

358. Diabetes places people with both Type 1 and Type 2 diabetes at increased risk for low magnesium levels, due to loss of the mineral in the urine. An adequate intake of magnesium is therefore important; it may also improve glucose metabolism and reduce cardiovascular disease.

359. Copper supplementation is not recommended for people with diabetes due to the tendency to have already high copper levels.

360. People with diabetes are at increased risk for zinc deficiency. An adequate intake has been shown to support normal immune system function.

361. Consuming low-fat dairy products as part of a diet high in fruits and vegetables and low in fat has been shown to decrease blood pressure as much as some blood pressure drugs.

362. Consuming adequate calcium, along with vitamin D, is necessary to maintain bone calcium stores and reduce the risk of osteoporosis and fracture.

363. Do not avoid calcium entirely if you have kidney stones; some types of kidney stones may actually be reduced by a high-calcium diet. Ask your doctor how much calcium you can consume of you have kidney stones.

364. Most adults with diabetes should not take iron supplements, as it may worsen blood glucose control.

365. Adequate vitamin C intake may improve iron absorption from vegetable sources.

VITAMINS IN FOOD AND SUPPLEMENTS

by Belinda O'Connell, M.S., R.D., L.D.

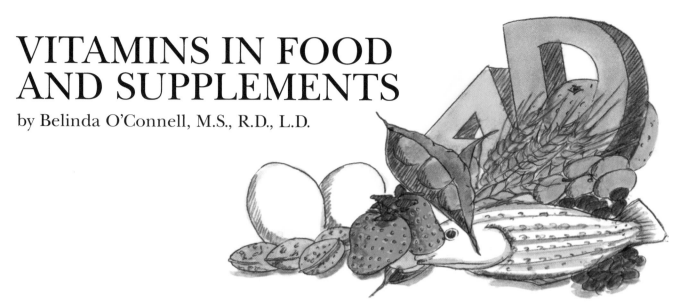

By now, just about everyone has heard that a diet high in fruits, vegetables, low-fat dairy products, and whole grains has health benefits, in part because such a diet is high in vitamins and minerals. But the percentage of Americans who actually eat enough of these foods remains quite low.

You may be one of those who is wondering if you should be taking a vitamin or mineral supplement to help fill in the gaps. Would a multivitamin be a good "insurance policy" for you? In addition, you may wonder if having diabetes changes your vitamin requirements, possibly meaning that a multivitamin or specific vitamin supplements would be good for you.

There's no simple answer to any of these questions, but this article examines what the research says about the role of vitamins in diet and health, the benefits and drawbacks of vitamin supplementation, and the possible roles of certain vitamins in diabetes management.

What are vitamins?

Vitamins are chemical compounds used by the body to perform basic functions necessary for good health. They act as important components of basic chemical reactions that produce energy, build tissue, and regulate body processes. With few exceptions, the body is unable to make vitamins itself, so they must be obtained through food or supplements on a regular basis. The body needs only small amounts of vitamins each day, but those small amounts are essential; even mild deficiencies can lead to serious disease states.

Vitamins are categorized as either water-soluble or fat-soluble. Water-soluble vitamins include vitamins B_6 and B_{12}, folate, thiamine, riboflavin, niacin, and vitamin C. These vitamins circulate in

the bloodstream, are filtered by the kidneys, and are excreted in urine. Fat-soluble vitamins such as vitamins A, D, E, and K also circulate in the bloodstream but are not excreted in the urine to a significant degree.

Supplements: help or hype?

Since vitamins are so important in promoting and maintaining optimal health, many people assume they need to take supplements to stay healthy. For the most part, this is not true. A diet high in fruits and vegetables, low-fat dairy products, and whole grains can provide all the vitamins and minerals most people need. What's more, this type of diet is associated with decreased rates of many diseases, including Type 2 diabetes, heart disease, and cancer.

People who attempt to compensate for poor-quality diets by taking vitamin and mineral supplements do not necessarily derive the same overall health benefits as those who follow healthy diets, even if their vitamin intake is comparable. In fact, a few studies suggest that high doses of certain vitamin supplements, such as beta-carotene and B vitamins, can actually be harmful. In addition, many nutrients, when consumed in very large amounts, can decrease the absorption of other nutrients, potentially causing new deficiencies.

The fact is, nothing is likely to be as good for you as eating a nutritious diet. But if you recognize that the quality of your diet is less than ideal, it is probably helpful to take a multivitamin that provides approximately 100% of the Daily Value for most vitamins and minerals while you work to improve your diet. (See "Choosing a Multivitamin" on page 205 for more information.)

There are some groups of people who have increased vitamin requirements, decreased ability

CHOOSING A MULTIVITAMIN

For most healthy people, a general multivitamin supplement will provide adequate levels of vitamins and minerals. As you shop and compare labels, keep in mind that more is not necessarily better when it comes to vitamins. Here are some tips to help you make your choice:

■ Choose a multivitamin that provides no more than 100% of the % Daily Value (%DV) for all nutrients included.

■ Avoid "high potency" formulations or supplements with megadoses of specific vitamins or minerals. Side effects are more likely, and high doses of many micronutrients can interfere with the absorption of others, causing secondary deficiencies.

■ The nutrients most important to have in your supplement are vitamins A, D, E, thiamine, riboflavin, niacin, B_6, B_{12}, folic acid, zinc, magnesium, calcium, and iron. Other nutrients such as potassium, phosphorus, biotin, and pantothenic acid are less important because they are either widely available in foods or not proven to be essential.

■ Generic and name-brand supplements are equally effective, so choose the one that is the most economical.

■ Avoid taking individual supplements of vitamins and minerals unless instructed to do so by your physician. The one exception to this rule is calcium. Many people need to take calcium as a single supplement to get adequate levels. It is generally safe for most people to use in levels up to 100% of the %DV (1,000 mg), but it is always a good idea to check with your doctor before starting any new supplement.

■ Most vitamin and mineral supplements are better absorbed with food and should be taken at mealtime. However, avoid taking calcium and iron supplements with other supplements or with meals because they may decrease the absorption of each other and of other nutrients.

■ Men and postmenopausal women who do not have a history of anemia generally do not need supplemental iron. Unless recommended by their physician, it is best for them to avoid using supplements that provide more than the %DV for iron. People with hemochromatosis should not take supplemental iron in any form.

■ Look for supplements that have the US Pharmacopeia (USP) symbol of quality. This ensures the supplement meets government quality guidelines.

■ Check expiration dates and follow storage guidelines for optimal potency of ingredients.

■ Do not remove childproof safety caps, and always leave original labels on all supplement containers in case of accidental overdose. Store all vitamins and supplements out of the reach of children. Accidental iron overdose is the most common cause of childhood death due to poisoning in the United States.

to absorb or process certain nutrients, or difficulty meeting nutrition guidelines with food sources alone. For these people, multivitamins or individual nutrient supplements may be necessary. People with increased risk of nutrition deficiencies or a clear need for supplementation include the following:

■ Older people, who often have a decreased appetite, loss of taste and smell, dental problems, and a decreased ability to absorb and process nutrients such as zinc, vitamin D, calcium, vitamin B_{12}, folate, and vitamin B_6, may need supplementation.

■ Pregnant and lactating women have increased requirements for many nutrients, including calcium, iron, and folate. It is recommended that these women meet their increased folate requirements by taking folic acid supplements or by eating foods fortified with folic acid. (Folic acid is the synthetic form of the vitamin folate and is more easily absorbed by the body.)

■ Premenopausal women also need supplemental folic acid and may benefit from iron and calcium supplements.

■ People who smoke have increased vitamin C requirements.

■ People who have excessive intakes of alcohol may have increased nutrient requirements due to alcohol's negative effects on the absorption and processing of some nutrients.

■ People using certain medicines often have increased requirements due to greater nutrient losses or decreased absorption.

■ Vegans (vegetarians who consume no eggs or dairy products) may require supplemental zinc, calcium, and vitamins D and B_{12}.

■ People on low-calorie diets (less than 1200 calories per day) may need supplementation.

■ People who avoid whole food groups—because of food allergies, for example, or food intolerances such as lactose intolerance or gluten intolerance, also called celiac disease—may need supplementation.

■ People who have significant gastrointestinal disorders or have had major gastrointestinal surgery may need supplementation.

In general, healthy people with diabetes have similar nutrient requirements to other healthy people and do not require vitamin and mineral supplements unless they fall into one of the above categories or have a poor-quality diet. However, there are several factors that can place people with diabetes at increased risk of developing nutrient deficiencies. Because vitamins and minerals are essential for normal glucose metabolism and because several key hormones involved in energy and glucose metabolism, including insulin, are known to affect body stores of vitamins and minerals, it is important that people with diabetes be aware of those factors.

A common cause of nutrient deficiencies in people with diabetes is frequent or chronic high blood glucose. When blood glucose levels are high, more glucose is filtered and excreted through the kidneys. Increased rates of urinary excretion leads to loss of water-soluble vitamins and some trace minerals. Over time, chronic high blood glucose can lead to depletion of the body's vitamin and mineral stores. So, along with eating a healthy diet, maintaining blood glucose levels in the desired range is a key factor in keeping stores of nutrients optimal.

Appropriate levels of insulin are necessary for normal metabolism of some nutrients. For example, insulin is used for the transport of the mineral magnesium into cells. When insulin levels are inadequate, intracellular stores of magnesium can become depleted. In addition to magnesium, zinc and vitamin A play a role in normal insulin production, secretion, and action. (While insufficient levels of some nutrients may impair insulin secretion, excessive levels of these same nutrients hinder insulin secretion.)

In some people with Type 1 diabetes, the autoimmune process that causes beta-cell destruction can also result in a reduced ability to absorb vitamin B_{12} and/or gluten intolerance. In the case of reduced vitamin B_{12} absorption, supplemental vitamin B_{12} is necessary. While gluten intolerance itself does not necessarily cause nutrition deficiencies, the need to restrict certain foods (including wheat and many processed foods) and malabsorption of nutrients during periods of inflammation increases the risk of them.

Many medicines are known to alter vitamin and mineral absorption, utilization, and excretion, including some commonly used by people with diabetes. Diuretics, for example, and the blood-glucose-lowering drug metformin (an active ingredient in Glucophage, Glucophage XR, and Glucovance) may have a negative impact on nutrient status. Conversely, some nutrients affect medicine absorption and function, so it is important that you discuss with your health-care team any multivitamin or individual nutrient supplements that you are taking.

How much is enough?

Vitamin and mineral supplements are beneficial only when a person does not get an adequate supply of a vitamin or mineral in his diet. Dietary supplements can cure an existing nutrition deficiency, but they do not further improve a person's health once body stores are adequate. In fact, vitamin and mineral supplements in doses greater than those needed by the body are generally just excreted in the urine, providing no benefit. Those that are not excreted in the urine have the potential to be toxic.

There are several different nutrition standards set by the government that can be helpful in determining how much of a specific nutrient is present in a food or supplement, how much you may need, and how much is too much.

The percent Daily Values (%DV), which are used on nutrition labels, were developed to help consumers select products that fit into a healthy diet. The %DV tells you the percentage of your nutrient requirements that is provided by one serving of the food or supplement. For instance ½ cup (4 ounces) of orange juice provides 60% of the Daily Value for vitamin C, or a little more than half of your daily vitamin C requirement. The %DV is the most useful standard for assessing how a particular food or supplement fits into your diet.

Other nutrition standards you might see are the Dietary Reference Intakes (DRIs), which include the Recommended Dietary Allowance (RDA) and the Tolerable Upper Intake Level (UL). The DRIs are standards for each nutrient that determine the minimum and maximum level of a nutrient needed in the diet to maintain optimal health.

The RDA is the level of nutrient intake believed to meet the nutrition requirements of 97% of healthy people in the United States. By definition, it is higher than many people's individual require-

IMPROVING YOUR DIET

The following tips suggest ways to increase your intake of fruits, vegetables, low-fat dairy products, and whole grains. Start by incorporating one or two ideas into your usual routine, then add one or two more as the others become habit.

■ If you work during the week, shop on weekends so you have healthful foods on hand during the week, when you may be short on time.

■ If you are retired or don't work traditional office hours, it may be more convenient to shop on weekdays, when the grocery store is less crowded.

■ Stock up on canned, frozen, or dried fruits and vegetables in addition to fresh so you don't have to worry about foods spoiling.

■ If you do not regularly drink milk or consume other low-fat dairy products, purchase calcium-fortified juices, cereals, grains, and rice when possible.

■ Set aside time (perhaps on the weekend) to prepare fresh vegetables in bulk so that they're ready when you are. Romaine lettuce that is washed and dried will last all week in a sealed plastic container in the refrigerator. Washed and cut-up carrots, peppers, broccoli, cauliflower, and green beans can also be kept in plastic bags in the refrigerator. They can be used in salads or stir-fries, added to tomato sauce for a hearty pasta dish, or cooked in the microwave for a quick side dish.

■ Even if you have trouble chewing, you may still be able to eat healthful foods such as canned fruits and vegetables, applesauce, bananas, vegetable juices and purées, and low-fat milk, yogurt, and cottage cheese.

■ Add canned beans, whole-grain pasta, nuts, canned or dried fruits, or frozen peas or corn to salads.

■ Stock up on nonperishable, boxed whole-grain and bean side dishes. Wild rice, bulgur, and rice and bean mixes are quick, easy to prepare, and come in a variety of flavors.

■ When you cook, prepare enough so that there are leftovers for tomorrow's lunch or dinner.

■ Bring healthful, nonperishable foods to work for lunches and snacks. Canned soups with vegetables and beans, instant rice dishes, chili, and oatmeal can be stored in a desk drawer and heated up in a microwave. Apples and oranges will hold for a week at room temperature. Whole-grain cereal can be stored at your desk and skim milk purchased at the cafeteria, vending machine, or corner store. The lunchroom refrigerator can store frozen dinners, a loaf of bread and turkey for sandwiches, or a week's worth of fruits, bagged lettuce, baby carrots, and low-fat yogurt.

---

ments, so intakes lower than the RDA are not necessarily deficient.

The UL is the highest intake of a nutrient that is not associated with significant side effects (although any intake above the RDA is more likely to cause side effects). If you are considering taking individual supplements or high-dose supplements, it's helpful to know both the RDA and the UL. You should never take more than the UL unless instructed to do so by your physician. You can find the RDA and UL of specific vitamins and minerals on the National Institutes for Health Office of Dietary Supplements Web site at http://dietary-supplements.info.nih.gov and http://ods.od.nih.gov.

If you choose to take a multivitamin, do not think of it as a substitute for a healthy diet. Many types of research have shown that diets high in fruits, vegetables, and whole grains can prevent and help treat many chronic diseases such as cancer, diabetes, cardiovascular disease, and hypertension. But research studies looking at the effects of nutrition supplements have not always shown the same benefits. Since we do not yet know how to duplicate the effects of a healthy diet in a pill, the best strategy is to obtain your nutrients from a wide variety of foods.

So how do you eat well if you're short on time, energy, or ideas? The most important thing to do when trying to make dietary changes is to plan ahead. Most of us would eat much better if we had healthy foods on hand when we were hungry. It is the thought of going to the grocery store, shopping, unpacking groceries, and then preparing dinner that sends most of us running for the fast-food drive-through. For some simple ideas on increasing the nutritional value of your meals, see "Improving Your Diet" above.

Vitamins in diabetes management

The American Diabetes Association (ADA) currently recommends the use of vitamin and mineral supplements only in cases where a deficiency can be demonstrated or where general guidelines for supplement use in the U.S. population apply, as in pregnancy. The ADA additionally recognizes that people with diabetes who are at increased risk for nutrient deficiencies may benefit from a multivitamin supplement.

That said, the potential therapeutic role of vitamins in diabetes treatment is a subject of much interest among the public and research scientists alike. Preliminary research suggests that in some instances, very high doses of certain vitamins and minerals may provide a therapeutic benefit for people with diabetes. In these cases, the nutrient is given in a pharmacological dose and acts more like a drug than a nutrient, and like a drug, it carries the risk of significant side effects.

Some of the vitamins that have generated interest as possibly beneficial to people with diabetes are the antioxidants vitamins E and C, the B vitamins, and vitamins D and A.

Antioxidants. High blood glucose levels appear to increase the production of *free radicals,* highly reactive chemical compounds that can damage many tissues. Though occurring in the body naturally, free radicals are toxic and are believed to play a role in the development of diabetes-related complications such as retinopathy, neuropathy, and cardiovascular disease.

Antioxidants, certain vitamins and other compounds present in fruits and vegetables, counteract the damaging, *oxidative* effects of free radicals. Common antioxidants include beta-carotene (found in dark green and dark orange fruits and vegetables), lycopene (found in tomatoes), and the vitamins C and E. Increased levels of free radicals and free-radical damage in people with diabetes suggests that people with diabetes may have increased antioxidant requirements.

At this time, increasing your intake of fruits and vegetables is the safest and most effective way to increase your overall antioxidant intake. The effects of antioxidants in supplement form are still uncertain. In fact, high doses of beta-carotene have been associated with increased rates of lung cancer in smokers. Even vitamins E and C, which have been studied extensively, can cause unwanted side effects at very high doses.

Vitamin E. Cholesterol molecules that have been oxidized are more *atherogenic,* or heart-disease promoting, than normal cholesterol molecules. Vitamin E is believed to protect cholesterol and other blood fats from oxidative damage. Increased intakes of vitamin E are associated with decreased incidence of heart attacks and cardiovascular disease. Vitamin E has also been shown to decrease

the "stickiness" of blood cells, thereby decreasing the likelihood of blood clots and heart attacks.

But not all of the research on the effects of vitamin E supplements is positive. The largest clinical trial examining the effects of vitamin E supplements in people with diabetes, the Heart Outcomes Prevention Evaluation (HOPE) study, found no beneficial effect of 400 International Units (IUs) of natural vitamin E on incidence of stroke, heart attack, or death. At this time, the ADA feels there is inadequate research to support the widespread use of vitamin E supplements by people with diabetes. For most people, vitamin E is needed in only small amounts and is conveniently found in small amounts in lots of foods, such as green vegetables, nuts, plant oils, whole grains, and some meat and seafood.

Because vitamin E can decrease the ability of blood to clot, potential side effects of supplementation include increased bleeding. For this reason, vitamin E supplements should not be used by those on blood-thinning medicines without the knowledge of their physician.

Vitamin C. People with diabetes often have increased urinary vitamin C loss and decreased plasma vitamin C levels. For this reason, vitamin C supplements have been suggested for people with diabetes as an antioxidant and to decrease complications of diabetes. However, there is inadequate scientific research to recommend vitamin C supplements for these concerns at this time. Smokers, however, have been found to have increased vitamin C requirements.

The DRI for vitamin C is 75 milligrams per day for women and 90 milligrams per day for men; for smokers, an additional 35 milligrams per day is recommended. The UL is 2,000 milligrams per day. Adequate intakes of vitamin C are achievable with a varied diet that is high in fruits and vegetables. Supplements of vitamin C are generally believed to be safe, although recent research suggests that in high doses, vitamin C may act as a *prooxidant,* increasing free radical production. This effect may be more pronounced in the presence of minerals such as chromium and iron. People who have an inherited disorder in iron metabolism called *hemochromatosis* should not take vitamin C (or iron) supplements. High doses of vitamin C may interfere with some laboratory tests, including tests of blood glucose level.

B vitamins. The B vitamins include thiamine, niacin, pyridoxine (also called vitamin B_6), riboflavin, folate, and B_{12}. These nutrients play numerous roles but are primarily involved in energy, carbohydrate, fat, and protein metabolism.

DAILY VITAMIN NEEDS

The Recommended Dietary Allowances (RDA) suggest daily nutrient levels that are adequate for healthy adults. (Levels for children and for pregnant or lactating women may be different.) The Tolerable Upper Intake Levels (UL) indicate the highest amount one can take in the form of supplements before experiencing adverse health effects.

VITAMIN	RECOMMENDED DIETARY ALLOWANCE (RDA)	TOLERABLE UPPER INTAKE LEVEL (UL)	GOOD FOOD SOURCES
Vitamin A	Men: 900 micrograms (mcg or µg) per day Women: 700 µg per day	3,000 µg per day	■ Fortified milk ■ Sweet potato ■ Carrot ■ Eggs ■ Spinach
Thiamine (B$_1$)	Men: 1.2 milligrams (mg) per day Women: 1.1 mg per day	Not determined	■ Whole grains, enriched grain products ■ Legumes ■ Seeds ■ Peas
Riboflavin (B$_2$)	Men: 1.3 mg per day Women: 1.1 mg per day	Not determined	■ Dairy products ■ Enriched grain products ■ Eggs ■ Spinach
Niacin (nico-tinamide, B$_3$)	Men: 16 mg per day Women: 14 mg per day	35 mg per day	■ Poultry, fish, beef ■ Peanuts/peanut butter ■ Legumes ■ Avocado
Pyridoxine (B$_6$)	Adults 19–50: 1.3 mg per day, Men over 50: 1.7 mg per day, Women over 50: 1.5 mg per day	100 mg per day	■ Chicken, fish, pork ■ Whole grains ■ Nuts ■ Legumes
Folic acid, (folate folacin, B$_9$)	400 µg per day	1,000 µg per day (from supplements and fortified foods)	■ Fortified grain products, wheat germ ■ Green leafy vegetables ■ Legumes, peanuts ■ Avocado
Vitamin B$_{12}$ (cobalamin)	2.4 µg per day	Not determined	■ Meat, poultry, fish, shellfish ■ Eggs ■ Dairy products ■ Fortified foods
Vitamin C (ascorbic acid)	Men: 90 mg per day Women: 75 mg per day Smokers: add an additional 35 mg per day	2,000 mg per day	■ Bell pepper (green, red, orange, yellow) ■ Oranges/ orange juice ■ Broccoli ■ Strawberries
Vitamin D	Adults 19-50: 5 µg (200 IU) per day, Adults 51-70: 10 µg (400 IU) per day, Adults 71 and older: 15 g (600 IU) per day	50 µg (2,000 IU) per day	■ Fortified milk ■ Fortified breakfast cereals ■ Egg yolks ■ Salmon and other fatty fish
Vitamin E	15 mg (22 IU natural, 33 IU synthetic) per day	1,000 mg per day (from supplements and fortified foods)	■ Vegetable oils ■ Nuts, seeds ■ Wheat germ ■ Spinach
Vitamin K	Men: 120 µg per day Women: 90 µg per day	Not determined	■ Tea ■ Soybeans, soybean oil ■ Egg yolks ■ Dark green vegetables

Vitamins in Food and Supplements

Because the B vitamins are water-soluble, frequent high blood glucose levels can cause increased urinary losses and deficiencies.

Deficiencies of many B vitamins have been associated with abnormal blood glucose metabolism, but research studies in human subjects have generally shown either weak or no beneficial effect of supplements. Research also does not support the use of pyridoxine or other B vitamins as a treatment for diabetic neuropathy. In fact, excessive intakes of vitamin B_6 can be toxic, causing symptoms of neuropathy.

Folic acid. Because folic acid supplementation has been shown to decrease the incidence of some types of birth defects, all women of childbearing age are advised to take 400 micrograms of folic acid per day in the form of a supplement. Folate may also be helpful in decreasing the risk of cardiovascular disease by decreasing *homocysteine* levels. High blood levels of homocysteine (an amino acid) are associated with increased risk of cardiovascular disease. Many people with cardiovascular and renal complications of diabetes have been shown to have increased levels of homocysteine. It is not known if elevated homocysteine levels cause these complications or occur as a result of them. There is some preliminary research indicating that metformin, a drug commonly used in the treatment of Type 2 diabetes, may decrease B_{12} and folate absorption, causing elevated homocysteine levels. However, folic acid supplements reversed this effect.

Folate in foods is absorbed less well than synthetic folic acid in supplements, so those at risk of deficiency are encouraged to take synthetic folic acid supplements in addition to consuming a healthy diet. The elderly, particularly, often absorb folate less efficiently because of lower stomach acid levels. The DRI for folic acid is 400 micrograms per day; the UL is 1,000 micrograms per day. High intakes of folic acid can mask the early symptoms of B_{12} deficiency, potentially causing increased incidence of neuropathy. Because of this, those at risk for B_{12} deficiency, including the elderly, vegans, and people with gastrointestinal disorders, should be screened for B_{12} deficiency if they take folic acid supplements.

Niacin. Pharmacological doses of niacin have been used as an effective treatment for low HDL cholesterol, high LDL cholesterol, and high triglycerides in people who don't have diabetes. However, some research suggests that high doses of niacin can worsen blood glucose control in people with Type 2 diabetes. More recent research, though, demonstrates that at more moderate doses (750–2,000 mg per day), significant benefits to HDL, LDL, and triglyceride levels are accompanied by only modest changes in blood glucose that are generally amenable to adjustments in diabetes therapy. Supplemental doses of niacin at these levels should only be used under the management of a physician.

The DRI for niacin and for nicotinamide is 14–16 niacin equivalents (NE) per day; the UL is 35 NE per day.

Vitamin D. One of a handful of fat-soluble vitamins, vitamin D is needed to properly absorb calcium and for normal bone development. Interestingly, vitamin D can be synthesized by the body in the presence of sunlight. Exposure to the sun for as little as 5 to 15 minutes per day is believed to be adequate, although sunscreens with SPF 8 or greater interfere with vitamin D synthesis.

Supplements of up to 400 IU per day may be appropriate for those at risk of vitamin D deficiency, such as the homebound, the elderly, and other individuals who are not exposed to the sun. However, vitamin D supplements should be used under the supervision of a physician because toxicity can occur at relatively low doses compared to most nutrients.

While there is no formal recommendation for vitamin D supplementation for people with diabetes, it is known that people with Type 1 diabetes have increased rates of osteopenia, or decreased bone density, and some studies have found decreased vitamin D levels in people with newly diagnosed Type 1 diabetes. In these cases, supplementation may be advised.

Vitamin A. Body stores of vitamin A in healthy people with diabetes are generally thought to be similar to that of other healthy people in the United States. Some researchers have noted increases or decreases in various forms of vitamin A in people who have diabetes, but these effects have been inconsistent.

In laboratory studies, vitamin A altered insulin secretion by beta cells: Low doses increased insulin secretion and high doses decreased insulin secretion. However, this effect has not been noted in clinical trials conducted in humans. High-dose vitamin A supplements should be avoided due to potential toxicity.

Food first

Vitamins are pretty remarkable substances, and research into vitamins continues to reveal interesting new facts about them and how they work. What research has not shown yet, however, is a need for all people who have diabetes to take supplements of any particular vitamin. But that doesn't mean that people with diabetes can forget all about vitamins and nutrition. To the contrary, since high blood glucose and other factors related to diabetes can place a person at an increased risk of nutrient deficiencies, awareness of what constitutes a healthful diet is that much more important when you have diabetes. Ultimately, the best insurance policy against nutrition shortfalls is a high-quality diet. □

MINERALS IN FOOD AND SUPPLEMENTS

by Belinda O'Connell, M.S., R.D., L.D.

Minerals, much like vitamins, are chemical compounds required by the body to perform basic functions such as energy production, carbohydrate metabolism, bone growth, oxygen transport, and heart contraction. Inadequate levels of minerals in the diet can lead to serious diseases.

In the United States we have access to a wide variety and adequate quantities of food, so severe mineral deficiencies are rare. However, this abundance of food choices does not mean that we are all eating nutritionally "rich" diets, and because of this, many groups of people are, in fact, at risk for mild vitamin and mineral deficiencies.

People with diabetes may be more likely to have certain vitamin and mineral deficiencies because of increased nutrient losses caused by high blood glucose. Older age, low-calorie diets, and limited food choices due to food intolerances also raise the risk of vitamin and mineral deficiencies.

The best way to be certain you meet your basic vitamin and mineral needs is to consume a wide variety of healthful foods. Let the United States Department of Agriculture Dietary Guidelines be your guide: Emphasize fruits, vegetables, whole grains, and fat-free or low-fat milk and milk products; include lean meats, poultry, fish, beans, eggs, and nuts in your food plan; and try to keep the foods you choose low in saturated fats, *trans* fats, cholesterol, salt, and added sugars.

If you find those guidelines challenging, you may want to consider taking a general multivitamin that provides 100% of the daily value for essential vitamins and minerals as you work on improving your diet. But remember that we haven't figured out exactly what all the healthful components in foods are, so multivitamins and other supplements cannot be used as a replacement for a healthy, varied diet. Because vitamin and mineral supplements are only helpful in correcting nutrition deficiencies, very high doses such as those found in "high-potency" supplements do not provide any increased benefit over a multivitamin. In fact, very high doses may be harmful.

People who have limited food intakes, increased nutrition needs, or increased losses of vitamins and minerals are more likely to have borderline or mildly deficient body stores of nutrients. These people may need specific vitamin, mineral, or multivitamin supplements. People more likely to have nutrient deficiencies include the following groups:

■ People with chronically high blood glucose. Chronic high blood glucose can lead to increased urination. In turn, increased urinary water loss leads to increased loss of water-soluble vitamins and many minerals.

■ People on low-calorie or vegetarian diets and people with food intolerances. When you limit the quantity of foods you eat or avoid whole food groups, it is difficult to get all the vitamins and minerals your body needs. The same is true if your diet is of poor quality or does not include a wide variety of foods.

■ People who use several medicines. People who have chronic diseases or are on many different medicines are more likely to have decreased absorption of nutrients, increased urinary losses of nutrients, or increased needs for some nutrients.

■ People with high nutrition needs. Some groups of people have increased nutrient needs due to normal changes such as growth or decreased nutrient absorption due to age. People who often have increased needs include growing children, pregnant or lactating women, and older people.

If you fall into any of these "at risk" categories, you should discuss your needs with the members of your health-care team. They can give you individual guidelines on food choices and use of supplements.

Key minerals in diabetes

Research has shown that diabetes can affect the metabolism of nutrients and, in some cases, mineral requirements. This section highlights some of the minerals thought to be important in glucose metabolism, in insulin production or utilization, and in maintaining good health. The information on recommended intakes is for adults (those 19 and over); it's important to note that children and pregnant or lactating women often have different requirements for nutrients.

Chromium

Chromium is an essential trace mineral required for normal glucose metabolism. Its role in glucose metabolism was first identified in the 1960's when hospitalized patients who were being fed intravenous nutrient solutions that did not contain chromium developed high blood glucose levels. Their blood glucose levels improved when chromium was added to the nutrient mixture. Additional studies since then have looked at the effects of chromium supplements in people with Type 2 diabetes, Type 1 diabetes, gestational diabetes (diabetes that is diagnosed during pregnancy) and in insulin resistance. Chromium is also important for normal blood fat (cholesterol) metabolism.

Chromium appears to act by enhancing or increasing insulin's actions. But while chromium is believed to help the insulin present in your body work better, it cannot replace insulin. Numerous studies have looked at the effect of supplemental chromium on blood glucose control in people with diabetes. Overall, the results of research studies are mixed, with some showing positive effects and others negative or unclear results.

In general, research studies using higher doses (1,000 micrograms [μg or mcg] per day or more) and more bioavailable forms of chromium, such as chromium picolinate, have shown more positive effects than studies using other forms of chromium such as yeast or chromium chloride. Studies where subjects were consuming low-chromium diets or had other risk factors for chromium deficiency were also more likely to show positive effects. (Because chromium is a nutrient, supplements would be expected to have positive effects only in those people with an actual chromium deficiency.)

The best support for the use of chromium supplements in Type 2 diabetes is provided by a well-designed clinical trial conducted in China. In this study, 180 people with Type 2 diabetes were randomly assigned to take a placebo (inactive treatment) or chromium picolinate supplements. Two different levels of chromium were tested: a low-dose supplement of 200 μg of chromium picolinate per day or a high-dose supplement of 1,000 μg of chromium picolinate per day. The study lasted for four months. Both groups receiving chromium supplements had lower glycosylated hemoglobin (HbA_{1c}) levels than study subjects who had received the placebo. Average HbA_{1c} levels in the placebo group were 8.5%; in the 200 μg group, 7.5%; and in the 1,000 μg group, 6.6%.

These decreases in HbA_{1c} are similar in size to those seen with many oral blood-glucose-lowering medicines. In addition, the high-dose supplement group had lower fasting blood glucose levels, lower cholesterol levels, and lower glucose and insulin levels after a glucose challenge. (A glucose challenge or glucose tolerance test is a common research test where a person is given a standard dose of glucose under experimental conditions. Researchers then closely monitor the person's blood glucose level over time to see how high it goes, how long it takes to return to normal, and other measures.)

The fact that this study was well designed and had clinically important and dose-dependent effects is encouraging, though questions still remain about the applicability of this study in the United States, where ethnicity, dietary chromium intakes, and average weight of people with diabetes differ from that of the Chinese study subjects.

Dietary chromium (Cr^{3+}) toxicity is believed to be low in comparison to other trace elements. But there is research in animals and test tubes that indicate it could be potentially dangerous. Low-dose supplements are unlikely to be harmful, but the safety of higher doses, which have been shown to be more effective, has not been established. People with liver or kidney disease are more likely to experience negative side effects with chromium supplements and should avoid them. (Cr^{6+}, a different chemical form of chromium not present in food, is a known cancer-causing agent. Exposure to Cr^{6+} in certain industrial work settings has occurred through inhaling Cr^{6+}-laden dust.)

Research is inadequate at this time to set a Recommended Dietary Allowance (RDA) or safe Tolerable Upper Intake Level (UL) for chromium. The RDA of a nutrient is the dietary intake level that should fulfill the requirements of 97% to 98% of healthy people in the group described. Adequate Intakes (AIs), recommended intakes assumed to be adequate for a group of healthy people, are given when there's not enough information to create an RDA. ULs describe the highest dietary intake of a nutrient that is likely to pose no risk for most people. Ingesting more than the UL poses a health risk that may increase as intake above the UL increases. The UL is not a recommended intake level, and consuming a nutrient in excess of an RDA has no recognized benefit.

AIs for chromium intake are 25 µg/day for women 19–50 years of age, 20 µg/day for women over 50, 35 µg/day for men 19–50 years of age, and 30 µg/day for men over 50. Actual chromium intakes in the United States are estimated to be about 15 µg per 1,000 calories. It is felt that chromium intakes in the United States are generally adequate, though the potential for deficiency is present with poor diets, strenuous exercise, and high blood glucose levels.

Vanadium

The trace element vanadium has not been established as an essential nutrient, nor has deficiency been seen in humans. Vanadium is believed to act by mimicking the actions of insulin, or by increasing activation of the insulin receptor and hormone communication pathways within the cell.

There are only a few small clinical trials that have looked at the effects of vanadium supplements in humans. These studies have focused primarily on Type 2 diabetes, though animal studies suggest vanadium may be beneficial in both Type 1 and Type 2 diabetes. In people with Type 2 diabetes, vanadium decreased glucose release by the

LABEL KNOW-HOW

Having nutrition information on food labels is great if you know how to use it. Not all information is equally helpful in figuring out how healthful a food really is. When reading labels, focus on the Nutrition Facts panel. This section of the label gives you the "hard facts" and is regulated by the Food and Drug Administration (FDA), so it is less likely to have confusing or misleading information. The Nutrition Facts panel contains a lot of information. When evaluating a food for its vitamin and mineral content, look at the serving size and the percent daily values (%DV). It is also helpful to read the ingredients list. As always, watch the fat, saturated fat, *trans* fat, cholesterol, carbohydrate, sodium, and fiber content to evaluate how well a food fits into your overall food plan.

Serving size. This tells you the serving size to which all of the other nutrition information on the label applies. If the amount you eat is larger or smaller than the serving size listed, you need to adjust the nutrition information accordingly.

Percent Daily Value (%DV). These numbers help you to evaluate how the food fits into a healthy diet. Specifically, they tell you what percent of the average American's nutrient needs a serving of this food provides. (Your individual nutrient needs may in fact be slightly more or less, but the %DV still provides a good estimate.)

Of all the vitamins and minerals, the FDA only requires manufacturers to list the %DV for vitamin A, vitamin C, iron, and calcium on labels, but some companies voluntarily provide information on others. Foods that are fortified or enriched with any other nutrients must include information on these additives. There are also %DVs for total fat, saturated fat, carbohydrate, sodium, cholesterol, and fiber on labels. The Nutrition Facts panel of the label lists the number of grams (or milligrams) of each of these in a serving of the food, as well as the %DVs for each.

The FDA also allows foods that provide 20% or more of the %DV for a nutrient to make the claim that it is "high in" that vitamin or mineral. This descriptive term on food labels is regulated and cannot be used in a misleading context.

liver, increased the use of glucose for energy, and increased insulin sensitivity in most studies. Very high doses of vanadium decreased fasting blood glucose levels, HbA_{1c} levels, and cholesterol levels. Overall, therapeutic doses of vanadium appear to have a mild effect on insulin sensitivity and glucose use in Type 2 diabetes. However, there is no information on the long-term effects of vanadium supplements in diabetes.

There is not enough information about vanadium to set a recommended level of intake, but as little as 10–30 µg/day is believed to be adequate for most people. Because vanadium is needed in such small quantities, relatively small doses have the potential for significant side effects with regular use. The UL for vanadium is 1.8 milligrams (mg) per day, but some researchers have recommended limiting daily vanadium intake to less than 100 µg/day. Researchers are currently working to develop forms of vanadium that are better absorbed and have fewer side effects.

Magnesium

The mineral magnesium functions as an essential part of over 300 enzymes in the body. It is essential for most energy-requiring reactions such as glucose transport into cells, the burning of food for energy, normal nerve function, and heart contraction. Magnesium deficiency has been associated with increased blood pressure levels, insulin resistance, glucose intolerance, dyslipidemia (abnormal blood fat levels), increased platelet aggregation (platelets are the cells in the body that form blood clots), cardiovascular disease, and complications of diabetes and pregnancy. It is not known if low body stores of magnesium actually cause these disorders or if they simply occur simultaneously.

Magnesium is one of the more common micronutrient deficiencies found in people with diabetes. Decreased blood magnesium levels and increased urinary magnesium losses have been measured in people with Type 1 diabetes and also those with Type 2 diabetes, and low dietary magnesium intake has been associated with increased occurrence of Type 2 diabetes in some studies. Poor magnesium status in people with diabetes is most likely due to increased urinary losses caused by high blood glucose levels. (Diabetic ketoacidosis, a condition that occurs in people with diabetes if insulin levels are low, also decreases magnesium levels.) Low-calorie and poor-quality diets are also more likely to be inadequate in magnesium content, and people using some types of blood pressure drugs and diuretics are at increased risk for deficiencies due to increased urinary magnesium loss. One small study found that only 25% of people with Type 2 diabetes met the RDA for magnesium.

The RDA for magnesium for women 19 to 30 is 310 mg/day and 320 mg/day for those over 30. For men, the RDA is 400 mg/day for those 19 to 30 and 420 mg/day for men over 30. Diets high in saturated fat, sugar, caffeine, and alcohol may decrease magnesium absorption or increase requirements. The UL for magnesium is 350 mg/day of supplemental magnesium in addition to usual magnesium intake from food.

Because only a very small amount of the body's magnesium is present in blood, important tissue stores of magnesium can get very low before any deficiency is able to be measured with common blood tests. This means that borderline deficiencies may exist in many people who have normal blood magnesium levels. The American Diabetes Association has recommended assessment of magnesium status in individuals at risk for deficiency. That includes people with high blood glucose levels, congestive heart failure, or ketoacidosis, people who abuse alcohol, women who are pregnant, and people with other nutrition deficiencies and low caloric intakes. Supplements are appropriate when deficiency can be documented. Magnesium is a relatively nontoxic substance in people with normal kidney function, but taking supplements can lead to dangerously high magnesium levels in people with decreased kidney function.

Copper

Copper is another essential trace mineral. It is important for normal energy production and iron metabolism, and it acts as a *cofactor* (a molecule necessary for the proper action of an enzyme) for one of the body's antioxidant defense systems. Copper deficiency has been associated with glucose intolerance. In most studies of people with diabetes, copper levels have been found to be normal or slightly elevated. Increased copper levels have been associated with increased occurrence of complications of diabetes, such as cardiovascular disease and retinopathy. Because of this, copper supplements are not recommended for people with diabetes.

The RDA for copper is 900 µg/day for adults, and the UL is 10,000 µg/day. Toxicity from dietary copper in the United States is rare. High levels of supplemental iron, zinc, molybdenum, and vitamin C can decrease copper absorption. High copper intake can have similar effects on absorption of other trace minerals, and low copper intake impairs iron metabolism.

Zinc

In animals, poor zinc status causes insulin resistance and decreases insulin release from the pancreas. Effects of zinc on insulin secretion are dose-dependent, with very low and very high levels causing decreased insulin secretion. Severe zinc deficiency can cause glucose intolerance. High-dose zinc supplements have not been shown to improve blood glucose levels in people with diabetes.

Zinc is important for normal immune system function, and zinc supplements have improved some measures of immune function in people with Type 2 diabetes. Early research suggests that zinc supplements may also improve healing of leg ulcers in older individuals and improve growth in children with Type 1 diabetes. Zinc has been promoted as a treatment for the common cold, but research to date has not consistently shown benefit.

Because a person's zinc status can be difficult to measure, the incidence of zinc deficiency in people with diabetes is uncertain. Some studies suggest that people with diabetes have lower zinc levels than people who don't have diabetes. Increased urinary zinc loss due to increased *glycosuria* (increased urinary glucose loss due to high blood glucose levels) and decreased intestinal zinc absorption may predispose people with diabetes to mild zinc deficiencies. A study of people with Type 2 diabetes found that fewer than 3% of women and 14% of men met the RDA for zinc intake. Potential risk for zinc deficiency is greater in people following vegetarian diets, in pregnant and lactating women, in children who are growing, in people with gastrointestinal disorders, in people with high blood glucose levels, in older people, and in people with low caloric intakes. High alcohol intakes and use of several medicines can also increase the risk of zinc deficiency.

The RDA for zinc is 8 mg/day for women and 11 mg/day for men. Dietary supplements of iron and calcium may decrease zinc absorption. Whole-grain products contain a form of zinc that is less well utilized by the body because they also contain compounds called phytates, which bind to zinc and decrease its absorption.

The UL for zinc is 40 mg/day for adults. Zinc toxicity is relatively rare and has generally occurred due to accidental exposure to high doses of zinc or through high-dose supplements. Zinc supplements of 100–300 mg/day can interfere with copper absorption. High-dose zinc supplements have caused unfavorable changes in blood cholesterol levels (increased LDL [the "bad cholesterol"] and decreased HDL [the "good cholesterol"]), impaired immune function, and anemia.

Calcium

Calcium is necessary for normal bone and tooth development, nerve impulse conduction, muscle contraction, and blood clotting. Increased rates of osteoporosis have been measured in older people with diabetes, and studies have found decreased levels of *bone-mineral density* (a measure of calcium stores in bone) in people with Type 1 diabetes and in those with Type 2 diabetes, and increased *bone turnover*—the normal process of bone breakdown and rebuilding—in people with Type 1 diabetes. Osteoporosis and poor bone mineral stores increase the risk of bone fractures.

Poor calcium status may increase blood pressure levels in some groups of people. Consumption of low-fat dairy products as part of a diet high in fruits and vegetables and low in fat decreased blood pressure levels as much as blood pressure drugs in the Dietary Approaches to Stop Hypertension (DASH) trial.

Bone calcium stores are built up during childhood and into a person's early 20's. After age 30 there is little accumulation of calcium in bone, and after menopause in women and age 65 in men, bone mineral stores significantly decline. Calcium intake in the early years, when bone is forming, and in older people, in whom bone calcium stores can decline rapidly, is very important. Dietary calcium intakes in adolescent girls, women, and people over 65 frequently do not meet the recommended guidelines. Calcium supplements up to 1,000–1,500 mg/day for people in these groups and others at risk for calcium deficiency, such as people with lactose intolerance, are recommended.

Calcium absorption and metabolism can be affected by other dietary factors. Vitamin D is necessary for calcium absorption (combination vitamin D and calcium supplements are available), and calcium absorption from dairy products is higher than from vegetable and grain sources. High dietary protein, sodium, and phosphorus intakes may decrease calcium stores in the body, and caffeine can also decrease calcium absorption. (The AI value set for vitamin D is 5.0 μg or 200 International Units [IU] per day for adults ages 19 to 50, 10 μg or 400 IU per day for adults 51 to 70, and 15 μg or 600 IU for those over 70.)

Calcium supplements should be taken at a different time from other vitamin and mineral supplements because high doses of calcium can decrease the absorption of some trace minerals.

Spreading your calcium intake out will also increase the ability of your body to absorb it. Two supplements of 500 mg each, taken at different times will be better absorbed than a single 1,000-mg supplement. Avoid supplements that contain calcium from dolomite, oyster shell, or bone meal because they may be contaminated with lead.

The AI for calcium is 1,000 mg/day for men and women 19 to 50 and 1,200 mg/day for men and women over 50. The UL is 2,500 mg/day. Calcium supplements are generally considered safe, although they may interfere with the absorption of certain drugs such as atenolol (a blood pressure drug), some antibiotics, fluoride, iron, and bisphosphates (drugs used to treat osteoporosis). In the past, people with kidney stones were counseled to avoid high calcium intakes, but more recent research indicates that high-calcium diets may actually decrease the risk of some types of kidney stones by binding to oxalates in the intestine and decreasing their absorption. (People with absorptive hypercalciuria, on the other hand, may experience increased stone formation with calcium supplements.)

Iron

The mineral iron is important for normal red blood cell development, oxygen transport, and energy production. People with diabetes appear to have similar iron requirements as the general U.S. population. Iron deficiency is most common in periods of rapid growth such as occurs in young children (6 months to 4 years), adolescence, and pregnancy. Women who are menstruating can experience high iron losses. Iron supplements are often recommended during pregnancy.

High iron stores in the body have been associated with cardiovascular disease in some studies. This relationship is far from clear, but it is probably prudent for men and postmenopausal women who have no history of anemia to avoid taking supplemental iron. The effects of iron on glucose metabolism under normal conditions is probably not great, but people with a genetic disorder called *hemochromatosis* (a condition which leads to excessive body stores of iron) often develop glucose intolerance. One study of people with diabetes who had elevated iron stores (but not hemochromatosis) measured improvements in blood glucose control with the use of an experimental drug that decreased blood iron levels.

The RDA for iron is 8 mg/day for men 19 and over. The RDA for women 19 to 50 is 18 mg/day, and women over 50 have an RDA of 8 mg/day. Iron from animal products (called *heme* iron) is better

absorbed than iron from vegetable sources. Vitamin C may also improve iron absorption from plant and dairy foods. The UL for iron is 45 mg/day.

Poisoning from iron supplements is the most common cause of death from accidental poisoning in young children. Supplements containing iron need to be stored in childproof containers and out of the reach of young children.

Manganese

Manganese is important for normal bone development, reproduction, nerve function, and antioxidant defenses of the body. Its role in glucose metabolism is uncertain. In animal models, manganese deficiency caused glucose intolerance, but supplements in people with Type 2 diabetes have had little or no effect. Manganese status of people with diabetes is poorly understood at this time, and supplements are not recommended. Manganese deficiency is not a concern because it is widely available in the food supply.

The AI for manganese is 2.3 mg/day for men and 1.8 mg/day for women. The UL is 11 mg/day for adults. Toxicity risk with manganese is relatively low and has generally occurred in humans as a result of accidental exposure to high levels through industrial dust or contaminated water.

Selenium

Selenium is a trace mineral that helps the body to neutralize *free radicals*. (Free radicals are chemical substances produced during normal cellular processes that can cause damage to cells when they occur in high levels. It is believed that damage from free radicals influences the development of many common diseases such as cancer, Alzheimer disease, and cardiovascular disease.) Selenium works in cooperation with other antioxidants such as vitamin E and glutathione.

In animals, selenium deficiency results in impaired insulin secretion and glucose intolerance. Selenium deficiency has also been associated with a rare form of cardiomyopathy (a disorder of the heart muscle). The amount of selenium in foods varies depending on the geographic region in which an animal was raised and soil selenium concentrations in which plants were grown, making the determination of an average American's selenium intake difficult. The selenium status of people with diabetes is not well characterized at this time, though there is no reason to think they have an increased risk for deficiency; thus, supplements are generally not recommended. The RDA for selenium is 55 µg/day for adults and the UL is 400 µg/day. Selenium toxicity is rare.

DAILY MINERAL NEEDS

The Recommended Dietary Allowances (RDAs) suggest daily nutrient levels that are adequate for healthy adults. (Levels for children and for pregnant or lactating women may be different.) Adequate Intakes (AIs) are recommended intakes assumed to be adequate for a group of healthy people when there's not enough information to create an RDA. The Tolerable Upper Intake Levels (ULs) indicate the highest amount of nutrient intake not associated with adverse health effects.

MINERAL	RECOMMENDED DIETARY ALLOWANCE (RDA) OR ADEQUATE INTAKE (AI)	TOLERABLE UPPER INTAKE LEVEL (UL)	FOOD SOURCES
Chromium	Men 19–50: 35 micrograms (mcg or µg) Men over 50: 30 µg Women 19–50: 25 µg Women over 50: 20 µg	No UL set, but previous Estimated Safe and Adequate Daily Dietary Intake (ESADDI) set by the government was 50–200 µg per day	Whole grains, mushrooms, broccoli, dried beans, seeds, wine and beer, brewer's yeast, American cheese, wheat germ
Vanadium	No RDA or AI set	1.8 milligrams (mg) per day	Buckwheat, oats, shellfish, parsley, mushrooms, dillseed
Magnesium	Men 19–30: 400 mg Men over 30: 420 mg Women 19–30: 310 mg Women over 30: 320 mg	350 mg per day	Whole grains, nuts, peanut butter, fish, legumes, dark green leafy vegetables, potatoes with skin
Calcium	Children under 18: 1,300 mg Adults 19–50: 1,000 mg Adults over 51: 1,200 mg	2.5 grams per day	Milk, yogurt, cheese, salmon (with bones), dark green leafy vegetables, almonds, tofu prepared with calcium, fortified foods such as cereals, grains, rice, snack bars, juices, and soy beverages
Iron	Men: 8 mg Premenopausal women: 18 mg Postmenopausal women: 8 mg	45 mg per day	Beef, eggs, fish, poultry, clams, fortified cereals and grains
Zinc	Men: 11 mg Women: 8 mg	40 mg per day	Meat, eggs, seafood, whole grains, wheat germ, nuts, legumes
Copper	900 µg	10,000 µg per day	Organ meats, seafood, cocoa powder, nuts, legumes, seeds
Selenium	55 µg	400 µg per day	Seafood, organ meats, whole grains, seeds
Manganese	Men: 2.3 mg Women: 1.8 mg	11 mg per day	Whole grains and cereal products, fruits and vegetables
Molybdenum	45 µg	2 mg per day	Content in foods is variable, with milk, beans, breads, and cereals the most common sources

NUTRITION RESOURCES

These resources provide accurate information on nutrition, vitamins, minerals, and nutritional supplements:

Newsletters

CENTER FOR SCIENCE IN THE PUBLIC INTEREST'S NUTRITION ACTION HEALTHLETTER
www.cspinet.org
A chatty, informative resource that gives the low-down on recent studies, dietary trends and fads, and consumer awareness. Includes practical tips for health-conscious consumers on shopping, food safety, analyzing food labels and advertising, and eating out. Features "Healthy Cook" recipes and a "Health Watch" column, which recommends one product to try and one to stay away from. Special $20 offer for new subscribers for 10 issues.

TUFTS UNIVERSITY HEALTH AND NUTRITION LETTER
http://healthletter.tufts.edu
(800) 274-7581
A monthly letter researched by the Tufts University School of Nutrition Science and Policy with the latest news on nutrition, wellness, and clinical trials. Content is developed largely from reader questions. Internet special of $18 for 12 issues.

Books

THE AMERICAN DIETETIC ASSOCIATION'S COMPLETE FOOD AND NUTRITION GUIDE
Revised & Updated 3rd Edition
Roberta Larson Duyff, M.S., R.D., F.A.D.A., C.F.C.S.
John Wiley and Sons
New York, New York, 1996

Organizations

THE AMERICAN DIETETIC ASSOCIATION
www.eatright.org
(800) 877-0877
Primarily an organization for health-care professionals, the ADA Web site includes articles on healthy lifestyles and a "Find a NUTRITION PROFESSIONAL" feature.

NATIONAL INSTITUTES OF HEALTH OFFICE OF DIETARY SUPPLEMENTS
http://dietary-supplements.info. nih.gov
This organization conducts research into the role of dietary supplements in improving health. The Web site offers fact sheets on dietary supplements and articles on the misuse or adverse effects of certain supplements.

Web Sites

NATIONAL COUNCIL AGAINST HEALTH FRAUD
www.ncahf.org
(978) 532-9383
This Web site is a private, nonprofit volunteer organization run by Stephen Barrett, M.D., and supported by an advisory board of health-care professionals. The Web site discloses fraudulent health claims or inaccurate labeling of products and advocates reliable health information for consumers. It offers a free weekly electronic newsletter, "Consumer Health Digest."

HEALTHFINDER
www.healthfinder.gov
A useful link to health information resources developed by the U.S. Department of Health and Human Services. For nutrition information, look up "nutrition" under "all topics" in the Health Library.

Food still the preferred route

As with vitamins, trace mineral requirements, except in select cases, are best obtained through food. Because risk for toxicity increases significantly with high intakes, use of individual high-dose vitamin or mineral supplements should generally be avoided. Older people, people who have poor-quality or low-calorie diets, and those who have other risk factors for vitamin and mineral deficiencies such as chronically high blood glucose should discuss ways to improve their intake of important nutrients through foods with their health-care team. In many cases, a simple multivitamin supplement that provides approximately 100% of the daily value for most nutrients is appropriate. Premenopausal women, teens, and pregnant women may also benefit from additional supplements such as iron or calcium. Older people and people with poor blood glucose control are at risk for several micronutrient deficiencies and should discuss this with their health-care team. □

ANTIOXIDANTS
Should You Supplement?

by Robert A. Jacob, Ph.D.

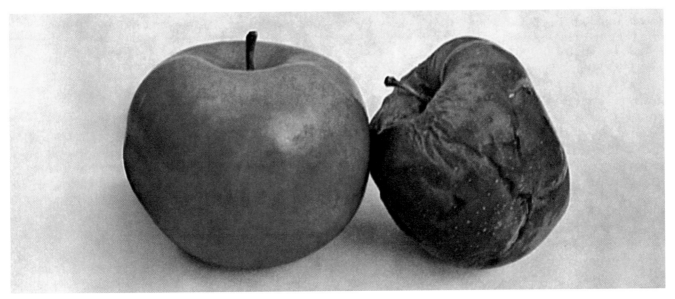

Oxygen is a Jekyll and Hyde element. We need it for critical body functions, such as respiration and immune response, but oxygen's dark side is a reactive chemical nature that can damage body cells and tissues. The perpetrators of this "oxidative damage" are various oxygen-containing molecules, most of which are types of *free radicals*—unstable, highly energized molecules that contain an unpaired electron.

Since stable chemical bonds require electron pairs, free radicals generated in the body steal electrons from nearby molecules, damaging vital cell components and body tissues. Oxidative damage in the body is akin to rusting of metal, the browning of freshly cut apples, or fats going rancid. Certain substances known as *antioxidants,* however, can help prevent this kind of damage. This article examines the special relationship between oxidative damage, antioxidant protection, diabetes, and complications of diabetes.

Oxidative damage

Free radicals and other "reactive oxygen species" are formed by a variety of normal processes within the body (including respiration and immune and inflammatory responses) as well as by elements outside the body, such as air pollutants, sunlight, and radiation. Whatever their source, reactive oxygen species can promote damage that is linked to increased risk of a variety of diseases and even to the aging process itself.

Oxidative damage to LDL (low-density lipoprotein or "bad") cholesterol particles in the blood is believed to be a key factor in the progression of heart disease. Oxidative damage to fatty nerve tissue is linked to increased risk of various nervous system disorders, including Parkinson disease. Free radical damage to DNA can alter genetic material in the cell nucleus and, as a result, increase cancer risk. Cataract formation in the eye may also involve free radical damage to lens proteins. Oxidative damage has also been linked to arthritis and inflammatory conditions, shock and trauma, kidney disease, multiple sclerosis, bowel diseases, and diabetes.

Antioxidant protection

As a defense against oxidative damage, the body normally maintains a variety of mechanisms to prevent such damage while allowing the use of oxygen for normal functions. Such "antioxidant protection" derives from sources both inside the body (endogenous) and outside the body (exogenous). Endogenous antioxidants include molecules and enzymes that neutralize free radicals and other reactive oxygen species, as well as metal-binding proteins that sequester iron and copper atoms (which can promote certain oxidative reactions if free). The body also makes several key antioxidant enzymes that help "recycle," or regenerate, other antioxidants (such as vitamin C and vitamin E) that have been altered by their protective activity.

Exogenous antioxidants obtained from the diet also play an important role in the body's antioxidant defense. These include vitamin C, vitamin E, carotenoids such as beta-carotene and lycopene, and other *phytonutrients,* or substances found in fruits, vegetables, and other plant foods that provide health benefits. Vitamin C (ascorbic acid), which is water-soluble, and vitamin E (tocopherol), which is fat-soluble, are especially effective antioxidants because they quench a variety of reactive oxygen species and are quickly regenerated back to their active form after they neutralize free radicals. Small amounts of these vitamins obtained from the diet provide a great deal of antioxidant protection, but research indicates that larger doses provide little additional protection. Vitamin C, which is abundant in fruits and vegetables, is concentrated in white blood cells that generate reactive oxygen species by using oxygen to burn bacterial and viral invaders; vitamin C may protect against DNA damage in the cell. Vitamin E, found in nuts, seeds, vegetable oils, and wheat germ, among other foods, protects unsaturated fat in cell membranes and fatty nerve tissue from oxidative degradation. Carotenoids, which are colored nutrients found in fruits and vegetables, provide their own unique antioxidant protection apart from vitamins C and E. Beta-carotene, the orange color in carrots, and lycopene, the red color in tomatoes, are effective quenchers of *singlet oxygen,* a form of reactive oxygen species that is not a free radical but is highly reactive.

Diabetes and oxidative damage

Normally, the body maintains a balance between the amount of reactive oxygen species generated and its antioxidant defense. This balance may be tipped, however, by conditions that greatly increase the generation of reactive oxygen species (such as cigarette smoke in the lungs) and/or lack of antioxidant defense due to malnutrition. Many diseases involve increased production of reactive oxygen species, including infections and inflammatory conditions such as arthritis and inflammatory bowel diseases.

There is substantial evidence that people with diabetes tend to have increased generation of reactive oxygen species, decreased antioxidant protection, and therefore increased oxidative damage. Hyperglycemia, or a high blood glucose level, has been shown to increase reactive oxygen species and end products of oxidative damage in isolated cell cultures, in animals with diabetes, and in humans with diabetes. Measurement of the end products of oxidative damage to body fat, proteins, and DNA are commonly used to assess the degree of oxidative damage to body cells and tissues. Most studies show that these measures are increased in people with diabetes.

The activities of key antioxidant enzymes are also found to be abnormal in people with diabetes. In some studies, these enzyme activities are seen to be lower than normal, suggesting a compromised antioxidant defense, while other studies show higher activity, suggesting an increased response to oxidative stress. Some studies indicate that oxidative damage is greater in people with Type 2 diabetes compared to those with Type 1, especially people with Type 2 diabetes and the metabolic syndrome, which involves central obesity, hypertension (high blood pressure), and high blood fat levels along with insulin resistance (decreased effectiveness of insulin in metabolizing blood glucose).

There is evidence that antioxidant protection is decreased and oxidative stress increased in some people even before the onset of diabetes. For instance, increased levels of oxidative stress have been found in people who have impaired glucose tolerance, or prediabetes.

Evidence for antioxidant protection

Overall, the evidence indicates that hyperglycemia creates additional oxidative stress, and that measures of oxidative damage are generally increased in people with diabetes. Therefore, the question arises as to whether antioxidant treatment may delay or prevent diabetes, or delay the onset of diabetes complications that include cardiovascular, kidney, nerve, and eye diseases. Cell culture and animal studies support the hypothesis that antioxidants can protect diabetic cells from some damage. However, two types of human studies must also be examined to answer the question: population studies and clinical trials.

Population studies. Population, or *epidemiologic,* studies have looked at the relationship between antioxidant intake and the development of diabetes. They have also examined the effects of antioxidant intake on a group of people with diabetes compared to a similar group without the condition.

Examination of the diets of some 4,300 Finnish adults (40–69 years old) without diabetes showed that those with low dietary intakes of vitamin E had a significantly greater risk of developing Type 2 diabetes over the next two decades. There was no relationship between intake of vitamin C and risk of future diabetes development. In another study of 81 male and 101 female Finnish adults at high risk for Type 2 diabetes, dietary carotenoids were associated with improved measures of glucose metabolism (fasting plasma glucose concentration and insulin resistance) in men but not women. In a third study, blood levels of five carotenoids were measured in 1,597 Australian adults who were healthy or had varying degrees of impaired glucose metabolism. Those with higher blood levels of the carotenoids had a healthier profile of glucose metabolism tests—fasting plasma glucose levels, insulin concentrations, and glucose tolerance levels.

Like carotenoids, *flavonoids* are a class of antioxidants found in fruits and vegetables and in some plant-based beverages including tea and red wine. To study the possible benefit of dietary flavonoids for preventing Type 2 diabetes in women, dietary flavonoid intake, as well as insulin resistance and inflammation, were measured in 38,018 healthy U.S. women over an average of nine years. The results showed no relationship between intake of flavonoids and risk of developing Type 2 diabetes. However, there was a modest benefit for consumption of apples and tea.

The relationship between vitamin C and E intake and diabetic retinopathy (eye disease) was assessed in two U.S. studies of populations of 998 and 1,353 adults with Type 2 diabetes. There were no significant associations for dietary intake or blood level of the vitamins with the occurrence of retinopathy. However, one of the studies showed that those taking supplements of the vitamins for more than three years had a reduced risk of retinopathy.

In summary, population studies have shown mixed results as to possible benefits of antioxidants to people with diabetes. Some show a benefit, others show no relationship, and none show harm.

Clinical trials. Population studies are limited in that they show only associations between dietary factors and medical conditions—they do not show cause and effect. For instance, high carotenoid levels in the blood are markers for high fruit and vegetable intake: Therefore, the beneficial effects on glucose metabolism associated with carotenoids in the Australian study noted above could actually be due to other substances in the fruits and vegetables rather than the carotenoids. To prove conclusively that a dietary factor has an impact on a

medical condition requires further clinical trials with better-controlled conditions. Ideally, studies to determine the potential benefit of antioxidant nutrients on disease prevention should be large and be carried out over many years. They should also be placebo-controlled (control subjects receive an inert pill which is indistinguishable from the antioxidant treatment pill) and double-blind (neither the subjects nor the investigators know who is getting the antioxidant or the placebo pills until the results are analyzed).

A number of smaller studies of people with diabetes have shown positive results with antioxidant treatments, while others have shown no benefit. Two Italian studies found that treatment of people with Type 2 diabetes with vitamin E decreased HbA_{1c}, a measure of long-term blood glucose control, and improved markers of heart function. However, Swedish investigators found that two years of antioxidant treatment in children with Type 1 diabetes (beginning at diagnosis) had no effect on blood glucose levels, HbA_{1c}, and insulin doses as compared to similar children receiving placebo treatment. And in a small study in Scotland, people with Type 2 diabetes who were given a low-flavonoid base diet enriched with large amounts of onions and tea (which are high-flavonoid foods) were found to have lower levels of oxidative damage to the DNA of white blood cells compared to the same subjects on the diet without the onions and tea.

In smokers and people with cardiovascular disease and/or hypertension (high blood pressure), vitamin C is known to improve the ability of blood vessels to relax and allow increased blood flow. This may be important to people with diabetes since they have a high rate of complications involving the blood vessels. In fact, studies have shown that intravenous infusion of vitamin C improves vascular relaxation in people with both Type 1 and Type 2 diabetes. However, oral consumption of large amounts of vitamin C by people with Type 2 diabetes in separate English and Swedish studies had no such effect. And treatment of 49 people with diabetes in the Boston area with combined vitamins C and E supplements for six months showed improvement in vascular function for people with Type 1 diabetes but not for those with Type 2.

Over the past two decades, large clinical trials of antioxidant supplements have been conducted with participants who had preexisting heart disease or some risk factors for heart disease such as smoking and diabetes. These studies focused primarily on the potential benefit of vitamins E, C, and/or the carotenoid beta-carotene for preventing cardiovascular disease. The studies did not specifically target diabetic populations, but the results are pertinent to people with diabetes because some were included in some of the studies and because the cardiovascular disease end points measured are some of the complications people with diabetes often develop.

A 1996 English study, the Cambridge Heart Antioxidant Study, found that vitamin E supplements given to 2,002 adults with preexisting heart disease significantly reduced the occurrence of heart attacks after one year of supplementation. These findings encouraged further studies of vitamin E. However, a number of subsequent studies did not show benefits for consumption of vitamin E supplements in amounts of 20 to 40 times the RDA (recommended dietary allowance, now 15 milligrams [mg] per day). More recently, a 2002 British study gave a trio of antioxidant supplements (vitamins E and C and beta-carotene) or placebo to 20,536 adults with cardiovascular disease or diabetes for five years. As compared to the placebo group, the people who took the supplements had substantially increased blood levels of the antioxidants, but the antioxidants had no effect on the occurrence of cardiovascular events (such as heart attack or stroke), cancer, or hospitalizations for nonvascular problems.

Some of the large antioxidant clinical trials enrolled enough people with Type 2 diabetes to assess the effects of antioxidant supplements in the diabetic group separately. In 2002, investigators from Canada, the United States, and Germany reported the effects of supplementing adults age 55 and over, who had either cardiovascular disease or Type 2 diabetes and an additional coronary risk factor, with vitamin E for an average of 4.5 years. For the group of 3,654 people with diabetes, vitamin E had no effect on incidence of heart attacks, strokes, or nephropathy (kidney disease)—all among the complications of diabetes. A 2003 Italian study tested vitamin E and low-dose aspirin for preventing heart disease and stroke in 4,495 adults age 50 and over with heart disease risk factors, including 1,031 people with diabetes. Over a median period of 3.7 years, there was no benefit found for vitamin E supplementation in either the subjects with diabetes or those without. (Low-dose aspirin was less effective for preventing cardiovascular events in the diabetic group as compared to the nondiabetic group.) Finally, a 2003 analysis and summary of 15 vitamin E and beta-carotene clinical trials (called a meta-analysis) concluded that the results showed no beneficial effect for various doses of the antioxidants in diverse

FOOD SOURCES OF ANTIOXIDANTS

While taking large doses of antioxidants in the form of supplements does not appear to prevent disease, getting enough in your diet is still important. Eating plenty of fruits and vegetables is the best way to make sure your body gets the antioxidants it needs. This is because fruits and vegetables provide a wide variety of antioxidants as well as other healthful nutrients, such as B vitamins and dietary fiber.

Vitamin C[*] (RDA is 90 mg/day for adult men and 75 mg/day for adult women)

FOOD, AMOUNT	VITAMIN C (mg)
Guava, raw, ½ cup	188
Red bell pepper, raw, ½ cup	142
Kiwifruit, 1 medium	70
Orange, raw, 1 medium	70
Orange juice, ⅓ cup	61–93
Green bell pepper, raw, ½ cup	60

Vitamin E[*] (RDA is 15 mg/day for adults)

FOOD, AMOUNT	VITAMIN E (mg)
Wheat germ oil, 1 tablespoon	20.3
Sunflower seeds, dry roasted, 1 ounce	7.4
Almonds, 1 ounce	7.3
Sunflower oil, high-linoleic, 1 tablespoon	5.6
Safflower oil, high-oleic, 1 tablespoon	4.6
Hazelnuts (filberts), 1 ounce	4.3

Beta-carotene
Good sources include dark orange, red, and dark green vegetables and fruits, such as apricots, broccoli, cantaloupe, carrots, leafy greens, papaya, sweet potato, and pumpkin.

Lycopene
Good sources include deep red fruits and vegetables, such as tomatoes and tomato products (sauce, paste, juice, ketchup, etc.), guava, watermelon, papaya, and pink grapefruit.

[*] Data on vitamin C and vitamin E adapted from the *Dietary Guidelines for Americans 2005*.

populations for the prevention of cardiovascular diseases. In fact, beta-carotene supplements were shown to slightly increase risk of death from cardiovascular and all causes.

Alpha-lipoic acid

Alpha-lipoic acid (also called ALA or *thioctic acid*) is a unique, sulfur-containing compound that is made in small amounts in the body but is not obtained from the diet. It neutralizes a variety of reactive oxygen species and can "recycle" vitamins C and E in the body. In people with diabetes, ALA appears to enhance insulin action and blood vessel circulation, protect against diabetic neuropathy (nerve disease), and inhibit protein glycation (a reaction between excess glucose and protein that impairs the protein's function and forms harmful end products in the body).

Some, but not all, studies have found that treating people with Type 2 diabetes with ALA improved blood glucose control and also reduced measures of oxidative stress that may contribute to diabetes complications. In one German study, people with Type 1 and Type 2 diabetes who were given 600 mg per day of ALA for 18 months had lower levels of two markers for diabetic kidney disease than a control group of people with diabetes that did not receive the ALA.

Most promising of the studies with ALA have been those that indicate benefits toward the symptoms of diabetic neuropathy. The studies have generally treated people with diabetes with 600 mg of ALA per day, either intravenously or orally, and have found improvement in both systemic and localized symptoms of neuropathy such as pain, numbness, burning sensation, foot problems, and heart rhythm problems. One specific study published in 2000 showed that both intravenous infusion and oral consumption of ALA enhanced blood vessel relaxation and improved circulation in small blood vessels in people with diabetic peripheral neuropathy. A 2004 article in the journal *Treatments in Endocrinology* reviewed the studies on ALA and diabetic neuropathy. The review included seven randomized clinical trials of ALA in people with diabetic neuropathy and concluded that short-term (3 weeks) intravenous infusion and long-term (4–7 months) oral consumption of ALA improved symptoms of neuropathy to a clinically meaningful degree while indicating a high safety profile for the drug.

The bottom line

Oxidative stress is strongly linked to the development of diabetes and its complications. While laboratory and animal studies show benefits from antioxidant treatments, human clinical trials of the major dietary antioxidants—vitamin E, vitamin C, and carotenoids—have been largely negative. While these natural antioxidants are generally safe, the evidence does not support their use for preventing or treating diabetic conditions. This conclusion is similar to that of the year 2000 report of the National Academy of Sciences panel on Dietary Antioxidants and Related Compounds, which states that the evidence does not warrant increased intakes of the antioxidants to protect against chronic degenerative diseases, including diabetes.

The negative findings for vitamin E, vitamin C, and carotenoids should not end the research on antioxidant protection for diabetes. Clinical trials that focus specifically on people with diabetes have not yet been conducted. Since the body limits the amount of natural antioxidants in tissue cells (including the insulin-producing pancreatic beta cells), some scientists have recently suggested that artificially created antioxidants designed to better enter the cells may provide protection against oxidative damage in people with diabetes. Others suggest that some drugs currently used to treat cardiovascular disorders, including statins, ACE inhibitors, and calcium channel blockers, provide antioxidant protection beyond their other mechanisms of action. Also, since most trials have only studied single antioxidants, studies with multiple antioxidants (such as combinations obtained from foods) should be considered.

Alpha-lipoic acid has been shown to be beneficial for safely treating diabetic neuropathy, and the recent development of an oral sustained-release form holds further promise (sustained-release forms maintain more even blood levels of a drug for a longer period of time). To help determine conclusively whether ALA is effective for treating diabetic neuropathy, a large multicenter trial is being conducted in North America and Europe to assess the effects of oral treatment with ALA on the progression of diabetic neuropathy. Despite some disappointing results so far, further research holds promise for providing clinically significant antioxidant protection against diabetes and its complications. □

AMYLIN
Insulin's Partner

by Wayne L. Clark

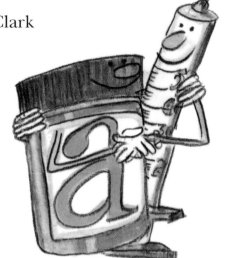

Diabetologist Steven V. Edelman is probably a little more conversant than the average physician on the subject of pramlintide (brand name Symlin), one of the newest diabetes drugs to receive U.S. Food and Drug Administration (FDA) approval. That's not only because he has been an investigator in some of the clinical trials of the drug, but because he has been taking it himself as a research subject in someone else's clinical trial for the past five years.

"I started off being an investigator," explains the Clinical Professor of Medicine at the University of California, San Diego and the San Diego VA Medical Center. "My patients were telling me all the good things that were happening to them, and I decided I wanted to try it. But you can't be in your own study, so I went to a colleague who was an investigator and became a subject."

Pramlintide is a synthetic analog of amylin, a neuroendocrine hormone that is absent in Type 1 diabetes and diminished in Type 2 diabetes. It's fitting that it might play a major role in diabetes management, because it comes from the same pancreatic beta cells that normally produce insulin. The beta cells release insulin and amylin in response to a rise in circulating blood glucose levels.

Amylin was first described in 1987, and the FDA approved the synthetic version pramlintide—marketed as Symlin by Amylin Pharmaceuticals of San Diego, California—in March 2005. It is currently approved for people with Type 1 diabetes and people with Type 2 diabetes who use insulin.

Dr. Edelman, who has had diabetes for 38 years, believes that pramlintide will be a boon for many people because it will help them even out the "peaks and valleys" in their blood glucose levels. "Pramlintide…replaces a hormone that should be present anyway," he notes, and he's "a big fan of replacing hormones that would normally be there."

How it works

Amylin's effects are many, but its primary action is on the release of insulin to the bloodstream following a meal. The postmeal (postprandial) blood glucose level is a critical part of overall blood glucose management that is generally underappreciated by most people who have diabetes and many physicians.

In people who don't have diabetes, the pancreatic beta cells release insulin in sync with the rise in blood glucose following a meal. Insulin levels generally reach their peak within 10 minutes. A chart showing insulin release and blood glucose levels in a person without diabetes reveals almost perfectly matched curves. Seldom does that person's blood glucose top 140 mg/dl in the hour or two after a meal.

In Type 2 diabetes, the release of insulin in response to rising blood glucose is both delayed and blunted. In Type 1 diabetes, there is no insulin release at all. In the absence of injected insulin (or an oral medicine that stimulates insulin release in people with Type 2 diabetes who still produce insulin), the result is a blood glucose level that rises to 300 mg/dl or more and remains high for several hours.

Compounding the problem, there also is an abnormal postprandial increase in release of the hormone glucagon from the alpha cells of the pancreas in people with diabetes. Glucagon stimulates the liver to release stored glucose into the bloodstream, which raises blood glucose levels. In fact, injectable glucagon is often used as a treatment for hypoglycemia (low blood glucose).

There are two general ways to control the amount of glucose in the bloodstream following a meal. One is to change the rate at which it enters, or "appears," in the blood, the other to change the rate at which it "disappears" from the blood. Diabetes creates dysfunction in both rates, so there is too much glucose entering and not enough leaving.

Dr. Edelman says, "Insulin works on the rate of glucose disappearance, allowing the cells of the body to absorb and use it. Amylin's role is to work in concert with insulin to limit the rate at which the glucose appears in the first place."

The mechanism of action of pramlintide is essentially threefold. First, it suppresses the appetite. This action is notable enough that the manufacturer has just begun a large clinical trial in people who are obese but do not have diabetes. The trials will help determine whether the drug might be used to treat obesity.

Second, pramlintide suppresses the postprandial release of the hormone glucagon. As mentioned earlier, glucagon stimulates the liver to release glucose and is inappropriately released after meals in people with diabetes.

Third, pramlintide controls how fast the stomach empties food into the small intestine, which is where glucose is absorbed as carbohydrates are broken down. Amylin slows down the muscle contractions of the stomach, slowing the progression of food into the next section of the gastrointestinal tract.

"So [by taking pramlintide] you have less food being consumed, a slower rate of absorption, and less glucagon being released," Dr. Edelman says. "Now, you have a balance. In fact, the balance works so well that you have to reduce your dose of fast-acting insulin by 30% to 50% when you start using pramlintide.

"Insulin has a very narrow therapeutic window," he notes. "If you give too little, you have hyperglycemia, and if you give too much, you have hypoglycemia. There's not much room for error. That's why people with diabetes have such a hard time regulating their blood sugar levels and why there's the roller coaster. Even with the insulin pump and the advantages it offers in fine-tuning control, you're still dealing with insulin alone and its narrow therapeutic window."

What's more, people with diabetes inject insulin into the subcutaneous tissue, while in people who don't have diabetes, insulin is released directly into the portal vein that serves the liver. Injected insulin therefore has a much lower and slower effect on the liver, in which glucagon is stimulating glucose production. There is less insulin to counteract this production, so the result—particularly after eating—is high blood glucose levels.

Problems with postmeal highs

Many experts believe that blood glucose levels that vary widely are even more harmful than a blood glucose level that stays steadily high. So high post-prandial blood glucose levels could be very harmful. Dr. Edelman points out that a person with diabetes may spend 12 hours a day (during waking hours) in the hyperglycemic postprandial state as opposed to the fasting state.

"Even for people with access to all the tools and experts," he says, "normalization or near normalization of the hemoglobin A_{1c} [HbA_{1c}]—which measures blood sugar control over time—is difficult. What's more, [even people] with a normal A_{1c} can have severe problems with wide and unpredictable glucose swings throughout the day and night. Their fasting blood sugar levels may not be that high, and yet they've lost the 'first-phase insulin release' that normally comes with a meal. So they can be lulled into a false sense of security by their [low] fasting blood sugar levels."

Because normal HbA_{1c} levels can conceal swings in blood glucose, Dr. Edelman recommends that people with Type 1 diabetes in particular monitor their blood glucose level two hours after meals, in addition to before meals. This way they may be able to catch a high postprandial blood glucose level in time to correct or at least mitigate it.

How serious a long-term issue is postprandial hyperglycemia? There is mounting evidence that it can contribute to a higher incidence of microvascular (kidney, eye, and nerve) complications and also to macrovascular (heart and blood vessel) complications.

It is believed that one of the primary causes of vascular complications in diabetes is increased "oxidative stress," a state of excess production of harmful "free radicals" (by-products of normal processes that can cause problems when they accumulate in high amounts). This process is driven by the excess glucose in the bloodstream that is characteristic of diabetes, and an increase in oxidative stress has been observed postprandially both in people with Type 1 diabetes and people with Type 2 diabetes.

A new study examined the effect of pramlintide on postprandial blood glucose levels and correlated it with markers of oxidative stress. The investigators in this small study report that levels of substances associated with oxidative stress were lower in people using pramlintide and that it may be a valuable tool to help reduce long-term complications.

Those complications and their correlation with postprandial blood glucose levels are a growing focus of research and treatment. The Honolulu Heart Study, for instance, showed that people who had higher blood glucose levels an hour after eating a standardized amount of glucose had a higher incidence of coronary artery disease.

The DECODE study, published in 1999, examined how mortality rates compared to fasting blood glucose levels and two-hour postprandial blood glucose levels. There was relatively little increase in risk among people with fasting blood glucose levels of about 140 mg/dl compared with those who had fasting levels around 110 mg/dl. But there was a striking increase in risk among people with postprandial blood glucose levels of 200 mg/dl or higher compared with those who had postprandial levels around 140 mg/dl. The investigators concluded that two-hour blood glucose levels could give a better indication of a person's risk for death than a fasting blood glucose alone.

The Kumamoto study in 2000 examined the two-hour postprandial glucose level, among other things. The investigators charted a tenfold increase in nephropathy (kidney disease) and a sixfold increase in retinopathy (eye disease) between when the values were 180 mg/dl and when they were 260 mg/dl.

To market, to market

The story of pramlintide's arrival on the market provides a glimpse into how difficult it is to bring a new drug from idea to reality. Clinical research on the drug began in 1995, when Amylin Pharmaceuticals partnered with Johnson & Johnson. Successful phase II trials were published in early 1997, and phase III data released in August 1997 showed some improvement in control in Type 1 diabetes but not in Type 2 diabetes. The company's stock price tumbled due to the much smaller potential market, and partner Johnson & Johnson pulled out of the project in 1998. Amylin persevered, however, and the FDA deemed pramlintide "approvable" in 2001. It took another four years to establish a safe dosage and gather enough clinical data to achieve final approval.

There were four double-blind, placebo-controlled studies that provided the main basis for the opinion that pramlintide is safe and effective. In these studies, participants who used pramlintide along with insulin achieved reductions in HbA$_{1c}$ levels on the order of 0.5% to 1.0% from their baseline values, and about 0.3% to 0.5% compared to placebo. When given along with insulin, pramlintide allowed a twofold to threefold increase in the proportion of people who were able to achieve ADA target levels of an HbA$_{1c}$ level of less than 7% compared to people using insulin alone. Total daily insulin doses also were generally lower for the people using pramlintide.

Participants also tended to either not gain weight (if they were of normal weight) or to lose weight (if they were overweight) as they lowered their HbA$_{1c}$ levels, an occurrence that was twice as common in those taking pramlintide. People with Type 1 diabetes who were overweight lost an average of 1.6 kilograms (3½ pounds), and those with Type 2 diabetes who were overweight lost an average of 2.4 kilograms (5 pounds). This finding accounts for the interest in pramlintide as an obesity treatment in people who don't have diabetes.

The primary concerns holding up pramlintide's approval were nausea and severe hypoglycemia experienced by some participants in the clinical trials, primarily people with Type 1 diabetes. Obviously, severe hypoglycemia is a cause for concern. The Health Research Group of the activist organization Public Citizen testified against FDA approval of pramlintide, citing that and other possible dangers.

Studies did reveal a transient increase in the occurrence of severe hypoglycemia, but it did not extend beyond the initial four weeks of treatment. Investigators like Dr. Edelman speculate that there is a period of adjustment when insulin doses need to be modified to account for the effects of pramlintide. Other side effects noted, such as nausea, anorexia (loss of appetite), and vomiting, also occurred early in the course of using pramlintide and resolved over time.

In the end, the FDA approved pramlintide, requiring it to have a strong warning on its label about its potential for causing hypoglycemia. Dr. Edelman believes that on balance pramlintide will prove to be a useful addition to the diabetes treatment arsenal and that "any tool with the potential to help the growing number of people with diabetes live more normal lives is valuable." □

EXENATIDE
From the Gila Monster to You

by Wayne L. Clark

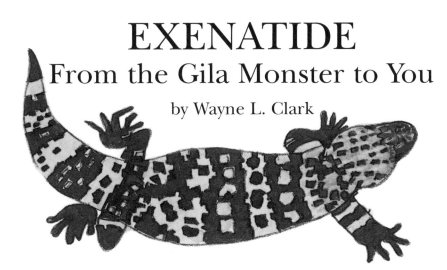

One of the most interesting parts of the story behind the Type 2 diabetes drug exenatide is its source: the saliva of the Gila monster, a large, arguably homely, poisonous lizard that inhabits the deserts of the American Southwest. The injectable drug (brand name Byetta) that is now being prescribed to some 3 million people with Type 2 diabetes is actually a synthetic version of the hormone exendin-4, found naturally in the Gila monster's saliva.

Exenatide is the first of a new class of drugs known as "incretin mimetics." Essentially, these substances enhance insulin secretion in response to elevated blood glucose levels. Exenatide also suppresses secretion of glucagon (a hormone that raises blood glucose levels) and slows the emptying of the stomach, both of which help improve blood glucose regulation. Studies have also shown that exenatide may decrease appetite.

Exendin-4 was isolated from the lizard's saliva by endocrinologist John Eng, M.D., of the Bronx Veterans Affairs Medical Center in New York City. But you shouldn't picture Dr. Eng trudging through the desert wrangling lizards. In fact, Dr. Eng didn't even see a live Gila monster until 12 years after he discovered the wondrous properties of the hormone in its saliva.

Two threads of research came together to produce exenatide. Dr. Eng had been studying hormones to determine if any of them might have pharmaceutical value. He followed up on earlier studies showing that some animal venoms could produce inflammation in the pancreas, and first among the venoms of interest was that of the Gila monster. So he ordered samples from a supplier in the Southwest and began to test them.

Meanwhile, other researchers were examining the hormone glucagon-like peptide-1 (GLP-1), which occurs naturally in the human gut. GLP-1 stimulates insulin secretion from the pancreas in response to high blood glucose levels. Exendin-4 had similar properties, and Dr. Eng put the two threads together. He found that exendin-4 had an important advantage over GLP-1. The human hormone is destroyed quickly in the bloodstream, while exendin-4 lasts several hours before being degraded.

Exendin-4 was a potential drug without a home until four years after its discovery, when Amylin Pharmaceuticals, Inc., of San Diego licensed it from Dr. Eng. Amylin joined forces with Eli Lilly and Company to bring the drug to market as exenatide injection, trade-named Byetta. They received FDA approval in April 2005 for the drug to be used by people with Type 2 diabetes who are unable to control their blood glucose levels with oral medicines.

Early speculation was that the drug could benefit millions of the estimated 20 million people with Type 2 diabetes in America alone, and could be worth $1 billion a year to its manufacturers.

More help for blood glucose control

The excitement about exenatide is due to the degree to which it helps people who use oral medicines stabilize their blood glucose levels. The major problem faced by people with diabetes in terms of their blood glucose levels is often the postprandial, or after-meal, increase in those levels. It's an effect that not only drives up blood glucose levels at that time but also contributes to keeping them high much of the day. The result is demonstrated by the high glycosylated hemoglobin (HbA_{1c}, a measure of long-term blood glucose control) levels experienced by many people with diabetes, despite their best efforts to manage their blood glucose levels.

In a person who does not have diabetes, the

beta cells in the pancreas release insulin in sync with the rise in blood glucose following a meal. Insulin levels generally reach their peak within 10 minutes. A chart showing insulin release and blood glucose levels in a person without diabetes reveals almost perfectly matched curves. Seldom does that person's blood glucose top 140 mg/dl in the hour or two after a meal.

In Type 2 diabetes, the release of insulin in response to blood glucose is both delayed and blunted. If the person does not inject insulin or take a drug that stimulates insulin release, eating can cause a blood glucose level that rises to 300 mg/dl or more and remains high for several hours. A rapid-acting insulin analog (aspart, glulisine, or lispro) can stop acting while the blood glucose level is still rising, especially if the person has delayed stomach emptying (gastroparesis), resulting in high blood glucose levels hours after a meal.

Exenatide acts like the naturally occurring hormone GLP-1 to in-crease insulin secretion in the presence of increased blood glucose. This is called the "incretin effect," which gives rise to the name of the drug class. Exenatide is called a "mimetic" because it mimics the natural incretins.

People with diabetes also experience a postprandial increase in excretion of the hormone glucagon from the alpha cells of the pancreas. Glucagon stimulates the liver to release glucose into the bloodstream, which raises blood glucose levels. Exenatide lowers the levels of glucagon circulating in the blood, further improving blood glucose control.

Exenatide has other beneficial effects, including appetite suppression, slower emptying of the stomach, and weight loss.

The primary clinical trials that led to the approval of exenatide consisted of three 30-week phase III trials. (Phase III trials are the late-phase studies required by the FDA to evaluate a drug's safety and efficacy before judging whether to approve it.) All three were randomized trials in which neither the investigators nor the participants knew whether they were getting exenatide or a placebo (sham treatment). Participants continued their current medicines and injected either 5 micrograms or 10 micrograms of exenatide (or the placebo) before their morning and evening meals.

The first trial enrolled people with Type 2 diabetes who had inadequate blood glucose control with use of the oral medicine metformin. Metformin suppresses glucose production by the liver and also increases tissue sensitivity to insulin.

Nearly half (46%) of the people who received 10 micrograms of exenatide in addition to met-

formin were able to reach an HbA_{1c} goal of 7% or less, compared with only 13% of the people receiving a placebo. The people who received the highest dose of exenatide also experienced modest weight loss (about 3% of their body weight) and did not experience more episodes of hypoglycemia than people taking the placebo, which is always a concern when a blood-glucose-lowering drug is introduced.

Another trial was conducted in people with Type 2 diabetes who were inadequately controlled while taking one of the sulfonylureas (glimepiride, glipizide, or glyburide). The sulfonylureas are oral medicines that bind to receptors on the beta cells and stimulate insulin secretion; they may also decrease glucose production by the liver.

The results were similar to the metformin trial, with 41% of people taking the higher dose of exenatide with a sulfonylurea achieving an HbA_{1c} of 7% of lower, compared with only 9% of the people receiving a placebo in addition to the sulfonylurea. The group using exenatide also experienced modest weight loss. There was a significantly higher incidence of hypoglycemia in the group taking exenatide—36% for those on 10 micrograms of exenatide and 14% for those on 5 micrograms—compared with 3% for the placebo group.

The third trial tested the effect of exenatide on people with Type 2 diabetes who were inadequately controlled on combination therapy of metformin and a sulfonylurea. Thirty-four percent of the people who added 10 micrograms of exenatide achieved an HbA_{1c} of 7% or less, compared with 9% of the people on placebo. This trial also found a higher incidence of hypoglycemia in the group receiving exenatide. (Twenty-eight percent of the group receiving 10 micrograms of exenatide experienced hypoglycemia, compared with 13% in the group receiving placebo.)

Researchers concluded that to reduce the increased risk of hypoglycemia when using exenatide with a sulfonylurea, physicians might consider reducing the dose of the sulfonylurea. Exenatide is labeled with that caution for people taking a sulfonylurea. There is no similar caution for metformin users.

The other notable side effect of exenatide is mild to moderate nausea, which affected 44% of the people in the clinical trials who received the drug, compared with only 18% of those who did not. The effect appears to be dose-dependent and decreases over time as the person becomes used to the drug.

Exenatide's developers were concerned that because the drug must be injected, it would not be

A WORD FROM OUR SPONSOR

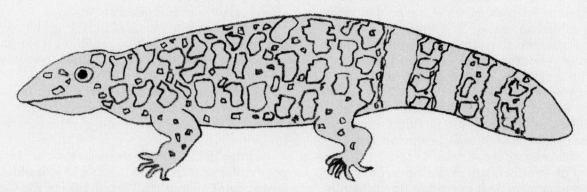

The Gila monster (*Heloderma suspectum*) is a poisonous lizard (one of only two known species of venomous lizards) that inhabits desert areas of the American Southwest and northern Mexico. It can reach up to 24 inches in length and can live for up to 30 years.

The Gila monster delivers its venom through its saliva as it chews on its prey, as opposed to injecting it as a snake does. The venom is not generally fatal to humans, but a Gila monster bite is described as extremely painful.

appealing to people who otherwise don't use injectable medicines (as opposed to those who already inject insulin and are used to the idea). So they developed a prefilled injector "pen" that holds a 30-day supply of the drug, to make it as easy as possible.

That other new drug

If the effects of exenatide sound somewhat familiar, that may be because another relatively new diabetes drug, pramlintide (Symlin, also marketed by Amylin Pharmaceuticals) has many of the same effects. The two drugs are different, however, with different mechanisms of action. Pramlintide is a synthetic version of a hormone that is coproduced and cosecreted with insulin in the beta cells of the pancreas and binds to receptors in the stomach and brain. It acts to suppress the appetite, slow the emptying of the stomach, and suppress glucagon secretion. The FDA has approved it for use in people with diabetes who use insulin, whether they have Type 1 or Type 2 diabetes.

By contrast, exenatide is a synthetic variant of a hormone produced in the intestine that binds to receptors in the pancreas, stomach, lung, and brain. Like pramlintide, it suppresses appetite, slows stomach emptying, and suppresses glucagon secretion, but it also stimulates the beta cells to produce insulin in response to blood glucose levels. Pramlintide does not stimulate the beta cells.

Exenatide is currently approved for use only in people with Type 2 diabetes, and only in those who take metformin, one of the sulfonylureas, one of the thiazolinediones, or a combination of metformin and one of the other two classes of drugs. It is not approved for use in people who take insulin; however, trials are in progress to study its use both as a stand-alone therapy and as an add-on to insulin therapy. A long-acting version of exenatide is in development, which would replace twice-daily injections with one injection a week.

In October 2007, the FDA issued a Medwatch warning about exenatide, due to 30 cases of acute pancreatitis in people taking the drug. The manufacturer is adding precautionary language to the packaging.

What's next?

Research results presented at the American Diabetes Association's 65th Annual Scientific Sessions in June 2005 provided evidence that exenatide might eventually be an alternative to insulin for people with Type 2 diabetes who are unable to control their blood glucose levels with oral medicines. The research compared exenatide with insulin glargine (a long-acting insulin analog) in people taking both metformin and a sulfonylurea. At the end of the study, people receiving insulin and people receiving exenatide had similar success in controlling blood glucose levels. Exenatide lowered HbA$_{1c}$ levels by 1.0% versus 1.1% for insulin, and 46% of the people receiving exenatide achieved an HbA$_{1c}$ level of 7% or less compared with 48% of those taking insulin.

The big difference between the two therapies was body weight—the people taking exenatide lost an average of 5.1 pounds, while the people taking insulin gained an average of 4.0 pounds. Weight gain is a common side effect of insulin therapy, and lowered body weight is generally helpful in controlling diabetes and preventing cardiovascular complications.

Some experts speculate that exenatide may have still other benefits yet to be fully investigated. For instance, because studies in animals have shown that exenatide can cause beta-cell regeneration and prevent beta-cell death, research is in progress to determine if exenatide has the same effect in humans. Promising results could have significant implications for both people with Type 1 diabetes and those with Type 2.

There are other incretin mimetics under development as well. Liraglutide, which is being developed by Novo Nordisk, and PC-DAC:Exendin-4, which is a product of ConjuChem, are long-acting GLP-1 analogs in the research pipeline.

Meanwhile, a new class of oral drugs has been introduced that produces a similar effect by saving the patient's own GLP-1 by inhibiting the enzyme that breaks it down. The DPP-IV inhibitor sitagliptin is approved for use by itself or in combination with metformin or a thiazolinedione. Another DPP-IV inhibitor, vildagliptin, is in development.

In June 2005, Dr. Eng was able to write the first prescription for exenatide, as his 13-year-old discovery came to market. With thanks to the Gila monster, he provided the medicine for one of his patients at the Bronx Veterans Affairs Medical Center in New York City. □

ORAL MEDICINES FOR TYPE 2 DIABETES

by Patti Geil, M.S., R.D., C.D.E., and Laura Hieronymus, M.S.Ed., A.P.R.N., B.C.-A.D.M., C.D.E.

A man's health can be judged by which he takes two at a time—pills or stairs
—Joan Welsh

Taking care of your diabetes is a bit like building a home. With input from your diabetes care team contractors, you begin by drafting a well-thought-out set of blueprints and assembling all the tools you need to control your blood glucose levels. Healthy eating and physical activity serve as a sturdy foundation for your house of diabetes care, while monitoring blood glucose provides you with feedback for changes to the existing plans.

Although eating well and exercising are always the first line of therapy for all types of diabetes, there may come a time when you and your healthcare team decide to intensify your Type 2 diabetes control by adding an oral blood-glucose-lowering medicine to your carefully crafted plan. Oral dia-

betes medicines are one tool that can give you a step up toward reaching your blood glucose targets and reinforcing your strong diabetes home.

What goes wrong

Type 2 diabetes is a complex condition, which means there are a multitude of options for successful treatment. In a person without diabetes, blood glucose rises whenever food is eaten. The pancreas quickly senses the glucose and produces insulin, which opens the doors of the muscle and fat cells so the glucose can be used for energy. People with Type 2 diabetes may release the proper amount of insulin in response to glucose, but the cells are "insulin resistant"; that is, they can't sense the insulin and don't take in much glucose. This leaves glucose in the bloodstream, which stimulates the pancreas to produce more insulin than would normally be necessary. Over the course of years, the pancreas may fail to keep up with the demand for insulin, leading to persistently elevated blood glucose levels and a diagnosis of Type 2 diabetes.

The liver is also involved in the process by tracking insulin levels in the blood. In a person without diabetes, both insulin and glucose levels are elevated at the same time after eating. If a person hasn't eaten for several hours (such as overnight), the liver senses the lack of insulin and responds by producing glucose from storage to keep the blood glucose level from dropping too low. When Type 2 diabetes sets in, the liver may fail to sense insulin levels properly and may produce more glucose than required.

In a nutshell, three areas "in need of repairs" characterize Type 2 diabetes: insulin resistance (muscle cells that don't easily take in glucose), insulin deficiency (a pancreas that doesn't make enough insulin), and increased hepatic glucose output (a liver that releases too much glucose). Fortunately, there are several options in the diabetes toolbox to make the needed repairs, including healthy eating, physical activity, and oral medicines.

The diabetes toolbox

Keeping blood glucose levels near to normal can reduce your risk of the chronic or long-term complications of diabetes such as retinopathy (eye disease), nephropathy (kidney disease), neuropathy (nerve damage), and cardiovascular disease. You and your health-care team should work together to draw up the blueprints for successfully reaching your individualized target blood glucose goals.

Many health-care providers and their patients choose to begin the path to intensified blood glucose control with oral medicines. It's important to note up front that oral medicines are not insulin. Insulin can't be given orally because digestive enzymes would destroy it. Control of Type 2 diabetes involves a stepwise approach that begins with identifying the proper treatment plan based on your age, weight, desired level of blood glucose control, and specific characteristics of the medicines being considered.

Often the plan begins with *monotherapy*, which is one blood-glucose-lowering oral medicine in addition to a healthy lifestyle. If this doesn't achieve the desired result, adding one or more additional medicines (*combination therapy*) may be considered.

Combination therapy may involve taking two or more individual pills, or it may be achieved with one of the newer combination pills, which have two drugs in one pill.

Research has shown that most of the oral diabetes medicines currently on the market lower glycosylated hemoglobin (HbA_{1c} or A1C) approximately 1% to 2%. The HbA_{1c} test is an indicator of average blood glucose control over the previous 2–3 months. The American Diabetes Association currently advocates an HbA_{1c} reading lower than 7% for most people with diabetes. The American Academy of Clinical Endocrinologists recommends an HbA_{1c} value below 6.5%. You and your health-care provider should agree on a target that is right for you. Higher HbA_{1c} levels are associated with the development of diabetes complications.

In general, certain classes of drugs, including the sulfonylureas, meglitinides, D-phenylalanine derivatives, and biguanides, are more potent in lowering blood glucose than are others, such as the thiazolidinediones, alpha-glucosidase inhibitors, or dipeptidyl peptidase-4 (DPP-4) inhibitors when used as monotherapy. (See "Effectiveness of Oral Medicines" on page 232 for a comparison.) However, there are limits to how much of any one drug can be taken. When a maximal dose of one drug isn't enough to keep blood glucose levels in the desired range, adding a drug from a different class can lower blood glucose further. The combination of oral diabetes drugs used is typically based on what drugs are approved by the Food and Drug Adminstration (FDA) for use with other forms of these drugs.

Injection therapies are another option for treating Type 2 diabetes. Many physicians recommend starting exenatide or insulin when combinations of oral medicines are not effective at keeping blood glucose under control. Exenatide or insulin may either be added to the current regimen of pills or used in place of one or more of the oral medicines a person has been taking. If you are taking a regimen of insulin that includes mealtime insulin and despite your best efforts your blood glucose is not well controlled, then another injectable, called pramlintide may be added to your mealtime insulin regimen. (See "What Are Exenatide and Pramlintide" on page 233.)

Type 2 diabetes involves several problems in metabolism, and oral medicines have been developed to provide solutions to each one. Seven distinct classes of oral drugs are now available for the treatment of Type 2 diabetes. "Oral Diabetes Medicines at a Glance" on pages 234–235 summarizes the important characteristics of each class. Each

EFFECTIVENESS OF ORAL MEDICINES

Some classes of diabetes drugs lower blood glucose more than others, but in some cases, two or even three classes of drugs can be combined for more effective treatment.

DRUG CLASS	EXAMPLES	AMOUNT IT DECREASES FASTING BLOOD GLUCOSE LEVELS	AMOUNT IT DECREASES HbA$_{1c}$
Alpha-glucosidase inhibitors	acarbose (**Precose**) miglitol (**Glyset**)	35–40 mg/dl	0.7% to 1.0%
Biguanides	metformin (**Glucophage**)	50–70 mg/dl	1.5% to 2.0%
DPP-4 inhibitors	sitagliptin (**Januvia**)	20–60 mg/dl	0.6% to 0.7%
D-Phenylalanine derivatives	nateglinide (**Starlix**)	65–75 mg/dl	0.5% to 2.0%
Meglitinides	repaglinide (**Prandin**)	65–75 mg/dl	0.5% to 2.0%
Sulfonylureas	glipizide (**Glucotrol, Glucotrol XL**) glyburide (**DiaBeta, Glynase, Micronase**) glimepiride (**Amaryl**)	60–70 mg/dl	0.8% to 2.0%
Thiazolidinediones	pioglitazone (**Actos**) rosiglitazone (**Avandia**)	25–50 mg/dl	0.5% to 1.5%

class has a different mechanism of action, which means that each contributes to blood glucose control in a different way.

Alpha-glucosidase inhibitors. This class of drugs, which includes acarbose (brand name Precose) and miglitol (Glyset), acts by inhibiting the breakdown and subsequent absorption of carbohydrates from the gut following meals, so it is most effective in controlling postprandial (after-meal) elevations in blood glucose.

Hypoglycemia (low blood glucose) generally does not occur when one of these pills is taken as monotherapy, but it can occur when one or the other is taken in combination with a blood-glucose-lowering drug that can cause hypoglycemia. It's important to note that because of the carbohydrate-blocking effect of alpha-glucosidase inhibitors, some traditional treatments for low blood glucose, such as fruit juice, aren't as effective at raising blood glucose as they normally would be. Sources of pure glucose, such as tablets or gel, are recommended. Gastrointestinal side effects such as abdominal discomfort, bloating, flatulence, and diarrhea may occur when using an alpha-glucosidase inhibitor.

Biguanides. Only one biguanide, namely metformin (Glucophage), is currently approved for marketing in the United States. Metformin is most effective in overweight or obese people who are insulin-resistant. It works by reducing liver glucose output, and it may also improve insulin sensitivity in the liver and muscle and fat cells. Metformin appears to suppress appetite and also lower cardiovascular risk factors without risk of hypoglycemia. Its major disadvantage is that it can cause gastrointestinal problems, particularly at higher doses.

A rare but serious side effect of metformin is lactic acidosis, in which lactic acid builds up in the bloodstream. People with heart, lung, kidney, or liver problems and those who drink alcohol heavily are more prone to developing lactic acidosis.

Sulfonylureas. This class of drugs—which includes glipizide (Glucotrol, Glucotrol XL), glyburide (DiaBeta, Glynase, Micronase), glimepiride (Amaryl), and the less commonly used chlorpropamide (Diabinese), tolazamide (Tolinase), and tolbutamide (Orinase)—works most successfully in those who have recently been diagnosed with Type 2 diabetes. Sulfonylureas are "pancreas stimulators" that cause the beta cells to release more insulin. They are generally inexpensive, and they reduce fasting blood glucose levels effectively.

Side effects associated with their use include weight gain and hypoglycemia.

Dipeptidyl peptidase-4 inhibitors. This drug class, which includes once-daily sitagliptin (Januvia), is used in Type 2 diabetes to block an enzyme that inactivates the hormones called glucagon-like peptide-1 (GLP-1) and glucose-dependent insulinotropic polypeptide (GIP). GLP-1 levels are decreased in Type 2 diabetes. When used alone or with other oral agents that do not cause hypoglycemia, the risk of hypoglycemia is low. As with other drugs, when used in combination with a secretagogue (which includes meglitinides and sulfonylureas), the risk for hypoglycemia may increase. The most common side effects reported include upper-respiratory tract infection, stuffy or runny nose, and sore throat and headache, as well as an occasional upset stomach and diarrhea. If you have kidney problems, your physician may prescribe lower doses of this drug. Your physician will likely recommend periodic blood tests to measure how well your kidneys are working.

Meglitinides and D-phenylalanine derivatives. There is one meglitinide on the market, repaglinide (Prandin), and one D-phenylalanine derivative, nateglinide (Starlix). These drugs are not sulfonylureas, but their mechanism of action closely resembles them. They stimulate the release of insulin from pancreatic beta cells, but they take effect more quickly, and their effects last for only a short amount of time. They are also most effective in people recently diagnosed with Type 2 diabetes, and they act to control postprandial blood glucose elevations.

Either drug should be taken immediately before a meal; if you skip a meal, don't take a pill or you will risk hypoglycemia. If you have trouble maintaining a regular eating pattern, you may have a problem remembering to take these pills.

Thiazolidinediones. Thiazolidinediones, often referred to as TZDs or glitazones, are insulin sensitizers, designed to help insulin work better in muscle and fat tissue while protecting insulin-producing beta cells from further damage. The first approved drug in this class, troglitazone (Rezulin), was removed from the market in 2000 due to reports of severe liver toxicity. The currently available TZDs, pioglitazone (Actos) and rosiglitazone (Avandia), have not been associated with this problem. Nonetheless, periodic liver function tests are still recommended for people taking either pioglitazone or rosiglitazone.

Because the TZDs don't increase insulin secretion, they do not carry the risk of hypoglycemia. People who already use insulin may find that

WHAT ARE EXENATIDE AND PRAMLINTIDE?

Exenatide (brand name Byetta) is an incretin mimetic used in the treatment of Type 2 diabetes which "mimics" the hormone glucagon-like peptide-1 (GLP-1) in the body. This drug is typically added to specific types of oral agents. Exenatide does not cause hypoglycemia, but when added to drugs that have hypoglycemia as a side effect, such as secretagogues, avoiding hypoglycemia is important.

Pramlintide (Symlin) is a synthetic form of amylin. Amylin is a naturally occurring hormone manufactured by the beta cells in the pancreas that works together with insulin to control blood glucose levels. While pramlintide does not cause hypoglycemia alone, when it is used with insulin, your premeal insulin dose may need to be lowered to avoid insulin-induced hypoglycemia.

adding a TZD to their diabetes regimen may help to significantly reduce their daily insulin requirement. However, TZDs are costly, and significant weight gain has been reported with their use.

Special considerations

Oral blood-glucose-lowering medicines are generally not recommended for use in Type 1 diabetes because of the total lack of pancreatic insulin production that characterizes this condition. However, research has shown that the alpha-glucosidase inhibitors may be helpful in controlling postprandial blood glucose in people with Type 1 diabetes due to the drug's ability to block the absorption of carbohydrate. Also, because of the insulin resistance that occurs in puberty, metformin has been shown to improve metabolic control in adolescents with Type 1 diabetes. This effect seems to be associated with improved insulin-induced glucose uptake by tissues. In both situations, oral medicines are not a substitute for insulin. They are used in addition to the insulin regimen. It should be noted that these are "off-label" uses of these drugs; neither is approved by the U.S. Food and Drug Administration for marketing as a treatment for Type 1 diabetes.

During pregnancy, insulin has always been the treatment of choice for diabetes because oral medicines have long been thought to increase the risk of damage to the fetus. However, research into

ORAL DIABETES MEDICINES AT A GLANCE

DRUG CLASS	DRUG NAMES	HOW IT WORKS
Alpha-glucosidase inhibitors	acarbose (**Precose**) miglitol (**Glyset**)	Slows down the digestion of certain carbohydrates in intestines
Biguanides[†]	metformin (**Glucophage, Glucophage XR, Riomet** [liquid formulation]))	Decreases production of glucose by the liver; improves insulin sensitivity in liver, muscle, and fat cells
Dipeptidyl peptidase-4 inhibitors	sitagliptin (**Januvia**)	Blocks the enzyme dipeptidyl peptidase-4 (or DPP-4) that inactivates the hormones called glucagon-like peptide-1 (or GLP-1) and glucose-dependent insulinotropic polypeptide (GIP)
D-Phenylalanine derivatives	nateglinide (**Starlix**)	Stimulates the pancreas to release more insulin
Meglitinides	repaglinide (**Prandin**)	Stimulates the pancreas to release more insulin
Sulfonylureas	chlorpropamide (**Diabinese**) glyburide (**Diabeta, Glynase, Micronase**) glipizide (**Glucotrol**) glipizide extended-release (**Glucotrol XL**) glimepiride (**Amaryl**)	Stimulates the pancreas to release more insulin
Thiazoli-dinediones[‡]	pioglitazone (**Actos**) rosiglitazone (**Avandia**)	Improves insulin sensitivity, decreases production of glucose in the liver; takes up to 4–6 weeks for full effect
Combination products	**Avandamet** (rosiglitazone and metformin) **Glucovance** (glyburide and metformin) **Metaglip** (glipizide and metformin) **Actoplus met** (pioglitazone and metformin) **Avandaryl** (rosiglitazone and glimepiride) **Duetact** (pioglitazone and glimepiride)	Drug actions include those for each type of medicine in pill.

The information in this table is based on drug package labeling.

[†]Liver and kidney function should be checked before starting metformin and periodically while taking it; discontinue before and for at least 48 hours after surgical procedures or radiocontrast dye studies.

Drugs and Dietary Supplements

WHEN TO TAKE	SIDE EFFECTS	COMMENTS
Take with the first bite of each meal.	Upset stomach, diarrhea, gas, bloating	Increase dose gradually; if hypoglycemia develops, use glucose gel or tablets for treatment; monitor liver function with acarbose; not to be used by people with inflammatory bowel disease.
Take with food to minimize side effects.	Nausea, diarrhea, gas, metallic taste, decreased absorption of vitamin B_{12}	May improve lipid (blood fat) levels; use only with normal kidney function due to risk of lactic acidosis. If lactic acidosis is suspected, call for medical help immediately; avoid alcohol.
Taken once daily.	Upper-respiratory tract infection, stuffy or runny nose, sore throat and headache, occasional upset stomach and diarrhea.	
Take 1 to 30 minutes before meals.	Hypoglycemia, weight gain, headache	Skip dose if meal skipped.
Take 15 minutes before meals.	Hypoglycemia, weight gain, headache	Skip dose if meal skipped; add dose if meal added.
Take with food.	Hypoglycemia, edema (swelling), low sodium	Long acting (up to 72 hours); avoid alcohol.
Take before a meal. Take 30 minutes before a meal. May be taken with a meal; do not crush or chew. Take before or with meals.	Hypoglycemia, weight gain, nausea, diarrhea, constipation, stomach pain, sun sensitivity, skin rash (can occur with glyburide, glipizide, glipizide extended-release, and glimepiride)	With all sulfonylureas, create a regular schedule to eat meals. Eat meals on time and do not skip.
Take with or between meals.	Headache, weight gain, anemia, edema (swelling)	May improve lipid (blood fat) levels.
Take as directed.	See side effects for each type of medicine in pill.	

‡Liver function tests must be done before starting a thiazolidinedione and periodically while taking it; caution is needed if a person has heart failure; may decrease effectiveness of birth control medicines or cause ovulation to resume.

certain oral medicines (particularly glyburide and metformin) has lead to their consideration as treatment for gestational diabetes and Type 2 diabetes during pregnancy. This is an area of controversy, however, and one in which a woman and her health-care team have to carefully weigh the risks and benefits together.

Getting the most from your medicines

Caring for your diabetes requires attention to detail in many areas, from meal planning to physical activity to monitoring of blood glucose. With everything else to consider, it's no surprise that some people occasionally forget to take their oral medicines. In fact, research shows that nearly one in three people with Type 2 diabetes who need oral medicines fail to take them daily. Unfortunately, this doubles the likelihood of hospitalizations for heart- or diabetes-related complications.

What should you do if you forget to take your diabetes pill or pills? As a general rule, you can take a missed dose of medicine as soon as you remember it. However, if it is almost time for your next scheduled dose, you may be advised to skip the missed dose and go back to your regular schedule. Do not take a double dose. Taking a missed dose of repaglinide or nateglinide between meals could result in hypoglycemia because these drugs stimulate the release of insulin from the pancreas. If you miss a dose of acarbose or miglitol, taking it between meals will have little effect, because its action is based on stopping the absorption of carbohydrate after eating. Instead, resume taking it at your next meal.

Treating diabetes is an art grounded in science. Work with your diabetes team to choose and use the oral medicine or combination of oral medicines that works best for your situation. You may want to consider the cost of the drug and the number of times per day you have to take it, as well as side effects and possible interactions with any other drugs you may take. Fortunately, today's diabetes toolbox is well stocked with options to help you reach your blood glucose targets! □

BLOOD PRESSURE DRUGS
What Are the Options?

by Laura Hieronymus, M.S.Ed., A.P.R.N., B.C.-A.D.M., C.D.E., and Stacy Griffin, R.Ph., Pharm.D.-C.

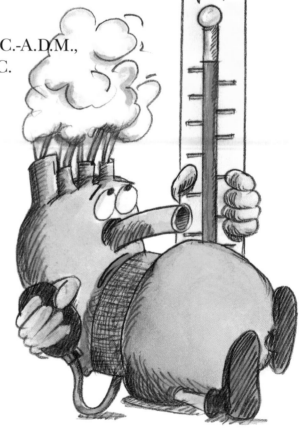

High blood pressure is often referred to as the "silent killer" because many people are not aware that they have it, but kill it can and does. According to the World Health Organization, high blood pressure is estimated to cause 1 in every 8 deaths in the world, making it the third leading cause of death worldwide. This article discusses current recommendations for treating blood pressure and presents information on the drugs available to control high blood pressure.

Hypertension is the medical term for high blood pressure. "Hyper" means "high," and "tension" refers to "strain, stress, or pressure." Hypertension is defined as a generally symptomless condition in which abnormally high pressure in the arteries increases the risk of problems such as stroke, aneurysm (an abnormal bulge in a blood vessel that may burst), heart attack, heart failure, and kidney damage.

Your heart is a pump that keeps blood circulating throughout your body. Blood is pushed through the arteries at pressures determined by a variety of factors, such as the demand for oxygen and nutrients carried in the blood, and can vary throughout the day. When you have high blood pressure, the pressure on your arteries stays too high and damages the artery walls. When arteries are damaged, cholesterol and other substances tend to stick to the walls, building up and causing blockages. If blockages occur in the arteries that supply blood to the heart muscle, a heart attack may result; likewise, blockages that occur in the arteries that supply blood to the brain can lead to strokes. High blood pressure can also cause "hardening" of the small arteries that supply blood to organs, such as the eyes and kidneys, contributing to an inadequate flow of nutrients.

Blood pressure is expressed as two numbers, systolic pressure and diastolic pressure. Systolic pressure, the first number, is the pressure on the arteries when the heart contracts. Diastolic pressure is the pressure on the arteries when the heart relaxes between beats.

In people who have diabetes, high blood pressure (defined by the American Diabetes Association as a blood pressure above 130/80 mm Hg) increases the risk of diabetes complications such as stroke, heart disease, peripheral vascular disease (narrowed arteries in the legs and sometimes the arms), retinopathy (eye disease), nephropathy (kidney disease), and perhaps even neuropathy (nerve damage). In people with Type 2 diabetes, high blood pressure is often part of a cluster of problems referred to as dysmetabolic syndrome (also called metabolic syndrome or syndrome X) that includes high blood glucose, blood fat disorders, obesity, and insulin resistance. In people with Type 1 diabetes, high blood pressure may indicate the possibility of kidney problems. In fact, depending on age, weight, and ethnicity, high blood pressure affects 20% to 60% of people with diabetes.

High blood pressure generally causes no symptoms, even while it may be causing damage to your body. Some symptoms that are commonly thought to be a result of high blood pressure, such as headaches, dizziness, a flushed face, and nosebleeds, are vague and occur as often in people who do not have high blood pressure as in those who do. Actual, serious symptoms of high blood pressure, such as shortness of breath, visual problems, and fatigue, are usually the result of damage to organs, such as the heart, brain, eyes, and kid-

QUESTIONS TO ASK YOUR DOCTOR

- What is my blood pressure reading in numbers? (Ask your health-care provider to write it down for you.)
- What is my blood pressure goal?
- Is my blood pressure under adequate control?
- Is my systolic pressure too high?
- What would be a healthy weight for me?
- Is there a diet to help me lose weight (if I need to) and lower my blood pressure?
- Is there a recommended healthy eating plan I should follow to help lower my blood pressure (if I don't need to lose weight)?
- Is it safe for me to start doing regular physical activity?
- What is the name of my blood pressure medicine? Is that the brand name or the generic name?
- What are the possible side effects of my medicines? (Be sure the doctor knows about any allergies you have and any other drugs you are taking, including over-the-counter drugs, vitamins, and dietary supplements.)
- What time of day should I take my blood pressure medicine?
- Should I take it with food?
- Are there any foods, beverages, or dietary supplements I should avoid when taking this medicine?
- What should I do if I forget to take my blood pressure medicine at the recommended time? Should I take it as soon as I remember, or should I wait until the next dose is due?

This list of questions was developed by the National Heart, Lung, and Blood Institute, which is part of the National Institutes of Health and the U.S. Department of Health and Human Services.

neys, from the presence of long-standing or untreated high blood pressure.

To prevent high blood pressure from causing any organ damage, it's important to recognize and treat it early. Your diabetes health-care team should check your blood pressure at every regularly scheduled visit. When they do, ask what your level is. Blood pressure monitoring goes hand in hand with blood glucose monitoring in preventing many diabetes complications.

New blood pressure targets

The seventh report of the Joint National Committee on Prevention, Detection, Evaluation, and Treatment of High Blood Pressure has recommended new guidelines for prevention and management of high blood pressure. These recommendations, which were published in the May 21, 2003, issue of *The Journal of the American Medical Association,* are as follows:

■ In persons over 50 years, systolic blood pressure of more than 140 mm Hg is a more important risk factor for cardiovascular disease than diastolic blood pressure.

■ Risk of cardiovascular disease begins at 115/75 mm Hg and doubles with each increment of 20/10 mm Hg. Individuals who have normal blood pressure at 55 years of age have a 90% lifetime risk of developing high blood pressure.

■ Individuals with a systolic blood pressure of 120 to 139 mm Hg and a diastolic of 80 to 89 mm Hg should be considered "prehypertensive" and should make health-promoting lifestyle modifications to prevent cardiovascular disease.

■ Thiazide diuretics should be used to treat most people with hypertension; however, certain high-risk conditions, such as diabetes, may also be better treated with the addition of other antihypertensive drugs such as angiotensin-converting enzyme (ACE) inhibitors, angiotensin-II receptor blockers, beta-blockers, or calcium channel blockers. (Note that not all experts on hypertension agree that diuretics are the best choice or should be the first choice for most people.)

■ Most people with high blood pressure need two or more antihypertensive drugs to achieve blood pressure goals (less than 130/80 mm Hg in persons with diabetes or chronic kidney disease).

■ If a person's blood pressure is higher than 150/90 mm Hg, his doctor should consider initiating therapy with two drugs.

■ The most effective therapy prescribed by the most careful clinicians will control high blood pressure only if the person is motivated to be a partner in the process.

Work with your health-care team to determine the best treatment plan for you. (See "Questions to Ask Your Doctor" on page 237.)

Healthy lifestyle habits

Maintaining a healthy lifestyle can help to control your blood pressure. When discussing plans to manage your blood pressure with your doctor, be sure to ask what sort of lifestyle modifications would help you the most. Your doctor or diabetes educator can help you to establish and maintain a plan that includes physical activity and, if needed, stress reduction and smoking cessation. A registered dietitian, ideally one who specializes in diabetes management, can help you design an individualized meal plan and set goals for weight loss, if necessary. Making healthy food choices such as fruits, vegetables, and low-fat dairy foods, as well as choosing and preparing foods with less sodium are key considerations that go hand in hand with counting carbohydrates for blood glucose control. If you drink alcoholic beverages, do so in moderation, which for most men is no more than two drinks per day, while most women and lighter-weight persons should consume no more than one drink per day. One drink is equivalent to 5 ounces of wine, 12 ounces of beer, or 1–1½ ounces of distilled spirits.

Drug therapy

Changing lifestyle habits may not be enough to lower your blood pressure to meet recommended goals. You may also need to take blood-pressure-lowering drugs. However, drugs should be added to, not substituted for, healthy lifestyle behaviors since exercising, eating right, and reducing stress will help your medicines work and may reduce the amount of medicine needed.

If your doctor prescribes medicines to treat your high blood pressure, you must take your drugs exactly as prescribed, even if you feel fine. Because some antihypertensive drugs can cause serious problems if stopped suddenly, you should never stop taking your medicine without first checking with your doctor. If you think the drugs may be causing some side effects, speak with your doctor immediately but don't stop taking the medicines without guidance. Some of the most common side effects are included in this article and the table "Common Blood Pressure Drugs by Class" on page 239. If you have any additional side effects that you think are related to these drugs, discuss these concerns with your doctor or pharmacist. If you are pregnant or planning to become pregnant, check with your doctor regarding the safety of your blood pressure medicine during pregnancy. If you are taking an "extended release" product to lower your blood pressure, you should swallow it whole. Do not crush, split, or chew it. Taking your medicine at the same time each day will help you remember to take it regularly and make your therapy more effective. (See "Tips to Help You Remember to Take Your Blood Pressure Drugs" on page 241.)

High blood pressure is a chronic disease that

COMMON BLOOD PRESSURE DRUGS BY CLASS

The following are some of the most common medicines used to treat high blood pressure. Many of them are also available as combination pills containing two antihypertensive drugs.

CLASS	CAUTIONS OR POSSIBLE CONTRAINDICATIONS
Alpha–beta blockers carvedilol (brand name Coreg) labetalol (Normodyne, Trandate)	Same cautions as alpha-blockers and beta-blockers (see below).
Alpha-blockers doxazosin (Cardura) prazosin (Minipress)	Rise from sitting position carefully; may cause dizziness.
Angiotensin-converting enzyme (ACE) inhibitors benazepril (Lotensin) captopril (Capoten) enalapril (Vasotec) fosinopril (Monopril) lisinopril (Prinivil, Zestril) moexipril (Univasc) perindopril (Aceon) quinapril (Accupril) ramipril (Altace) trandolapril (Mavik)	Avoid during pregnancy. May increase blood potassium levels. May not be appropriate for people with impaired function of or blood flow to the kidneys or those who are blood-volume-depleted such as people on dialysis or using intensive diuretic therapy.
Angiotensin-II receptor blockers (ARB) candesartan (Atacand) irbesartan (Avapro) losartan (Cozaar) olmesartan (Benicar) telmisartan (Micardis) valsartan (Diovan)	Avoid during pregnancy. May increase blood potassium levels. May not be appropriate for people with impaired function of or blood flow to the kidneys or those who are blood-volume-depleted such as people on dialysis or using intensive diuretic therapy.
Beta-blockers atenolol (Tenormin) bisoprolol (Zebeta) metoprolol (Lopressor, Toprol XL) nadolol (Corgard) pinbutolol (Levatol) propranolol (Inderal)	Report any symptoms of shortness of breath, swelling, wheezing, extremely slow heartbeat, cold hands and feet, blue fingernails, or confusion. Should be used with caution in people with congestive heart failure, heart block, chronic obstructive pulmonary disease, or asthma. Rise from sitting position carefully; may cause dizziness.
Calcium channel blockers ■ *Dihydropyridines* amlodipine (Norvasc) felodipine (Plendil) isradipine (Dynacirc CR) nicardipine (Cardene, Cardene SR) nifedipine (Adalat CC, Procardia XL) nisoldipine (Sular)	Do not take if you have severe hypotension (low blood pressure). Immediate-release nifedipine has been associated with an increased risk of heart attack.
■ *Nondihydropyridines* diltiazem (Cardizem, Cardizem CD, Tiazac) verapamil (Calan, Covera-HS, Isoptin, Verelan PM)	Do not take if you have severe congestive heart failure or have had a recent heart attack. Report dizziness, leg swelling, or shortness of breath.
Direct vasodilators hydralazine (Apresoline) minoxidil (Loniten)	Do not use if you have symptomatic chest pain or severe coronary artery disease. Hydralazine is not recommended for use in people with lupus erythematosus.
Thiazide diuretics hydrochlorothiazide (HydroDIURIL) indapamide (Lozol) metolazone (Zaroxolyn)	May cause decreased blood potassium levels. Should be used with caution in people with gout.

generally requires taking medicines for a long period of time, possibly for the rest of your life. Blood-pressure-lowering medicines work in various ways, with many people needing at least two different blood pressure drugs to reach optimal goals. In fact, 29% of participants in the United Kingdom Prospective Diabetes Study required three or more blood pressure drugs to achieve blood pressure levels in the goal range. (The results of the United Kingdom Prospective Diabetes Study, published in 1998, demonstrated that blood pressure control is as important as blood glucose control in preventing diabetic complications.)

Thiazide diuretics. These drugs are often called water pills because they help to rid the body of excess sodium and water through the urine. The resulting reduced fluid volume in the blood vessels lowers blood pressure. Sodium is also flushed out of the blood vessel walls, allowing the blood vessels to widen. Side effects may include changes in blood sugar levels, blood fats (cholesterol and triglycerides), blood electrolytes, energy level, and uric acid levels (which can cause symptoms in people with gout), as well as impotence and dizziness. Thiazide diuretics may also cause increased sun sensitivity, which can result in redness, peeling, hives, blisters, or scaly patches.

If you take a drug in this class, it helps to take it early in the day to reduce the chances of having to get up at night to go to the bathroom. If you are taking more than one dose a day, take the last dose no later than 6 PM unless otherwise directed by your doctor. If the medicine upsets your stomach, it may be taken with food or a glass of milk. If you notice any sun sensitivity, reduce your sun exposure or cover up before heading outdoors.

ACE inhibitors. ACE inhibitors block conversion of the hormone angiotensin I to angiotensin II, the active form that causes blood vessels to narrow. This helps the arteries to relax so that blood pressure goes down. ACE inhibitors have also been found to be very beneficial for people with diabetes because they have protective effects on the kidneys, even if your blood pressure is within normal range. Side effects may include a dry cough, skin rash, high blood potassium levels, and taste disturbances. Your doctor may monitor your blood potassium levels periodically. Some people are unable to take ACE inhibitors due to the dry cough.

Angiotensin-II receptor blockers. These drugs, called ARBs for short, block the angiotensin II hormone that causes blood vessels to narrow. This also helps the arteries to relax, and blood pressure goes down. They also prevent the kidneys from retaining salt and water. ARBs have also been found to be very beneficial for people with diabetes because they have protective effects on the kidneys, even in people with blood pressure in normal range. ARBs appear to have fewer and less severe side effects than ACE inhibitors. Side effects include high potassium levels and cough. Your doctor may monitor your blood potassium levels periodically if you are taking a drug in this class.

Beta-blockers. Beta-blockers reduce the number of nerve impulses that occur in the heart and blood vessels. The effects of adrenaline are reduced, which helps the heart to beat less frequently and with less contracting force. Many beta-blockers are also used to prevent the heart-related chest pain or pressure associated with angina pectoris (a condition often occurring during exertion where too little blood reaches the heart). Side effects may include bronchospasm, masking of low blood sugar symptoms, insomnia, tiredness, decreased exercise tolerance, increased triglyceride levels, increased blood sugar levels, and decreased sex drive. They may also cause weight gain. It is important not to stop taking beta-blockers abruptly because your condition could worsen.

Calcium channel blockers. Calcium channel blockers can be divided into two classes based on their chemical structures: nondihydropyridine drugs and dihydropyridine drugs. Medicines in the nondihydropyridine class help to keep muscle cells in the heart and blood vessels from taking up calcium, which helps the blood vessels to relax, causing blood pressure to go down. Dihydropyridine medicines are more specific drugs that have no direct effect on the heart but do help to keep calcium out of muscle cells in the peripheral blood vessels. The nondihydropyridines have been shown to reduce the risk of further cardiac events in some people when taken after an initial heart attack. For people with high systolic blood pressure but normal diastolic blood pressure the long-acting versions of dihydropyridine calcium channel blockers have been shown to have favorable effects on reducing the risk of stroke. Calcium channel blockers have shown some protective effects on the kidneys for people with diabetes; although this protection is less than the protection offered by ACE inhibitors, a calcium channel blocker could provide some useful kidney protection for people who cannot tolerate ACE inhibitors or ARBs. Side effects may include constipation, ankle swelling, headache, flushing, and changes in the gums.

TIPS TO HELP YOU REMEMBER TO
TAKE YOUR BLOOD PRESSURE DRUGS

■ Take your drugs at the same time every day. Try to link taking them with something else that you do regularly, like brushing your teeth. If your doctor told you to take your pills with food, try taking them at the same time as you have your meal every day.

■ Write it down. Put a reminder note on the refrigerator, by the phone, on the medicine cabinet, or even on the bathroom mirror. Change the message frequently, using different colors to get your attention, or moving the notes to a different spot.

■ Keep a chart or calendar to write down when you take your drugs. Keep this calendar posted so you can quickly see if you've taken your drugs. Use colored pens to help you keep track of more than one type of medicine.

■ Try using a special pillbox that helps keep your pills organized. You can buy these containers at most drugstores or pharmacies.

■ Ask for help. Family or friends can be a great support system. Put together a team. If you have friends who also take medicines, help remind each other.

■ Put a favorite picture of yourself or a loved one on the refrigerator with a note that says, "Remember to take your high blood pressure medicine."

■ Ask a friend or relative to call your telephone answering machine to remind you to take your high blood pressure drugs, and do not erase the message.

■ Take your high blood pressure drugs right after you brush your teeth and keep them with your toothbrush as a reminder.

■ If you use the telephone company's voice mail service, record a reminder for yourself, and the service can automatically call you every day at the same time.

■ Establish a buddy system with a friend who also is on daily medication and arrange to call each other every day with a reminder to "take your medicine."

■ Ask one or more of your children or grandchildren to call you every day with a quick reminder. It's a great way to stay in touch, and little ones love to help the grown-ups.

■ If you have a personal computer, program a start-up reminder to take your high blood pressure drugs, or sign up with one of the free services that will send you reminder e-mail every day.

■ Remember to refill your prescription. Each time you pick up a refill, make a note on your calendar to order and pick up the next refill one week before the medicine is due to run out.

This list of tips was developed by the National Heart, Lung, and Blood Institute, which is part of the National Institutes of Health and the U.S. Department of Health and Human Services.

Alpha-blockers. These drugs reduce nerve impulses to the blood vessels, relaxing the muscle tissue in blood vessels, which allows the blood to pass through more easily; however, this class of medicines has not been shown to decrease the risk of long-term complications of high blood pressure. Favorable effects include decreasing total cholesterol and increasing HDL cholesterol. They also may improve glucose tolerance. These drugs should be taken at bedtime to lessen the chance of lightheadedness or drowsiness. When taking this type of drug, do not stand up suddenly after sitting, stand for long periods, or exercise too vigorously, especially in hot weather.

Alpha–beta blockers. Alpha–beta blockers work the same way as alpha-blockers but also slow heart rate the way beta-blockers do. Side effects include those common to both types of blood pressure medicines.

Direct vasodilators. These cause blood vessels to widen by relaxing the muscle in the vessel walls, causing a decrease in the blood pressure. Side effects include rapid heart rate, water retention, head-ache, stuffy nose, nausea, and fatigue. One of the drugs in this class, minoxidil, may cause undesirable hair growth.

Some people with high blood pressure may also have another condition that may make some types of medicines more appealing or restrict their use. Drug choice may also be influenced by the fact that many medicines that treat high blood pressure also treat other conditions. If two or more conditions exist, it can be helpful to use one medicine that benefits both conditions. For example,

ACE inhibitors also have protective effects on the kidneys in people with diabetes, so it would be logical to consider them for a person with high blood pressure and diabetes.

Just as some drugs lower blood pressure, others can raise it. Check with your doctor or pharmacist before using any medicines that may increase blood pressure. Some prescription items that may cause an increase in blood pressure include birth control pills, albuterol (used to treat bronchospasm in people with asthma), nonsteroidal anti-inflammatory drugs, and steroid therapy. Women who have high blood pressure and take birth control pills may be advised to try other birth control options. Over-the-counter products that can raise blood pressure such as ibuprofen, naproxen, nasal decongestants (pseudoephedrine), appetite suppressants, and herbal products such as ma huang (ephedra), goldenseal, and licorice may need to be avoided. (Ephedra is now considered by most to be a dangerous drug and should not be used.)

Monitoring blood pressure at home

If you are an adult with diabetes and high blood pressure, you may want to consider monitoring your blood pressure at home. By doing so, you can collect information on what your blood pressure typically is at certain times of day and how it responds to various activities or to any changes in your blood pressure medicines. Home blood pressure monitoring is important because a number of studies have shown that high blood pressure readings found during regular morning blood pressure checks at home are more predictive of complications such as death or kidney disease than a high blood pressure measurement found at a clinic visit. It may be to your advantage to record your blood pressure readings along with your blood glucose readings. If you monitor your blood pressure, make sure you understand how to use your equipment properly. The nurse at your diabetes clinic or doctor's office (or another member of your diabetes-care team who is trained in blood pressure monitoring) can show you how or help with your technique.

Blood pressure monitors come in several basic models. Automatic monitors with a cuff that is wrapped around the upper arm are easier to use than manual or semiautomatic models, and are usually cheaper than models that monitor blood pressure at the wrist. Wrist monitors tend not to be as accurate as models that encircle the upper arm and are not recommended for people with diabetes who also have circulatory problems. Blood pressure cuffs are not one-size-fits-all. Using a cuff that is too big or too small can give incorrect readings, so read the instructions carefully and talk to your health-care provider for help in determining the right size for you. Your health-care team should also help you calibrate your home blood-pressure- monitoring device for accuracy once a year.

The cost of a home blood pressure monitor starts at about $30. Call your health insurance company or talk with your pharmacist about the possibility of insurance coverage for blood pressure equipment.

Reduce your risk now

The good news is that if you have been diagnosed with high blood pressure, you can still take steps to prevent damage from occurring. Damaged arteries can repair themselves if blood pressure returns to normal before there is extensive damage. In the United Kingdom Prospective Diabetes Study, each 10 mm Hg decrease in mean systolic blood pressure was associated with reductions in risk of 13% for any diabetes-related complications, 11% for heart attack, and 15% for deaths related to diabetes.

When you have diabetes, it is to your benefit to be aware of your blood pressure to assure it is within recommended goals. Work with your health-care team to get the most out of your treatment plan. After all, a healthy blood pressure is an essential part of a healthy you! □

Diabetes Complications

Tips 366–463 245

Keeping On Top of Neuropathy 252

Dealing With Constipation 255

Urinary Tract Infections 259
Treatment and Prevention

Cardiac Rehabilitation 262

Treating Heart Failure 265

Stroke Rehabilitation. 270
Offering Hope and Help

Say Yes to Intimacy. 274
Treatment Options for Erectile Dysfunction

Sexual Wellness 280

Protecting Your Kidneys 283

Treating Gastroparesis. 288

Diabetic Ketoacidosis. 293
A Preventable Crisis

6

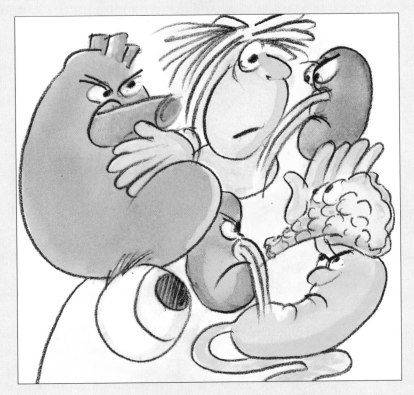

Diabetes Complications Tips

366–463

366. Going a day without a bowel movement does not signify constipation; each person's digestive system has its own natural time frame. A problem is present if you have difficulty or pain passing a stool or extreme infrequency in doing so.

367. Constipation can be caused or worsened by a sedentary lifestyle and a diet low in fiber and high in fat. Exercise improves muscle tone throughout the body, including the digestive tract.

368. Not responding to the urge to have a bowel movement can cause the stool to dry out in the colon, resulting in constipation.

369. Medicines and supplements that can cause constipation include calcium, iron, diuretics, antidepressants, and some pain medicines. Various other medicines can cause fluid loss that results in constipation.

370. To help prevent constipation, increase fluid intake, exercise regularly, avoid laxatives unless prescribed, and eat more whole grains, fruits, and vegetables.

371. Try to get a mix of soluble and insoluble fiber from your diet. Soluble fiber (meaning that it dissolves in water) slows stomach emptying, delays the release of glucose into the bloodstream, and reduces unhealthy cholesterol levels. Insoluble

fiber stimulates muscular contractions that keep the digestive process moving. Both soluble and insoluble fiber can soften and add bulk to the stool, easing constipation.

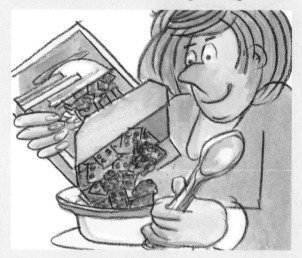

372. To increase your fiber intake, try starting the day with a high-fiber cereal and eating fruit for snacks. Limit foods with almost no fiber such as cheese, meat, ice cream, and many processed foods.

373. If you are not used to eating high-fiber foods, add them gradually to your diet to limit gas, bloating, or diarrhea.

374. Fiber works together with fluid in the digestive system; make sure to increase your nonalcoholic, noncaffeinated fluid intake along with your fiber intake unless you already drink plenty of fluids.

375. Chemical laxatives can be harmful because the colon begins to rely on the chemical stimulation to pass a bowel movement, losing the ability to do so as well when the chemicals are not present. Fiber supplements used as laxatives do not cause this problem.

376. If constipation occurs soon after you start a new drug, or if it accompanies fever, blood in the stool, or unexplained weight loss, see your doctor.

377. If you experience constipation because of gastropathy, a form of neuropathy that causes delayed stomach emptying, avoid high-fat and high-fiber foods, and follow general nutritional recommendations from your health-care provider.

378. Although it may be very difficult to be optimistic, a diagnosis of heart disease can be seen as an opportunity to make a commitment to changing lifestyle habits for the better.

379. Cardiac rehabilitation is a proven method to lower the risk of death and disability and improve the quality of life after a heart attack or heart-related diagnosis or surgery. Almost anyone with heart disease can benefit from some type of cardiac rehab.

380. The American Heart Association recommends cardiac rehab as a helpful option for anyone with several modifiable risk factors for heart disease, including obesity, physical inactivity, diabetes, smoking, high stress level, high blood pressure, and high cholesterol. Cardiac rehab programs can be found not just in hospitals, but in community settings like Y's, as well.

381. If you have heart disease, talk to your doctor about the possibility of enrolling in a cardiac rehab program; a doctor's recommendation can encourage enrollment and may even be necessary for some programs.

382. An individualized exercise program, as offered in cardiac rehab, can instill confidence and good exercise habits so that exercising and its benefits are maintained.

383. Developing a detailed healthy-eating plan with a dietitian can help people lower their cholesterol and blood pressure, keep blood glucose levels in check, and help in weight loss.

384. Depression after a heart attack can impair recovery. If you feel depressed because of your medical condition, support from mental-health professionals can help both your emotional and physical well-being.

385. Some rehab programs offer support groups or classes for the whole family; explore this option if you or your family are interested.

386. If you enroll is a cardiac rehab program, taking an active role in your own care is

necessary; the success of any program requires a mixture of good guidance and a commitment to following it.

387. For people who do not live near a cardiac rehab program or have other reasons not to travel, home-based rehab programs may be an option. Talk to your doctor about it.

388. If you are choosing among cardiac rehab programs, make the decision based on convenience, the range of services offered, and affordability, including what is covered by your insurance. Ask if a program is certified by the American Association of Cardiovascular and Pulmonary Rehabilitation, indicating that it has met patient care and staff expertise standards.

389. Some medical experts recommend that people with Type 2 diabetes have their glomerular filtration rate, an indicator of kidney function, measured through a blood creatinine test because a microalbuminuria test may miss cases of diabetic kidney disease.

390. Drugs called ACE inhibitors and ARBs can reduce blood pressure and help prevent kidney damage; ask your doctor about drug options if you believe you may be at high risk for kidney disease.

391. Dietary protein restriction to slow the progression of kidney disease remains controversial, although it has been shown effective in some cases. Ask your doctor whether you should limit your protein intake for this reason, and if so, plan out your meals with a dietitian.

392. Overuse of over-the-counter analgesics such as aspirin, acetaminophen and ibuprofen can lead or contribute to chronic kidney failure. Use these products as directed on the label, do not combine them, and do not use them regularly or for prolonged periods. If you have kidney disease, ask your doctor before using any of these drugs.

393. A lack of sexual desire may result from depression or from a common class of antidepressant drugs called selective sero-

tonin reuptake inhibitors (SSRIs). High blood glucose can also cause sluggishness that results in reduced sexual desire.

394. Diabetic neuropathy may be a cause of sexual problems, including erectile dysfunction and orgasm disorders.

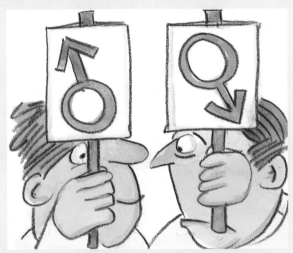

395. Men with diabetes as young as 45 are twice as likely to have a low testosterone level as men without diabetes, often leading to reduced sexual desire. Testosterone deficiency can be treated.

396. Vaginal dryness in women, which can result in painful intercourse, may be worsened by high blood glucose levels.

397. High blood glucose can cause infection in the urinary tract or vagina.

398. Controlling blood pressure may reduce the severity or prevent the progression of erectile dysfunction and other sexual disorders.

399. Sexual problems can lead to emotional problems as well if they persist, which can also have ramifications for someone's partner. Even though seeking help may be difficult, treatment can greatly improve one's well-being.

400. Fatigue, shortness of breath, a cough that produces a frothy discharge, and swollen legs and ankles may signify heart failure. If you have these symptoms, see a doctor; a variety of treatments are available for heart failure.

401. Tight blood glucose control can limit damage to the blood vessels, reducing

the likelihood of developing coronary artery disease and heart failure.

402. Obesity or overweight has been found to be a significant independent risk factor for heart failure, in addition to diabetes.

403. It is much easier to prevent heart failure than to treat it, so maintaining blood glucose control, normal blood pressure, and normal blood lipid levels is essential.

404. It only takes two hours for a harmful level of acidic ketones to build up in the bloodstream if your body runs out of insulin, since most of the body can no longer use glucose as fuel and must break down fats (which creates ketones in the process).

405. Diabetic ketoacidosis, characterized by an extremely high blood glucose level and a toxic level of ketones in the blood, is a medical emergency with possible symptoms of extreme thirst and urination, vomiting, fever, paleness, elevated heart rate, nausea or abdominal pain, fruity or acidic smelling breath, shortness of breath, and lethargy.

406. Although most cases of diabetic ketoacidosis occur in people with Type 1 diabetes, it can occur in people with Type 2 daibetes, as well.

407. During periods of illness or infection, people with diabetes should perform either a urine or blood ketone test to check for diabetic ketoacidosis.

408. Check for ketones if your blood glucose level is over 250 mg/dl twice in a row, or even only once if you intend to exercise soon.

409. Perform a ketone test if your insulin pump malfunctions and causes an interruption in insulin delivery, if you experience traumatic stress, or if you have any symptoms of ketoacidosis such as increased urination, stomachache, or dry mouth.

410. General treatment guidelines for ketones include drinking plenty of water, taking insulin to bring down the blood glucose level, and rechecking for ketones as well as checking blood glucose every three to four hours. If the ketone level does not go down, or if it goes up, go to the hospital—this constitutes a medical emergency.

411. Urine ketone strips are available in individually-wrapped packets, which last longer than those that come packaged together once the package is opened. Since they may be used only sporadically, this can help ensure that they are not wasted.

412. It is possible to have extremely elevated blood glucose without ketones, especially in people with Type 2 diabetes who are dehydrated. This is called hyperosmolar hyperglycemic state, and its symptoms include excessive thirst, hallucination, sensory loss, rapid eye movement, paralysis on one side of the body, and seizure. It may be mistaken for a stroke.

413. Symptoms of a urinary tract infection include possible burning upon urination, the need to urinate frequently or urgently, and lower abdominal pain. Urine may look milky or cloudy, or possible even reddish from blood.

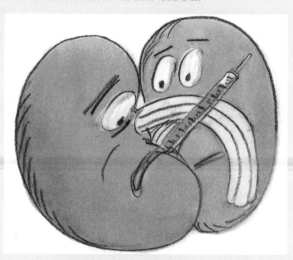

414. A fever, pain in the back or side below the ribs, nausea, or vomiting along with symptoms of a urinary tract infection may indicate that the infection has reached the kidneys.

415. Frequent urinary tract infections may be a sign of other diabetic complications such as neuropathy, which can affect nerves to the bladder.

416. Elevated blood glucose raises the risk of infection, including urinary tract infections.

417. Holding urine in the bladder for a long period of time raises the risk of bladder and urinary tract infections, a risk already elevated in people with diabetes. This risk is higher for women than for men.

418. If you suspect that you have a urinary tract infection, see your doctor so that he can order a urinalysis and make a diagnosis. Treatment consists of antibiotics; if the kidneys are infected, hospitalization may be required.

419. If you have a urinary tract infection, in addition to your prescribed course of treatment, drink plenty of fluids and avoid caffeine, spicy foods, alcohol, and citrus juices, which can irritate the bladder.

420. Drinking plenty of fluids regularly, and urinating regularly, can help prevent urinary tract infections.

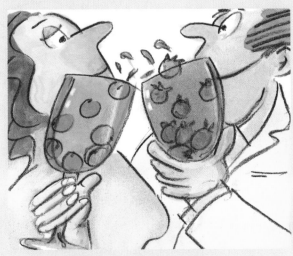

421. Some evidence suggests that consuming cranberry and blueberry juices and vitamin C may help prevent urinary tract infections.

422. To reduce the risk of urinary tract infections, women should wipe in a front-to-back motion after a bowel movement.

423. Women should avoid douches and "feminine hygiene" sprays, which can irritate the urethral tissue and increase the risk of urinary tract infections.

424. Baths may carry a higher risk of urinary tract infections than showers, since prolonged contact with soap can irritate the urethral tissue.

425. Women prone to urinary tract infections should urinate following sexual activity to rid the urethral area of bacteria. If this does not help, prescribed antibiotics may be taken following intercourse.

426. People with diabetes have two to four times the risk of having a stroke as people without diabetes; tight blood glucose control, however, can reduce this risk.

427. Normalizing blood pressure and blood lipid levels reduces the risk of stroke.

428. Rehabilitation is vital to regaining physical and mental function after a stroke.

429. Most physical therapists can teach family members of the recovering individual how to assist with exercises and help with daily activities; this can greatly help recovery.

430. An occupational therapist can be vital to helping an individual who has had a stroke adapt to daily life again.

431. A speech-language pathologist can help someone who has communication problems after a stroke recover language skills and learn alternative ways to communicate when recovery is not possible.

432. New diabetes care equipment may be necessary after a stroke, including insulin dosers that require only one hand and alternate-site blood glucose meters with large displays, or with sound if vision is impaired.

433. If preferred diabetes equipment is not covered by insurance after a stroke, write a letter of appeal to the company explaining the needs of the individual.

434. Angled mirrors on poles and sponges on poles for applying lotion may help with foot care after a stroke if mobility is impaired.

435. A rehabilitative staff member should assess the home of someone recovering from a stroke to ensure safety. Precautions should include proper lighting, tacked-down carpets, clear walkways,

removal of scatter rugs, and possibly installation of grab bars in the bathroom.

436. Special provisions for meal preparation and easy access to a phone or lifeline in case of emergency should be made for people recovering from a stroke who live alone.

437. Erectile dysfunction, or impotence, is not a normal part of aging; it is usually caused by disease, injury, or a drug, and it can be treated.

438. High blood glucose levels can contribute to the blockage or narrowing of blood vessels, which can restrict blood flow to the penis and cause erectile dysfunction. High blood glucose can also lead to neuropathy, damaging the nerve signals needed for an erection to occur.

439. Getting exercise and controlling blood pressure and blood glucose levels can preserve and even improve sexual function in both men and women.

440. An erection lasting more than four hours, a relatively rare side effect of drug treatment for impotence, requires immediate medical attention to prevent permanent damage to the penis.

441. For men, to decrease the risk of impotence, control blood glucose levels as your diabetes plan directs and don't drink alcohol in excess, smoke, or use illicit drugs. Impotence can also result from certain drugs used to treat high blood pressure and heart disease, from cardiovascular disease itself, or from several other factors.

442. It can be crucial to the treatment of impotence to determine whether the cause is mainly physical or psychological; to determine this, doctors may discuss the patient's feelings toward intimacy or administer a physical test.

443. Over the last few years, several new drug treatments for impotence have been developed; if you decide to seek treatment, the chances of success are now greatly improved.

444. If drug treatments for impotence fail, other options such as vacuum devices and penile implants may prove helpful.

445. A penile implant should be only a last-resort treatment for impotence, since it carries surgical risks and permanently alters the internal structure of the penis.

446. Anxiety about sexual performance can compound physical problems. Talk therapy with a psychiatrist, sex therapist, or social worker can help men overcome psychological barriers to intimacy.

447. If you are a man who has impotence, consider seeing a doctor with your partner. Although the causes of your impotence may be physical, communication with your partner can also help improve intimacy.

448. Even though treatment of neuropathy lags behind knowledge of how to diagnose it, knowing you have it is valuable because it allows you to take steps to prevent more serious complications.

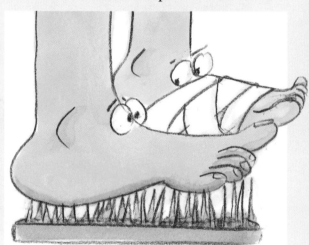

449. If foot pain occurs in one foot due to neuropathy, the other foot may present a greater risk because sensation in it could be diminished, increasing the risk of unnoticed injury and infection.

450. Most people with diabetes should examine their feet daily to check for sores and ulcers. If you have diminished foot sensation because of neuropathy, what you see must replace pain as the indicator that something is wrong with them.

451. The American Diabetes Association recommends that every person with diabetes have a foot examination at least every year. Those with neuropathy should have

an examination at every visit with a health-care professional that includes a test for loss of sensation.

452. Diabetes should not be assumed to be the cause of peripheral neuropathy; making this conclusion could lead to a different underlying cause being ignored. Neuropathy due to diabetes is usually symmetrical and gets worse going closer toward the foot.

453. Some studies have found 63% fewer amputations in people with diabetes among those who regularly see a professional for foot care.

454. Wearing appropriate shoes or inserts can greatly reduce the likelihood of developing an ulcer or other foot injury.

455. Sexual dysfunction, delayed stomach emptying, diarrhea, and difficulty urinating may indicate autonomic neuropathy, or neuropathy affecting the body's internal systems.

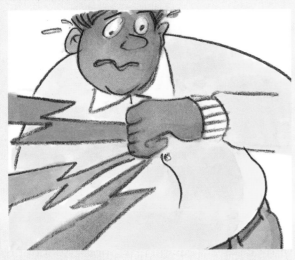

457. Symptoms such as heartburn, difficulty swallowing, low blood glucose after a meal followed by high blood glucose, alternating between constipation and diarrhea, and weight loss may indicate gastroparesis, or delayed stomach emptying due to nerve damage.

458. Even if symptoms of gastroparesis disappear, it is unlikely that the underlying problem is also gone.

459. If left untreated, gastroparesis can cause serious problems including a mass of undigested material in the stomach called a *bezoar*, which typically requires medical intervention to remove followed by a liquid diet for several months.

460. Special nutritional supplements are usually necessary for someone who follows a liquid diet; consult a dietitian for advice on getting adequate nutrients.

461. It may help to divide a liquid diet into six small meals taken throughout the day.

462. Intensive blood glucose control, as well as a specialized diet and exercise, can lessen symptoms of gastroparesis.

463. Many drug treatments, some recently developed, are available to treat gastroparesis. Numerous medical options exist when drug treatments fail.

456. Many doctors recommend regular heart-rate variability tests in people with autonomic neuropathy to check for specific heart rhythm problems, which may then be corrected.

KEEPING ON TOP OF NEUROPATHY

by Wayne Clark

Most people with diabetes have heard of the diabetic nerve damage called neuropathy, though apparently many aren't fully aware of its dangers, which include impotence, heart-rhythm abnormalities, and amputations. Neuropathy affects 90% of people who have had either Type 1 or Type 2 diabetes for more than 10 years, although the symptoms can be subtle or even absent. Most commonly thought of as a foot-care issue, neuropathy actually has several forms and can affect many parts of the body. New tests make diagnosing neuropathy easier, yet long-available, simple tests are still effective and underused weapons.

Even though current knowledge of treating neuropathy lags behind knowledge of how to diagnose it, knowing you have neuropathy is valuable because it allows you to take steps to prevent more serious complications. This article describes two general forms of neuropathy, peripheral and autonomic, and some of the tests used to diagnose them.

Peripheral neuropathy

Peripheral neuropathy, which affects the feet, legs, and, less commonly, the hands, is dangerous because its symptoms can be so subtle. In fact, the "symptomless" foot is most likely to have a problem.

"Pain is what takes most people to the doctor's office," says John B. Perry, D.P.M., a podiatrist in Portland, Maine, who specializes in diabetic foot care. "If it *doesn't* hurt, you don't come in. The problem is, people with diabetes don't have the same sensations in their feet. You have to check and have them checked when they don't hurt.

"I tell people with neuropathy that the nerves in their feet aren't sending information anymore," he says, "and that they have to use their brain and their eyes and their fingers to save their feet."

The damage and the danger from diabetic peripheral neuropathy comes from two basic problems: loss of nerve function and loss of blood supply. Both are caused by the primary dysfunction of diabetes: too much glucose in the blood.

The damage that high blood glucose levels do to the nerves is a complex and still not fully understood cascade of cellular events that is often described as a "dying back" of the nerve fibers. The nerve fibers, the insulating layer that surrounds them, and the cell bodies that supply the nerve with food and fuel, die off. The damage begins at the ends of the longest nerves—those that go to the toes—first, but can eventually affect any and all parts of the peripheral nervous system.

Diabetes also reduces blood flow to the nerves and to the extremities. This contributes to neuropathy and injury, and also affects the body's ability to heal injuries.

Foot disease caused by neuropathy is the most common complication leading to hospitalization of people with diabetes, but according to the National Institutes of Health, only half of people with diabetes check their feet daily. Each year, some 86,000 Americans with diabetes have a lower-extremity amputation, and up to 85% of those losses could have been prevented.

The first and most important step to protecting the feet is preventing injury, whether or not neuropathy has been diagnosed. The most common cause of injury to the feet is improperly fitting footwear. People who do not have neuropathy respond to repetitive stress or pain in their feet by shifting their weight or posture, adjusting their gait, or fixing their shoes. A person with neuropathy does not have the same sensations of pain or discomfort, so the stress goes unrelieved and progresses to a blister or sore, which can develop into an ulcer that requires medical attention. People with diabetes are particularly prone to foot problems as they age, so vigilance becomes ever more important.

"Even without diabetes," Dr. Perry says, "the feet have wear and tear from aging. The toes contract and become less flexible, and where a flexible toe moves with shoe gear, a rigid toe rubs against it. Our arches flatten as we age, and the foot widens. Without diabetes, someone can feel the effects of these changes. With diabetes, they don't feel them, and they're at risk for a blister or a callus.

"Visual deficits from aging might prevent someone from seeing a blister or a cut on his foot," he says. "Loss of flexibility might make it harder to look at the bottom of the feet. Even a diminished sense of smell, a normal part of aging, can prevent someone from smelling an infection."

Diagnosing peripheral neuropathy

The American Diabetes Association recommends that all people with diabetes have a foot examination every year. Those with diagnosed neuropathy should have a foot examination at every visit with a health professional. That examination should include at least a crude test for loss of sensation, and some professionals believe that more sophisticated tests should be included as well.

There are several relatively simple ways to assess the loss of protective sensation that signals peripheral neuropathy. Among the simplest and easiest to administer is the Semmes–Weinstein 5.07 (10-gram) monofilament test. The monofilament is a piece of nylon that is designed to bend as its tip is pressed against the foot.

The test is simple: the person lies down or sits barefoot, with legs extended and supported. The examiner presses the monofilament against four to ten locations on each foot and records whether the person feels the pressure. The filament bends at 10 grams of force, which can be felt by most people with intact nerve function. A secondary but equally important benefit to the monofilament test is that it causes the examiner to take a close look at the feet.

Vibration testing with a tuning fork is another simple test for loss of sensation. The fork is struck and applied to various parts of the foot or leg. The person having the test reports his perception of both the start of vibration and the cessation of vibration.

A professional can also test pain perception by pricking a person's skin with a sterile needle.

An annual examination should also include checking pulses in each foot to check the blood supply to the feet. If a problem is found, more complicated studies can be done to pinpoint the cause.

Joseph C. Arezzo, Ph.D., Professor of Neurology and Neuroscience at the Albert Einstein College of Medicine in New York City, cautions that while the monofilament and other simple tests for sensation have value, they fall short of a complete assessment.

"For a rapid and simple screening, it's a useful technique," he says, "but it can only tell you gross abnormality. That's important because if you're diabetic and have neuropathy, it's almost immediately assumed that it's due to diabetes. In fact, you could have an asymmetric neuropathy, or a slipped disk, or a nerve root disease. In other words, people with diabetes can have anything else that can go wrong with anyone. If you assume the loss of sensation is due to diabetes, you could miss the other problems."

Diabetic peripheral neuropathy is symmetrical, so Dr. Arezzo says that a screening should determine if the loss of sensation is worse on one side than the other, which might indicate a different condition. Likewise, diabetic peripheral neuropathy is usually worse the further you go toward the foot, so if it is not, that could also indicate the need to look for another problem.

"You need to look at the progression and severity, which can be done as simply as adding different monofilaments that bend at lower forces," he says, "and you should test not just both feet, but both ankles and both knees."

The "gold standard" for assessing neuropathy is to assess a person's *electrophysiology* by directly measuring nerve conduction and the strength of nerve signals. A nerve conduction study tests the response of muscles to mild electrical shocks, which are delivered through pads placed on the skin. The person indicates when he feels a tingling sensation, which may or may not be painful. A more invasive examination involves inserting thin needles into the muscle to measure the nerve conduction and does not involve electricity. The only pain associated with this test is that of the actual insertion of the needle through the skin.

"Electrophysiology is getting simpler and more likely to be available in the primary practitioner's office," Dr. Arezzo says. "There is a handheld device that is available now. Sensory evaluations are also going to become more practical, more computerized, and simpler to do."

Another approach is quantitative sensory testing, which measures and evaluates responses to stimuli such as hot and cold, vibration, and pain. Computerized analysis and standardized threshold levels have made these tests much more useful, and people with diabetes are more and more likely to see them in their physicians' offices.

There are shortcomings to sensory testing, and so researchers continue to look for more sensitive and definitive measures of nerve function. For instance, electrophysiological exams assess myelinated fibers (nerves within a sheath), but it may be that neuropathy is evident first in small, unmyelinated nerve fibers, such as certain nerves that feed the blood vessels in the skin.

"These smaller fibers escape the attention of a standard electrophysiological test," says Aaron I. Vinik, M.D., Ph.D., Director of the Diabetes Research Institute of the Strelitz Diabetes Institutes at Eastern Virginia Medical School in Norfolk, Virginia. "Diminished blood flow in the skin, which is regulated by these small, unmyelinated nerve fibers, is one of the earliest abnormalities you can detect in diabetes."

There are several means of measuring the status of these nerves, including laser Doppler measurement of blood flow. "It's going to take a long while before this becomes standardized and can be used in clinical practice," Dr. Vinik says, "but it's easy to perform, it's not invasive, and it can be done in a doctor's office in 10 or 15 minutes."

Other, more esoteric, measurement methods used by researchers to evaluate nerves include *microdialysis* and *iontophoresis,* but Dr. Vinik believes they will remain research tools only.

Another technique called a *skin punch biopsy* continues to be of interest as a potential clinical tool. The technique is available to clinicians now, though it is not routinely recommended.

Active participation is foremost

Diabetes care is a team effort, and in the prevention of foot disease, the individual with diabetes who is educated and aware is the most effective member of the team.

"The more you know, the better," Dr. Perry says. "Here in Maine, we've documented a 51% increase in the utilization of podiatrists after a patient goes to Ambulatory Diabetes Education classes. Some studies have found a 63% improvement in amputation avoidance when the patient sees a professional for foot care, so the potential benefit of education to patients is tremendous.

"There is a tremendous amount of denial about foot problems, especially in men over 50. They're afraid of what it means, that if they report a problem they're going to lose their foot. Some of that is, frankly, justified, because the surgical approach—amputation—is still the first resort of many medical professionals. But amputation is *not* inevitable. Our first goal is to save the foot."

The science of wound care has improved greatly in the past few years, along with the science of prevention. Ulcers that once were certain to lead to amputation can now be healed, and there are many simple, noninvasive ways to prevent ulcers in the first place.

"We have a lot of tools at our disposal," Dr. Perry says. "The right shoes, inserts, physical therapy, and stretching, for instance. We might be able to recommend prophylactic surgery to straighten a contracted toe that would otherwise be at risk, or lower limb bypass surgery to improve blood flow. We know a lot more about wound care today,

TIPS FOR FOOT CARE

When it comes to protecting your feet from injury, you're on the front lines. Here are some tips to help you keep your feet healthy:

■ Don't walk barefoot, even indoors or on the beach.

■ Shake out your shoes before you put them on.

■ Visually inspect and feel your feet every day. If you have a significant other, ask him or her to help you.

■ Keep your feet clean and well-moisturized; dry, cracked skin is an entryway for germs. Apply lotion daily, except between your toes, where extra moisture can lead to breakdown of the skin.

■ Cut your toenails straight across (or following the natural curve of your toes) and not too short. File the edges.

■ Never buy tight shoes—and take any shoes to your foot doctor for a fit check before you wear them. The best choices are leather shoes with low heels, worn with cotton or wool socks. The most problematic choices are plastic shoes, shoes with pointed toes, and high heels.

■ Consider inserts for your shoes, as recommended by a foot-care professional.

■ Keep the blood moving through your feet by exercising regularly and keeping your feet elevated when sitting. Avoid sitting with your legs crossed.

■ Don't smoke. In addition to an increased risk for lung cancer and cardiovascular disease, smoking is linked to worsened blood flow.

■ Work with your health-care team to keep your blood sugar level in your goal range.

and there are new medications that actually help regrow skin to cover wounds."

Autonomic neuropathy

Less well known, and perhaps more dangerous even than peripheral neuropathy, is autonomic neuropathy. This condition affects the autonomic nerves, the nerves that regulate involuntary body functions and systems such as the digestive system, the sexual organs, the urinary tract, the heart, and the sweat glands. Symptoms come in a wide variety of forms, including sexual dysfunction, delayed emptying of the stomach, diarrhea, and difficulty urinating.

Cardiac autonomic neuropathy, an important

factor for cardiovascular mortality in people with diabetes, may cause "silent" heart attacks because people with this form of neuropathy don't feel cardiac pain. Moreover, neuropathy may affect the ability of the heart to vary its rate in response to exercise or a change in position. This loss of heart-rate variability is predictive of serious cardiac problems.

"I believe that measurement of heart-rate variability will become a standard of care in due course," says Dr. Vinik. "It was very difficult to do in the early days, but now there are several machines available that can do it in the doctor's office in 10 or 15 minutes. You get a standardized report that gives you a number, and I believe that this number will be known as commonly as those for cholesterol, blood glucose, or hemoglobin A_{1c}.

"In our practice," he says, "every person with autonomic neuropathy gets a heart-rate variability test, as does every person who has had diabetes more than five years. Every person with Type 2 diabetes gets the test on the first day we see them because they may have had diabetes for seven or eight years already. There are a number of treatment options for improving heart-rate variability."

Another form of autonomic neuropathy and a debilitating late-onset complication of diabetes is *gastroparesis,* a paralysis or dysfunction of the stomach that causes food to move through the digestive tract either too slowly or not at all. Serious cases are readily diagnosed, but more commonly, gastroparesis (or gastropathy) is subtle, causes unpleasant symptoms, and interferes with blood sugar control because food absorption is delayed.

At one time, the only way to diagnosis gastroparesis was with a complicated procedure that examined the different phases of contraction of the stomach and could only be done in a research laboratory. Then researchers developed the *electrogastrogram,* which is similar to an electrocardiogram. They found that the stomach could be subject to rhythm disturbances much like those of the heart: tachygastria (fast contractions), bradygastria (slow contractions), or gastric arrhythmia (irregular contractions).

"Unfortunately, there is no specific therapy for stomach arrythmias as yet," Dr. Vinik says, "but we're hopeful that they will be developed."

Measurement and diagnosis of both peripheral neuropathy and autonomic neuropathy continues to advance. Right now, as always, the vigilance of the individual who has diabetes and the rest of the health-care team is the best prevention. □

DEALING WITH CONSTIPATION

by Judy Giusti, M.S., R.D., L.D., C.D.E.

It's 7 AM, and you have just enough time to pull up to the drive-through window of the local fast-food place for a cup of coffee and a breakfast sandwich before heading off to work. No time to eat at home and certainly no extra bathroom time.

Did someone say bathroom? We all use it, but few of us care to discuss what goes on in there—or what doesn't. Yet everyone experiences constipation at one time or another. Constipation is embarrassing, uncomfortable, and in most cases, preventable. Perhaps a little talking about it would do some good.

What it is

Constipation is the condition of having painful, difficult, or infrequent bowel movements. Many people believe they are constipated if they do not have a daily bowel movement. However, each person's digestive tract has its own time frame for digesting food and removing waste. Having infrequent bowel movements is not a concern as long as the individual is not having pain or difficulty passing stools. Three bowel movements a day may be normal for one person; for someone else, three times a week is normal.

To understand constipation, it is important to understand how food is digested and absorbed. Digestion begins in the mouth when we chew. Saliva, excreted from the salivary glands, softens and binds food together to make it easier to swallow and provides enzymes that begin the process of digesting starches in the mouth. Swallowing begins as a voluntary process then continues automatically as *peristalsis,* the wavelike, rhythmic contraction of the gastrointestinal tract muscles, propels food through the esophagus to the stomach.

In the stomach, food is mixed with gastric juices, which break up the food, and churned into a uniform substance that can be passed into the small intestine for digestion. Most nutrients are absorbed into the body from the small intestine.

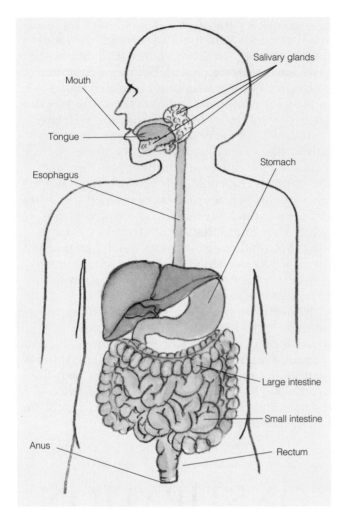

Mouth
Salivary glands
Tongue
Esophagus
Stomach
Large intestine
Small intestine
Anus
Rectum

What material is left then passes into the colon, or large intestine, where water and salts are absorbed into the body. Stools are the solid waste products of the digestive process that collect in the colon and eventually are excreted.

A person becomes constipated when the stools remain too long in the colon because of sluggish gastrointestinal movement, inadequate fiber intake, or poor bowel habits. The longer the stools remain in the colon, the more water is absorbed, and the harder and drier the stools become.

The human digestive tract is often sensitive to external factors such as traveling, which disrupts normal routines, or periods of stress. During these times, it is important to follow the recommendations for preventing constipation.

Causes

Over 4 million Americans are constipated most or all of the time, making it the most common gastrointestinal complaint. This condition most often results from a sedentary lifestyle and a low-fiber, high-fat diet. Being sedentary can lead to prob-

lems with elimination because poor muscle tone weakens normal gastrointestinal tract *motility*, or movement. Regular exercise, on the other hand, improves muscle tone in all parts of the body, including the digestive tract.

Having a hectic schedule and poor bowel habits can also contribute to chronic constipation. For a number of reasons, people often do not respond to the urge to have a bowel movement. They may feel too busy, be reluctant to use a public facility, or be unable to find an available facility when the need arises. When the urge to defecate is ignored, water continues to be absorbed from stools, making them small and hard and causing constipation.

Some medicines can also cause constipation. Calcium supplements, iron supplements, diuretics, antidepressants, and some pain medicines can affect the muscles and nerves of the colon, resulting in a slower movement of the stool. Some medicines can also cause fluid loss, leaving the stool hard and dry.

Prevention and treatment

In most cases, the same treatment and prevention recommendations apply no matter what the cause of constipation: increase fluids; get regular exercise; eat more whole grains, fruits, and vegetables; and avoid laxatives unless they are prescribed by a physician. However, if constipation is caused by an underlying condition such as *gastropathy*, or slowed stomach emptying (discussed later in this article), these suggestions may not apply.

Nutrition plays a major role in helping to prevent constipation and keep the gastrointestinal system functioning smoothly. An important part of a healthy diet is fiber. The American Diabetes Association and The American Dietetic Association recommend that most Americans eat 20 to 35 grams of fiber a day. However, the average American eats about 10 to 15 grams of fiber daily.

Fiber is the part of a plant food that the body cannot digest; fiber is not found in animal products. There are two kinds of fiber: insoluble and soluble. Insoluble fiber, or "roughage," helps to keep the waste products of digestion moving by stimulating muscular contractions in the gastrointestinal tract. It does not dissolve in water. Insoluble fiber is found in whole grains, fruits, and vegetables. Wheat bran is an excellent source of insoluble fiber and very effective at easing constipation. A half-cup serving of Original General Mills Fiber One cereal, for example, provides 14 grams of fiber. Adding a couple of tablespoons of Fiber One to your favorite cereal is a good way to increase your fiber intake gradually.

Soluble fiber, which dissolves in water and

forms a gel in the stomach, has numerous health benefits. The gel slows down stomach emptying and helps delay the release of glucose into the bloodstream, which assists with blood glucose control. In addition, a diet high in soluble fiber has been shown to lower blood cholesterol levels. Soluble fiber is found in fruits, oats, and legumes (dried beans, peas, and lentils). A medium apple contains 4 grams of fiber, and a half-cup serving of kidney beans provides 6 grams of fiber.

Together, soluble and insoluble fiber add bulk to the stool, stimulating peristalsis, and absorb water, softening the stool to make passage easier and prevent constipation. For good sources of both soluble and insoluble fiber, see "Fiber Facts" on this page.

Another potential benefit to increasing your fiber intake is improved blood glucose control. A recent study in people with Type 2 diabetes showed that eating a high-fiber diet may help to bring down blood glucose levels. In the study, published in the May 11, 2000, issue of *The New England Journal of Medicine*, seven people with Type 2 diabetes followed a diet containing 24 grams of fiber per day for six weeks while six others followed a diet containing 50 grams of fiber per day. After six weeks the two groups switched diets, and the study continued for another six weeks. In both groups, the higher-fiber diet caused a blood glucose level decrease of about 10%, the equivalent of an additional dose of oral diabetes medicine.

To increase your daily fiber intake, try starting the day with a high-fiber cereal at breakfast. In contrast to a typical breakfast sandwich, which has only 1 gram of fiber, a one-cup serving of a high-fiber cereal such as Raisin Bran topped with a banana contains about 10 grams of fiber. Choose whole-grain bread instead of white bread at lunch, snack on a piece of fruit between meals, and be sure to have vegetables every day with meals. Not all vegetables are fiber-rich, however. Iceberg lettuce and cucumbers, for instance, are mostly water and contain only about 1 gram of fiber per cup. Eating a wide variety of fresh vegetables, particularly asparagus, broccoli, Brussels sprouts, cabbage, carrots, and green beans, is a healthy way to obtain fiber and essential nutrients. Limit foods that contain little or no fiber, such as cheese, meat, ice cream, and processed foods.

The Nutrition Facts panel on food packages is an excellent resource to determine whether you are getting enough fiber. Good sources of fiber are foods with 3 or more grams of fiber per serving. When reading food labels, don't forget to check the serving size; all the information on a food label is based on one serving, not the entire package.

FIBER FACTS

Dietary fiber comes in two varieties, soluble and insoluble. Soluble fiber delays stomach emptying and glucose absorption and lowers blood cholesterol. Insoluble fiber promotes gastrointestinal motility and adds bulk to the stool.

GOOD SOURCES OF SOLUBLE FIBER
Apples
Barley
Citrus fruits
Legumes
Oats
Strawberries

GOOD SOURCES OF INSOLUBLE FIBER
Vegetables
Wheat bran
Whole-grain breads and cereals

HOW TO INCREASE YOUR FIBER INTAKE

For most people, adding more fiber to the diet is a good idea. (For people with gastropathy, or delayed stomach emptying, increasing fiber intake is not recommended.) To avoid unpleasant side effects such as gas while adding more fiber to your diet, add it gradually, using the following tips:
■ Drink plenty of liquids.
■ Eat a variety of high-fiber foods every day.
■ Eat whole fruit in place of juice.
■ Eat the skin on fruits and vegetables.
■ Add beans to casseroles, soups, and salads.
■ Choose whole-grain cereals, breads, and crackers.
■ Substitute wheat flour for part of the white flour when baking.

Fiber is included as part of the total carbohydrate on a label. Since it is neither digested nor absorbed, however, it will not raise your blood glucose level. When counting carbohydrate, subtract the grams of fiber from the total carbohydrate of a food serving to determine the grams of carbohydrate being absorbed.

If you are not used to eating high-fiber foods it is important to add these foods to the diet gradually to allow your gastrointestinal system to adjust to a higher fiber intake. This will help to prevent gas, bloating, or diarrhea.

Since fiber works together with fluid to improve bowel function, it is also important to drink plenty of fluid each day. Fiber attracts the fluid that provides bulk and makes the stool soft, which stimulates muscle contraction in the colon. Increasing fiber intake without increasing fluid intake can actually cause hard, dry stools and constipation. General recommendations are to drink 8 glasses of fluid (preferably water) each day. Alcohol and liquids containing caffeine, such as coffee and some soft drinks, may have a dehydrating effect by stimulating more frequent urination, so it's best to stick to nonalcoholic, decaffeinated beverages.

Adding some prunes to your diet may also help. Prunes contain a chemical called *dihydroxyphenyl isatin*, which has been shown to help increase intestinal motility. Eating prunes at night can help with elimination the next morning. (Three prunes or one-third of a cup of prune juice is about the equivalent of one carbohydrate choice, or 15 grams of carbohydrate.)

In addition to increasing fiber and fluid intake, keeping physically active can help prevent constipation. Try increasing your level of physical activity by walking 20 to 30 minutes each day, taking the stairs instead of the elevator or escalator when possible, parking farther away from your workplace or from stores, or walking around the mall before starting to shop. Check with your doctor before starting a formal exercise program.

Having regular mealtimes and allowing time in your day to have a bowel movement are also important to help prevent constipation.

Laxatives

Laxatives or enemas should not be used on a regular basis to treat constipation because they can be habit-forming: The colon can become dependent on these methods and become unable to contract and move stools along naturally. Laxatives and enemas can also disrupt the fluid, salt, and mineral balances in the body. Check with a doctor before taking a laxative. Occasionally, doctors may recommend a fiber supplement to act as a bulking agent. Fiber supplements absorb water and make the stool softer. Drugs called stool softeners can also ease problems with constipation.

When to see a doctor

Occasionally, constipation is a cause for serious concern. It can be a sign of problems with the colon or rectum, such as an intestinal obstruction, tumors, cancer, diverticulosis, or scar tissue. Irritable bowel disease, or spastic colon, can cause symptoms alternating between diarrhea and con-

PREVENTING CONSTIPATION

Constipation is not inevitable. Here are a few simple things you can do to stay regular:

■ Get regular exercise.
■ Drink plenty of fluids.
■ Do not ignore the urge to have a bowel movement.
■ Set aside time to go to the bathroom after breakfast or dinner.
■ Do not take laxatives unless they are recommended by a doctor.
■ Check with a doctor if a significant change in bowel habits occurs.

stipation. If constipation occurs immediately after you start a new drug or vitamin supplement or occurs together with fever, blood in the stool, or unexplained weight loss, see a doctor.

Constipation can also be caused by gastropathy, a form of diabetic neuropathy. When the nerves to the stomach are damaged by prolonged high blood sugar, the stomach and intestinal muscles do not function properly, and the transit of food from the stomach is delayed. In addition to constipation, gastropathy can also cause nausea, vomiting, diarrhea, and cramps, and it tends to make blood sugar levels erratic and hard to control. People who have gastropathy (or symptoms of gastropathy) should check with their doctor or dietitian for specific nutrition recommendations. Since fiber and fat also delay stomach emptying, high-fiber and high-fat foods are not recommended for people with gastropathy. Tight blood glucose control can help to relieve symptoms. Certain drugs may also be prescribed for this problem.

Making changes

Constipation, while uncomfortable, is temporary, treatable, and rarely a cause for alarm. However, it is often an indication that your diet and lifestyle are not as healthful as they could be. Dealing with a bout of constipation could be a good time to examine your habits and make some improvements.

Getting regular exercise; eating more fiber-rich whole grains, legumes, fruits, and vegetables; drinking plenty of water; and setting regular times for meals and bathroom use will not only prevent constipation and digestive problems, but they will contribute to overall good health and well-being. □

URINARY TRACT INFECTIONS
TREATMENT AND PREVENTION

by Eduardo Randrup, M.D., and Neil Baum, M.D.

Urinary tract infections (UTIs) are a serious health problem affecting millions of people each year. They are of particular interest to people with diabetes because both the incidence of UTIs and the incidence of serious UTI complications appears to be higher among people who have diabetes. What's more, having frequent UTIs can be a sign of certain diabetes complications. For these reasons, it's important to know about the signs and symptoms of UTIs and to seek medical attention promptly if you experience them.

What is a UTI?

The urinary system is composed of the kidneys, ureters, bladder, and urethra. The kidneys, a pair of fist-size organs located below the ribs near the middle of the back, remove waste products from the blood in the form of urine, maintain a balance of salts and minerals in the blood, and produce several hormones, including one that stimulates the production of red blood cells. The ureters are tubes that carry urine from the kidneys to the bladder, an expandable storage organ for urine in the lower abdomen. Urine is emptied from the bladder through the urethra.

Every day, the average adult passes about a quart and a half to two quarts of urine. The amount of urine that is passed depends on the person's diet as well as the temperature and humidity.

Normally, urine contains fluids, salts, and waste products, but it is sterile, free of bacteria, viruses, and fungi. When microorganisms gain entry to the urinary system through the opening of the urethra, they can multiply and cause an infection. Most UTIs are caused by *Escherichia coli (E. coli)* bacteria, which normally live in the large intestine.

In most cases, the bacteria that can cause a UTI enter through the urethra. An infection limited to the urethra is called *urethritis*. From there, bacteria can spread to the bladder, causing a bladder infection, or *cystitis*. If the infection is not treated promptly, bacteria may travel up the ureters to the kidneys; an infection of the kidneys is called *pyelonephritis*.

Bacteria called *Chlamydia* and *Mycoplasma* may also cause UTIs, but the infections they cause tend to remain limited to the urethra and reproductive system. *Chlamydia* and *Mycoplasma* are usually sexually transmitted, so these infections require treatment of both partners.

In addition to the immune system's protection, the urinary system's physical structure helps prevent most infections. The ureters and bladder normally prevent urine from backing up toward the kidneys, and the flow of urine from the bladder helps wash bacteria out of the urethra. Men have added protection because the prostate gland produces secretions that slow bacterial growth. Obstructions to the flow of urine can contribute to the development of a UTI. Such problems include kidney or bladder stones and an enlarged prostate gland.

Higher risk for women

Women are more prone to having UTIs than men, except perhaps in the neonatal period and in the late stages of life, when both sexes appear to have an almost equal risk of acquiring this type of infection. One reason for this higher risk is simply anatomical. In women, the urethral opening is located about two inches from the rectum, which is believed to be the major source of the bacteria that cause UTIs. In men, this distance is much greater. The distance between the urethral opening and the inside of the bladder in women is about two inches; in men, this distance is four to five times greater, making it more difficult for bacteria to gain access to the bladder in men.

Women also tend to have a somewhat larger bladder capacity than men, a fact possibly linked to social situations or upbringing. For example, many women are reluctant to use public bathrooms for fear of contamination due to unsanitary environments. As a result, these women hold urine in their bladder for longer periods of time. This raises the risk of infection because bacteria have more time to establish themselves in the urinary tract because they are not being washed out as frequently by urine.

Pregnant women may be at higher risk of contracting a UTI or at least have a higher risk of having a UTI spread to the kidneys. Frequent passing of small amounts of urine is a hallmark of pregnancy as the expanding uterus presses on the bladder and tricks the body into sensing a full bladder, but because the frequent need to urinate may also be a sign of a UTI, pregnant women should be cautious and may need periodic testing of their urine. Treating a UTI during pregnancy is important to prevent problems such as premature delivery or high blood pressure.

Women who use a diaphragm or spermicidal foam for birth control may be at higher risk of contracting UTIs. Women who are past menopause may also have a greater risk, possibly because of changes in vaginal and urinary tissues caused by loss of the hormone estrogen.

Diabetes connection

One of the characteristics of diabetes is a greater vulnerability to infections in various systems of the body, including the urinary tract. Various factors contribute to this phenomenon. One of them is that infection-fighting white blood cells have impaired function in people with diabetes. Normally, when an infection occurs somewhere in the body, white blood cells migrate through the blood to the area where the infection is taking place. This response is typically slow and imperfect in a person who has diabetes.

Diabetes also affects very small blood vessels, or capillaries, causing a decrease in the amount of blood delivered to the tissues. This interferes with the body's ability to fight invading microorganisms such as bacteria.

Diabetes can also cause neuropathies, impairments of the function of nerves, which can result in decreased performance of various organ systems. Neuropathy of the nerves to the bladder can cause problems such as reduced sensations of bladder fullness and incomplete bladder-emptying when urinating. Urine remaining in the bladder can provide a breeding ground for bacteria, especially if one's blood glucose is frequently high, resulting in excess glucose in the urine. Having more than two bladder infections per year could be a sign of diabetic nerve damage that may require evaluation by your physician.

These and other abnormalities in diabetes make a person more prone to acquiring an infection and make it easier for an infection to become more severe or more widespread once it has started.

Diagnosis

Symptoms of a UTI may range from nonexistent to severe burning upon urination, a need to urinate frequently or urgently, and lower abdominal pain. The urine itself may look milky, cloudy, or

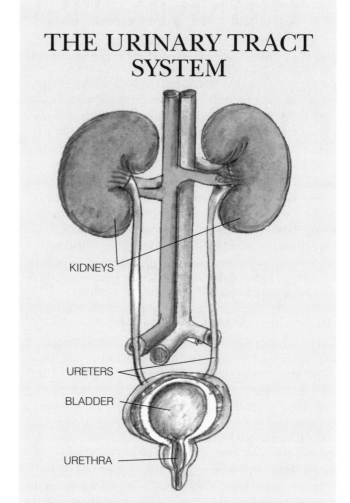

THE URINARY TRACT SYSTEM

KIDNEYS

URETERS

BLADDER

URETHRA

The kidneys produce hormones, regulate the body's balance of salts and fluid, and create urine from the wastes and fluid they filter from the blood. Urine travels to the bladder through the ureters and is expelled from the body through the urethra.

even reddish if blood is present. A fever may indicate that the infection has reached the kidneys. Other symptoms of a kidney infection include pain in the back or side below the ribs, nausea, and vomiting.

If you suspect you have a UTI, see your doctor so he can order a urinalysis. This laboratory test examines the urine specimen under a microscope. If there is an infection, there will be evidence of bacteria, white blood cells, red blood cells, and mucus in the sediment.

Another useful test is a urine culture. In this test, a urine sample is placed in a culture medium, which is ideal for bacteria to grow and reproduce, along with some antibiotic disks. Examination of the bacteria and their reactions to the various antibiotics identifies the bacteria and the antibiotics that would best treat the infection. The urine culture report usually takes two days to receive, and it indicates the most appropriate antibiotic therapy. Physicians do not need to wait for the culture results before they initiate treatment, but they may modify the choice of antibiotic when the results of the culture are available.

Radiologic methods, such as x-rays or ultrasound, are not initially used to diagnose UTIs. These methods are used to assess the urinary tract in people with frequent or recurrent infections, which may indicate the presence of urinary stones, an obstruction, anatomic abnormalities of the urinary tract, or severe infections of the kidneys.

Treatment

The treatment of a UTI consists of a course of antibiotics. Several classes of antibacterials are effective in eradicating bacteria from the urinary tract. Trimethoprim–sulfamethoxazole (160 mg and 800 mg, respectively, in one tablet, twice a day) is a classic choice, which is successful and relatively inexpensive. However, people who use sulfonylureas, including glyburide (brand names DiaBeta, Glynase, Micronase), glipizide (Glucotrol), glimepiride (Amaryl), and chlorpropamide (Diabinese), should only use the trimethoprim because the combination of sulfur-containing antibiotics and sulfonylureas can cause a sharp decrease in blood glucose levels.

The fluoroquinolones, such as ciprofloxacin (250 mg twice a day) or levofloxacin (250 mg or 500 mg once a day), are excellent but more expensive. Nitrofurantoin macrocrystals (100 mg twice a day) is a good choice, especially in women, and has the advantage of not inducing a concomitant overgrowth of vaginal yeast, which may occur with prolonged antibiotic treatments. Ampicillin, amoxicillin, cephalosporins, and other betalactam antibiotics are also possible choices. For severe UTIs involving the kidneys, the aminoglycosides (gentamicin or amikacin) are a possibility, as are the cephalosporins.

The duration of the antibiotic treatment can be limited to three days for routine, uncomplicated infections of the urinary tract. In more severe or complicated UTIs, a 7–10 day course may be required. Kidney infections may require hospitalization for several days followed by 3–4 weeks of antibiotic therapy.

In addition to taking antibiotics, a person with a UTI should drink plenty of fluids. It can also help to avoid caffeine, spicy foods, alcohol, and citrus juices because they can irritate the bladder and exacerbate the frequent or urgent need to urinate.

Prevention

Drinking fluids is not just part of the cure; it's also part of a good UTI-prevention strategy. Drinking six to eight glasses of water a day can help you to keep hydrated and to urinate regularly, which can prevent bacteria from gaining a foothold. There is also some evidence that cranberry juice and blueberry juice contain chemicals that make it difficult for *E. coli* to adhere to cells in the urinary tract. Drinking these juices or taking vitamin C supplements can also cause the urine to be more acidic, which inhibits bacterial growth. If you actually get a UTI, though, you may wish to avoid citrus juices and vitamin C supplements if the acidic urine is painful to pass.

Attention to personal hygiene may also help prevent UTIs. It is important that women wipe from the front to the back when cleaning after a bowel movement. Doing the reverse—wiping with a forward motion—can move bacteria toward the genital area. This places potentially infecting bacteria closer to where they can cause an infection.

Other simple prevention methods include the following: urinating when you feel the urge to do so; avoiding the use of douches and feminine hygiene sprays, which can cause irritation of urethral tissue and give bacteria an easier entry; and taking showers instead of baths because baths can prolong contact of urethral tissues with irritating soaps and microorganisms.

Sexual hygiene. In some women, UTIs are clearly related to sexual activity. In these cases it is believed that the mechanical aspects of intercourse push the bacteria into, or close to, the urethral opening, giving them access to the urinary tract. Women prone to infections following intercourse should urinate following sexual activity to rid the urethra of any potentially invading bacteria.

Women prone to UTIs may be prescribed a dose of an antibiotic to take right after intercourse and a second dose 12 hours later. These two doses are usually sufficient to inhibit bacterial growth and prevent any intruding bacteria from causing a UTI.

Recurring UTIs. Some physicians recommend that women with recurrent UTIs use a prophylactic antibiotic every night for three months to several years. In this situation, it is common to use low doses of trimethoprim–sulfamethoxazole or nitrofurantoin. This regimen keeps a minimum amount of antibiotic always present in the urine, which converts it from a growth-supporting medium to a growth-inhibiting medium with a minimum of antibiotic use.

Alternatively, some physicians prescribe a stock of antibiotic pills so that the woman can start treatment on her own initiative as soon as the first symptoms of a UTI occur. These treatment courses are usually only for three days. The use of an over-the-counter home UTI test kit may be recommended to confirm the presence of infection. Patient-initiated treatment should be done under a doctor's supervision.

On the horizon

In the future, scientists may develop vaccines that can prevent UTIs from recurring. Researchers have found that children and women who tend to get UTIs repeatedly are more likely to lack certain forms of proteins called antibodies, which fight infection. Children and women who do not get

UTIs are more likely to have normal levels of antibodies in their genital and urinary tracts. There is some urgency in the need for such vaccines since bacterial strains that are resistant to many common antibiotics are becoming increasingly prevalent.

A vaccine administered through a suppository in the vagina has helped some women develop resistance to recurrent infection and is also under development. Investigators are also testing a vaccine that prevents *E. coli* from attaching to the lining of the bladder. More studies are needed to determine the long-term effects of these vaccines.

Keeping UTIs at bay

People with diabetes may be more prone to having a UTI, but it's not inevitable. The urinary system was built to take care of itself, and you can help to keep it healthy and free of infection. Practicing good hygiene and keeping your diabetes under control can help prevent a UTI. □

CARDIAC REHABILITATION
by Linnea Hagberg, R.D.

This year, an estimated 1.1 million Americans will have a heart attack. Although an attack proves fatal to many, more than half (55%) survive. It may take some optimism to see the silver lining, but surviving a heart attack or being diagnosed with another form of heart disease *can* be viewed as an opportunity to evaluate your lifestyle habits and commit to making needed changes.

One proven method to help in this evaluation is participation in a cardiac rehabilitation program, which can also help you to acquire the tools and support necessary to initiate a heart-healthy lifestyle. Cardiac rehabilitation can enhance recovery from an acute problem such as a heart attack or heart surgery, control symptoms such as angina, and help people with heart disease learn lifestyle strategies to reduce the likelihood of future problems. Participating in a cardiac rehab program can, literally, be life-saving. In a country where coronary heart disease is the leading cause of death of both men and women, studies show that participating in cardiac rehabilitation can lower the risk of premature death, reduce disability, and improve the quality of life for people with heart problems.

Helping to mend a broken heart

Cardiac rehabilitation, or cardiac rehab as it's commonly called, is a comprehensive, individualized program of exercise and education. Cardiac rehab programs emerged in the 1960's, when doctors began to realize that encouraging people hospitalized for heart problems to move about and gradually resume some regular activities under medical supervision offered a better route to recovery than prolonged bed rest. Early rehab programs focused heavily on exercise, usually conducted under carefully monitored conditions.

Today's rehab programs take a two-pronged approach. The first branch, prescribed for nearly all participants, is designing an individualized, graduated exercise program that helps people learn how to exercise safely and improve their strength and stamina. The second branch consists of an array of services designed to educate and counsel people with heart disease to improve their cardiovascular well-being and teach heart-healthy habits. Doctors, nurses, exercise specialists, dietitians, psychologists or other behavioral therapists, and physical and occupational therapists may all be involved. Services offered include diet counseling, smoking cessation and stress management guidance, and social and psychological support.

All people with heart disease are not alike, of course, so a cardiac rehab team will look for the right mix of services to address each person's needs. The overall goal of cardiac rehabilitation is to help participants restore and maintain their optimal physical, psychological, social, and occupational standing.

Who benefits?

Cardiac rehab programs are not just for those who have had a heart attack; people with other heart problems can benefit as well. For example, the American Heart Association suggests that cardiac rehab be considered for people who have several modifiable risk factors for coronary disease. Modifiable risk factors for heart disease are obesity, physical inactivity, diabetes, smoking, stress, high blood pressure, and high cholesterol. Because diabetes is a risk factor for heart disease, it is extremely important for people with diabetes to keep their blood sugar in check and be zealous in addressing their other cardiac risk factors.

Other candidates for cardiac rehab include those who have had coronary artery bypass surgery, a heart transplant, heart valve surgery, or angioplasty, and those with controlled heart failure and stable angina. Recommendations from the National Institutes of Health note that almost everyone with heart disease, regardless of age or gender, can benefit from some type of cardiac rehab.

Beginning rehab

People who have been hospitalized for a coronary problem such as a heart attack or heart surgery are likely to receive some initial cardiac rehab while still in the hospital. Monitored short walks and stretching exercises under the supervision of medical staff may be offered. Hospital staff may also provide some preliminary lifestyle counseling (for smokers, this is a great time to commit to quitting) and offer information about recovering from and living with a heart condition.

Because hospital stays have become so short, however, the bulk of cardiac rehabilitation occurs after discharge, with a physician's approval. Coordinated cardiac rehab programs often take place in hospitals or medical centers and may even be offered in community settings such as Y's.

It isn't often that people are afforded the type of comprehensive, personalized, holistic care provided in cardiac rehab. Unfortunately, and in spite of well-documented evidence that rehab programs are successful, only a fraction of those potentially eligible for cardiac rehab avail themselves of the opportunity to enroll in a program. One factor that encourages people to enroll in a program is a recommendation from their doctor. That's why it's important for people with heart disease to talk with their doctor about the possibility of attending a rehab program, and to initiate the conversation if their doctor doesn't.

The ABC's of cardiac rehab

Once the decision to attend a cardiac rehab program is made, the next step is to locate a program (see "Choosing a Cardiac Rehab Program" on page 264) and begin the process. What follows is an overview of what might occur in a typical program:

Initial evaluation. When beginning a rehab program, the first step is a thorough evaluation of a person's current state of health and a medical history review. This evaluation may include a physical exam, an exercise tolerance test, any pertinent lab testing, and a psychosocial assessment. Blood pressure, weight, cholesterol levels, management of diabetes, and any current diet plans will be considered, and medication will be reviewed. The goal of this evaluation is to pinpoint areas of cardiovascular risk.

Once areas of concern are identified, participants meet with a nurse or other cardiac rehab staff member to review these areas of concern and develop a care plan to address them. These meetings are likely to continue on a regular basis throughout the rehabilitation process to record and monitor progress.

With the help of a variety of experts on the rehab staff, participants then begin the work of helping themselves recover and learning new strategies to address identified problems.

Exercise program. Exercise offers a number of benefits. It increases blood flow to the heart and strengthens the heart's contractions so that it can pump more blood with less effort. Exercise training improves the ability to perform physical activity. Exercise also helps people achieve and maintain a healthy weight; control diabetes, high blood pressure, and high cholesterol; and reduce stress.

Each person will receive an individualized exercise prescription. In cardiac rehabilitation, exercise programs often start out slowly under close medical supervision and gradually become more intense. Both aerobic, heart-strengthening exercises, such as walking, and resistance training to strengthen muscles may be included. Over time,

CHOOSING A CARDIAC REHAB PROGRAM

There is no single model for the delivery of cardiac rehabilitation services. In some cases, rather than attending a rehab program in a central location, your doctor or other medical personnel may arrange a set of services conducted by different, independent practitioners. For example, you may participate in a guided exercise plan at one location and visit a dietitian separately. People at low risk may receive instruction in an exercise plan that they can do at home rather than at a rehab facility, although experts still recommend periodic face-to-face sessions with a physician.

Doctors are also experimenting with home telephone electrocardiogram-monitored programs. With these systems, the telephone connects the patient to a central monitoring system that measures heart rate and rhythm, providing an extra, at-home safety net during exercise.

For some people, home-based rehab can be a blessing. Not everyone lives near a cardiac rehab program. Others may prefer to exercise independently. It's important to realize, however, that a full mix of services should still be obtained whenever possible. Studies indicate that while exercise alone is effective in reducing coronary risk, exercise in combination with dietary changes is more effective. A combination of diet and exercise, for example, is the best route to lowering LDL (bad) cholesterol while raising HDL (good) cholesterol. Benefits are also intertwined—diet and exercise together enhance weight loss, which in turn can help control diabetes or lower high blood pressure.

When available, there is also something to be said for the coordinated care provided by a rehab center staffed by experts who make it their job to help people with heart disease.

For those who can choose from a variety of formal rehab programs, the goal is to find a program you are comfortable with, since your willing participation is the key factor to success. Your doctor or nurse may recommend a specific program, or you may be told about a cardiac rehab program at the hospital where you received treatment.

Here are some factors to consider in choosing a cardiac rehab plan, based on recommendations issued by the National Institutes of Health:

■ Is the program offered at a convenient time for you?

■ Is it easy to get to? Is parking or public transportation available? Programs may have several sessions a week, and a long commute may discourage your attendance. You may also wish to avoid encountering heavy traffic or parking problems that might induce stress.

■ Does the program offer a wide range of services? More important, does the program provide services in the areas you need help with, such as quitting smoking?

■ Is the program affordable? Will you incur any costs not covered by insurance? Your insurance may cover all or part of the cost of some cardiac rehab services but not others. Find out what will be covered and for how long.

You may also wish to determine if the program has received certification from the American Association of Cardiovascular and Pulmonary Rehabilitation (AACVPR). AACVPR certification means that the program is staffed by qualified experts and meets rigorous patient care standards.

---

participants will build up both the intensity and duration of their exercise and will be given assistance in making the transition to exercising safely on their own.

Participating in a cardiac rehab exercise program can give the extra measure of security many people may need to feel confident about exercising on their own. Too often, people with heart disease limit their activity out of fear. This in turn can increase disability and hamper recovery. Learning to exercise in a supervised setting such as that offered by many cardiac rehab programs can offer valuable reassurance.

Diet and nutrition consultation. The right diet plays a central role in lowering cardiovascular risk, particularly when it occurs in tandem with an exercise program. A healthful eating plan can help people lower their cholesterol and blood pressure, keep blood sugar in check, and aid in weight loss.

A meeting with a dietitian may be part of the initial evaluation people experience upon entering rehab. Most people also work privately with a dietitian to address their individual needs and create an eating plan they can stick with. Group sessions that cover the basics of heart-healthy nutrition may also be offered.

Smoking. Smoking is a major risk factor for heart disease. According to the American Heart Association, smoking is so widespread and significant a risk factor that a Surgeon General of the United States has called it "the most important of the known modifiable risk factors for coronary heart disease in the United States." In addition to increasing the risk of heart disease by itself, when combined with other factors, it greatly increases risk. Smoking increases blood pressure, makes it more likely that blood will clot, lowers exercise tolerance, and increases low-density lipoprotein (LDL) cholesterol, the "bad" cholesterol.

No one says that quitting is easy, but attending a smoking cessation program can help. A hospital or rehab center may have its own smoking cessation program, or program staff may help participants find a suitable program.

Emotional well-being. Depression in the aftermath of a heart attack is a common occurrence. Being depressed, in turn, can affect recovery, making it difficult to find the energy and determination necessary to make effective changes. The initial evaluation process can help people identify their state of mind. Psychologists or other mental-health staff will then provide necessary support.

Stress also contributes to the risk of heart disease. So-called type A personalities and others who experience a lot of stress or anger can learn to manage these emotions during rehabilitation.

People who have experienced a life-threatening event such as a heart attack and others with serious heart disease may also be anxious or concerned about its impact on their lives or have questions about how to manage their condition. To address these issues, rehab programs often offer general education classes centered on living with heart disease or access to group support programs for participants and their families.

Sticking with the program

A cardiac rehab program may last anywhere from six weeks to six months or more. Ideally, participation in a supervised program should last until it is reasonably certain that independent exercise is safe and people are fully versed in the basics of managing their own risk factors. Of course, rehab is really a lifelong commitment since lifestyle changes need to be permanent.

When participating in a cardiac rehab program, it is important that each person take an active role in his own care. Remember, while many health-care professionals may be involved in a cardiac rehab care team, the most important member of the team is the person with heart disease. When it comes down to getting out to walk on a chilly morning, forgoing extra helpings at dinner, or following other heart-healthy practices, there is only one person who can take the measures necessary to benefit his own health. □

TREATING HEART FAILURE
by Wayne L. Clark

It may begin as a subtle fatigue, a general weakness, and a shortness of breath that is easy to dismiss as part of normal aging. As it progresses, you may notice that you have difficulty breathing when lying down, and that your legs and ankles swell from fluid retention.

These can be symptoms of a number of conditions, but for five million Americans, they are the symptoms of heart failure. Up to 10% of those over age 75 can expect to develop heart failure. The prevalence is less than 1% for those under age 50, but for that 1% it is devastating.

People with diabetes are at special risk: A third or more of those with heart failure have diabetes. The link between diabetes and heart failure was described in the Framingham (Massachusetts) Heart Study as early as 1974. Today, it is estimated

that people with diabetes, whether Type 1 or Type 2, have anywhere from a two- to eight-fold increased risk of developing heart failure. Women with diabetes have a greater risk than men with diabetes.

Moreover, the incidence of heart failure in African-Americans is 50% higher than that of the general population. African-Americans are also 1.6 times more likely to have diabetes, so heart failure and other complications are significant risks for this population.

In an age of major advances in the treatment of heart disease, heart failure is the only major cardiovascular disorder that is increasing in prevalence. Ironically, this may be a result of people surviving heart attacks and other illnesses—such as diabetes—and living longer. Hospitalizations for heart failure have doubled in the past 20 years, and the condition now accounts for 5% of the total health-care costs of the United States.

Heart failure is a serious condition. Less than 50% of people with severe heart failure survive five years from diagnosis; less than 25% survive eight years.

The term "heart failure" covers a number of more specific conditions, but they are all characterized by the heart's "failure" to pump blood efficiently. The most common cause of heart failure is a loss of function of the left ventricle, the lower chamber on the left side of the heart. Oxygen-rich blood from the lungs fills the left atrium, the chamber above the left ventricle, which empties the blood into the left ventricle. The left ventricle then contracts, pumping the blood out to the body.

Heart failure can also occur on the right side of the heart, which receives the oxygen-depleted blood from the body. This blood fills the right atrium, which empties into the right ventricle, which pumps the blood to the lungs for a new supply of oxygen.

The left ventricle's pumping action can be affected in two ways. In systolic failure, the left ventricle loses its ability to contract, so it cannot pump enough of the blood it receives from the lungs out into the body. The walls of the chamber become thin, large, and floppy, in an attempt to compensate for the loss of power with an increase in volume. The result can be a backup of blood in the lungs, causing fluid to leak into the lungs. This is the cause of one of the symptoms of advancing heart failure, a cough that brings up frothy sputum.

In diastolic failure, which represents 20% to 40% of cases, the left ventricle cannot relax and fill completely with blood, leading to fluid accumulation in the lower extremities. In this instance, the walls of the ventricle have become thickened and stiff and unable to relax sufficiently.

Symptoms are similar in right-side heart failure. If the right ventricle cannot pump enough of the blood that is returned to it, the result is congestion in the veins that return the blood. This can cause the veins to expand and the internal organs to distend, or swell. Failure of the right ventricle can occur by itself or as a consequence of failure on the left side of the heart.

The increased risk faced by people with diabetes is due largely to the fact that they are at higher risk for the two most common contributing causes of heart failure: coronary artery disease, or atherosclerosis, and hypertension, or high blood pressure. These are the same reasons that people with diabetes have a 2–4 times higher risk of heart attack and stroke.

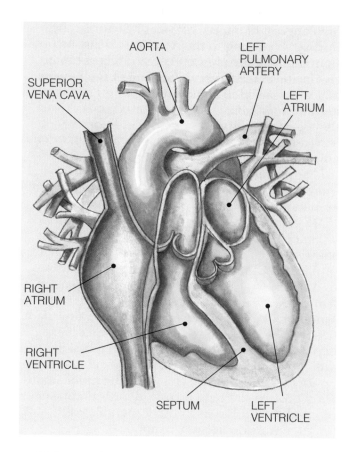

Diabetes affects the cells that line the blood vessels. These cells are key to regulating blood flow, coagulation, and the status of the smooth-muscle cells in the vessel walls. Anything that compromises the vessel lining accelerates thickening of the walls, limits the flexibility of the vessel, increases the likelihood of clots, and ultimately leads to atherosclerosis.

Atherosclerosis creates blood clots that can block off the blood vessels to the heart, and even if the clots are not serious enough to cause a full-blown heart attack, they can destroy and weaken the heart muscle by depriving it of oxygen. The damaged tissue can lose its strength and flexibility, and heart failure is the result.

Hypertension can be caused by the loss of production of vasodilators (chemicals in the body that relax blood vessels) as well as an increase in the production of vasoconstrictors (chemicals that constrict blood vessels), both of which are more likely in diabetes.

Obesity and overweight, which are often associated with diabetes, have been found to be strong and independent risk factors for heart failure. Data from the Framingham Heart Study revealed that women who are obese are twice as likely to develop heart failure, and men have a 90% increased risk. Among both men and women who

Diabetes Complications

are overweight, there is a 34% higher risk. Overweight is generally defined as a body-mass index above 25, obesity as a body mass index above 30.

For these and other reasons, the presence of diabetes is by itself considered to be a risk factor for heart failure.

"Statistically, diabetes is an independent risk factor for heart failure," says Douglas Sawyer, M.D., Ph.D., Assistant Professor of Medicine at Boston University Medical Center. "In large epidemiological studies, the risk from diabetes is independent of other risk factors. At a molecular and physiological level, diabetes has effects on cardiac structure that are independent of the effects of coronary artery disease and hypertension."

This direct damage to the heart tissue likely accounts for what is called *diabetic cardiomyopathy.* Cardiomyopathy, or disease of the heart muscle, can be caused by a number of disorders, and there is still some debate as to whether the condition has a different form in people with diabetes.

"The existence of a specific diabetic cardiomyopathy is more accepted in the research world," Dr. Sawyer says, "because there are diabetic animal models of cardiomyopathy in which all other causes have been controlled. Clinically, it's more difficult because all the risk factors are so intertwined.

"Certainly we can say that if there isn't a true diabetic cardiomyopathy, there are unique features of the diabetic heart that make it more susceptible to heart failure as well as atherosclerosis."

Another sign that suggests a distinct diabetic cardiomyopathy is the finding that diastolic heart failure often occurs in people with diabetes who have no symptoms or signs of atherosclerotic disease. The supposition is that in these cases, the heart failure is due to diabetic cardiomyopathy, caused by damage to the smaller blood vessels in the heart muscle and in changes at the cellular level. A variety of structural changes in the heart tissue of people with diabetes have been documented, including thickening of the walls of small blood vessels and microaneurysms, or bulges in the walls of the vessels.

Yet another factor that may raise the risk of heart failure in people with diabetes is *cardiac autonomic neuropathy.* Neuropathy is generally thought of as a lack of sensation in the extremities, particularly the legs, but autonomic neuropathy affects organs and involuntary bodily processes. Autonomic neuropathy affects the heart in 17% of people with Type 1 diabetes and in 22% of people with Type 2 diabetes. Its devastating effects on the nerves around the heart may contribute to a loss of left ventricular function.

Research has found that blood sugar control is directly related to the risk of heart failure, underscoring both the added risk that diabetes poses and the importance of good control. In one study, at the Kaiser Permanente Medical Care Program of Northern California, researchers found that each 1% increase in HbA_{1c}, a measure of blood sugar control over time, was associated with an 8% increased risk of heart failure—regardless of age, sex, ethnicity, education, smoking status, alcohol use, hypertension, obesity, use of beta-blockers and angiotensin-converting enzyme (ACE) inhibitors, type and duration of diabetes, and incidence of heart attack.

Diagnosis and treatment

Most people with heart failure first learn of their diagnosis after going to see their doctor because of problems with fatigue or shortness of breath. In addition to a decreased tolerance for exercise, heart failure may result in swollen ankles, weight gain from fluid buildup, and difficulty breathing even when lying down.

Diagnosis is often difficult because the symptoms of heart failure are similar to those from other causes. Sometimes, heart failure is discovered in the course of treating another cardiac problem, such as a heart attack.

A definitive diagnosis can be made by adding the results of one or more tests to the symptoms. A chest x-ray, for instance, can reveal an enlarged heart and fluid buildup in the lungs. An electrocardiogram will show changes in the heart's electrical activity and the thickness of the chamber walls.

Doctors can use echocardiograms to measure the size of the heart with sound waves and measure its movement as it relaxes and contracts. From these measurements, they can calculate the *ejection fraction,* a measure of how much of the blood in the ventricle is pumped out, or ejected, during each contraction. In a healthy heart, the ejection fraction is 50% or higher. In heart failure, the ejection fraction is often less than 40%.

If appropriate, a catheter can be inserted into an artery and threaded through to the heart, where it can measure the pressures during contraction and relaxation. The same procedure, with a different catheter, can inject contrast dye into the coronary arteries to detect atherosclerosis on x-rays.

Heart failure usually cannot be cured, but it can be managed. The American College of Cardiology and the American Heart Association have developed extensive treatment guidelines for heart failure. To reduce the risk of developing heart failure in people at high risk for it (such as people with high blood pressure and people with diabetes), the guidelines call for treating high blood pressure, lowering cholesterol, quitting smoking, increasing exercise, limiting alcohol and illicit drugs, controlling heart rhythm disturbances, and treating thyroid disease. They also recommend the use of angiotensin-converting enzyme (ACE) inhibitors or angiotensin receptor blockers (ARBs) in some members of this high-risk group, including people with diabetes, and the use of beta blockers to control blood pressure.

ACE inhibitors block the formation of a substance that constricts blood vessels and causes the heart to work harder. ACE inhibitors are often standard therapy for people with diabetes even without heart failure, because they also help protect the kidneys. ARBs thwart the same vessel-constricting substance, but do it by preventing it from working.

If physicians detect structural changes in the heart, but there are no symptoms of heart failure, the treatment becomes more aggressive. Recommendations include using all of the above approaches, plus using beta-blockers if there has been a heart attack or if the person's ejection fraction is low.

If symptoms of heart failure are present, another layer of medical treatment is added. This can include the use of diuretics to remove excess fluid and digitalis to increase the force of the heart's contraction. Drugs that can cause problems in people with a weakened heart, such as nonsteroidal anti-inflammatory drugs (such as ibuprofen), antiarrhythmia drugs, and calcium channel blockers are withdrawn.

In advanced and "end stage" heart failure, more aggressive control of fluid levels is recommended, and interventions such as heart transplant may be considered.

New treatments, new hope

ACE inhibitors are the constant in treating most forms of heart failure. Some people who cannot tolerate them may be given a combination of nitrates and other vasodilators to accomplish much the same result, or in some cases an angiotensin-II receptor blocker may be used. The advent of ACE inhibitors and beta-blockers alone has been responsible for a 50% reduction in mortality in the past 40–50 years. A new study, however, challenges the usefulness of these drugs.

Several high blood pressure drugs were compared in the Antihypertensive and Lipid-Lowering Treatment to Prevent Heart Attack Trial (ALLHAT). A diuretic, or "water pill," was found to reduce blood pressure more effectively than an

ACE inhibitor, an alpha-blocker, or a calcium channel blocker. It also significantly lowered the risk of heart failure and other cardiac complications in people with hypertension. The findings of ALLHAT may lead to using the more effective (and less expensive) diuretic as a first-line treatment for high blood pressure, particularly in people at risk for heart failure.

However, the ALLHAT trial has come under substantial fire since its publication. It was immediately challenged by many cardiologists due to alleged flaws in the study design, and a subsequent Australian study concluded that ACE inhibitors are slightly (11%) better. A study validating ALLHAT, published in 2007, reached the conclusion that diuretics were, indeed, the best first-line therapy. The controversy is still not settled, but scientists from both sides recommend that physicians make decisions based on each individual's situation. African-Americans, for example, don't respond well to ACE inhibitors, so a diuretic may be a good first choice.

ACE inhibitors have held their own in other studies. The Omapatrilat Versus Enalapril Randomized Trial of Utility in Reducing Events (OVERTURE) trial compared a new type of drug called a vasopeptidase inhibitor with the standard ACE inhibitor enalapril. Omapatrilat blocks the angiotensin-converting enzyme as an ACE inhibitor does, but also blocks neutral endopeptidase, an enzyme that breaks down substances beneficial to the heart. It was hoped that the drug would control blood pressure and perhaps work even better in people with both heart failure and high blood pressure. The latest studies produced equivocal results, though, and there were questions about some increased side effects with omipatrilat. The drug or others in its class may be back in clinical trials at some point.

A relatively new addition to heart failure treatment is spironolactone. It inhibits aldosterone, which promotes salt retention (and therefore water retention) and has other effects that are harmful in heart failure. In a trial that added spironolactone to the standard regimen of ACE inhibitors, diuretics, and/or digoxin, a 30% reduction in hospitalization or death caused investigators to declare the trial a success and end it early. There have since been concerns about the drug's carcinogenicity and effect on the kidneys, but it remains an option, especially in severe heart failure.

Anemia is a troublesome feature of heart failure for many people, exacerbating symptoms of fatigue and shortness of breath. Many experts are advocating treating the anemia with erythropoi-

BODY-MASS INDEX

Body-mass index (BMI) is one of several tools used to assess whether a person is at a healthy weight. A BMI of 18.5 to 25 is considered normal. People with a BMI between 25 and 30 are considered overweight, and people with a BMI over 30 are considered obese.

HEIGHT	WEIGHT IN POUNDS					
5'0"	128	153	179	204	230	255
5'1"	132	158	185	211	238	264
5'2"	136	164	191	218	246	273
5'3"	141	169	197	225	254	282
5'4"	145	174	204	232	262	291
5'5"	150	180	210	240	270	300
5'6"	155	186	216	247	278	309
5'7"	159	191	223	255	287	319
5'8"	164	197	230	262	295	328
5'9"	169	203	236	270	304	338
5'10"	174	209	243	278	313	348
5'11"	179	215	250	286	322	358
6'0"	184	221	258	294	331	368
6'1"	189	227	265	302	340	378
6'2"	194	233	272	311	350	389
6'3"	200	240	279	319	359	399
6'4"	205	246	287	328	369	410
BMI	**25**	**30**	**35**	**40**	**45**	**50**

etin, which stimulates the production of more oxygen-carrying red blood cells, based on the strength of early trials.

Of particular interest to many people with diabetes, metformin's role in heart failure is being debated. Metformin is the first-line medication for Type 2 diabetes, and had long been believed to increase the risk of heart failure. However, recent evidence suggests that it is not harmful to people with diabetes and heart failure, and that it may, in fact, be helpful.

There are also mechanical and surgical interventions for heart failure. For instance, implantable cardioverter defibrillators (ICDs), which monitor heart rhythms and can correct abnormal rhythms, have improved survival for people with heart failure who have had previous heart attacks. ICDs are not currently recommended for people at high risk of heart failure but with no symptoms.

More recently, a therapy called "cardiac resynchronization therapy (CRT)" or "biventricular pacing" has used what is basically an enhanced implantable pacemaker to synchronize the contractions of the left and right ventricles, which, in heart failure, can become uncoordinated and therefore inefficient. People in advanced stages of heart failure have shown improvement in function and in quality of life with resynchronization, and the therapy is now recommended for people with severe disease.

One trial investigated the comparative benefits of medical treatment only, medical treatment with resynchronization therapy, and medical treatment with resynchronization therapy and an ICD. The trial was ended early because of the striking positive results of the combination of medical treatment, resynchronization, and ICD.

A new surgical procedure may help people who

develop heart failure because of a heart attack that affects the front of the heart. Surgical ventricular restoration involves cutting the left ventricle wall, overlapping the edges of the incision, and using a patch to close the incision. The idea is to restore the ventricle, which is often distended in heart failure, to a normal shape and size. It is performed on people already undergoing an open heart procedure.

People with serious, life-threatening heart failure may be candidates for the use of a Left Ventricular Assist Device (LVAD). The LVAD is a mechanical pump that is implanted under the ribs and essentially replaces the left ventricle's function. It is currently used as a "bridge" therapy for people awaiting heart transplant and is being considered as a permanent therapy for those not eligible for transplant and even as a replacement for transplant.

Heart transplantation is an alternative for a few very sick people. However, there are only about 2,000 donor hearts in the United States each year, so the potential of the therapy is very limited.

On the leading edge of cardiac research, scientists are investigating a way to actually replace the muscle cells damaged by a heart attack. Heart muscle cells do not replicate, so researchers are attempting to transplant either muscle cells from other parts of the person's body or bone marrow cells from the person into scarred regions of the heart. Preliminary results have been very encouraging, with improvements in function following the transplants.

In another approach to saving heart muscle, researchers are looking for ways to cause new blood vessels to grow in portions of the heart muscle at risk of dying. The science of *angiogenesis,* or new blood vessel growth, holds promise for treating not only heart failure but atherosclerosis as well.

It is much easier to prevent heart failure than to treat it, and Dr. Sawyer reminds us that the lifestyle advice all people with diabetes receive is still the best way to prevent heart failure—as well as other complications.

"Exercise, blood glucose control, blood pressure control, blood lipids control, and good, regular preventive care are the key," he says. "We recommend them to our patients over and over again, because they're so important." □

STROKE REHABILITATION
OFFERING HELP AND HOPE

by Jeffrey Larson, P.T., A.T.C.

Although stroke is the third leading cause of death in the United States (behind heart disease and cancer), most people who have a stroke survive, but they are often left with some physical or cognitive impairments. Stroke is of particular concern to people with diabetes because they have two to four times the risk of having a stroke as people who don't have diabetes. Depending on its severity, a stroke can be so damaging that it leaves a person permanently disabled, or it can be mild and lead to problems that, while hindering, do not prevent a person from returning to work or enjoying his old routines. Rehabilitation cannot reverse the brain damage done by a stroke, but it has an important role in helping people who have had strokes to regain as much physical and mental function as possible.

People with diabetes are at a higher risk of stroke because over time, high blood glucose levels damage blood vessels, making the walls thicker and less elastic, which can increase blood pressure. Diabetes also makes blood "stickier," or more viscous, and prone to clotting. Higher blood glucose levels can also cause high blood fat levels. These fats (or lipids) build up on blood vessel walls along with other blood components, a vessel-narrowing condition called atherosclerosis. Higher blood pressure, more viscous blood, and narrowed blood vessels set the stage for stroke.

Impaired blood flow to any portion of the brain that is serious enough to damage tissues is called a stroke, or cerebrovascular accident. Stroke is usually caused by a blood clot that forms or lodges in the arteries supplying blood to the brain. (Stroke can also be caused when a blood vessel ruptures in the brain.)

In the United States, approximately 150,000 people die each year from strokes. However, nearly 4 million people in the United States have survived a stroke and are living with the aftereffects. Depending on the severity of a stroke, rehabilitation can begin while recovering in the hospital within two days after the stroke has occurred. When the person has progressed to a point where he is ready to leave the hospital, rehabilitation continues with home therapy or outpatient therapy. People with more severe problems are transferred from the hospital to a long-term care facility that provides therapy and skilled nursing care.

The goal for stroke rehabilitation is to improve function so that the person can become as independent as possible. Rehabilitation, much like diabetes care, is centered around a team, one that consists of physicians; rehabilitative professionals such as physical, occupational, and speech therapists; and the person who has had a stroke and his family. The team meets regularly to discuss the progress of treatment. The team approach allows everyone to work together and to address all the different aspects of the recovery process.

Physical therapy

Physical therapists work with people who have had strokes to improve their mobility, balance, and coordination. They teach exercises and techniques that improve walking, getting in and out of a bed or a chair, and balance. This may include instruction on the use of assistive devices such as a walker or a cane. If the team decides the goal of the rehabilitation is eventually to see the individual return home, it is important that family members who will be living with the individual learn how to assist with exercises. The physical therapist may also teach family members how to assist the person to perform daily activities such as walking and getting from his bed to a chair.

One of the major goals in rehabilitation is to decrease and overcome uncontrollable muscle tightness in a leg or arm. This involuntary muscle contraction (spasticity) is a common physical response to the brain injury caused by stroke, one that can cause pain and affect movement. In a healthy person, the brain tells skeletal muscles when to relax and when to contract to move a limb. In a person with spasticity, the muscle does not obey the nervous system's order to relax, so it remains contracted.

Spasticity is commonly seen in the arm, producing a characteristic posture of a clenched fist and bent elbow, with the arm pressed against the chest. When spasticity is present in the leg, it usually

INDEPENDENT LIVING AIDS

A stroke can affect your mobility and vision, making routine tasks and diabetes care more challenging. An occupational therapist will likely be able to give you many good suggestions for Web sites and catalogs that sell assistive devices; we include a small selection here.

ACTIVEFOREVER.COM
(800) 377-8033
www.activeforever.com
This site's assistive devices, including long-handled mirrors and devices for washing feet or applying lotion, are helpfully grouped by department and by medical condition.

DISABILITYPRODUCTS.COM
(800) 688-4576
www.disabilityproducts.com
This site offers a variety of helpful products, such as a long-handled adjustable mirror, to make daily life safer and more comfortable for people with disabilities.

GOLD VIOLIN
(877) 648-8400
www.goldviolin.com
This company aims to sell stylish versions of independent living products. You can call to order or request a catalog. AARP members can receive a small discount from Gold Violin.

INDEPENDENT LIVING AIDS, INC.
(800) 537-2118
www.independentliving.com
Although it specializes in products for the blind or visually impaired, this mail-order company offers a wide variety of devices that people with mobility difficulties may appreciate, including pill organizers and "talking" pill bottles, kitchen and bath aids, and mirrors on poles for helping to check your feet. Order online or request a catalog.

causes a stiff knee and pointed foot, interfering with an individual's ability to walk. Ultimately, an individual and his physician will decide which treatments are appropriate for his situation, but a muscle-stretching program is considered basic management for spasticity and is performed at least one or two times daily. Physical therapists instruct the person and his family members on specific stretches that can be performed independently or with assistance. Other techniques to decrease spasticity include applying cold packs, using oral or injected medicines, or even surgery.

Occupational therapy

After having a stroke, people often discover that they can no longer perform certain activities the way they used to. Occupational therapy involves teaching new techniques to accomplish daily activities such as eating, bathing, using the toilet, dressing, writing, and cooking and possibly more complex tasks such as getting in and out of a vehicle or work-related responsibilities. Occupational therapists show people new ways to carry out affected functions and how to use adaptive devices such as a special long-handled shoehorn to help with dressing.

If stretching alone is not sufficient to treat spasticity, an occupational therapist can create specially designed casts and splints to improve the range of motion of the affected limb. Physical and occupational therapists work closely together to ensure that problems with both upper and lower extremities are met.

Speech-language therapy

A stroke can potentially cause damage to the area of the brain responsible for language, causing difficulties with communication. After a stroke, some individuals are unable to understand spoken words or speak, while others may be able to understand but cannot be understood by others when they try to speak. Some people can no longer read or write, while others may have only slight difficulty pronouncing words. Such communication problems can be frightening for both the affected person and his family.

If these problems are severe, the rehabilitation team often requires the addition of a speech-language pathologist. Speech-language pathologists help people recover language skills and learn alternative ways to communicate when speech recovery is not possible. They also teach the person's family how to help him improve his communication skills.

Speech-language pathologists also work with individuals who have developed a swallowing dysfunction known as dysphagia. They can also help the person cope with memory loss or other cognitive problems such as difficulty with numbers and calculating.

Diabetes care

People with diabetes who have a stroke may experience increased difficulty keeping their blood glu-cose level under control during and after recovery from a stroke. A decline in fine motor control and vision, a tremor, or muscle spasticity can affect a person's self-care routine. If the side of the body affected by the stroke is the dominant side (that is, if a right-handed person's right side was affected), it will take a lot of practice to relearn diabetes care habits. The occupational therapist and nursing staff may introduce new techniques and technology that can assist in tasks such as administering insulin and monitoring blood glucose.

Insulin dosers or vial holders may make injecting insulin easier if the stroke has caused problems with vision or fine motor skills. Insulin dosers use replaceable cartridges of insulin or come prefilled and have either a large dial or display screen for easier viewing of the dose being dialed. To assist those with low vision, the Innolet makes audible clicks while the dial is being turned to help with accurate dosing (it is currently the only device approved for the visually impaired). Insulin pens require two hands to use, and although some make clicking noises when dialed, pen manufacturers do not recommend relying on these sounds for dosing. Although it's not available in retail stores (it can be ordered through online retailers), Insulin-Aid, a sturdy insulin vial holder that attaches to metallic surfaces with a magnet, can help vial and syringe users who are unable to use both hands well.

Newer blood glucose meters also offer features that people with disabilities may find useful. For example, some meters have alternate-site testing capability, so fingers don't always have to be pricked for a blood drop (which can be helpful if a person only has use of one hand), large display screens for people with vision problems, and the ability to take the meter and test strip to the blood sample rather than moving the lanced body part to a level meter. A few meters use preloaded drums or cartridges of test strips, eliminating the need to handle individual strips or to insert strips into a slot in the meter yourself. The Precision Sof-Tact goes even further, with lancing and transfer of the sample to a strip accomplished by pushing one button. Strip technology has also improved such that some brands allow users to add more blood to the strip if the initial drop was inadequate. Diabetes educators often have a wide variety of diabetes tools on hand for people to try, so it's very helpful to visit one to see firsthand what might work best. If a person's preferred meter is not covered by his insurance, he can write a letter of appeal to the company explaining his needs after the stroke.

In addition to the gadgets that help people with impaired mobility with daily tasks such as picking

FOR HELP AND INFORMATION

The following organizations offer information and other links to resources.

THE AMERICAN OCCUPATIONAL THERAPY ASSOCIATION, INC.
(301) 652-2682
TDD: (800) 377-8555
www.aota.org
The AOTA offers helpful "Tips for Living" that you can view online or download. The tips cover topics such as recovering from a stroke, aids for people with diabetes, suggestions for safely enjoying activities such as travel and gardening, and returning to work.

AMERICAN PHYSICAL THERAPY ASSOCIATION
(800) 999-APTA (2782)
(703) 684-APTA (2782)
TDD: (703) 683-6748
www.apta.org
Learn more about physical therapy, search for a physical therapist by location or specialty, or find out how your insurance may work with physical therapy.

AMERICAN SPEECH-LANGUAGE-HEARING ASSOCIATION
(800) 638-8255
www.asha.org
ASHA's Web site offers information on the swallowing disorder dysphagia and can help you find a speech-language pathologist or support group in your area.

AMERICAN STROKE ASSOCIATION
(888) 4-STROKE (478-7653)
www.strokeassociation.org
A division of the American Heart Association that offers explanations of the injury and recovery process, rehabilitation suggestions, and information about local stroke support groups.

NATIONAL INSTITUTE OF NEUROLOGICAL DISORDERS AND STROKE
(800) 352-9424
TTY: (301) 468-5981
www.ninds.nih.gov
Part of the National Institutes of Health, NINDS provides information and publications on a variety of neurological disorders and provides a link to the Clinicaltrials.gov site for information on clinical trials involving people who have had a stroke.

NATIONAL STROKE ASSOCIATION
(800) STROKES (787-6537)
www.stroke.org
The Web site offers online ordering of books and brochures for the affected individual and his family (also available by phone) and information on prevention, recovery, and rehabilitation. The Web site is also available in French and Spanish.

---

objects off the floor, there are devices that can help with your foot-care routine. Some of the foot-care devices include angled mirrors on poles to help you examine the bottoms of your feet and sponges on poles that can help you to apply lotion to your feet to keep them from drying and cracking. An occupational therapist or a certified diabetes educator should be able to refer you to Web sites or catalog companies that carry such items. (A short list is on page 271.)

In addition to changes in physical abilities, there are some other ways in which having a stroke can affect a person's blood glucose control. Anger or frustration with the lasting effects of stroke can lead to higher levels of stress hormones, which increase blood glucose level. Depression, which affects a number of people who have had a stroke, can cause people to neglect their self-care and allow blood glucose levels to fluctuate. Depending on factors such as a change in activity levels after a stroke or swallowing difficulties, people may also need to develop and adjust to a new diet with the help of a registered dietitian.

Setting goals

Throughout the rehabilitation process, the team works together to achieve specific goals determined at the start of the program. Goals are an important part of rehabilitation and can include being able to walk 60 feet with a four-legged cane in three weeks with minimal assistance from the therapist or being able to comb one's hair without difficulty. Rehabilitative goals depend on the severity of the stroke and the individual's previous activity level. Goals may also need to be modified throughout the rehabilitation process as some are achieved more quickly than anticipated and others take longer than expected.

The team also needs to make sure that the goals are realistic. If goals are set too high, they may leave a person feeling frustrated and defeated. If they are too low, the person may not get all the services that would benefit him because he was not challenged to his full potential. If the goals do not match a person's interests, he may become bored and may not be willing to spend time and energy achieving them.

Going home

Once the majority of goals set while recovering in the hospital or care facility have been met, many people are able to return home; however, decisions about rehabilitation and planning to return home are often difficult. Social workers can help by making arrangements for necessary support services and providing or arranging for counseling (individual and family) to help with emotional adjustments. One or more members of the rehabilitative staff usually conduct a home assessment at or before the time of transition from the hospital or care facility. Safety is a key issue, with special attention given to proper lighting, tacked-down carpets, clear walkways, and removal of scatter rugs. Other physical improvements that may be recommended include getting furniture designed to be easier to get in and out of and installing grab bars in the bath or shower and beside the toilet.

The recovery process does not simply end at a person's front door. The transition back home only means that the individual is now ready to live independently while continuing to strive for and achieve rehabilitation goals. The physical therapist may intensify exercises that were initiated in the hospital, while the occupational therapist addresses the needs specific to the individual's home. Continued rehabilitation through outpatient clinics or a home health service, along with nursing care, can help the individual to function safely and to his best ability at home.

For people who live alone, special provisions may need to be in place before the return home. Common concerns include the preparation of meals, maximizing safety within the home to prevent falls, and the availability of a phone or lifeline to summon assistance in an emergency.

Hard work and rewards

With guidance from a team of rehabilitation professionals, people who have had a stroke are able to tap into their potential to have the best quality of life possible. Fatigue and discouragement at times is normal, but the important thing is to recognize the progress made and take satisfaction in each achievement, however large or small.

Another point to remember is that there are organizations such as the American Stroke Association that can provide information and support. For contact information for this and other help organizations, see "For Help and Information" above.

Rehabilitation can be a long, hard journey, but having a team means coordinated, complete care. It also means not having to go through the process alone. □

SAY YES TO INTIMACY
Treatment Options for Erectile Dysfunction
by Donna Rice, B.S.N., R.N., C.D.E.

It is a well-known fact that chronic illness can cause problems with sexual function. Today, erectile dysfunction, also called impotence, affects an estimated 30 million men in the United States. It is a problem that often leads to frustration, embarrassment, loss of self-esteem, isolation, and depression. It can also lead to strain in a relationship, particularly if a man withdraws from his partner rather than communicating openly about what he is experiencing. Men with diabetes have a higher incidence of erectile dysfunction, yet it is often ignored and left untreated.

Men willing to seek help, though, find that erectile dysfunction is treatable. Today, there are many options that work well and have restored erectile function to many men.

Erectile dysfunction

Erectile dysfunction has a variety of definitions and forms, but the one discussed in this article is "the persistent inability to get or maintain an erection sufficient for sexual intercourse." It is usually

DRUGS AND DEVICES
FOR ERECTILE DYSFUNCTION

There are a number of drugs, devices, and implants that can help men and their partners overcome erectile dysfunction. The table below can help you to compare these options.

DRUG NAME	MAXIMUM USAGE OR DOSE	TIME IT TAKES TO ACT	HOW LONG EFFECTS LAST
Alprostadil penile injection (Caverject Impulse)	May be used up to three times a week at effective dose	5–20 minutes	1 hour
Alprostadil urethral suppository (MUSE)	May be used up to twice a day at effective dose	5–10 minutes	30–60 minutes
Sildenafil (Viagra)	100 mg daily	½–2 hours (median: 1 hour)	4 hours
Tadalafil (Cialis)	20 mg daily	½–6 hours (median: 2 hours)	36 hours
Vardenafil (Levitra)	20 mg daily	½–2 hours (median: 1 hour)	4 hours
DEVICE TYPE	TIME IT TAKES TO BE EFFECTIVE	HOW LONG THE DEVICE CAN BE USED AT ANY ONE TIME	MAXIMUM USAGE
Constriction band	varies	Must be removed within 30 minutes	Allow at least an hour between applications
Vacuum device with constriction band	minutes	Constriction band must be removed within 30 minutes	Allow at least an hour between applications
Penile splint	minutes	no limit	no limit
Surgical implant	minutes	no limit	no limit

caused by disease, injury, or a drug and is not a normal part of the aging process.

An erection normally occurs when sexual stimulation causes nerves in the penis to release certain chemicals that start a cascade of reactions, resulting in the widening of blood vessels entering the penis and a narrowing of vessels leaving the penis. The increased blood flow allowed by the widened arteries fills the spongy tissues of the penis, causing the penis to thicken and lengthen. The engorged tissues compress the veins that take blood out of the penis, further narrowing them, which limits blood outflow and maintains the erection.

There are many complications associated with diabetes; however, the two complications that have a direct effect on erections are blood flow problems and nerve problems (neuropathy). High blood glucose levels can contribute to blockages or narrowing of blood vessels. Better known for causing problems such as atherosclerosis and periph-

eral artery disease (narrowing of the blood vessels supplying the legs and arms), this process can also affect blood vessels that supply blood to the penis.

Diabetic neuropathy also contributes to erectile dysfunction. Nerves are involved in signaling the blood vessels of the penis to widen or narrow (dilate or constrict). Over time, high blood glucose levels damage nerves, and as a result, they cannot properly signal the vessels to open and close, making an erection difficult to achieve.

Most often, erectile problems in men with diabetes are a result of problems with both blood flow and nerve function. However, getting regular exercise, controlling one's blood pressure, and controlling one's blood glucose, in addition to being good for controlling one's diabetes, can prevent or delay neuropathy and vascular problems and help improve sexual function. For men already experiencing erectile difficulties, though, there are several treatment options.

The three main categories of treatment are drugs, mechanical devices, and surgery. Drugs can be taken orally, as a suppository, or as an injection. Mechanical devices cause more blood to enter the penis (vacuum devices), prevent blood from leaving the penis (constriction bands), or support the penis to make it more rigid (splints). Surgical treatment involves implanting a device into the penis. Some men have to try several of these options before finding the one that works best for them and their partners.

Throughout this process, communication is key. The man and his partner need to talk about the pros and cons of each option to find a mutually satisfying solution. Health-care providers can give information, advice, and options, but ultimately it is the couple who must use and be satisfied with the treatment they choose.

Medicines

Although they are taken differently, the drugs described here are all basically vasodilators that increase the amount of blood that can enter the penis. They mainly differ in side effects, time to onset of action, and convenience.

Pills. Sildenafil (Viagra) took the market by storm several years ago, bringing sexual dysfunction out of the closet and getting men into doctors' offices to deal with it. The overwhelming response to sildenafil and the increased awareness of erectile dysfunction as a real problem for millions of men enticed two new contenders into the market: vardenafil (Levitra) and tadalafil (Cialis). The introduction of these new drugs increases the choices for treating this problem.

The main difference between the three drugs is that tadalafil can last up to 36 hours compared with 4 hours for sildenafil and vardenafil. However, it has not been studied whether a man can achieve multiple erections per dose of tadalafil, and tadalafil may have a greater potential for drug interactions because of its longer period of effectiveness.

The actions of all three drugs are similar in that they increase blood flow to the penis. They work by stopping the degradation of the vessel-widening chemicals that are produced in response to sexual stimulation; with their degradation stopped, the chemicals are free to continue allowing more blood into the penis. Because these drugs don't produce vessel-widening chemicals themselves, the user must have some sexual stimulation to start the release of such chemicals and achieve an erection. The three drugs all start to work in as little as 30 minutes. (See the table on page 275.)

Each medicine can be taken daily and each has the following possible side effects: headaches, flushing, upset stomach, visual disturbances, and prolonged erections. (Prolonged erections lasting more than four hours require immediate medical attention to prevent permanent damage to the penis.) Tadalafil may also cause muscle aches or back pain while its competitors don't, but it is also less likely than its competitors to cause so-called "blue vision," a condition in which users temporarily experience a blue tinge to their vision while using the drug. Sildenafil has been around longer than its competitors and therefore has a more proven safety profile. Sildenafil should be taken on an empty stomach or with a light (low-fat) meal; the others can be taken with food or on an empty stomach. Alcohol may be used in moderation with any of these medicines.

All three drugs have similar precautions. You should not use these drugs if you are taking a drug that contains nitrate or an alpha-blocker (with one exception for tadalafil), which is used to treat high blood pressure or an enlarged prostate gland. Tadalafil may be taken with 0.4 milligrams of once-daily tamsulosin (Flomax).

Again, it's important to note that erections won't happen automatically with these drugs. Sexual stimulation is a must for these medicines to be effective, so if the mood isn't right, a man may not get an erection, even if he has successfully used the pill before.

Urethral suppository. A urethral suppository containing the drug alprostadil (MUSE) hit the market a year before sildenafil. Like the oral medicines, the alprostadil suppository is a vasodilator that allows blood to enter the penis. About the size of a grain of rice, the suppository is placed into the urethral opening at the tip of the penis. (The urethra is the tube in the penis that allows urine to flow out of the body.) It dissolves inside the urethra where it is then absorbed into the blood. Proper insertion of the suppository is important; education and practice are critical to obtain the desired results. An erection that lasts for about one hour will usually occur in about 5–15 minutes. A man first takes the drug in his doctor's office for instruction, safety, and determining the proper dose for him.

Potential side effects of the alprostadil suppository include mild dizziness, a burning sensation in the urethra, prolonged erection, and aching and pain in the penis and testicles. Minor urethral bleeding or spotting due to improper administration can occur. Sexual stimulation will enhance the effect of the drug.

Diabetes Complications

Penile injections. Alprostadil can also be injected into the penis to treat erectile dysfunction. Penile injection therapy was introduced in 1995. Although it is a highly effective therapy, fear or reluctance to give an injection into the penis and the convenience of taking a pill have allowed the oral drugs to dominate the market. Men using penile injections have reported that this therapy gives good results and very natural looking erections (alprostadil, whether injected or used as a urethral suppository, often enables a man to achieve a firm head to his penis, while other therapies can result in a soft head). Unlike the other medicines listed before, penile injections require very little sexual stimulation to result in an erection.

The drug is injected with a syringe and needle (similar to insulin injections), causing blood vessels to dilate, which brings more blood into the penis. An erection occurs in about 5–20 minutes and can last up to an hour. This treatment requires practice to correctly administer the medicine. As with the alprostadil suppository, a man's first dose is taken in the doctor's office to ensure safety, learn proper technique, and find the proper dose. Penile injection therapy can be used three times per week, with at least 24 hours between each dose.

Potential side effects include pain, infection, and scarring. Too large of a dose can cause prolonged, painful erections, but education and careful dosing can prevent this problem.

Mechanical devices

Before there were drugs, mechanical devices were the main treatment for erectile dysfunction. Although drug companies have the financial muscle to advertise the latest medicines, these little-heralded devices are still useful and effective.

Constriction bands. Some men, especially men with diabetes, are able to get an erection but are unable to maintain it because of venous leakage. The blood flows out as fast as it comes in. With position changes or with penetration, men with leakage can lose their erections. This is where a constriction band can help. There are a number of bands on the market made in a variety of materials, sizes, and shapes. A man uses a band by placing it at the base of the penis after an erection is attained to prevent blood from leaving the penis. Some men use constriction bands in conjunction with alprostadil or the oral erectile dysfunction treatments.

To prevent tissues from becoming oxygen-starved, the constriction band should be left on for no more than 30 minutes, and there should be about an hour's time between applications. In

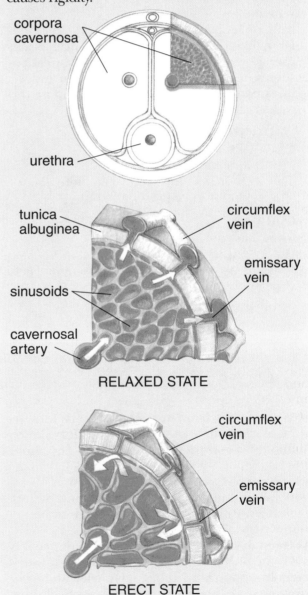

HOW AN ERECTION OCCURS

The illustrations below show a cross section of the penis. In the relaxed state, blood flows from the artery that feeds each of the corpora cavernosa, through the sinusoids, and empties via the emissary veins that lie within the tunica albuginea. In the erect state, the smooth-muscle walls of the sinusoids relax, allowing blood to expand the sinusoids, which results in swelling of the penis and compression of the emissary veins. Any further flow of blood into the penis causes rigidity.

corpora cavernosa

urethra

tunica albuginea

circumflex vein

emissary vein

sinusoids

cavernosal artery

RELAXED STATE

circumflex vein

emissary vein

ERECT STATE

FOR MORE INFORMATION

For more information about erectile dysfunction, treatments for it, and sexuality in general, the following resources may be of interest.

SEXUALITY AND IMPOTENCE

www.urologyhealth.org
This Web site from the American Urological Association has pages on several topics related to sexual function and infertility. It can also help you find a urologist, and you can sign up for a free e-mail or print newsletter.

THE NEW MALE SEXUALITY

Bernie Zilbergeld, Ph.D.
Bantam
New York City, 1999
Dr. Zilbergeld draws on his experiences as a sex therapist to give advice on a variety of relationship issues. This revised edition also includes information on how sildenafil can help men with erectile dysfunction.

DRUG TREATMENTS

CAVERJECT IMPULSE
www.caverjectimpulse.com
This Web site can help you learn more about alprostadil for injection.

CIALIS
www.cialis.com
(877) CIALIS-1 (242-5471)
Visit this Web site to learn more about tadalafil (Cialis).

LEVITRA
www.levitra.com
Also available in a Spanish version, this Web site has information on vardenafil (Levitra) that you can view online or have sent to you in the mail or through e-mail.

MUSE
www.vivus.com
(888) 367-6873
Information about the alprostadil urethral suppository (MUSE), including instructional videos.

VIAGRA
www.viagra.com
(888) 4-VIAGRA (484-2472)
Sildenafil's (Viagra) official site. The Web site is also available in a Spanish language version.

MECHANICAL AND IMPLANTABLE DEVICES

AMERICAN MEDICAL SYSTEMS
www.visitams.com/mens_erectile_restoration.html
(800) 328-3881
Makers of medical devices such as penile implants, including 3-piece (700 Series), 2-piece (Ambicor), and noninflatable (Malleable and DURA) varieties.

REJOYN
www.rejoyn.com/Rejoyn.html
(888) 473-5696
Find out more about the Rejoyn family of products, including a vacuum device (Vacuum Therapy System), a constriction band (Support Ring System), and a penile splint (Support Sleeve System).

TIMM MEDICAL TECHNOLOGIES, INC.
www.timmmedical.com
(800) 438-8592
Makers of a vacuum device (ErecAid).

---

some cases, the band may also compress the urethra, blocking the emission of ejaculatory fluids (although a constriction band is not—and should not be used as—a contraceptive device). A man who has a reduced ability to sense pain in his penis should not use a constriction band because pain is a warning that the device needs to be removed.

Vacuum devices. An external vacuum device was once the only treatment available for men with erectile dysfunction. Today, it is a tried and true treatment used by many men. It is relatively inexpensive and does not require injections or medicines to be successful. These devices can be bought over the counter or with a prescription, and they are often covered by insurance plans, including Medicare.

The device consists of a plastic cylinder, a pump (either handheld or battery-operated), a set of constriction bands, and a water-soluble lubricant. The lubricant is applied to the base of the penis to help form an airtight seal. Then the cylinder is placed over the flaccid penis and held tight against the pelvis. The pump is activated to create a vacuum within the cylinder, drawing blood into the penis. Once the penis is engorged with blood, a constriction band is rolled off the cylinder to near the base of the penis. The cylinder is removed, and the penis is left erect. The constriction band must be removed within 30 minutes.

Some possible side effects include a bluish color to the penis (from bruising or the tourniquet-like effect of the band), discomfort or pain (from pumping with too much pressure or from a constriction band that is too tight), coolness of the penis, and wobbliness of the penis near the base (the portion of the penis beyond the constriction band is still soft, so to minimize this problem, the band should be applied as far toward the base of the penis as possible). These problems can be lessened with practice and education.

Vacuum therapy is very effective, but it takes time and patience to use with ease. Statistics show that with practice, all men can find a level of success. Your physician or health professional can help with understanding and effectively applying the technique.

Penile splint. The penile splint (Rejoyn Support Sleeve System) is a relatively new and inexpensive treatment for men with erection problems. It allows men to have intercourse with a flaccid or semi-erect penis. The penis is placed in a tubular "splint" and a condom is applied over the penis. Penile splints allow for insertion and can produce a satisfying experience for both partners. These products can be purchased over the counter and can be used as frequently as you choose.

Surgery

Penile implants are considered a last resort, both because surgery is necessary to place them and because the surgery permanently changes some internal structures of the penis. As a result, if removal of the device becomes necessary for some reason, other erectile dysfunction treatments will not work. Those who choose penile implants, however, find they can create a natural-looking erection. There are several different models on the market, but the most common and most effective is the three-piece inflatable implant. (Other varieties include a two-piece inflatable implant and a noninflatable implant.) It consists of two cylinders placed in the penis, a pump placed in the scrotum next to the testicles, and a fluid reservoir placed in the abdomen. Squeezing the pump transfers the fluid from the reservoir to the cylinders, creating an erection. Because this is a surgical procedure, it usually involves an overnight hospital stay. Recovery is complete in about six weeks and involves some pain, bruising, and tenderness. As with any surgery, infection is a possibility, but measures are taken before, during, and after surgery to minimize the risk.

There is a reported high satisfaction rate among men and their partners with implants. Because the penis does not become engorged with blood, it can stay erect all day with no harm, and lovemaking can be prolonged as long as desired. It is important to be aware that any mechanical device can fail due to wear. The statistics show about a 10%–12% failure rate over about 10 years. If a mechanical failure occurs, the implant can usually be replaced. Be sure to discuss all of these issues with your doctor before having surgery.

Getting help

Today, men who have erectile problems do not need to accept them as permanent. There are options that address a variety of needs and circumstances. If you're one of those men, speak to your doctor about what might work well for you, and bring your partner in on the discussion. Couples who work together tend to have the best success with treatment. Depending on the cause of your erectile dysfunction, your doctor may be able to treat you himself or may refer you to a urologist or other specialist. But you can only get the help you need by asking for it, so the sooner you take that first step, the sooner you'll be saying yes to sexual intercourse. □

SEXUAL WELLNESS

by Laura Hieronymus, M.S.Ed., A.P.R.N., B.C.-A.D.M., C.D.E., and Lawrence Maguire, M.D.

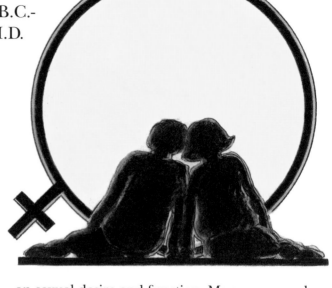

Intimacy is being seen and known as the person you truly are.
–Amy Bloom

Researchers believe that up to 50% of people with diabetes will experience some sort of sexual dysfunction at some point. But even if diabetes doesn't directly cause sexual dysfunction, other diabetes-related health issues can influence your sexual desire and may be a threat to intimacy within a relationship. It is important for you to be educated and aware of these issues, both to prevent health or sexual problems as much as possible and to be prepared to cope if they arise.

Types of sexual problems

Sex experts have divided sexual dysfunction disorders into four categories: desire disorders, arousal disorders, orgasm disorders, and pain disorders. One type of disorder can and often does coexist with another. None of these types of disorders is unique to people with diabetes, but diabetes can contribute to some of them. Sexual problems can occur at any stage in a person's life and can occur suddenly or gradually over time.

Desire disorders. Decreased libido, or a persistent lack of desire for sexual activity, is called a desire disorder. Common predisposing factors include changes in testosterone production (in both men and women) and a decrease in estrogen level in women, most commonly associated with menopause. Psychological or relationship problems can also lead to desire disorders.

Testosterone is a sex hormone that plays an important role in puberty. In men, testosterone is produced primarily in the testes, the reproductive glands that also produce sperm. As men age, their testosterone level tends to decrease, along with their sex drive. In men with diabetes, however, a decrease in testosterone production may occur at a much younger age. Men with diabetes as young as 45 are twice as likely to have a low testosterone level as men who don't have diabetes.

In women, small amounts of testosterone are produced primarily by the ovaries and adrenal glands. While the role of testosterone in women is poorly understood, it is believed to have an effect on sexual desire and function. Menopause and certain medical conditions may cause a woman to have a low testosterone level, possibly contributing to lowered sexual desire.

Women with polycystic ovary syndrome (PCOS), a disorder characterized by menstrual irregularities and infertility, however, tend to have the opposite problem: a high testosterone level. Like Type 2 diabetes, PCOS is associated with insulin resistance, in which the body is unable to use insulin efficiently. In fact, about 50% of women with PCOS eventually develop Type 2 diabetes.

A high testosterone level in a woman—whether or not she has PCOS—can cause development of male sex characteristics, including an increase in body hair and facial hair, a deepening of the voice, male-pattern baldness, and clitoral enlargement. High testosterone is not directly associated with a lack of sexual desire, but the physical changes it can cause can affect a woman's self-esteem and cause her to feel unattractive and sexually undesirable.

The decline in estrogen levels that occurs with menopause similarly may not directly affect a woman's level of sexual desire, but other aspects of menopause, such as hot flashes, may affect how she feels about sex. In some women, hot flashes can contribute to fatigue and sleep deprivation. In others, hot flashes can alter mood and consequently affect the quality of their sexual relationship.

In addition to these hormonal changes, the following can contribute to lack of sexual desire:
■ Physical changes that often occur with aging, including lack of energy, loss of strength, and stiffness with body movement, can affect both sexual function and sexual desire.

■ Fatigue or tiredness, whatever its cause, can profoundly affect a person's interest in sexual activity.

■ Pregnancy and the tiredness, discomfort, changes in body image, and changes in hormone levels that go with it can lower sexual desire.

■ A well-known side effect of antidepressants in the selective serotonin reuptake inhibitor (SSRI) class is reduced sexual desire in both men and women. The SSRIs include fluoxetine (brand name Prozac), sertraline (Zoloft), and paroxetine (Paxil).

■ Depression can contribute to a lack of interest in sex or lack of energy associated with sexual desire. Depression is common among those living with a chronic illness such as diabetes.

Arousal disorders. The inability to become aroused or to maintain sufficient sexual excitement is called an arousal disorder. In women, sexual arousal disorder involves an inability to attain or maintain swelling and lubrication of the genitals. In men, it involves difficulty attaining or maintaining an erection. Arousal disorder may appear to stem from an avoidance or aversion to sexual contact with a partner. But in fact, the roots of the problem can be physical as well as psychological.

Orgasm disorders. A persistent delay in or absence of orgasm following a normal sexual excitement phase can occur in both men and women. Use of SSRIs commonly contributes to this problem. (If you have been prescribed one of these drugs, however, do not discontinue it without first consulting your prescriber.) Diabetic neuropathy (nerve damage associated with diabetes) may also contribute to the lack of ability to achieve orgasm.

Pain disorders. Pain associated with sex is more common in women than in men, but it can affect both sexes. Its causes can be physical, psychological, or both. In some cases, women experience pain with intercourse because of *vaginismus,* an involuntary spasm of the vaginal wall muscles. While the cause of vaginismus is not clear, trauma such as rape or abuse may play a role.

Poor lubrication and vaginal dryness can also contribute to painful intercourse in women. The possible causes of poor lubrication and vaginal dryness are many, and they include the hormonal changes that occur with pregnancy and breast-feeding. With menopause and the accompanying decrease in estrogen production, the vaginal lining becomes thinner, which can cause vaginal dryness and pain with sexual activity. In women with diabetes, these symptoms can often be exaggerated, especially during periods of less than ideal blood glucose control.

If you or your partner is experiencing pain during sex that appears to be related to vaginal dry-

ness or irritation, your health-care professional may suggest taking time for adequate stimulation prior to intercourse, using a vaginal estrogen cream or water-based lubricant, and avoiding contraceptive foams and creams that may be irritating to the vaginal lining.

Is it my diabetes?

The physical health issues that are commonly associated with diabetes can contribute to sexual problems, so when any form of sexual dysfunction develops in a person with diabetes, it should be considered as a possible cause. However, diabetes should not automatically be assumed to be the problem; other potentially relevant health issues, many of which are not diabetes-specific, should be examined as well.

Most diabetes complications are related to high blood glucose, and sexual problems are no exception. In the short term, high blood glucose can negatively affect your energy level as well as your mood, which can cause any relationship to suffer. Your body's cells require glucose for energy; high blood glucose levels usually indicate that glucose is not being moved into your body's cells, and you therefore have less energy than usual. The higher your blood glucose levels, the more tired you will typically feel.

In addition, when blood glucose levels are high, you may feel irritable or cranky. Other symptoms of high blood glucose such as frequent urination, feeling thirsty, and having blurry vision can be annoying and preoccupying, keeping you from any preferred behavior, including spending time with your partner.

Persistent high blood glucose levels can increase the likelihood of infections in the urinary tract, vagina, and penis, which can obviously put a damper on intimate moments.

Over the long term, blood glucose levels that remain high and uncontrolled contribute to neuropathy (nerve damage) and blood vessel damage leading to impaired blood circulation. Both of these can affect the body's response to sexual stimulation, leading to erectile dysfunction in more than one in three men with diabetes as well as lubrication problems related to sexual function in up to 60% of women with diabetes.

Impaired circulation. High blood glucose, high blood pressure, and high cholesterol all raise the risk of developing atherosclerosis, or an accumulation of fatty material under the inner lining of the arteries. Atherosclerosis raises the risk of having a heart attack or stroke, and it can also lead to impotence and problems with arousal and orgasm (in men and women) if it impedes blood flow to the genital region.

Neuropathy. As many as 50% of people with diabetes eventually develop some type of nerve damage. While damage to the peripheral nerves is associated with burning, tingling, or numbness in the feet, damage to the nerves that regulate involuntary functions, such as those that relate to response or excitement from sexual stimulation, can contribute to sexual problems. The function of nerve fibers plays a vital role in one's ability to experience sexual pleasure.

Prevention

Preventing diabetes complications, including sexual complications, involves controlling your blood glucose, blood pressure, and blood lipid levels. If your glycosylated hemoglobin (HbA_{1c}) level is currently higher than 7% (or higher than the HbA_{1c} goal recommended by your diabetes care provider), your blood pressure higher than 130/80 mm Hg, your low-density lipoprotein (LDL) cholesterol 100 mg/dl or above, or your triglyceride level 150 mg/dl or above, speak to your provider about bringing these levels into the recommended ranges.

Take a proactive role in your diabetes health by monitoring your blood glucose levels, taking action when they are too high (based on medical advice), and communicating regularly with your diabetes care team. Maintaining excellent health takes hard work, but the payoffs are many, including feeling better mentally and physically.

Getting help

If you're experiencing persistent sexual difficulties, speak to your diabetes care provider about it. Based on your description of the difficulties you're having as well as your previous medical history, including any drugs you may be taking, your provider may be able to rule out some possible causes or identify some likely ones. He may choose to treat you himself or may refer you to a specialist such as a urologist for care. If your diabetes control appears to be a contributing factor, your provider may recommend changes in your treatment plan or refer you to an endocrinologist or possibly to a diabetes educator for education and skills training. If your sexual problem appears to be primarily psychological in nature or your provider believes you may be experiencing depression, he may refer you to a mental health care provider such as a psychiatrist or psychologist for therapy and, if needed, antidepressant drug therapy.

No matter what their cause, sexual problems

READ MORE ABOUT IT

When it comes to sex and sexuality, being informed can only help.

MEDLINE PLUS
Female Sexual Dysfunction
www.nlm.nih.gov/medlineplus/
femalesexualdysfunction.html
Read articles from respected publications on various aspects of female sexual dysfunction.

SEXUALITYANDU.CA
Canadian Web site about sexuality covers various forms of sexual dysfunction as well as relationship issues, contraception, sexually transmitted infections, and more.

UROLOGYCHANNEL
www.urologychannel.com
Read about erectile dysfunction, female sexual dysfunction, and other subjects related to the reproductive system and urinary tract.

tend to have profound effects on emotional well-being and on relationships. Talking with a licensed psychotherapist or seeking the help of a marriage and family therapist can help you cope as you seek medical help or adjust to changes in your sexual function. In many cases, psychological counseling along with treatment of physical factors contributing to sexual problems offers the best solution to management.

Maintaining your relationship

While you seek medical help or mental health care, it's important to keep the lines of communication open with your partner. Talking frankly about the problems you're experiencing and your feelings about them, as well as listening to what your partner has to say, will most likely bring you closer. When you talk, keep in mind that what makes a relationship satisfying for the people involved is really up to them—not to some notion about what intimate relationships should be.

Recognizing the fact that women and men commonly have different perspectives regarding intimate relationships may be helpful. Men typically want a partner who is willing and interested in a sexual relationship, and they often associate intimacy with sexual contact. Women, on the other hand, tend to feel closer to a partner who listens to them and most often connect sexual intimacy with love.

So let that special person see and know who you truly are, as well as what you want within the relationship. People who understand the needs of their partners—and recognize that those needs might be different from their own—have the best chance for creating longer-lasting, more satisfying, intimate relationships. □

PROTECTING YOUR KIDNEYS

by Robert S. Dinsmoor

Diabetic nephropathy (kidney disease) is the leading cause of kidney failure in the United States. That's the bad news. The good news is that the outlook for protecting your kidneys has gotten much brighter over the past decade or so. There are now a number of measures you can take that have been scientifically proven to protect your kidneys and lower the risk of developing diabetes-related kidney disease. Here's what the research shows.

When good kidneys go bad

Your kidneys, which are each about the size of your fist, are located near the middle of your back, just below the rib cage. By no coincidence, they are shaped like kidney beans. One of their jobs is to filter waste products and extra water from the bloodstream. This waste and excess water, in the form of urine, flow through tubes called ureters and into the bladder. The bladder stores urine until it is full enough to create the urge to urinate.

How does this filtering process work? Each kidney is made up of about one million tiny filtering units called *nephrons.* Tiny blood vessels called *arterioles* deliver blood to the nephrons. Within each nephron, the blood vessels form a complex called a *glomerulus.* It is within these glomeruli that the filtering activity actually takes place. The filtered blood leaves through another arteriole and is eventually carried back to the heart. Meanwhile, the material filtered from the blood passes through a tubule, where it is converted to urine, and then carried to the bladder through the ureters.

Diabetes sets the stage for kidney damage. Chronic high blood glucose levels, often in combination with high blood pressure, damage the glomeruli and progressively diminish kidney function. (High blood pressure alone is the second-leading cause of kidney failure behind diabetes.) This type of kidney dysfunction is known as diabetic nephropathy. In its earliest stages, it has no symptoms; however, the "silent" damage going on behind the scenes can still pave the way for kidney failure.

In the first stage of diabetic nephropathy, called *hyperfiltration,* the kidneys filter larger quantities of blood than usual in an attempt to compensate for damaged nephrons. Hyperfiltration is the first stage of the problem, but it does not necessarily lead to kidney failure. In fact, some people may stay in this stage and not progress further, especially if they maintain control of their blood glucose and blood pressure levels.

If damage from high blood glucose levels (and high blood pressure) continues for many years, this may lead to the second stage, called *microalbuminuria.* Normally, the kidneys do not allow significant amounts of proteins from the bloodstream into the urine. However, once they become damaged, tiny amounts of protein leak into the urine. The appearance of small amounts of the protein albumin in the urine indicates the start of diabetic nephropathy. (Albumin in the urine can also signal the possibility of glomerular disease or chronic high blood pressure, while the presence of other types of protein would raise suspicions of other types of kidney disease.) Laboratory tests can detect this small amount of albumin while kidney disease is still fairly treatable. However, your doctor must specifically request a microalbumin test of your urine, because standard urine tests are not sensitive enough to notice these small amounts of albumin.

As in hyperfiltration, some people may develop microalbuminuria but not progress to later stages of kidney disease, especially if it is caught and treated early. However, even if nephropathy does not develop, the presence of microalbuminuria is itself a risk factor for cardiovascular diseases in people with Type 2 diabetes.

In the third stage (sometimes called overt diabetic nephropathy or nephrotic syndrome), large amounts of albumin spill into the urine (a condition called *macroalbuminuria*), which can be detected even on routine urine tests. As more

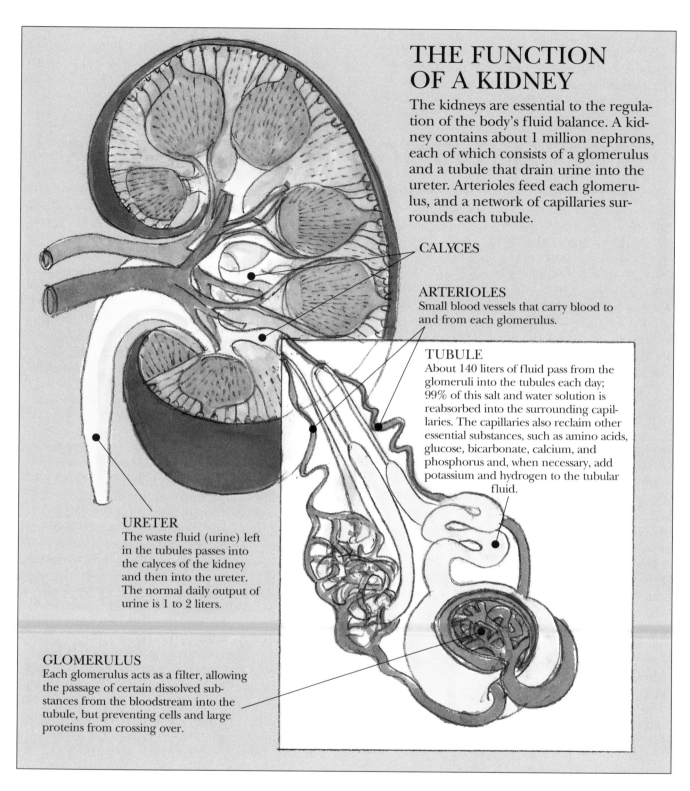

THE FUNCTION OF A KIDNEY

The kidneys are essential to the regulation of the body's fluid balance. A kidney contains about 1 million nephrons, each of which consists of a glomerulus and a tubule that drain urine into the ureter. Arterioles feed each glomerulus, and a network of capillaries surrounds each tubule.

CALYCES

ARTERIOLES
Small blood vessels that carry blood to and from each glomerulus.

TUBULE
About 140 liters of fluid pass from the glomeruli into the tubules each day; 99% of this salt and water solution is reabsorbed into the surrounding capillaries. The capillaries also reclaim other essential substances, such as amino acids, glucose, bicarbonate, calcium, and phosphorus and, when necessary, add potassium and hydrogen to the tubular fluid.

URETER
The waste fluid (urine) left in the tubules passes into the calyces of the kidney and then into the ureter. The normal daily output of urine is 1 to 2 liters.

GLOMERULUS
Each glomerulus acts as a filter, allowing the passage of certain dissolved substances from the bloodstream into the tubule, but preventing cells and large proteins from crossing over.

albumin passes into the urine, less remains in the bloodstream. Since these proteins normally help to retain fluid in the bloodstream, their loss allows fluid to begin leaking out of the arteries and capillaries. This fluid tends to build up in the tissues, a condition known as *edema.* Excess fluid can collect in the legs and feet and later even in the chest (*pleural effusion*), around the heart (*pericardial effusion*), and in the abdomen (*ascites*), causing symptoms such as fatigue, chest pain, and shortness of breath. Also at this stage, people tend to develop high blood pressure if they do not have it already (people who already have high blood pressure will find it worsens).

Diabetes Complications

In the fourth stage, called advanced clinical nephropathy, the kidneys can no longer remove most of the body's waste products. Toxins begin to build up in the bloodstream, and anemia (low red blood cell count) may develop, causing fatigue.

In the fifth stage, called kidney failure, the kidneys barely function at all, causing *uremia*, the buildup of urea and other waste products in the blood. Uremia causes symptoms such as nausea, vomiting, and fatigue. In 50% of people who have Type 1 diabetes and overt nephropathy, kidney failure develops within 10 years. Among people with Type 2 diabetes and overt nephropathy, 20% progress to kidney failure in 20 years. People with kidney failure require dialysis, a treatment that takes over the function of the kidneys by filtering waste products and removing water from the blood. In some cases, people with kidney failure can get a kidney transplant, but most must wait for a long time for a suitable donor kidney to become available.

If you work with a nephrologist (a physician who specializes in kidney diseases) to treat problems with diabetic nephropathy, he may refer to different stages than the ones described here because the National Kidney Foundation (NKF) has its own five-stage classification system for chronic kidney disease. The NKF bases its system on kidney filtering function alone, so it does not differentiate between the initial causes of the kidney disease. In the NKF's model, people with diabetic nephropathy who show microalbuminuria would usually be grouped in "stage 1 chronic kidney disease." Kidney failure occurs in "stage 5 chronic kidney disease."

Screening

One of the best screening tools for the earliest stages of diabetic kidney disease is the urine microalbumin test, which can be done in one of three ways and also involves a check of urinary creatinine levels. (Creatinine is a by-product of normal muscle breakdown.) To monitor your albumin levels, your health-care team can order a one-time in-office check of urine (a "random spot collection," often done first thing in the morning), a 24-hour urine collection (analyzing all the urine you produce in 24 hours), or a timed collection (analyzing all the urine you produce over a certain number of hours). The 24-hour sample is supposed to give the most accurate results (and may still be recommended for certain people with unusual protein intakes or extreme muscle loss), but because it can be a hassle and because the shorter tests offer good accuracy when corrected by checking creatinine lev-

els, many health-care providers simply use the shorter tests. (Several companies sell home test kits that allow people to mail urine samples to a laboratory for microalbumin testing; however, you should discuss this option with your health-care team before trying one.)

If a test shows the presence of albumin in the urine, the physician usually orders one or two repeat tests to confirm the result (because albumin levels in urine can vary from day to day). To reach a firm diagnosis of microalbuminuria, a person needs to have certain levels of albumin in the urine on at least two of three tests in three to six months. The more albumin that is in the urine, the more severe the kidney disease.

Currently, the American Diabetes Association (ADA) recommends starting to screen for microalbuminuria in people who have had Type 1 diabetes for 5 years and at the time of diagnosis in people with Type 2 diabetes (since diabetes may have been developing and causing problems for many years before diagnosis). All people with diabetes should be screened annually after their first microalbumin test (or have repeat testing within six months if a test result is positive for microalbuminuria).

While microalbuminuria may be a very sensitive test in people with Type 1 diabetes, there is evidence that testing for microalbuminuria alone may miss many cases of diabetic kidney disease in people with Type 2 diabetes. In a study reported in the June 25, 2003, issue of *The Journal of the American Medical Association*, researchers studied data from 1,197 people with Type 2 diabetes who were 40 years or older. In addition to testing for microalbuminuria, they tested participants' glomerular filtration rate (GFR), a measure of how well the kidneys are able to filter waste from the blood. GFR is considered the best gauge of kidney function (and is the measure the NKF uses to divide up its five-stage kidney disease classification system), and a persistently low GFR indicates kidney disease. Of those study subjects who had a low GFR, 55% did not have microalbuminuria. So some medical experts now recommend that people with Type 2 diabetes also have their GFR tested annually to catch early nephropathy that a microalbumin test may miss.

GFR cannot be measured directly. Currently, it is closely approximated, in part, by using the blood concentration of creatinine. Healthy kidneys excrete creatinine in the urine, so a buildup of creatinine in the blood shows that the kidneys aren't working well. By measuring the concentration of creatinine in the bloodstream and using it in an equation that takes into account the person's weight, age, sex, and race, doctors can estimate the GFR and get a sense of kidney function. The higher the blood creatinine level, the lower the GFR. Some physicians also use the blood creatinine level and GFR calculation to track the decline of kidney function and to gauge any benefits of treatment.

Prevention and treatment

At least two large studies have shown beyond a shadow of a doubt that tight blood glucose control can significantly lower the risk of developing microalbuminuria and diabetic kidney disease. The glycosylated hemoglobin (HbA_{1c}) test gives a measure of one's long-term control of blood glucose and hence one's risk for diabetic complications. The ADA currently recommends that people with diabetes have an HbA_{1c} test two to four times each year and strive for an HbA_{1c} level under 7%.

Controlling blood pressure is important not only for reducing the risk of cardiovascular disease but also for protecting the kidneys. According to the ADA, both high systolic blood pressure (the pressure at the moment of the heart beat) and high diastolic pressure (the pressure between beats) can speed up the progression of diabetic kidney disease, and aggressive treatment of high blood pressure can greatly decrease the rate of fall in GFR. Treating high blood pressure has also been shown to raise life expectancy and reduce the need for dialysis and transplantation once diabetic kidney disease has developed. According to the ADA, people with diabetes should strive to maintain a systolic blood pressure under 130 mm Hg and a diastolic pressure under 80 mm Hg.

In some cases, initial therapy for high blood pressure should consist of lifestyle modifications, such as losing weight, cutting back on sodium and alcohol consumption, and getting more exercise. One of the most effective lifestyle changes would be to follow the DASH (Dietary Approaches to Stop Hypertension) eating plan, which is a diet low in saturated fat, total fat, and cholesterol that emphasizes fruits, vegetables, and low-fat dairy products. The DASH diet is most effective when combined with a reduction in sodium intake. You can download a copy of "Your Guide to Lowering Your Blood Pressure with DASH," which includes a week's worth of menus, from www.nhlbi.nih.gov/ health/public/heart/hbp/dash or call (301) 592-8573 for a free copy.

For treating high blood pressure in people with diabetes—or for treating anyone with diabetes and microalbuminuria or overt nephropathy—specific

ANALGESICS AND KIDNEY HEALTH

Over-the-counter analgesics, such as aspirin, acetaminophen, ibuprofen, ketoprofen, and naproxen, are usually safe when taken as directed. However, if taken in excess or over too long a period of time, they can harm the kidneys. According to the National Kidney Foundation, as many as 3% to 5% of new cases of chronic kidney failure each year may be caused by the overuse of these painkillers. Products in which two or more painkillers are combined may be especially harmful to kidneys when used to excess.

The National Kidney Foundation recommends that these products be used only under a doctor's supervision in people with kidney disease, heart disease, high blood pressure, or liver disease; in people over 65; or in people taking diuretics. Their effects can be monitored through a number of simple blood tests, such as BUN (blood urea nitrogen) and serum creatinine levels. Sometimes a urine test is used to check for protein in the urine (a sign of kidney damage as well as diseases such as diabetic nephropathy). The National Kidney Foundation offers other tips for the safe use of analgesics:

■ Do not use them for more than 10 days for pain or more than 3 days for fever. If these conditions persist be-yond those periods, see your doctor.

■ Avoid prolonged use of products that contain mixtures of painkillers.

■ If you are taking analgesics, be sure to drink six to eight glasses of fluid a day.

■ If you have kidney disease, consult your doctor before using an analgesic.

■ Make sure your doctor knows about all the drugs you are taking, including over-the-counter products and dietary supplements.

■ Make sure you read the warning label before using any over-the-counter analgesic.

blood-pressure-lowering drugs called angiotensin-converting enzyme (ACE) inhibitors and angiotensin-II receptor blockers (ARBs) are the drugs of choice. ACE inhibitors include quinapril (Accupril), perindopril (Aceon), ramipril (Altace), captopril (Capoten), benazepril (Lotensin), trandolapril (Mavik), lisinopril (Prinivil, Zestril), and enalapril (Vasotec). ARBs include candesartan (Atacand), irbesartan (Avapro), olmesartan (Benicar), losartan (Cozaar), valsartan (Diovan), telmisartan (Micardis), and eprosartan (Teveten). These drugs appear to have a protective effect on kidneys above and beyond blood pressure control.

ACE normally converts a hormone called angiotensin I to a related hormone called angiotensin II, which constricts blood vessels, increases sodium and water retention, activates the sympathetic nervous system, stimulates fibrosis (stiffening) of the heart and blood vessels, and promotes heart cell growth. The immediate net effect of these changes is to raise blood pressure, but over time this hormone can cause damage to the heart and kidneys. ACE inhibitors block the action of ACE, thus decreasing the amount of angiotensin II and in turn minimizing its effects.

ARBs also work to decrease the effects of angiotensin II, but at a different point in the process. For angiotensin II to exert its effects throughout the body, it must bind to certain receptors (much as a key fits into a lock) on cell surfaces. ARBs prevent angiotensin II from binding to its receptors and thus reduce its effects.

Large numbers of studies have shown that in people with diabetes, ACE inhibitors can have a number of beneficial effects, including preventing or delaying the progression of nephropathy in people with microalbuminuria or overt diabetic nephropathy, decreasing the risk of heart attack and stroke, and decreasing mortality, so people with diabetes and hypertension are routinely prescribed ACE inhibitors.

Like ACE inhibitors, ARBs decrease levels of albumin in the urine and have been shown to effectively prevent progression of nephropathy in people with microalbuminuria or overt diabetic nephropathy. If an ACE inhibitor or ARB used alone is not sufficient to lower blood pressure, other blood-pressure-lowering drugs such as diuretics may need to be added; ACE inhibitors and ARBs can even be used together.

The effectiveness of dietary protein restriction in protecting the kidneys remains somewhat controversial. Dietary protein restriction has been shown to slow the progression of kidney disease in some animal models. Small clinical studies in people with diabetic kidney disease have shown that people who were able to restrict their dietary protein to 0.8 grams per kilogram of body weight per day (which is actually also the Recommended Dietary Allowance of protein for adults) were able to modestly slow the rate of fall in GFR. That level of protein consumption works out to about 54 grams of protein per day for a person weighing 150 pounds.

In a study reported in the March 18, 2003, issue of *Annals of Internal Medicine,* researchers studied dietary protein and kidney function in women with either normal kidney function or mild kidney disease. Female nurses, 42–68 years old, reported on their eating habits over a period of 11 years, after which their GFR was measured. In women with normal kidney function at the start of the study, there was no association between protein intake and GFR. Yet, in women with mild kidney disease at the start of the study, GFR declined as they ate more protein—especially nondairy animal protein. Experts now recommend a protein intake of 0.8 grams per kilogram of body weight per day in people who have overt nephropathy—and perhaps lower if this has a beneficial effect on the GFR. Protein-restricted diets should be designed by a registered dietitian, who can take into consideration all aspects of nutrition and dietary management of diabetes.

Risk reduction steps

Diabetic nephropathy is the leading cause of kidney failure in the United States. Yet with proper screening and diagnosis, some lifestyle changes, and good control of blood glucose and blood pressure with appropriate medicines, you can greatly reduce your chances of developing advanced kidney disease. The other good news: These same measures can also protect your heart, blood vessels, eyes, and nerves. □

TREATING GASTROPARESIS

by Kathryn Feigenbaum, R.N., M.S.N., C.D.E.

Although the term gastroparesis may be new to some, the symptoms of this ailment, in which the stomach's ability to move food into the small intestine is impaired, can be all too familiar, as up to 50% of people with diabetes will develop gastroparesis. The slow stomach emptying characteristic of this condition can cause nausea, vomiting, a feeling of fullness after eating a small amount of food, bloating, discomfort in the upper abdomen, and a lack of appetite. These symptoms can also be accompanied by erratic blood glucose levels, requiring frequent blood glucose checks and injections of insulin.

Symptoms and complications

The most common cause of gastroparesis is damage to the nerve fibers that control the movements of the stomach, branches of a major nerve known as the vagus nerve. The exact cause of the nerve damage is not completely understood, but the most widely accepted theory is that insulin deficiency, high blood glucose levels, or both gradually damage the vagus nerve.

Symptoms associated with gastroparesis include heartburn, reflux of food and liquids into the esophagus, difficulty swallowing, hypoglycemia (low blood glucose) after a meal followed by high blood glucose, constipation alternating with diarrhea, and weight loss. Other consequences and complications include the erratic absorption of medicines taken by mouth, foul breath, dehydration, electrolyte imbalance (electrolytes include salts such as sodium and potassium), and potentially even coma and death.

Gastroparesis can be diagnosed by special studies that evaluate how well the stomach and small intestine are digesting food. The common tests used for diagnosis are listed on page 289.

At times, the symptoms of gastroparesis may improve or even disappear. However, the actual delay in stomach emptying time does not seem to correlate very well with the symptoms a person experiences. Additionally, the severity of nerve damage does not match the intensity of the symptoms.

Some people with gastroparesis develop bacterial infections in their stomach or small intestine, and others form a mass of undigested food in the stomach called a bezoar. This retained undigested material can worsen a person's nausea and vomiting and can sometimes even develop into a complete blockage between the stomach and the small intestine.

Treatment for bezoars may include taking papaya juice or an enzyme known as cellulase orally or via injection to aid digestion. More serious bezoars may require the placement of a tube through the nose into the stomach so that the stomach can be flushed with Coca-Cola or a medicine called acetylcysteine, both of which can help dissolve the mass. Sometimes the undigested material can be broken up and taken out through the mouth using special equipment or through an incision into the stomach. Following any type of bezoar treatment, people must typically stick to a liquid diet for several months to help minimize the accumulation of undigested material in the stomach.

Managing blood glucose and nutrition

Having to follow a liquid diet for a prolonged period can be difficult for some people. However, individual preferences and tastes can be incorporated into the diet to make meals more palatable. Special consideration is needed to make sure that required nutrients, vitamins, minerals, and electrolytes are included in the diet. For example, people with gastroparesis are sometimes deficient in vitamins and minerals such as vitamin B_{12}, vitamin D, and iron, and may therefore need supplements containing these micronutrients. Stomach irritants such as nicotine and caffeine should be avoided.

It's also important for a person to take in enough calories and nutrients to maintain his body weight. Meals should have a low fat and fiber content and be small in volume. Daily consumption may therefore be divided into six small meals taken throughout the day. Liquids and solid foods that have been pureed in a blender are encouraged. Some examples of recipes for liquid meals begin on page 291.

All people with gastroparesis are advised to monitor their blood glucose frequently. Intensive blood glucose control that keeps levels stable and as close to normal as possible appears to reduce the severity of gastroparesis symptoms. High blood glucose, on the other hand, can worsen the slow movement of food through the gastrointestinal

DIAGNOSTIC TESTS FOR GASTROPARESIS

TEST	EXPLANATION
Gastric Emptying Scan	The person eat a meal containing a small, safe amount of radioactive material. The amount of radioactivity in the stomach is monitored to determine how quickly food leaves the stomach.
Gastric Manometry	A thin tube is inserted through the mouth into the stomach. A wire in the tube takes measurements of the stomach's electrical and muscular activity as it digests food, indicating whether the stomach is contracting in an efficient manner.
Magnetic Resonance Imaging (MRI)	A body scan is done using a magnetic field and radio waves to take three-dimensional pictures of the gastrointestinal tract.
Upper Endoscopy	After sedation, a flexible, lighted instrument with a very small camera attached (Gastroscopy) is inserted through the mouth to the stomach and first part of the small intestine. This enables the doctor to see any abnormalities in the esophagus, stomach, and small intestine. This test can rule out causes of gastroparesis other than diabetes.
Barium X-Ray	After fasting for 12 hours, the person drinks a shake containing barium, which makes the stomach visible on x-ray. The stomach is then x-rayed to see if any food is present.

tract. A continuous glucose monitoring system, which uses a sensor to measure glucose levels in fluid under the skin as often as every few minutes, can be a useful tool for tracking trends in glucose levels.

Checking blood glucose levels after meals is especially important to determine whether either food intake or the timing or size of insulin doses needs to be adjusted to maintain blood glucose within goal range. Some people who use rapid-acting insulin such as lispro (brand name Humalog), aspart (NovoLog), or glulisine (Apidra) administer their injection after they've finished eating a meal so they can better match the timing of food absorption. People who use an insulin pump can use the extended bolus or square-wave bolus features, which spread the delivery of an insulin dose over a selected period of time. A person's health-care provider can assist with determining the percentage of insulin to be delayed and the duration of the bolus infusion. Oral diabetes medicines may also be considered by the health-care team for use alone or together with insulin.

Medical treatments

In addition to blood glucose control, certain drugs or other treatments can also help reduce the symptoms of gastroparesis. For a list of the drugs, see page 290. Total parenteral nutrition. People who do not improve with medicines and who cannot get the proper nutrition through eating are often hospitalized so they can benefit from intravenous fluids that provide calories, minerals, vitamins, and nutrients, a type of treatment known as total parenteral nutrition. A tube may be threaded through the person's nose into the stomach to drain fluid and air.

Enteral nutrition. An alternative to total parenteral nutrition is enteral nutrition, in which the necessary medicines and nutrients are provided directly into the gastrointestinal tract via a tube placed into the stomach or small intestine. The tube can also be used to drain liquid and air from the gastrointestinal tract. Both total parenteral nutrition and enteral nutrition treatments may last for a long period of time, depending on when the

MEDICINES TO TREAT GASTROPARESIS

MEDICINE	HOW IT WORKS
Bethanechol (Urecholine)	Increases muscle contractions in the gastrointestinal tract.
Cisapride (Propulsid)	Increases the contractions of the gastrointestinal tract. In the United States, this drug is restricted to people who meet certain eligibility requirements due to its effects on the heart.
Domperidone (Motilium)	Increases stomach contractions, accelerating emptying of solid foods. This drug also lessens nausea and vomiting. There is a potential undesired effect on the heart. This drug is only available in Europe, Mexico, and Canada.
Erythromycin	Increases stomach contractions, decreasing the amount of time the stomach needs to empty.
Metaclopramide (Reglan)	Normalizes contractions of stomach muscles and decreases nausea and vomiting.
Octreotide (Sandostatin)	Improves contractions of the gastrointestinal tract. May also enhance effects of erythromycin.
Tegaserod (Zelnorm)	Decreases stomach emptying time, moving food into the intestine and reducing the chance of bezoar formation.

stomach is able to handle solid food again.

Gastric electrical stimulation. When a person has not responded to drug treatment or other conservative treatments such as changing the amounts or types of food in the diet, gastric electrical stimulation may be tried. This technique uses mild electrical pulses produced by a gastric pacemaker to stimulate the nerves of the lower stomach. These pulses are transmitted by means of electrodes that are surgically placed in the wall of the lower stomach. The settings of the device can be adjusted with an external programming system based on individual circumstances, such as the number of times a person becomes nauseated and vomits. Gastric electrical stimulation can be temporarily stopped by the health-care provider if a person needs to undergo magnetic resonance imaging (MRI), radiation therapy, defibrillation, or other medical procedures. This therapy may be used in conjunction with specific medicines to decrease gastroparesis symptoms.

Potential side effects, though rare, may include infection, unwanted movement of the device, a hole in the gastrointestinal tract, an undesirable change in stimulation (due to movement of the electrodes, for example), bleeding, bruising, pain at the site of an electrode, allergic reaction, pneumonia, and dehydration.

Botox. Injections of *Botulinum* toxin (Botox) at the connection between the stomach and small intestine have recently been used to increase the emptying of food from the stomach. This method works because the muscle that controls the opening of the stomach into the small intestine, when injected with Botox, becomes paralyzed by the Botox and allows food to pass through continuously.

Experimental treatments. One treatment for gastroparesis that is currently under investigation is the use of nitric oxide to normalize the movements of the gastrointestinal tract. Acupressure therapy is also being considered as a way to relieve the nausea, vomiting, and bloating that can be caused by gastroparesis.

Getting help

People who have gastroparesis should speak to their health-care team about creating a treatment plan that best fits their individual needs. Keeping a logbook with records of blood glucose levels, meal times and amounts, symptoms, exercise times and amounts, and medicine doses and schedules can help the health-care team make adjustments in the medical plan and also help the person with gastroparesis make daily decisions about his insulin and carbohydrate needs. Coping with gastroparesis can be frustrating, but it is important to remember that blood glucose monitoring, a balanced diet, and regular exercise can all help treat this condition. □

RECIPES FOR A LIQUID DIET

Sometimes it's necessary to follow a liquid diet if solids are not being digested properly. These recipes are tasty and nutritious.

Fruity yogurt sipper

1 large, ripe banana or 2 medium peaches,
  peeled and pitted
1½ cups whole milk
1 carton (8 ounces) vanilla yogurt
1–2 tablespoons powdered sugar
½ cup ice cubes

Cut fruit into chunks. Blend all ingredients except ice in a blender until smooth. Add ice one cube at a time, blending until smooth.

With banana:

Yield: 2 cups
Serving size: 1 cup
Per serving:
  Calories: 330
  Carbohydrate: 37 g
  Protein: 12 g
  Fat: 10 g
  Saturated fat: 5 g
  Cholesterol: 34 mg
  Sodium: 125 mg
  Fiber: 3 g
Carbohydrate choices: 2½

With peaches:

Yield: 2 cups
Serving size: 1 cup
Per serving:
  Calories: 310
  Carbohydrate: 32 g
  Protein: 13 g
  Fat: 10 g
  Saturated fat: 5 g
  Cholesterol: 34 mg
  Sodium: 125 mg
  Fiber: 2 g
Carbohydrate choices: 2

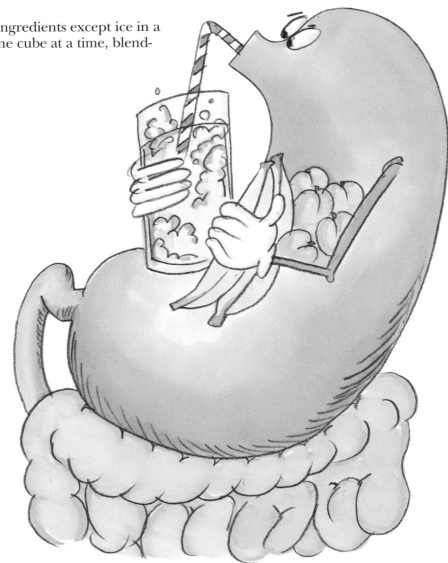

High-protein shake

1 cup protein-fortified, reduced-fat (2%) milk
½ cup regular ice cream
½ teaspoon vanilla extract
2 tablespoons butterscotch sauce, chocolate sauce, or fruit syrup

Put all ingredients in a blender. Blend at low speed for 10 seconds. For variety, try adding ½ cup banana or 1 tablespoon smooth peanut butter with 2 teaspoons sugar.

With butterscotch sauce:

Yield: 1½ cups
Serving size: 1 cup
Per serving:
    Calories: 252
    Carbohydrate: 39 g
    Protein: 9 g
    Fat: 8 g
    Saturated fat: 3 g
    Cholesterol: 35 mg
    Sodium: 209 mg
    Fiber: 0 g
Carbohydrate choices: 2½

With chocolate sauce:

Yield: 1½ cups
Serving size: 1 cup
Per serving:
    Calories: 276
    Carbohydrate: 36 g
    Protein: 10 g
    Fat: 11 g
    Saturated fat: 6 g
    Cholesterol: 35 g
    Sodium: 201 mg
    Fiber: 0 g
Carbohydrate choices: 2½

With banana and chocolate sauce:

Yield: 1½ cups
Serving size: 1 cup
Per serving:
    Calories: 317
    Carbohydrate: 49 g
    Protein: 10 g
    Fat: 8 g
    Saturated fat: 5 g
    Cholesterol: 35 mg
    Sodium: 201 mg
    Fiber: 1 g
Carbohydrate choices: 3

With peanut butter, sugar, and chocolate sauce:

Yield: 1½ cups
Serving size: 1 cup
Per serving:
    Calories: 367
    Carbohydrate: 43 g
    Protein: 10 g
    Fat: 14 g
    Saturated fat: 10 g
    Cholesterol: 35 mg
    Sodium: 248 mg
    Fiber: 1 g
Carbohydrate choices: 3

With fruit syrup:

Yield: 1½ cups
Serving size: 1 cup
Per serving:
    Calories: 257
    Carbohydrate: 40 g
    Protein: 8 g
    Fat: 8 g
    Saturated fat: 5 g
    Cholesterol: 35 mg
    Sodium: 113 mg
    Fiber: 0 g
Carbohydrate choices: 2½

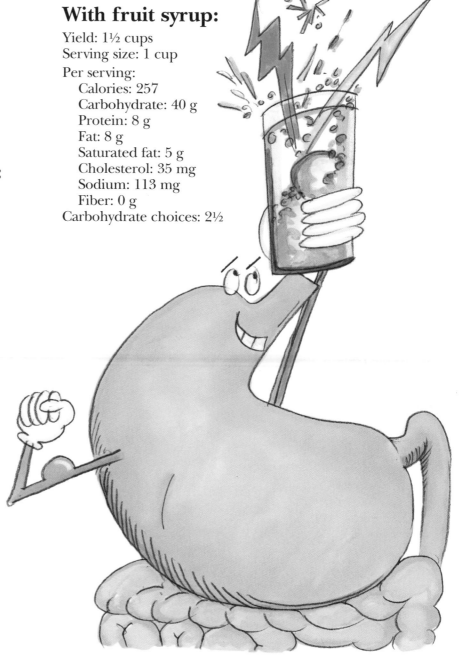

DIABETIC KETOACIDOSIS
A Preventable Crisis

by Jan Chait

People who have had diabetic ketoacidosis, or DKA, will tell you it's worse than any flu they've ever had, describing an overwhelming feeling of lethargy, unquenchable thirst, and unrelenting vomiting.

"It's sort of like having molasses for blood," says George. "Everything moves so slow, the mouth can feel so dry, and there is a cloud over your head. Just before diagnosis, when I was in high school, I would get out of a class and go to the bathroom to pee for about 10–12 minutes. Then I would head to the water fountain and begin drinking water for minutes at a time, usually until well after the next class had begun."

George, generally an upbeat person, said that while he has experienced varying degrees of DKA in his 40 years or so of having diabetes, "…at its worst, there is one reprieve from its ill feeling: Unfortunately, that is a coma."

But DKA can be more than a feeling of extreme discomfort, and it can result in more than a coma.

"It has the potential to kill," says Richard Hellman, M.D., past president of the American Association of Clinical Endocrinologists. "DKA is a medical emergency. It's the biggest medical emergency related to diabetes. It's also the most likely time for a child with diabetes to die."

DKA occurs when there is not enough insulin in the body, resulting in high blood glucose; the person is dehydrated; and too many ketones are present in the bloodstream, making it acidic. The initial insulin deficit is most often caused by the onset of diabetes, by an illness or infection, or by not taking insulin when it is needed.

Ketones are your brain's "second-best fuel," Hellman says, with glucose being number one. If you don't have enough glucose in your cells to supply energy to your brain, your body breaks fat down into small pieces so that it can be used as fuel. Ketones are formed during that process. Everybody has ketones in their bloodstream at some point, even people who don't have diabetes. Your body sometimes uses them for fuel when you restrict your food intake, when you haven't eaten for a while—even overnight, in very tiny amounts—and when you exercise.

The problem comes when you have diabetes and lack sufficient insulin to move glucose from your bloodstream into your body's cells. Your body believes it isn't getting enough food, so it reacts in two ways: It instructs the liver to turn glycogen (stored glucose) into glucose and release it into the bloodstream, and it begins to use fat for energy. The higher your blood glucose rises, the more fat is used—and the more ketones are formed.

"When you run out of insulin, ketone production becomes excessive," Hellman says. "It takes approximately two hours after you run out of insulin for excessive ketone accumulation to occur."

Ketones accumulate in your blood and, from there, go into the urine. That causes excessive urination, which is added to the increased urine production from high blood glucose. You then begin to become dehydrated.

At the same time, the increase in ketone production begins to change your body's chemistry, and it becomes more acidic. The increased acidity changes the delicate mechanisms that regulate your body—changes that can affect your heart and, perhaps, your brain. In addition to urinating more, your body also tries to get rid of the excess acid by exhaling it, so your breathing becomes shallow and rapid and smells like acetone, or fingernail polish remover. Badly needed fluids may not be retained because of vomiting. Because your body isn't getting the "food" it needs for energy, you have an overwhelming feeling of sleepiness. And you experience abdominal pain. In fact, Dr. Hellman says, DKA is sometimes misdiagnosed as appendicitis.

The treatment can be as simple as restoring fluids and insulin to the body, or as complicated as doing that plus bringing the body's chemistry back into balance, something that can only be done in a medical setting such as an emergency room or hospital.

Not just for Type 1 diabetes

Historically, DKA was thought of as a condition experienced only by people with Type 1 diabetes, but recent research is noting that DKA can occur in people with Type 2 diabetes as well, although it is generally not as severe in people with Type 2.

"A significant proportion of DKA occurs in patients with Type 2 diabetes," said one study, published in the September 27, 2004, issue of *Archives of Internal Medicine*. In that study, conducted in Dallas,

SIGNS AND SYMPTOMS

- Unexplained blood glucose level higher than 250 mg/dl
- Presence of ketones in blood or urine
- Fruity smelling breath
- Dry mouth
- Nausea
- Vomiting
- Fever
- Abdominal pain
- Low blood pressure
- Shortness of breath
- Dehydration
- Increased heart rate
- Pale or clammy skin
- Coma

Texas, nearly 22% of people with DKA who were identified as having diabetes had Type 2 diabetes.

Another study, conducted in the Bronx, New York, and published in the February 2007 issue of *Metabolism,* found that 32% of the subjects studied had Type 2 diabetes. This study focused on hospital admissions for DKA among ethnic minorities, primarily African-Americans and Hispanics. It concluded that African-Americans with Type 2 diabetes may be particularly susceptible to developing DKA.

How to check for ketones

Either a blood test or a urine test can check for ketones. The American Diabetes Association recommends that doctors use a blood test. Blood ketone testing equipment also is available for home use.

Why test blood rather than urine? First of all, because ketones enter the bloodstream first and then travel to the urine, ketones can be measured earlier in the blood. In addition, there are three types of ketones: acetoacetic acid, acetone, and beta-hydroxybutyric (β-OHB) acid. Urine ketone strips measure only acetoacetic acid and acetone, while blood ketone tests measure β-OHB, "the strongest and most prevalent acid in DKA," according to the 2004 ADA position paper "Hyperglycemic Crises in Diabetes."

Among people who are accustomed to checking their blood glucose, measuring blood ketones is widely accepted, according to a study published in the March 2006 issue of the British journal, *Diabetic Medicine.* In the study, 123 people 3 to 22 years old and their families were educated on sick-day care. Some were then given a meter that can measure blood ketones, and others were given urine ketone strips. While more than 90% of the subjects reported checking for blood ketones during illnesses, stress, or when blood glucose was elevated, only slightly more than 61% measured ketones in their urine. Hospital visits among those who checked for blood ketones were nearly half that of those who checked for urine ketones.

Two home meters are available to measure ketones in the blood: Abbott Diabetes Care's Precision Xtra (www.abbottdiabetescare.com) and CardioChek (www.cardiochek.com), which is made by Polymer Technology Systems, Inc. The Precision Xtra can also be used to check blood glucose levels, and CardioChek can also measure glucose, lipid, and creatinine levels.

While testing blood for ketones is the preferred method, the test strips are more costly than urine ketone strips, and it requires a meter that can check for blood ketones.

Urine ketone testing is done by dipping a reagent strip in urine, urinating on the strip, or, in the case of very young children, pressing the strip against a wet diaper. After a specified amount of time, the color on the strip is compared to a color chart on the container to determine the amount—if any—of ketones present. Ketones in the urine are measured in terms of the amount present: negative (no ketones), trace, small, moderate, or large.

Several brands of urine ketone strips are available, including Ketostix, Keto-Diastix (which also check for glucose in the urine), and Clinistix. Ask your pharmacist if ketone strips are available individually wrapped in foil packets. While the initial cost is higher, they last longer than the ones that are loosely packaged in vials. However, they may need to be specially ordered.

When to check for ketones

Don't wait for an emergency to happen before learning when to check for ketones and what to do if you detect ketones in your blood or urine. Talk to your doctor or diabetes educator in advance. In general, ketones should be checked for in the following situations:

- You have an unexplained blood glucose level over 250 mg/dl two times in a row.
- You are sick (with a cold, a sore throat, the flu, a stomach virus, suspected food poisoning, or anything else that makes you feel ill).
- You are planning to exercise and your blood glucose level is over 250 mg/dl.

HYPEROSMOLAR HYPERGLYCEMIC STATE

Dr. Richard Hellman, past president of the American Association of Clinical Endocrinologists, remembers once seeing a man whose blood glucose level was 2,400 mg/dl. "Basically," he said, "his blood looked like syrup."

However, the man was not experiencing diabetic ketoacidosis (DKA). Instead, he had a condition called hyperosmolar hyperglycemic state, or HHS. Like DKA, HHS is characterized by very high blood glucose levels, but unlike in DKA, people with HHS do not generally have ketones in their blood or urine.

Nonetheless, HHS can be deadly. According to the American Diabetes Association (ADA), while DKA has a death rate of less than 5%, that figure can reach around 15% for HHS.

Luckily, HHS is rare. The ADA says the annual rate for DKA ranges from 4.6 to 8 episodes per 1,000 people admitted to the hospital. HHS accounts for less than 1% of hospital admissions related primarily to diabetes.

HHS is most common in elderly people with new-onset Type 2 diabetes, particularly those who live in nursing homes, or in older people who have been diagnosed with Type 2 diabetes but who are unaware that their blood glucose is high or who haven't had enough fluid intake. Compounding the problem is that the thirst mechanism can be impaired in older people, and they're more apt to have kidney problems, Dr. Hellman says. When a person's thirst mechanism is impaired, the kidneys—which normally work to remove excess glucose from the blood—begin to conserve water. That leads to a higher glucose concentration in the bloodstream.

In many people, HHS begins with an infection, such as a urinary tract infection or pneumonia. Unlike DKA, which develops relatively quickly, HHS develops over several days, or even weeks.

"Diagnosis is sometimes a problem," Dr. Hellman says. "People with HHS look like they're suffering a stroke and may be vomiting. They have mental alterations that may look like a stroke or dementia."

The ADA says HHS can be prevented if nursing home staff and family members are vigilant about preventing dehydration in those who are unable to recognize or treat the condition themselves. Treatment of HHS generally involves using insulin to bring high blood glucose levels down.

Symptoms of HHS include the following:
- Dehydration
- Excessive thirst
- Low blood pressure
- High blood glucose level
- Hallucinations
- Sensory deficits, or impairment of one of the five senses, such as partial or total loss of hearing or vision, loss of sensation in some part of the body, or a loss of sense of balance
- Rapid eye movements
- Paralysis on one side of the body
- Seizures
- A partial or total loss of the ability to comprehend spoken or written language and express ideas

- You have symptoms of DKA, such as increased urination, a stomachache, and dry mouth.
- Your insulin pump has malfunctioned, causing an interruption in insulin delivery.
- You have experienced a traumatic stress.
- You are pregnant, in which case you should check for ketones every morning before breakfast and any time your blood glucose level is over 250 mg/dl. Pregnant women who have ketones in the morning are advised to eat more carbohydrate late in the evening or during the night.

If you detect ketones in your blood or urine, general treatment guidelines include drinking plenty of water or other calorie-free fluids to help flush ketones out of the body, taking insulin to bring your blood glucose level down, and rechecking both your blood glucose level and ketone level every three to four hours. Additional insulin may be needed to bring your blood glucose level down if ketones are present.

If ketone levels are not coming down, or are going up, treat the incident as a medical emergency and go to a hospital.

With proper vigilance, having ketones appear in your blood or urine won't escalate into a medical emergency, and your life won't be in peril. □

Foot Health

Tips 464–532 299

Taking Steps Toward Healthy Feet. 304

Wound Healing for Foot Ulcers 309

Foot Care 315
Drugstore Do's and Don't's

How to Choose Footwear 318

7

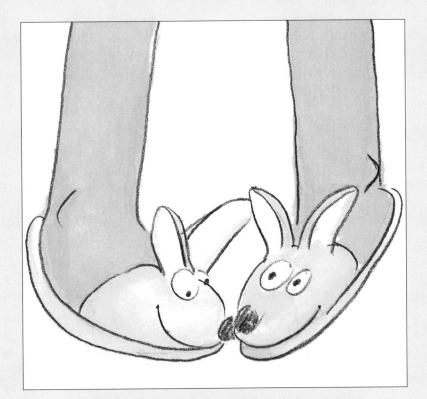

Foot Health Tips

464–532

464. Seek medical attention for foot or leg ulcers as soon as possible. Inadequately treated ulcers can result in infections and gangrene, which may eventually lead to the need for amputation.

465. People with peripheral neuropathy or with peripheral vascular disease, especially if they have limited joint mobility in the foot or a foot deformity, should check their feet regularly and carefully and wear more than one pair of shoes each day to reduce the risk of foot irritation.

466. Signs of peripheral vascular disease include leg pain that occurs only during movement, pain in the foot even while it is at rest, loss of hair on the lower legs and feet, skin that appears tight and shiny on the affected area, and reduced size of foot muscles.

467. Putting topical disinfectants such as iodine, acetic acid, or hydrogen peroxide on a foot or leg ulcer may actually impair wound healing. Do not add any steps to wound treatment that are not part of the plan developed with your health-care provider.

468. Take necessary steps to remove stress or pressure from an injured limb; this is necessary for healing to occur. Many devices

can assist in keeping pressure off of a wound.

469. Regular follow-up examinations for people with diabetic ulcers are an important part of treatment, even after they have healed; approximately 30% of ulcers recur.

470. Nutrition counseling from a dietitian can help provide a diet that aids the healing of ulcers and other wounds. This may include a diet high in protein.

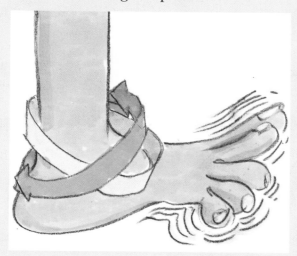

471. Try wiggling your toes and rotating your ankles for a few minutes every day to promote blood flow to your feet.

472. Never walk with bare feet or with just socks on, especially if your feet are numb, to reduce the risk of foot injury.

473. Do not soak your feet unless you're instructed to do so; this can dry out the skin and increase the risk of injury and infection.

474. Do not use commercial products to remove corns and calluses, strong antiseptics, or heating pads on your feet. All can cause irritation that increases the risk of foot complications.

475. Give feet a daily inspection for cuts and abrasions.

476. Ask your doctor to examine your feet periodically for any signs of nerve damage, such as loss of sensation, or reduced blood flow, such as coldness or hair loss on the feet and legs.

477. Wash your feet with warm or tepid water and soap every day.

478. If it's hard to see your feet, run your fingers over them to feel for calluses or sore spots.

479. The backs of your hands are sensitive to heat and can be run over your feet to find hot spots, which can indicate infection.

480. Apply a moisturizing lotion to your feet once or twice a day to help keep your skin healthy and moist.

481. Choose thick lotions over thin, "watery" lotions.

482. Don't put lotion between your toes, since the skin between toes tends to stay moist naturally; adding lotion there would over-moisturize that area and cause problems.

483. If you have troublesome calluses or corns on your feet, see your podiatrist for advice and treatment. Never use an acid product on any part of your feet.

484. Avoid even acid-free callus and corn home treatments, as well as pumice stones and files, which are not sterile and can cause breaks in the skin if you rub too vigorously or remove too much skin. Never take a sharp blade to your feet.

485. To treat a minor wound, first wash your hands with soap and water, then cleanse the wound with soap and water, rinse thoroughly, pat dry, and apply a thin layer of antibiotic ointment with a cotton swab (such as a Q-tips cotton swab) and an adhesive bandage. If you see no appreciable improvement in a treated wound within 24 hours, consult your doctor or podiatrist immediately.

486. Cut toenails straight across or following the natural curve of the toe, and not too short; this will avoid ingrown toenails.

487. Cutting toenails just after a shower or bath can make the job easier.

488. Gently smooth toenails with an emery board after clipping to keep them from snagging on socks.

489. When clipping or using an emery board on your toenails, never "dig" into the sides of your nails. Doing so can break the skin, opening the door to fungal or bacterial infections.

490. It may be a good idea to have your toenails cut regularly by a podiatrist if you cannot see or reach your toenails easily, if your nails are hard to cut because they're thick or you have a fungal nail infection, if the sides of your toenails curve into your skin, if you frequently have trouble clipping your toenails, or if you have reduced sensation or circulation in your feet. Toenail trimming every two or three months is usually recommended.

491. If you want a pedicure, buy your own inexpensive nail instrument set and bring it with you to your pedicurist. Make sure the technician knows never to cut your skin. For infection control, make sure the facility washes the basins that your feet may be placed in.

492. Don't use over-the-counter ingrown toenail remover products from the drugstore. If you have an ingrown toenail, see your podiatrist for treatment. If you see your toenail looking red or swollen, or you see drainage, blood, or pus on your toe, consult your podiatrist immediately. This is an emergency.

493. Because foot soaks can dry your skin, do not routinely soak your feet every night. Do not use alcohol or hydrogen peroxide as antiseptics on your feet; they will also dry your skin.

494. Capsaicin cream or ointment can sometimes reduce pain associated with diabetic neuropathy if used regularly over the course of several weeks. It can also relieve arthritis pain in some cases.

495. People with diabetes can safely use over-the-counter athlete's foot creams, and all athlete's foot creams are equally effective. To use an athlete's foot cream, wash your feet and dry well between your toes and on the bottoms of your feet. Rub the medicated cream in twice a day. If you see no improvement in five days, call your podiatrist. It might not be an athlete's foot fungus after all.

496. Make sure you have your doctor examine your feet at least once a year to check for the presence of foot problems and to

assess your risk of developing problems in the future. If you have neuropathy or peripheral arterial disease, your feet should be carefully inspected at every office visit.

497. Optimal blood glucose control can be beneficial in keeping your blood vessels and circulation healthy and helping the body resist, as well as fight off, infections.

498. If you smoke, your risk for foot problems increases; lowering your risk, obviously, involves quitting. Several options are available to assist with smoking cessation such as individual or group counseling and use of nicotine products or certain prescription medicines.

499. Call your diabetes care team if you experience high blood glucose levels for which you can determine no cause; this may be a sign of infection.

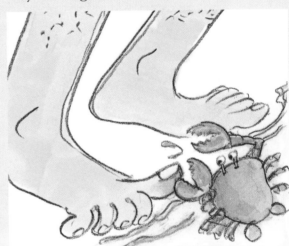

500. Don't forget to keep up your foot care even when your routine changes, such as when you're on vacation, a time when you may be tempted to walk barefoot in the sand or by the pool.

501. Shoes or slippers should always be worn to protect your feet; however, many foot ulcers start with rubbing from ill-fitting shoes, so it's important that your shoes fit well and don't cause any abnormal pressure on your feet.

502. Have your feet measured every time you buy shoes because feet change in size and shape over time.

503. It's better to be fitted for shoes in the afternoon or evening rather than first thing in the morning; walking around all day causes your feet to spread, so getting fitted when your feet are at their largest can help you to ensure a comfortable fit.

504. If you have complications that affect your feet, you may need special assistance selecting shoes or may need custom-made shoes.

505. If you have any lack of sensation in your feet (because of neuropathy, for example), you may want to seek the help of a certified pedorthist in selecting shoes.

506. People with lack of sensation in the feet, other changes in the feet caused by diabetes, or a history of foot ulcers may be candidates for orthotics, or specially designed insoles that are worn inside the shoes. If orthotics don't do the trick, it may be necessary to get custom-made shoes. To qualify for depth-inlay shoes, custom-molded shoes, or shoe inserts under Medicare Part B, your physician must certify that you have diabetes and are being treated, that you need the insert or shoe because you have diabetes, and that you have a condition such as an amputation, foot ulcers, calluses, poor circulation, or foot deformity.

507. Always wear socks with shoes to prevent blisters. Wear socks that fit well (tight socks impair circulation) and are seamless (to prevent blisters). Socks should be made of breathable material such as cotton or wool, ideally blended with a material that draws moisture away from the skin, such as acrylic.

508. To make sure your doctor checks your feet at each checkup, take off your shoes and socks before your doctor comes into the room.

509. File corns and calluses gently with an emery board or pumice stone. Do this after your bath or shower.

510. Always wear socks or stockings to avoid blisters. Do not wear socks or knee-high stockings that are too tight below your knee.

511. Wear shoes that fit well. Shop for shoes at the end of the day when your feet are bigger. Break in shoes slowly. Wear them 1 to 2 hours each day for the first 1 to 2 weeks.

512. Before putting your shoes on, feel the insides to make sure they have no sharp edges or objects that might injure your feet.

513. Choose a shoe with a toe box long enough so that the toes don't hit the front end of the shoe, spacious enough so that the toes can wiggle a little, and wide enough so as not to pinch the ball of the foot. However, it should not be so wide that the foot slides from side to side.

514. Choose a shoe with a toe box made of breathable materials, such as leather or cloth, which allows sweat to evaporate and helps keep feet drier throughout the day. Perforations in leather shoes make them even more breathable.

515. People with loss of sensation in their feet or with very delicate skin may be better off choosing shoe styles with no seams in the toe box.

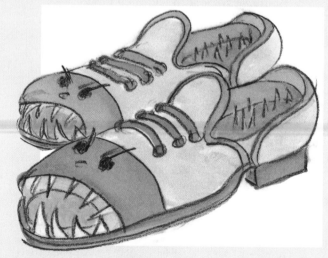

516. To avoid purchasing a shoe with a toe box that could irritate your feet, feel inside the shoes with your hand for stiff or scratchy seams or any rigid, well-defined structure. If you can feel any of these potential irritants, put the shoe back and try another model.

517. A shoe's tongue should be wide enough

and padded enough so that the laces don't dig into the top of your foot.

518. Any custom insert you buy should have at least three layers—a soft layer of foam on top and two stiffer layers on the bottom to provide some resilience.

519. To make sure that you choose a shoe with an arch that is strong enough, hold the shoe by the heel and push the toe box slightly up and toward the back of the shoe. The shoe should bend at the joint of the toes the way a foot does when pushing off. If it instead bends at the arch, don't buy it.

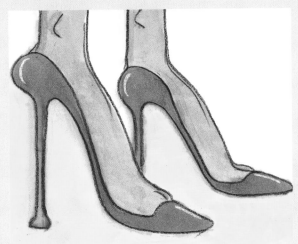

520. Avoid high-heeled shoes; they put increased pressure on the ball of the foot, place the back of the foot in an unstable position, and increase the movement of foot tissues in opposite directions, a primary cause of calluses, blisters, and ulcers. Heels should be less than one inch in height.

521. Avoid slip-on loafers, which provide inadequate foot support.

522. Avoid sandals with straps between the toes. These straps can cause irritation.

523. Many people have one foot that's larger than the other, so have both feet measured.

524. To get an accurate measurement, stand naturally with your weight divided evenly between both feet.

525. If you have narrow feet, choose shoes with wide-set eyelets to allow you to pull the laces tighter, if necessary. If you have wide feet, shoes with closely set rows of eyelets may work better.

526. When trying on shoes, make sure you are wearing the type of sock or stocking you normally wear, and don't forget to also bring any orthotics or inserts you will be wearing in the shoe.

527. There should be some room, preferably ½ inch to ⅝ inch, between the tip of your longest toe and the front of the shoe.

528. Walk around, and make sure that your arch is fully supported and that the break or bend of the shoe is located at the ball of your foot.

529. A properly fitted shoe should slip slightly in the heel, particularly when new, but it should not move excessively or slide off the back of the foot.

530. Roll your feet to the insides as if you were trying to flatten your arches, then to the outsides, as if to roll over onto your ankles. The shoe should feel like it is trying to restrict these motions, but it should not feel like it is placing excessive pressure against any one spot on the foot.

531. If it is suggested that your shoes need to be broken in, stretched, or otherwise modified, do not purchase the shoes, because they are the wrong ones for your feet.

532. Hard plastic or metal eyelets can irritate the top of the foot, so choose shoes with loops or punched-out holes whenever possible.

TAKING STEPS TOWARD HEALTHY FEET

by Laura Hieronymus, M.S.Ed., A.P.R.N., B.C.-A.D.M., C.D.E., and Belinda O'Connell, M.S., R.D., C.D.E.

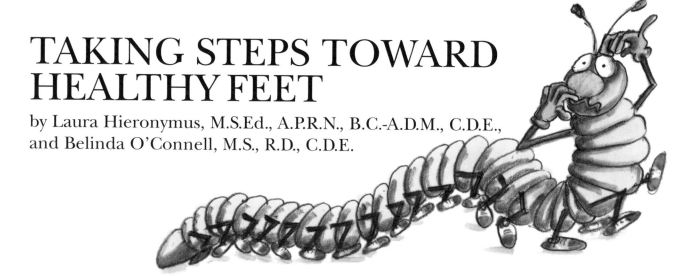

Diabetes is notorious for causing foot problems. In fact, it is the number one cause of lower limb amputations in the United States. In 2001, the latest year for which statistics are available, some 82,000 amputations—over half of all performed—were caused by diabetes.

But it doesn't have to be this way. You don't have to end up losing a limb because you have diabetes. It is estimated at least 50% of the amputations that occur each year in people with diabetes could be prevented through proper care of the feet and legs. By learning about the risks for foot problems and ways to take proper care of your feet, you raise your chances of keeping them for a lifetime.

Are you at risk?

The American Diabetes Association (ADA) has identified an increased risk of ulcers and amputations in the following groups of people with diabetes:

■ Those who have had diabetes for ten years or longer
■ Men
■ People whose blood glucose control is less than optimal
■ People who already have other diabetes complications, such as cardiovascular (heart) disease, retinopathy (eye disease), or nephropathy (kidney disease)
■ People with a history of smoking, because smoking is associated with early development of vascular (blood vessel) complications in diabetes.

In addition, the ADA associates the following foot-related complications with an increased risk of amputation:

■ Nerve damage (neuropathy) that has caused diminished sensation in the feet (ability to sense heat, cold, pressure, or pain)

■ Alterations in the normal structure and movement of the foot in the presence of neuropathy
■ Evidence of increased pressure on a part of the foot, such as redness, bruising, or bleeding under a callus
■ Bone deformity in the foot
■ Peripheral vascular disease that has caused a decrease or absence of pulses in the feet
■ Disease, damage, or deformity of the toenails.

Make sure you have your doctor examine your feet at least once a year to check for the presence of foot problems and to assess your risk of developing problems in the future. A commonly used test for detecting peripheral neuropathy (damage to the nerves supplying the feet, legs, hands, and arms) involves the physician pressing a Semmes–Weinstein monofilament, a flexible piece of nylon, against several places on the foot. The inability to sense the pressure of the filament at several points indicates neuropathy. To test for peripheral arterial disease, physicians examine the strength of the pulses in the feet and evaluate a person's ankle–brachial index, which is the ratio of the blood pressure in the calves to the blood pressure in the arms. If you have neuropathy or peripheral arterial disease, your feet should be carefully inspected at every office visit. Your diabetes care team can also advise you on steps you can take to maintain good foot health and keep your risk of foot problems as low as possible.

Risk reduction plan

Here are some of the most important steps you can take now to prevent diabetes-related foot complications:

Blood glucose control. The development of peripheral neuropathy is one of the most important predictors of foot ulcers and amputation. Peripheral neuropathy usually manifests itself as numbness, pricking, or tingling in the fingers or toes, and it can spread up the limb and affect muscles and sweat glands as well. Neuropathy can be prevented or delayed significantly by keeping blood glucose levels as near to the normal range as possible. Optimal blood glucose control can also be beneficial in keeping your blood vessels and circulation healthy and helping the body resist, as well as fight off, infections.

The ADA currently recommends keeping blood glucose levels before meals between 90 mg/dl and 130 mg/dl and keeping blood glucose levels one to two hours after meals below 180 mg/dl for most people. (Both of these ranges assume a meter that gives plasma glucose readings.) Your diabetes care team may recommend slightly different blood glucose goals for you based on personal characteristics such as your age and other health conditions you may have. Be sure you know what your personal blood glucose target range is.

Controlling blood fats. High blood levels of low-density lipoprotein (LDL) cholesterol (the so-called bad cholesterol) and the fats called triglycerides can contribute to atherosclerosis (hardening of the arteries) and heart disease. Atherosclerosis is also a contributor to the development of peripheral arterial disease, which itself increases risk for foot complications by interfering with the healing of wounds. Peripheral arterial disease can be symptomless or it can manifest itself in a number of ways including coolness of the fingers or toes, loss of hair on the hands or feet, or intermittent claudication (pain in the legs or buttocks that starts with activity and subsides with rest).

People with diabetes tend to have LDL levels similar to those of people who don't have diabetes, but diabetes often causes decreased levels of high-density lipoprotein (HDL) cholesterol (the so-called good cholesterol) and increased levels of triglycerides. The ADA recommends that people with diabetes achieve LDL levels below 100 mg/dl, triglycerides below 150 mg/dl, and HDL levels above 40 mg/dl (some experts recommend that women aim for HDL levels above 50 mg/dl). Depending on your levels and symptoms, your health-care team may recommend dietary changes, including lowering your intake of saturated and trans fats, exercise, and medicines.

Controlling blood pressure. High blood pressure is a major contributor to heart disease, the leading cause of death for people with diabetes. It also increases risks for peripheral arterial disease and impaired circulation to the feet. The ADA advises people with diabetes to attain blood pressures below 130/80 mm Hg. Dietary changes such as

WHAT CAN I DO TO TAKE CARE OF MY FEET?

■ Wash your feet in warm water every day. Make sure the water is not too hot by testing the temperature with your elbow. Do not soak your feet. Dry your feet well, especially between your toes

■ Look at your feet every day to check for cuts, sores, blisters, redness, calluses, or other problems. Checking every day is even more important if you have nerve damage or poor blood flow. If you cannot bend over or pull your feet up to check them, use a mirror. If you cannot see well, ask someone else to check your feet.

■ If your skin is dry, rub lotion on your feet after you wash and dry them. Do not put lotion between your toes.

■ File corns and calluses gently with an emery board or pumice stone. Do this after your bath or shower.

■ Cut your toenails once a week or when needed. Cut toenails when they are soft from washing. Cut them to the shape of the toe and not too short. File the edges with an emery board.

■ Always wear shoes or slippers to protect your feet from injuries.

■ Always wear socks or stockings to avoid blisters. Do not wear socks or knee-high stockings that are too tight below your knee.

■ Wear shoes that fit well. Shop for shoes at the end of the day when your feet are bigger. Break in shoes slowly. Wear them 1 to 2 hours each day for the first 1 to 2 weeks.

■ Before putting your shoes on, feel the insides to make sure they have no sharp edges or objects that might injure your feet.

This list of tips was developed by the National Diabetes Information Clearinghouse, a service of the National Institute of Diabetes and Digestive and Kidney Diseases. To order publications from the clearinghouse, including the booklet "Prevent Diabetes Problems: Keep Your Feet and Skin Healthy," call (800) 860-8747 or read it online at www.diabetes.niddk.nih.gov.

decreasing the sodium in your diet, exercising, and medicines are all possible treatments for high blood pressure.

Smoking cessation. As mentioned earlier, smoking is related to early development of vascular complications in people with diabetes. If you smoke, therefore, your risk for foot problems increases; lowering your risk, obviously, involves quitting. Several options are available to assist with smoking cessation such as individual or group counseling and use of nicotine products or certain prescription medicines. Your diabetes care team may be able to offer guidance on choosing an option for you.

Daily foot inspection. Take time to inspect your feet every day. Look at the tops and bottoms of your feet as well as between your toes. Rubbing the back of your hand (which is especially sensitive to temperature) along your foot can help you to detect cool spots, which may indicate impaired circulation, or unusually warm areas, which could be signs of inflammation and infection. If you examine your feet every day, you are likely to notice if something has changed. Check with your diabetes care team if you find a change that concerns you or if you notice any of the following in your feet and legs: redness, swelling, or increased warmth; any change in size, odor, or shape; pain, either at rest or when walking; any open sores; sores that do not heal; ingrown toenails; and corns or calluses (especially if there's any skin discoloration). In addition, call your diabetes care team if you experience high blood glucose levels for which you can determine no cause; this may be a sign of infection.

Foot care habits. In addition to inspecting your feet every day, practice the healthy foot care habits listed on page 305. Like your blood glucose control regimen, foot care is a daily process. Don't forget to keep up your foot care even when your routine changes, such as when you're on vacation, a time when you may be tempted to walk barefoot in the sand or by the pool.

Evaluating footwear. Shoes or slippers should always be worn to protect your feet; however, many foot ulcers start with rubbing from ill-fitting shoes, so it's important that your shoes fit well and don't cause any abnormal pressure on your feet. It may be helpful to have your feet measured every time you buy shoes because feet change in size and shape over time. It's also better to be fitted for shoes in the afternoon or evening rather than first thing in the morning; walking around all day causes your feet to spread, so getting fitted when your feet are at their largest can help you to ensure a comfortable fit.

Properly fitted shoes should fit both the width and length of your feet, allow room for the free movement of your toes, and be well-cushioned. High-heeled footwear or shoes with pointed toes can constrict or place undue pressure on parts of the foot, so they should be avoided. Sandals with straps between the toes can cause irritation or injury. Walking or athletic shoes, which offer padding and support, can be good choices, but people with diabetes who have complications that affect their feet may need special assistance selecting shoes or may need custom-made shoes.

If you have any lack of sensation in your feet (because of neuropathy, for example), it may be difficult to judge how well your shoes fit or sense whether any areas of your feet are being rubbed or irritated by shoe (or even sock) seams. You may want to seek the help of a certified pedorthist in selecting shoes. (See "For More Information" on page 308 for help in locating a certified pedorthist.)

Some people with lack of sensation in the feet, other changes in the feet caused by diabetes, or a history of foot ulcers may be candidates for orthotics, or specially designed insoles that are worn inside the shoes. Such insoles can be customized and modified to help control the way your foot moves or support the foot to avoid pain and pressure in a certain area. Some special shoes have extra depth to accommodate the placement of inserts. If orthotics don't do the trick, it may be necessary to get custom-made shoes. Many health insurance plans, including Medicare Part B, offer some coverage for orthotics or custom-made shoes. To qualify for depth-inlay shoes, custom-molded shoes, or shoe inserts under Medicare Part B, your physician must certify that you have diabetes and are being treated, that you need the insert or shoe because you have diabetes, and that you have a condition such as an amputation, foot ulcers, calluses, poor circulation, or foot deformity.

Socks should always be worn with shoes to prevent blisters. People with diabetes should wear socks that fit well (tight socks impair circulation) and are seamless (to prevent blisters). Socks should be made of breathable material such as cotton or wool, ideally blended with a material that draws moisture away from the skin, such as acrylic. (The nylon in stockings or pantyhose is not a breathable fabric, so these should be worn as little as possible.)

Diabetes and foot problems

Even common foot problems such as small cuts, calluses, or ingrown toenails can open the door to serious problems in a person with diabetes, particularly if his blood glucose is not in control. Because such problems can lead to infections and even foot ulcers, don't ignore even seemingly minor wounds, and don't hesitate to seek the advice of your health-care provider if a wound doesn't heal promptly.

Dryness. If not resolved, dry skin can crack, allowing germs to get under the skin, which can lead to infection.

Fungal infections. Athlete's foot and other fungal infections are more common in people with diabetes. Athlete's foot can cause cracking of the skin that can allow germs to enter the body.

Calluses. Calluses usually occur as the result of pressure or rubbing in an area of the foot. If not treated, they can sometimes lead to ulceration of the skin tissue underneath. Never try to trim a corn or callus with a razor or knife. Over-the-counter chemical callus removers should also be avoided. See your doctor or podiatrist if you have trouble with thick calluses.

Bone deformity. Diabetes increases the risk of problems such as hammertoe (sometimes called mallet toe or claw toe), which is a change in the position of the toe, causing it to appear curved. Hammertoes increase the likelihood for callus or corn formation due to pressure on the deformed toe. A bunion is a deformity that occurs in the joint of the big toe. The toe is turned inward, causing the joint to protrude outward. A bunion can contribute to pain in the foot, as well as poor fit of shoes, again contributing to abnormal pressures. Charcot foot is a severe deformity in which the arch and normal foot structure break down. Usually, Charcot foot is caused by severe neuropathy. Prompt evaluation and treatment are necessary.

Seeing a specialist

If your feet need special attention, your physician may refer you to one of the following types of specialist:

Neurologist. Neurologists are doctors (M.D. or D.O.) that treat diseases of the nervous system. Tight control of your blood glucose is the best way to prevent or slow the progression of neuropathy, but a neurologist can also help if neuropathy is causing you pain or if you're experiencing muscle weakness. Neurologists are also able to detect early signs of neuropathy.

Orthopedist. Orthopedists (also M.D. or D.O.) are concerned with the diagnosis, care, and treatment of musculoskeletal disorders. The orthopedist's scope of practice includes disorders of the body's bones, joints, ligaments, muscles, and tendons. Orthopedists treat problems such as bunions and hammertoes.

Pedorthist. A certified pedorthist (C.Ped.) has training and certification to design, manufacture, modify, and fit footwear to alleviate lower limb

HOW CAN I GET MY DOCTOR TO HELP ME TAKE CARE OF MY FEET?

■ Tell your doctor right away about any foot problems.

■ Ask your doctor to look at your feet at each diabetes checkup. To make sure your doctor checks your feet, take off your shoes and socks before your doctor comes into the room.

■ Ask your doctor to check how well the nerves in your feet sense feeling.

■ Ask your doctor to check how well blood is flowing to your legs and feet.

■ Ask your doctor to show you the best way to trim your toenails. Ask what lotion or cream to use on your legs and feet.

■ If you cannot cut your toenails or you have a foot problem, ask your doctor to send you to a foot doctor. A doctor who cares for feet is called a podiatrist.

This list of tips was developed by the National Diabetes Information Clearinghouse, a service of the National Institute of Diabetes and Digestive and Kidney Diseases. To order publications from the clearinghouse, including the booklet "Prevent Diabetes Problems: Keep Your Feet and Skin Healthy," call (800) 860-8747 or read it online at www.diabetes.niddk.nih.gov.

problems. A pedorthist is not a doctor, but some podiatrists are also certified as pedorthists.

Physical therapist. Physical therapists (P.T.) are health professionals who treat movement disorders. They often help people recover from a stroke or injury and also teach people how to avoid injuries. Physical therapists can help people with leg casts (to help ulcers heal), an amputation, neuropathy, or foot deformities to improve their mobility.

Podiatrist. Doctors of podiatric medicine (D.P.M.) are physicians and surgeons who practice on the lower extremities, primarily the feet and ankles. They treat problems from calluses and nail fungus to tumors, fractures, and deformities. They can fit orthotic inserts and design custom-made shoes.

Vascular surgeon. Vascular surgeons (M.D. or D.O.) specialize in treating diseases of the blood vessels. If you develop peripheral arterial disease

FOR MORE INFORMATION

Taking care of your feet requires learning about and addressing risk factors before they become problems. These resources can help you to take better care of your feet.

AMERICAN LUNG ASSOCIATION
www.lungusa.org
(800) LUNG-USA (586-4872)
The Web site of the American Lung Association. Click on "Quit Smoking" for information on quitting smoking, legislation against smoking, and smoking and pregnancy.

AMERICAN PHYSICAL THERAPY ASSOCIATION
www.apta.org
(800) 999-APTA (2782)
TDD: (703) 683-6748
Click on "For Consumers" to learn more about physical therapy, find physical therapists in your area, read information on a variety of conditions that can be helped by therapy, and how physical therapy works with your insurance.

AMERICAN PODIATRIC MEDICINE ASSOCIATION
www.apma.org
(800) FOOTCARE (366-8227)
The APMA's Web site can help you to find a podiatrist in your area and to learn more about ulcers and how diabetes affects the feet.

THE AMERICAN BOARD FOR CERTIFICATION IN ORTHOTICS, PROSTHETICS & PEDOTHOTICS
www.cpeds.org
(703) 836-7114
Use this Web site to locate a certified pedorthist in your area. Information for consumers was not yet available on the site when this article was written.

FEET CAN LAST A LIFETIME
http://ndep.nih.gov/resources/feet
Primarily aimed at health-care professionals, this booklet is also available offline by calling the National Diabetes Information Clearinghouse at (800) 860-8747. Also available from this site or through their ordering number, (800) 438-5383, is "Take Care of Your Feet for a Lifetime," a sheet of foot-care tips for people with diabetes.

LEGS FOR LIFE
www.legsforlife.org
Started by the Society of Interventional Radiology and now backed by a number of organizations, Legs for Life is a national program that provides free screenings for peripheral vascular disease. Visit the Web site to find a participating site or an interventional radiologist near you.

LOWER EXTREMITY AMPUTATION PREVENTION PROGRAM
www.hrsa.gov/leap
The LEAP program works to reduce the number of lower extremity amputations in people with diabetes. Visit the Web site or call to order your own free, reusable LEAP filament and instructional brochure to check your own feet for loss of sensation.

SMOKEFREE.GOV
www.smokefree.gov
(877) 44U-QUIT (448-7848)
TTY: (800) 332-8615
Created by a branch of the National Cancer Institute, this guide to quitting smoking offers brochures, a step-by-step quit guide, telephone numbers for local and state quitlines, and even an instant messaging service so you can chat with a staff member online.

---

that affects your feet, a vascular surgeon can perform an angioplasty, place a stent (a device that is placed in a blood vessel to keep it open after an angioplasty has widened it), or perform a bypass operation to improve blood flow to your feet.

The nature of your foot problems will determine which specialist's expertise may be necessary. In addition to these, there may be a time when another specialist's assistance is needed.

An ounce of prevention

When it comes to diabetes and foot-care management, an ounce of prevention is worth a pound of cure. Daily attention to your feet, visiting your diabetes care team as recommended, efforts toward reducing your risks for foot problems, and proper treatment when necessary, are all important parts in getting your feet to last your entire lifetime. □

WOUND HEALING FOR FOOT ULCERS

by Jeffrey A. Stone, D.O., M.P.H., and Leon R. Brill, D.P.M.

There are approximately 20 million people with diabetes in the United States, and an estimated 15% of them will develop an ulcer of the foot or leg at some point in their lives. Diabetic complications, including nerve damage in the extremities (called peripheral neuropathy), development of structural deformities in the foot, reduced immune function, and diminished blood flow in the extremities (called peripheral vascular disease), increase the risk of developing a lower-extremity ulcer. Men are more likely than women to develop an ulcer, and the risk for people of both sexes increases with age. Despite the gloomy statistics, though, there are things you can do to reduce your risk of ulcers and their complications, which include amputation.

Impact of diabetic ulcers

Although most diabetic ulcers heal when treated with a comprehensive wound management program, some develop into chronic, nonhealing ulcers. Inadequate treatment of chronic ulcers can lead to the development of infections and *gangrene* (tissue death), and many people with such severe complications ultimately undergo amputation of the affected limb. The risk of lower-extremity amputation in people who have diabetes is 15 times higher than that of people who do not have diabetes, and the risk increases with age: It is seven times greater in people over 65 than in people under 45.

Approximately 86,000 amputations are performed in people with diabetes annually (85% are preceded by an ulcer), accounting for more than half of the total number of surgically performed lower-extremity amputations in the United States each year. The risks of amputation of the other leg or foot or further amputation of the same limb are increased in individuals with diabetes who have undergone an amputation.

Lower-extremity problems due to diabetes have significant effects on health-care resources. More in-hospital days are spent treating diabetes-related foot infections than any other complication of the disease. The costs of treating nonhealing lower-extremity diabetic ulcers are substantial—possibly more than $5–6 billion annually in the United States, a total that includes treatment, hospital stays, decreased productivity because of related illness, disability, and premature death.

With proper care, however, many lower-extremity diabetic ulcers can be prevented, thereby potentially reducing the number of amputations. One objective of the U.S. Department of Health's Healthy People 2010 program is to reduce the rate of amputation in individuals with diabetes by 55% by the year 2010. To meet this objective, health-care professionals and people with diabetes must work together. People with diabetes can do their part by learning about proper foot care and about the complications associated with lower-extremity diabetic ulcers so that they know to seek prompt medical care when complications of the legs or feet occur. A delay in the treatment of ulcers is a major factor leading to amputation.

How and why ulcers form

The combination of peripheral neuropathy, peripheral vascular disease, and mechanical abnormality is the major contributing factor to the formation of diabetic foot ulcers. Although peripheral neuropathy or peripheral vascular disease alone increases the risk for an ulcer, their combination with structural abnormalities in the foot is what ultimately leads to increased pressure and stress on the tissues of the foot. Over time, this increased pressure can cause tissue breakdown and ultimately ulceration.

Peripheral neuropathy. Peripheral neuropathy may affect up to 60% of people with diabetes. Approximately 20% of people with diabetes develop neuropathy within 10 years of diagnosis, and up to 50% develop neuropathy within 25 years. The cause of neuropathy is poorly understood and is most likely the result of a number of diabetic metabolic changes.

Peripheral neuropathy is characterized by numbness in the feet, legs, hands, and arms; feelings of burning or tingling, and weakness in the extremities. It may cause muscle wasting in the feet, leading to loss of the stabilizing force of the toes and resulting in *contractures,* or deformities such as hammertoes.

Another type of neuropathy, called autonomic

neuropathy (damage to the nerves that regulate involuntary body functions), can cause changes such as the loss of blood vessel tone and loss of the sweating mechanism. These changes can contribute to the vulnerability of the foot to injury and ensuing ulceration and infection.

Peripheral vascular disease. Peripheral vascular disease has been estimated to be 20 times more prevalent in people with diabetes than in those who don't have diabetes. People with peripheral vascular disease are almost nine times more likely to have a foot amputation than those who do not have it. Peripheral vascular disease also has a major role in delayed wound healing and the development of gangrene.

The classic signs and symptoms of peripheral vascular disease include *intermittent claudication* (pain in the calves that occurs when walking but stops at rest) and *rest pain* (pain in the foot that occurs even when not walking). Others include loss of hair on the lower legs and feet, skin that appears tight and shiny, and wasting of the small muscles of the foot. Some of these signs and symptoms are similar to those of neuropathy.

Diagnosing peripheral vascular disease remains an inexact art. One way to assess circulation in the legs and feet is to determine the ankle–brachial index, the ratio of the systolic blood pressure in the ankle to that in the arm. An ankle–brachial index of 1 or 1.1 is considered normal; an ankle–brachial index below about 0.45 is a sign of severe narrowing of the blood vessels in the leg. However, in people with diabetes, the ankle–brachial index may be misleading, because hardened arteries, a condition that is common in diabetes, can give rise to an artificially high result.

Measuring transcutaneous oxygen pressure ($TcpO_2$), which is the pressure of oxygen at the skin, is also useful in determining the existence of *ischemia* (reduced blood flow to an area). Oxygenation is an important factor in wound healing. The $TcpO_2$ measurement gives an indication of the amount of oxygen being delivered to the skin by the blood. However, room temperature and the test administrator's technique can affect results.

A third examination technique, Doppler waveform analysis, which measures the velocity of blood, may give a more accurate picture of the blood supply to an area when done in addition to the ankle–brachial index and $TcpO_2$.

If the physician has any doubt about the presence and level of ischemia, the gold standard of *angiography* (x-rays of blood vessels taken after the injection of a dye, or contrast material) is often used. However, this test is not without risks. The contrast material used in angiography can cause allergic reactions and kidney damage.

Mechanical alterations of the foot. Muscle wasting and loss of muscle function due to neuropathy often leads to development of foot deformities. In fact, foot deformities are found in 50% of individuals with diabetes. One common deformity, ham-

HAMMERTOE

A hammertoe is a deformity of the foot in which a toe buckles, placing increased pressure on the ball of the foot, the tip of the toe, and the top of the toe, and raising the risk of ulceration in these areas.

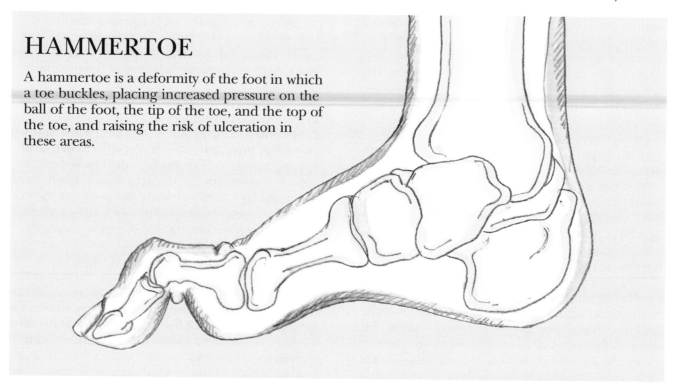

mertoe, results in increased pressure on the ball of the foot, raising the risk of ulceration in that area.

Another complication of diabetes, limited joint mobility, is thought to be a significant contributing factor to the heightened pressures on the foot and the development of ulcers. Limited joint mobility is thought to develop from the attachment of glucose molecules to proteins in the skin, soft tissue, and joints. However, limitation of joint motion alone does not appear to cause ulceration; rather, limited joint mobility combined with neuropathy increases the risk for ulceration.

How a wound heals

The body's normal wound-healing response consists of three distinct, yet overlapping, phases: inflammation, proliferation, and remodeling. The wound-healing process may continue for many months before healing occurs, particularly when the process is impaired by infection or disease.

Inflammation. When the body sustains an injury, nearby blood vessels release fluid into the wound to clear debris and dilute any potentially harmful substances. Blood particles called platelets gather at the site to start a clot and stop blood loss. Platelets also secrete several growth factors—including platelet-derived growth factor, epidermal growth factor, and transforming growth factor-beta—that have an important role in initiating the wound-healing response.

Following the formation of a blood clot, inflammatory white blood cells are rapidly recruited to the wound site. Among the first white blood cells on the scene, *neutrophils* function primarily to protect against bacterial infection. Other white blood cells, called *macrophages,* remove dead or damaged tissue, ingest bacteria, and serve as an important source of growth factors that sustain the wound-healing response.

Proliferation. Growth factors produced by macrophages and neutrophils attract *fibroblasts* (cells that generate the collagen fibers that make up part of the *extracellular matrix,* the substance in which cells are embedded) to the site of injury and stimulate their proliferation. At this point, the density of cells in the wound increases and the proliferative phase, which usually lasts several weeks, begins.

Once the number of inflammatory cells and macrophages at the wound site begins to decrease, other cells, including fibroblasts, *endothelial* cells (the cells lining the insides of blood vessels), and *keratinocytes* (the cells that produce skin), begin to produce growth factors that stimulate cellular proliferation, synthesis of extracellular matrix pro-

teins, and the formation of new blood vessels.

Remodeling. When cellular proliferation and the growth of new blood vessels decreases and the initial scar forms, the wound enters the remodeling phase, which can last up to two years. During this phase, a balance is reached between the production of extracellular matrix and its degradation by some of the body's natural enzymes. Growth factors also have important functions in the remodeling stage.

Determining the roles of growth factors in the wound-healing process has led researchers to speculate about their potential therapeutic use in chronic, nonhealing wounds, such as diabetic ulcers, pressure ulcers, and venous ulcers. With recent advances in molecular biology and protein chemistry, it is now possible through recombinant DNA technology to produce copious amounts of purified growth factors that can be applied topically to wounds. Results of animal studies suggest that topically applied growth factors, rhPDGF-BB (sold as becaplermin, brand name Regranex) and TGF-beta in particular, are able to promote or enhance wound healing. Several clinical trials of recombinant growth factors have been conducted. Most of these studies have examined the usefulness of becaplermin in healing diabetic and pressure ulcers.

Managing diabetic ulcers

Comprehensive wound management involves wound assessment, rigorous wound care, and follow-up and education. Thorough assessment of ulcers involves determination of cause, location, size, depth or stage of development, presence of *exudate* (liquid leaking from the wound), presence of dead tissue, presence of infection, and blood flow to the area.

The most important therapeutic interventions in treating nonhealing wounds are adequate *debridement* (removal of dead tissue from a wound), control of infection, off-loading of pressure, and appropriate topical management. The recent approval of becaplermin for treating diabetic foot ulcers has provided an important addition to the wound-healing armamentarium.

Debridement. Ulcers must be clean and free of infection and dead tissue to heal. Wound healing is impaired when any of the following is present: *eschar* (sloughed-off dead tissue), pus, infection, or large areas of dead tissue. To promote wound healing, these areas of devitalized or otherwise compromised tissue must first be removed by debridement, preferably sharp (surgical) debridement, provided the person can tolerate the procedure. Ulcers in a person with neuropathy can often be debrided

FOOT CARE GUIDELINES

When it comes to foot care, prevention and early detection are the names of the game.
These tips will help you to sidestep infections, cuts, and other breaks in the skin and to
notice any problems that do develop early, so you can get prompt treatment.

WHAT TO DO	WHY TO DO IT
Keep your blood sugar in your target range as much of the time as possible.	To prevent infection, speed healing, and prevent further damage to blood vessels and nerves.
Do not smoke.	Carbon monoxide and nicotine impair blood circulation.
Every day, wash your feet with mild soap and warm water; dry carefully. Pay special attention to the areas between toes and around nail beds.	To prevent fungal infections (such as athlete's foot) and other infections.
Inspect your feet carefully every day. Use a mirror if necessary.	To detect any problems such as cuts, blisters, red spots, or swelling early.
Cut toenails straight across (or following the natural curve of the toe) and not too short. A 1/16-inch to 1/8-inch rim of white nail beyond the pink nail bed should be clearly visible all the way across the top of the toenail. Have a podiatrist trim your nails if you cannot trim them yourself.	To avoid ingrown toenails and to avoid cutting your toes.
Be more active. Wiggle your toes and rotate your ankles for a few minutes several times a day.	To promote blood flow to your feet.
Never walk anywhere, even indoors, in bare feet or with socks only, especially if your feet are numb.	To protect feet from being injured by small or sharp objects and to prevent toes from being stubbed.
Take off your shoes at every doctor's visit.	Your doctor or nurse should check your feet.
Don't cross your legs when you sit.	To maintain good circulation.

aggressively and promptly without anesthesia because of the person's inability to feel pain in the area. When a person has feeling in the area, appropriate pain management steps can be used.

Debridement can be performed in one of four ways or in a combination of these four. Surgical debridement is the most efficient and selective method of removing devitalized tissue and is considered the method of choice by many clinicians. Enzymatic debridement is the use of enzymes to degrade dead tissue. Enzymatic agents are often used on people for whom sharp debridement is not a good option, but they have a very limited use in the treatment of lower-extremity diabetic ulcers. Autolytic debridement involves allowing the body's natural processes to remove dead tissue, a process physicians can help along by using

moist wound dressings. Mechanical debridement involves applying wound-adhering dressings to remove dead tissue. A drawback to this method is that such dressings may remove some healthy tissue along with the dead tissue.

Control of infection. Deep, lower-extremity diabetic ulcers are associated with an increased risk of bacterial infection. Infections interfere with the wound-healing process and may result in local *abscesses* (pockets of pus), *septicemia* (systemic bacterial infection), *cellulitis* (inflammation of connective tissue), and *osteomyelitis* (inflammation of bone and marrow cavity caused by infection).

Systemic antimicrobial treatment is called for when cellulitis, septicemia, or osteomyelitis is present. A physician can choose a specific therapy based on deep-tissue cultures of bacteria taken

WHAT TO DO	WHY TO DO IT
Do not soak your feet unless your health-care provider has prescribed this for a particular reason.	Soaking removes natural oils, causing feet to dry and crack. In addition, skin is soft and easily injured immediately following soaking.
If skin on feet is dry, apply lotion to the tops and bottoms.	To prevent skin from cracking.
Do not apply lotion between the toes. (You may apply powder between the toes if desired.)	To prevent fungal infections by keeping the area dry.
Never use commercial corn or callus removers or strong chemical antiseptics. Never perform "home surgery" with sharp cutting tools, and don't use hot water bottles or heating pads on feet.	To prevent burns, cuts, and skin erosion.
Shop for shoes late in the day, when your feet are most swollen, and make sure they fit well.	To avoid injuries when "breaking in" shoes and prevent chronic rubbing from ill-fitting shoes.
Check the insides of shoes daily before putting them on. Use your hand to check for cracks, irregularities, and loose objects.	Any object or rough edge in your shoe can cause blisters or breaks in the skin.
Wear socks that keep your feet dry. Avoid knee-high stockings or socks with tight elastic. Change socks often if your feet perspire heavily.	Wet feet are a breeding ground for bacteria. Tight socks constrict circulation.
Contact your doctor, nurse, or podiatrist immediately when you discover a problem.	Most foot problems are much easier to treat when they are attended to promptly.

from the wound, the blood, or a bone biopsy.

Topical disinfectants, such as povidone-iodine, acetic acid, hydrogen peroxide, and sodium hypochlorite, are toxic to fibroblasts and may actually impair wound healing.

Off-loading of pressure. Removing pressure and stress from the injured limb (called "off-loading") is as important as debridement and infection control. Without adequate off-loading, any progress that has been made in the treatment of the wounded foot will be halted or reversed.

There are many devices to off-load affected limbs, ranging from wheelchairs, crutches, and walkers to total-contact casts, total-contact sandals, short leg walkers, and Darco wedge shoes. Therapeutic footwear such as running shoes, extra-depth shoes, and custom-molded shoes should be reserved for a foot that has healed. Total contact casts are useful for off-loading the forefoot but less useful for off-loading the heel. They require specialized techniques in casting and leave little room for error. Any movement of the foot within the cast may produce new wounds.

Hyperbaric oxygen therapy. At normal atmospheric pressure, much of the oxygen in the blood is carried by hemoglobin, with a minimal amount of additional oxygen dissolved in plasma. Administration of high concentrations of oxygen at greater than atmospheric pressure (referred to as hyperbaric oxygen therapy) increases the amount of dissolved oxygen carried in the bloodstream by approximately 500%. Hyperbaric oxygen is used as an adjunctive therapy for wounds that are difficult to heal, such as diabetic foot ulcers.

Hyperbaric oxygen therapy enhances wound healing by increasing delivery of oxygen to the site of the wound. Studies suggest that hyperbaric oxygen therapy stimulates the growth of new blood vessels, although the precise mechanism has yet to be elucidated. In a 33-month study of 501 people with diabetes who had ischemic wounds, 119 received hyperbaric oxygen therapy and 382 were given standard, conservative treatment alone. In general, those people placed on hyperbaric oxygen therapy had larger and more wounds than those treated with standard care. However, more people in the hyperbaric oxygen group (72%) regained use of the affected limb(s) than those in the standard treatment group (53%).

The particulars of treatment with hyperbaric oxygen depend on the severity of the wound. In the absence of infection, for example, once-daily treatment with hyperbaric oxygen for 90 to 120 minutes is sufficient for stimulation of wound healing. Although treatment sessions are brief, tissue oxygen levels can remain elevated for several hours after treatment.

Wound dressings. Dressings for wounds are designed either to allow moisture to escape or to retain moisture (occlusive dressings). For diabetic ulcers, nonocclusive saline-gauze dressings are often placed directly in the wound. Before the gauze is removed, it is rewetted with a salt solution to facilitate removal and to avoid damage to healthy tissue. This type of dressing is inexpensive, easy to apply, and may aid in wound debridement by facilitating the removal of residual bits of dead tissue. A disadvantage of using saline dressings is that they may require more frequent changing than other dressings.

Follow-up examinations. Regular follow-up examinations for people with lower-extremity diabetic ulcers are an important component of treatment. An individual with a lower-extremity ulcer that is resistant to treatment or that will take a long time to close because it is large requires follow-up care. Complications following debridement or infection can include reinfection, further deterioration of the ulcer, or development of new ulcers. Even people whose ulcers heal must be reevaluated at regular intervals because approximately 30% of ulcers recur.

Follow-up care should also involve nutrition counseling with a registered dietitian to design a diet that will encourage wound healing and also aid in blood glucose control. Diets high in protein have been shown to aid in healing; protein is necessary for the body to produce the collagen of the extracellular matrix. For blood glucose control,

controlling the total amount of carbohydrate eaten per day and spreading carbohydrate consumption evenly across the day are often useful.

Since decreased blood flow to the extremities often contributes to the development of ulcers, follow-up care may include seeing a vascular surgeon, who can evaluate blood flow to (and oxygenation of) the feet. If there are blockages in the arteries leading to the feet, some sort of vascular surgery may be in order to improve it.

Smoking is a major contributor to peripheral vascular disease, so those who smoke should quit. If you smoke, speak with your physician about your desire to quit. He may recommend using a prescription pharmaceutical aid such as a nicotine inhaler or the drug bupropion (brand names Zyban and Wellbutrin), or may be able to recommend a "quit smoking" program. Because smoking also affects your blood glucose control, quitting may result in lowered insulin or diabetes medicine needs as well as improved vascular health.

When feasible, walking or other forms of physical activity are encouraged for those who have had diabetic ulcers. However, it's important to talk to your physician about which forms of exercise will be safe for you to perform, to wear well-fitting athletic or walking shoes when exercising, and to inspect your feet regularly for areas of pressure or irritation.

A person who has had a diabetic ulcer should monitor his blood glucose level regularly and take steps to keep it as close to normal as possible. Frequent or chronic high blood glucose has been linked to an increased risk of infection. The rate of infection decreases when blood glucose levels are better controlled.

Ulcer prevention

Keeping your blood sugar level in control and inspecting your feet every day are important steps that can reduce your risk of lower-limb ulceration and amputation. In addition, your health-care provider should examine your feet regularly for the presence of neuropathy, vascular problems, and deformities or changes in the shape of the foot.

The simplest and least expensive test for sensory neuropathy is Semmes–Weinstein aesthesiometry, in which a monofilament is touched to parts of the foot and the person reports whether he can feel it. If neuropathy is suspected, the diagnosis should be confirmed with objective tests using heat and vibration. Signs of wasting, weakness, or absent tendon reflexes are indicative of motor neuropathy. Reduced sweating, changes in skin texture, and distended foot veins suggest the presence of autonomic neuropathy. These findings may be confirmed with electrophysiologic tests (for motor neuropathy) or a quantitative sweat test and noninvasive Doppler (for autonomic neuropathy) if necessary.

Assessing foot pulses and noting skin temperature and pallor may provide an indication of the vascular status of the affected limb, although more precise tests, such as Doppler stethoscope, may be necessary to thoroughly assess vascular function.

Deformities of the toes, such as bunions, or Charcot foot, in which several bones and joints of the foot are affected, often contribute to abnormal stress patterns in the foot. It may be necessary to confirm structural abnormalities with x-rays.

If a lower-extremity diabetic ulcer does occur, it is best managed by a multidisciplinary team that includes nursing, medical, surgical, and rehabilitative services. The person with the ulcer and his family members are important team members, too. Communication among all team members is essential. To avoid amputation, work with your team, ask questions, and make sure you understand how you can best help promote the healing process. □

FOOT CARE
DRUGSTORE DO'S AND DON'T'S

by J. C. Tanenbaum, D.P.M.

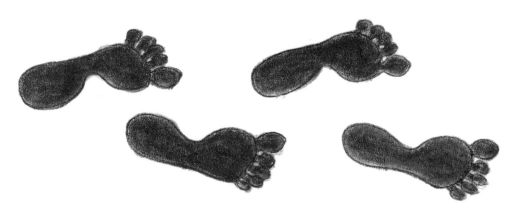

Even with diabetes, your feet can last a lifetime, and they stand a better chance of doing so if you treat them with tender, loving care. That includes giving them a daily inspection for cuts and abrasions as well as asking your doctor to examine them periodically for any signs of nerve damage, such as loss of sensation, or reduced blood flow, such as coldness or hair loss on the feet and legs.

The tools or products you use on your feet at home can have profound effects on their health, particularly if you have any degree of nerve damage or reduced blood flow in your feet. Using the right products can help to keep your skin—and feet—intact, while using the wrong ones can lead to breaks in the skin, which can allow bacteria to enter and, in the worst-case scenario, lead to foot ulcers.

Here, then, is your guide to over-the-counter foot products, including some that are safe to use and some to avoid.

Soap

Washing your feet with warm or tepid water and soap every day keeps them clean and gives you a good chance to do that daily inspection. (If it's hard to see your feet, run your fingers over them to feel for calluses or sore spots. The backs of your hands are sensitive to heat and can be run over your feet to find hot spots, which can indicate infection.)

There must be at least 50 varieties of soap on the shelves of most drugstores—liquid soaps, solid bar soaps, scented soaps, unscented soaps, etc. Which to choose? In general, bar soaps are a better choice than liquid soaps, and soaps that have moisturizing lotion in them are the best choice of all. The compound in soap that gives it its lather is a fatty acid called lanolin, and the more lather, the softer the soap. In most cases, bar soaps have more lather than liquid. The moisturizer is important because dry skin can lead to cracking and the entry of bacteria into the skin. It is much safer to be moist than dry.

If a soap feels gritty or granular, don't use it; you never want to use an abrasive on your feet. Perfumed soaps may cause skin reactions in some people, resulting in redness and swelling, so for these people, unscented soaps are best.

Moisturizing lotion

Applying a moisturizing lotion to your feet once or twice a day can also help keep your skin healthy and moist. In general, thick lotions do a better job of moisturizing than thin, "watery" lotions, but it's important not to overdo it with moisturizer. Skin that is too soft and moist can break down or become a breeding ground for infections. Putting lotion between your toes is generally discouraged, since the skin between toes tends to stay moist naturally; adding lotion there would overmoisturize that area.

Callus, corn, and wart removers

Even with the best foot care, it would be hard to go through life without developing a callus or corn on your feet. Both calluses and corns are thickened areas of skin that result from pressure and friction on a part of the foot. Ill-fitting shoes are a common cause of calluses and corns. To a certain degree, calluses and corns protect the foot; without that layer of thickened skin, pressure or friction might cause an open wound. But very thick calluses and corns can press into the foot, causing pain. And in a person with diabetes, a callus or corn can actually be a thin layer of hard skin covering a much deeper wound or ulceration.

With that in mind, it seems like a good idea to remove calluses and corns, but the drugstore is not the place to start. The active ingredient in over-the-counter corn and callus removers— whether packaged as a liquid or a medicated pad—is acid, and acid can eat away live skin as well as dead. If your skin tends to heal slowly, even one application of these products can lead to the creation of a wound that can take months or even years to heal. If you have troublesome calluses or corns on your feet, see your podiatrist for advice and treatment. Never use an acid product on any part of your feet.

Even acid-free callus and corn home treatments are not recommended for people who have diabetes. Pumice stones and files are not sterile and

can cause breaks in the skin if you rub too vigorously or remove too much skin. And whatever you do, don't take a sharp blade to your feet. It's just too easy to slip and cut yourself.

What if you develop a wart on your foot? Warts are caused by viruses that enter the skin directly. Warts that grow on the bottoms of the feet are often called plantar warts. Plantar warts may occur one at a time, or there can be hundreds of small warts on a person's foot. Many times, warts resemble calluses, but they can often be distinguished by small black dots in the body of the wart. While most warts will eventually go away with no treatment, a wart on the bottom of your foot can make walking painful, so you may be eager to remove it. Just like callus and corn removers, however, over-the-counter wart removers contain acids and are not recommended for use by people with diabetes. Instead, ask your podiatrist about other options for getting rid of a plantar wart.

Wound care

The drugstore is a good place to pick up two first-aid essentials: antibiotic ointment and adhesive bandages (such as Band-Aids). To treat a minor wound, first wash your hands with soap and water, then cleanse the wound with soap and water, rinse thoroughly, pat dry, and apply a thin layer of antibiotic ointment with a cotton swab (such as a Q-tips cotton swab) and an adhesive bandage. If you see no appreciable improvement within 24 hours, consult your doctor or podiatrist immediately. Even if a wound appears to be closing up, if you see signs of infection, such as redness, swelling, or pus, see your doctor or podiatrist.

As long as you are not allergic to latex, either fabric or plastic bandages will do. If your skin is very fragile, however, your doctor may advise you to use a gauze pad and paper tape in place of adhesive bandages or to cover wounds with a gauze bandage, taping the gauze to itself, rather than to your skin.

It is not necessary to buy any particular brand of antibiotic ointment; most have the same active components. However, when applying antibiotic ointment, it's much better to use a cotton swab than your fingers. Using your fingers can contaminate both the wound and the tube of antibiotic ointment.

Toenail care

For many people, the regular toenail trimmers or clippers sold at the drugstore are safe for home use. Toenails should be cut straight across or following the natural curve of the toe. Gently smoothing the toenails with an emery board after clipping can keep them from snagging on socks. When clipping or using an emery board on your toenails, never "dig" into the sides of your nails. Doing so can break the skin, opening the door to fungal or bacterial infections. Improper clipping can also lead to ingrown toenails, which can also become infected and painful.

If you cannot see or reach your toenails easily, if your nails are hard to cut because they're thick or you have a fungal nail infection, if the sides of your toenails curve into your skin, if you frequently have trouble clipping your toenails, or if you have reduced sensation or circulation in your feet, it may be a good idea to have your toenails cut regularly by a podiatrist. Toenail trimming every two or three months is usually recommended. In many instances, proper professional foot care can prevent problems from ever happening.

If you want a pedicure, buy your own inexpensive nail instrument set and bring it with you to your pedicurist. Make sure the technician knows never to cut your skin. For infection control, make sure the facility washes the basins that your feet may be placed in.

It's only logical that drugstores would stock ingrown toenail remover products next to the toenail clippers, but are they an option for people who have diabetes? No, they are not. Just like callus, corn, and wart removers, they contain acids, which work by eating away the skin, in this case on the sides of the toenail. Eroding the skin allows bacteria to penetrate, which can lead to an infection.

No matter how clean a person is, all toenails have bacteria and fungus growing on them. When an ingrown toenail digs into the skin, it pushes this bacteria into the deeper tissues of the affected toe. If the body cannot fight off the bacteria, it multiplies, and an infection results. Putting an acid on skin that is already broken simply makes the opening for bacteria larger.

If you have an ingrown toenail, see your podiatrist for treatment. If you see your toenail looking red or swollen, or you see drainage, blood, or pus on your toe, consult your podiatrist immediately. This is an emergency.

You can help to prevent ingrown toenails by learning to trim your toenails properly, wearing shoes with a wide enough toe box, and wearing socks that are not too tight.

Antiseptics

If you have had a wound or ingrown toenail treated by a podiatrist, he may recommend that you soak your foot or feet in a solution of Betadine (or generic povidine iodine) while the wound is healing. This widely used antiseptic helps prevent against infection with bacteria, fungi, and viruses. Use two capfuls of Betadine solution in a big basin of lukewarm water (never use it straight from the bottle). Soak your feet for a maximum of 20 minutes, then dry them well.

Anyone who is allergic to iodine should use Epsom salts in place of Betadine. When a foot soak is necessary, dissolve two tablespoons of Epsom salts in a big basin of lukewarm water, soak for no more than 20 minutes, and dry your feet well afterward. Soaking in Epsom salts is also a good way to reduce inflammation and pain.

Because foot soaks can dry your skin, do not routinely soak your feet every night. And do not use alcohol or hydrogen peroxide as antiseptics on your feet; they will also dry your skin.

Capsaicin products

A potentially useful drugstore purchase for people with diabetic neuropathy in their feet is capsaicin cream or ointment, which is sold under the brand names ArthriCare, Capzasin, Zostrix, and others. This topical medicine made from hot peppers can sometimes reduce pain associated with diabetic neuropathy if used regularly over the course of several weeks. It can also relieve arthritis pain in some cases.

When you first begin using capsaicin, it's normal to experience a warm, stinging, or burning sensation where you've applied it. This feeling should diminish with continued use. Capsaicin can also cause stinging and burning if it gets in your eyes or mucous membranes (such as your nose or mouth), so be sure to wash your hands thoroughly after applying it to your feet.

Athlete's foot products

Athlete's foot is a fungal infection that usually causes itching, cracking, and redness between the toes or on the bottoms of the feet. It's important to take care of it right away because any breaks in the skin can allow bacteria to enter and cause an infection. The good news is that as a rule, people with diabetes can safely use over-the-counter athlete's foot creams and that all athlete's foot creams are equally effective.

To use an athlete's foot cream, wash your feet and dry well between your toes and on the bottoms of your feet. Rub the medicated cream in twice a day. If you see no improvement in five days, call your podiatrist. It might not be an athlete's foot fungus after all.

When to seek professional help

You can do a lot to keep your feet healthy. In addition to protecting the skin on your feet by making smart drugstore purchases, you can extend their life by maintaining blood glucose control, following a heart-healthy diet, getting regular exercise, and wearing shoes that fit well. However, if you develop foot pain, wounds that don't heal quickly, or any other foot problem in spite of your best efforts, don't hesitate to call your podiatrist or another member of your diabetes care team. Foot problems that are caught early have the best chance of successful treatment. □

HOW TO CHOOSE FOOTWEAR
by Roy H. Lidtke, D.P.M., C.Ped.

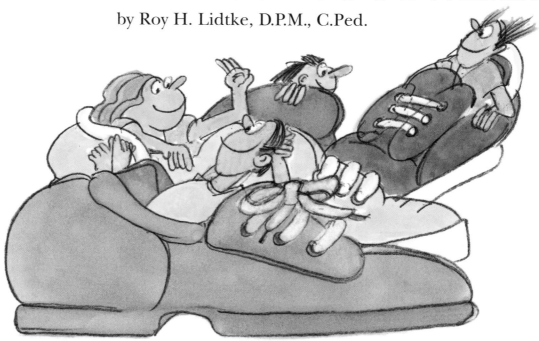

Ask 10 people what they look for in a pair of shoes, and you may well get 10 different answers. But ask 10 podiatrists what they recommend in shoes for people with diabetes, and you'll probably get about the same answer 10 times, with "good fit" near the top of most lists.

People with diabetes are at high risk of developing both impaired circulation to the feet and nerve damage in the feet. Impaired circulation causes wounds on the feet to heal more slowly, raising their risk of becoming infected. Nerve damage can cause loss of sensation in the feet, which means a person may not feel heat, cold, or pain in his feet. He may not notice that his shoes are rubbing or pinching or even that he is walking on small objects such as paperclips that have fallen into his shoes.

The combination of impaired circulation and nerve damage sets the stage for foot ulcers. When you add ill-fitting shoes to the mix, the risk of developing an ulcer goes even higher. But finding shoes that fit well is not impossible, and they don't have to be ugly, either.

Characteristics of a good shoe

Many people with diabetes can wear off-the-shelf shoes with no modifications. However, people who have foot deformities such as bunions, hammertoes, or Charcot joint (a form of joint breakdown) may need special inserts or specially made therapeutic shoes. In addition, people who have certain diabetes complications, such as a previous ulcer, and who have Medicare Part B may qualify for therapeutic shoes or inserts paid for in part by Medicare. (For more on this, see page 320.) Talk to your health-care provider about whether you need customized shoes or inserts or whether you can safely wear unmodified shoes.

Assuming you can wear off-the-shelf shoes, here are some shoe characteristics to keep in mind when shopping for and trying on shoes.

Toe box. The toe box is the part of the shoe that covers the toes and the ball of the foot. It should be long enough so that the toes don't hit the front end of the shoe, spacious enough so that the toes can wiggle a little, and wide enough so as not to pinch the ball of the foot. However, it should not be so wide that the foot slides from side to side. A toe box made of breathable materials, such as leather or cloth, allows sweat to evaporate and helps keep feet drier throughout the day. Perforations in leather shoes make them even more breathable.

Seams (where two pieces of material are stitched together) are stiffer than uncut materials and can be irritating if they rub against the feet. For this reason, people with loss of sensation in their feet or with very delicate skin may be better off choosing shoe styles with no seams in the toe box. Manufacturers commonly reinforce the toe box with plastics or fiberboard to make the area more durable. These materials can also be a source of friction, especially for people who have hammertoes or other changes in foot shape that cause the toes to rub against the top of the shoes.

To avoid purchasing a shoe with a toe box that could irritate your feet, feel inside the shoes with your hand for stiff or scratchy seams or any rigid, well-defined structure. If you can feel any of these potential irritants, put the shoe back and try another model.

Tongue. The tongue should be wide enough and padded enough so that the laces don't dig into the top of your foot. Some tongues have two slits in the middle through which you can thread the laces. Doing so helps hold the tongue in place so it does not slip to one side or the other.

Throat. The throat is the opening where your foot enters the shoe. Make sure that the rim of the throat, known as the collar, is well padded and low enough that it does not rub your anklebones.

Heel counter. This part of the shoe cups the heel. Because it needs to be stiff to control motion at the back of the foot, manufacturers often embed rigid materials here as well. However, there should also be adequate padding in this area to keep hard materials from rubbing against the foot.

The higher the heel counter, the more control it will provide. This is generally a good thing, as long as it does not dig into or rub against the back of the foot, anklebone, or Achilles tendon (the tendon that joins the calf muscles to the heel bone). Shoes with a high heel counter usually have a notch for the Achilles tendon so this does not occur.

Sock liner (insole). The foot sits directly on the sock liner which, in off-the-shelf shoes, is generally made of a single layer of foam. Buying shoes with

ANATOMY OF A SHOE

Heel counter · Throat · Eyelets · Upper · Toe box · Outsole · Midsole · Rockers

a removable sock liner makes it possible to replace the liner with one that is custom-made to fit your foot or an off-the-shelf product that provides more cushioning or a better fit. A custom insert should have at least three layers—a soft layer of foam on top and two stiffer layers on the bottom to provide some resilience.

Midsole. The midsole is the middle portion of the sole, which serves to cushion the foot. It can be difficult for the average shopper to evaluate the quality of a shoe's midsole, but a knowledgeable shoe fitter should have information about the types of midsoles that come with various shoe styles and their relative merits.

Several years ago, a trend started where manufacturers began removing foam from the arch area of the midsole to reduce the weight and cost of the shoe. The logic was that since people don't walk on their arches, they shouldn't need support in this area. The problem with this thinking, however, is that the shoe becomes weaker, and therefore more flexible, when material is removed. The more flexible the center of a shoe, the more stresses it produces across the middle of the arch because the shoe bends in a place the foot does not. Manufacturers quickly became aware of this problem and began reinforcing the arch area with stiffer plastics.

To make sure that you choose a shoe with an arch that is strong enough, hold the shoe by the heel and push the toe box slightly up and toward the back of the shoe. The shoe should bend at the joint of the toes the way a foot does when pushing off. If it instead bends at the arch, don't buy it.

MEDICARE THERAPEUTIC SHOE PROGRAM

In an effort to prevent foot ulcers in people with diabetes who are at risk, Medicare will help pay for therapeutic shoes. For those who qualify, Medicare will pay 80% of the allowed amount for one pair of shoes and up to three pairs of molded innersoles per year. (The allowed amount varies depending on the kind of footwear you need.) Most secondary insurers will help pay the other 20%.

Who qualifies? Not everyone with diabetes needs special shoes. To qualify, you must be under a comprehensive diabetes treatment plan and have one or more of the following:

■ Partial or complete amputation of the foot
■ Previous foot ulceration
■ History of preulcerative callus
■ Peripheral neuropathy with evidence of callus formation
■ Foot deformity
■ Poor circulation

Who does not qualify? People with diabetes who do not have one of the above conditions. It is not enough to just have diabetes.

What paperwork is required? The physician treating you for your diabetes must certify that you have diabetes, that you have one or more of the foot problems just mentioned, that you are under a comprehensive diabetes treatment plan, and that you need the special shoes. Medicare has a form for this certification. You will also need a prescription for the shoes.

Who prescribes the shoes? A prescription is required from a podiatrist or physician who knows how to fit shoes and inserts for people with diabetes. The prescription should indicate a particular type of footwear, such as shoes, inserts, or modifications.

Who supplies the shoes? The footwear must be fitted and furnished by a podiatrist or other qualified individual, such as a pedorthist, orthotist, or prosthetist. The certifying physician may not furnish the footwear unless he or she practices in a defined rural area or area where there is a shortage of health professionals. The prescribing podiatrist may be the supplier.

What do you get? Coverage is limited to one of the following per calendar year:

■ One pair of off-the-shelf extra-depth shoes and three additional pairs of special inserts that your podiatrist will select for you. Extra-depth shoes have room to accommodate innersoles or orthotics.

■ One pair of off-the-shelf extra-depth shoes including a modification, and two additional pairs of inserts.

■ One pair of custom-molded shoes and two additional pairs of special inserts.

I have diabetes and need new shoes. Why shouldn't I get them free from Medicare? Remember that there is no such thing as a free lunch—and there is no such thing as a free pair of shoes. There are over 16 million people with diabetes in the United States. Many of them are of Medicare age. If every Medicare beneficiary with diabetes gets special shoes, there will be no money left for the other important aspects of the Medicare program. If we abuse the shoe benefit, Medicare suffers—and everyone who depends on Medicare will suffer as well.

Outsole. This part of the shoe, usually made from carbon rubber, comes in direct contact with the ground, so it needs to be resilient and flexible.

Rocker bottom. A rocker-bottom shoe has the sole angled up from the ground at the heel and toe. This type of sole can help reduce pressure on the feet in a number of ways. It is a particularly helpful feature for people who have limited joint mobility (a condition in which the tissue around the joints be-comes stiff and inflexible) because the rocker replicates the normal rolling motion of the foot, sparing the stiff joints from moving as much as they otherwise would have to. This also reduces the stress across the skin of the feet. Rocker bot-

toms additionally keep the feet continually moving forward, facilitating the normal heel-to-toe rolling motion and reducing the amount of time that pressure is applied to the bottom of each foot.

To check whether the shoe you have selected has a rocker bottom, place it on a flat surface and push down on the heel. If there is a rocker in the heel, it will make the toe rise off the ground. Likewise, push down on the top of the shoe in the toe area. If there is a rocker in the toe, it will make the heel rise off the ground.

The amount and angle of the rocker changes from shoe to shoe, so the best way to test the one on the shoes you are looking at is to try the pair on and walk around the store. If the rocker is in the correct place for your foot, you will feel as if the shoe is pushing you in the direction you are walking. Because of this sensation, it may take some time to get used to walking in shoes with rockers. Also, because rocker soles have less contact area with the ground than regular soles, it is important to be cautious on uneven terrain.

What not to buy

Although there are a wide variety of shoes that are suitable for people with diabetes, there are also a few styles that should be avoided. High-heeled shoes fall into this category. High heels put increased pressure on the ball of the foot and place the back of the foot in an unstable position. They also increase *shear,* or the movement of foot tissues in opposing directions. Shear is a primary cause of calluses, blisters, and ulcers. A suitable heel will be less than one inch in height.

Slip-on loafers are another style that is best left in the store. Because there is very little of the shoe covering the top of the foot, these shoes provide inadequate support. They are also typically made of un-padded, rigid leather, which can be a source of friction.

Sandals that have straps between the toes are unsuitable as well, since the straps can cause irritation.

Shoe size

Having your feet measured each time you buy shoes is an important part of making sure the shoes you select fit your feet. Feet tend to change shape and size over time, so few people can wear the same shoes at age 50 as they did in high school. In addition, many people have one foot that's larger than the other, so you should have both feet measured. The tool used for determining shoe size is called the Brannock Device. It measures the width, taken across the ball of the foot; the arch length, measured from the heel to the ball of the foot; and the overall length from heel to toe. To get an accurate measurement, stand naturally with your weight divided evenly between both feet. Remember that your feet tend to swell the longer you are on them, so it is a good idea to shop for shoes toward the end of the day.

Ideally, the size for the arch measurement and the size for the heel-to-toe measurement should match. If they don't, the size is usually based on the longer of these two measurements. But these numbers don't tell the whole story, because even shoes with the same numerical size can vary in shape, height of the toe box, and overall depth. A person with a very thick foot or with joint changes in the foot may require an "extra-depth" shoe to accommodate the bulk of the foot or special shoe inserts. An expert shoe fitter will measure the height of the foot and the circumference of the foot around the arch, and use these numbers to match the foot with the appropriate shoe.

If you have narrow feet, shoes with wide-set eyelets will allow you to pull the laces tighter, if necessary. If you have wide feet, shoes with closely set rows of eyelets may work better.

A test run

Once your feet have been measured and you have chosen a shoe style, the real test is how they feel on your feet. Make sure you are wearing the type of sock or stocking you normally wear, and don't forget to also bring any orthotics or inserts you will be wearing in the shoe.

Put on both shoes and attach the laces, buckles, or straps, then stand up. There should be some room, preferably ½ inch to ⅝ inch, between the tip of your longest toe and the front of the shoe. Walk around, and make sure that your arch is fully supported and that the break or bend of the shoe is located at the ball of your foot. Check how the width accommodates the ball of your foot—if the upper portion of the shoe is bulging out over the midsole, the shoe is too narrow and you should ask for a larger width. As you walk, note whether your heel moves around in the shoe. Try rising up onto your toes (holding onto something for support) and notice whether the heel slips off the back of your foot. A properly fitted shoe should slip slightly in the heel, particularly when new, but it should not move excessively or slide off the back of the foot. Make sure the sides of the shoe aren't hitting your anklebones when you stand still or walk. Roll your feet to the insides as if you were trying to flatten your arches, then to the outsides, as if to roll over onto your ankles. The shoe should feel like it is trying to restrict these motions, but it should not feel like it is placing excessive pressure against any one spot on the foot. Walk around the store for as long as you need to make sure the shoe is comfortable and supportive. Shoes should not need to be broken in, stretched, or otherwise modified. If this is suggested, do not purchase the shoes, because they are the wrong ones for your feet.

It is a good idea to look for a shoe store with certified shoe fitters or certified pedorthists on staff. (You can get a list of certified pedorthists in your area by contacting the American Board for Certification in Orthotics, Prosthetics & Pedorthics at

LACING PATTERNS

Shoes should fit comfortably off the shelf, without any need for breaking in. However, you can fine-tune the fit by adjusting the lacing pattern.

A. If your feet are narrow, choose shoes with wide-set eyelets, so you can pull the laces tighter.

B. For feet that are wide, select shoes with closely set eyelets.

C. If the front of your foot is wide and your heel is narrow, or if your foot swells significantly during the day, use two sets of laces and adjust them independently.

D. You can handle a bump or high arch by stringing the laces straight up to the next eyelet in the area of the bump or arch.

E. Another way to accommodate a bump or high arch is to weave the laces straight across the tongue of the shoe, rather than diagonally.

F. If you need more room in the toe area, string one end of the lace from the bottom eyelet to the top eyelet on the opposite side, then pull the lace to lift the front of the shoe.

G. For a heel that is narrow or slipping inside the shoe, you can loop the laces through one another at the top before tying them.

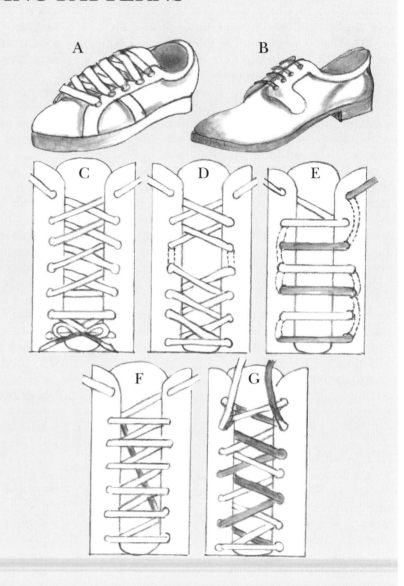

[703] 836-7114 or by visiting www.abcop.org.) A knowledgeable staff person will know the subtle differences in the sizes and shapes among brands and even among models within a brand. This kind of information and the help of a professional can be especially useful if you have any loss of sensation in your feet that prevents you from being able to tell whether a shoe is rubbing. A store with certified staff on board will generally also be happy to special order shoes for you if they do not have your size.

Lacing options

Although shoes should fit comfortably off the shelf, with no need for breaking in, you can fine-tune the fit by adjusting or changing the laces and lacing patterns.

Generally, round laces tend to stretch more than flat laces, making them a good choice for walking shoes. As you walk, your foot changes shape. Shoes and laces with some give, or flexibility, can accommodate those changes, while rigid shoes and inflexible laces will create pressure against your skin. The amount of give in a shoe is also influenced by the type of eyelets the laces go through. As a general rule, fabric or leather loops give more than plastic or metal eyelets, and eyelets give more than punched-out holes. However, hard plastic or metal eyelets can irritate the top of the foot, so choose shoes with loops or punched-out holes whenever possible.

Lacing patterns can be altered to accommodate a variety of foot shapes. For example, there is a tendency for the front of the foot to widen as a result of neuropathy, a flattening arch, or simply increasing age. If the front of the foot is wide and the heel is narrow, or if the foot swells significantly during the day, two sets of laces can be used so the bottom tie can be loosened, allowing for more room in the front of the shoe (see "Lacing Patterns" on page 322).

A person who has a high arch or a bump on the top of his foot can skip the crisscross lacing pattern in the area near the arch or bump and instead string the laces straight up to the next eyelet. Another way to deal with a high arch is to weave the laces straight across the tongue of the shoe, rather than diagonally. If more room is needed in the toe area, try stringing one end of the lace from the bottom eyelet to the top eyelet on the opposite side, then pulling the lace to lift the front of the shoe and increase room in the toe box. If the heel of the foot is narrow or is slipping inside the shoe excessively, the laces can be looped through one another at the top before being tied.

How do they look?

The key to finding a comfortable, attractive shoe is to find a store with a wide selection. Stores that have footwear from around the world are a good place to start; there are many well-designed shoes from Europe and New Zealand. Take your time selecting a pair, and ask about the return policy just in case the style you select turns out not to be the right one for you. And remember this process—you will need to repeat it whenever you get a new pair of shoes, which should be every 6 to 12 months. □

Exercise

Tips 533–594 327

Exercise Myths and Facts 332

Get Moving With Yoga 337

The High Price of Inactivity 341

Improving Your Balance 345

Stretching 352

Biking 101 358

8

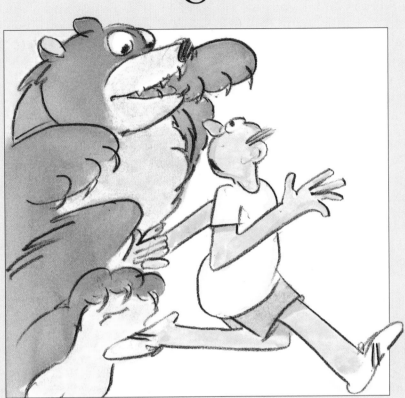

Exercise Tips

533–594

533. Try to do balance exercises every day, because the benefits only last as long you do the exercises. If you stay consistent, you should see improvements in just a few weeks.

534. Whenever you exercise, try to work to the point where you feel warm and slightly out of breath. If you do, then you can be sure that you're doing the best you can to burn lots of fat and glucose, increase your level of fitness, and improve your health.

535. Lift weights all you want, whenever you want. The more muscle you have, the more glucose you can burn, and the better your diabetes control may be.

536. The best time to exercise is the time you are most likely to do it. If exercising at night fits your schedule better, then by all means do it then. If getting a workout first thing in the morning makes you feel more energetic, all the better.

537. If you're trying to lose weight, an exercise program that includes aerobic activity as well as some type of calisthenics or weight lifting will probably help you the most.

538. Proper hydration, or fluid replacement, should begin before you exercise and continue during and after the activity. The amount of water you drink should

approximately equal the amount of fluid lost in sweat and urine.

539. Don't rely on thirst as an indicator of hydration status, because by the time you feel thirsty, you may already be dehydrated.

540. To get a sense of how much fluid you need, weigh yourself nude before and after exercise and drink 2 cups of water for every pound lost.

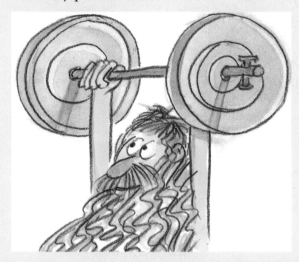

541. It's never too late to start lifting. Strength training helps increase bone mass, reduce the risk of falling, and preserve greater independence.

542. If you're unhappy about always having to eat before or during exercise to prevent or treat low blood sugar, speak to your doctor or diabetes educator about lowering your insulin doses on days you exercise.

543. To find the right yoga class for you, start by asking around for personal recommendations. Mention that you're looking for a yoga class in casual conversation; you'll probably be surprised by how many coworkers, friends, and acquaintances do or have done yoga and can either recommend or steer you away from certain classes or instructors.

544. If you live in a small town or suburban area, try your local YMCA, health clubs, or community centers for yoga classes. Most metropolitan areas have a number of yoga studios. If you're not ready to sign

up, ask about observing a class or even taking a trial class to see if you like it.

545. If you can't find a yoga class that suits you in your area, or if you'd prefer beginning at home, yoga videos offer an excellent—and inexpensive—alternative to live instruction.

546. Find yoga videos at your public library or local video rental store, or you can try browsing Internet yoga sites and online bookstores and reading reviews of yoga videos to find one that sounds right for you.

547. Dress for yoga in loose or stretchy, comfortable clothing that allows you to move easily.

548. Ask your yoga teacher about alternatives to practicing barefoot, such as wearing nonslip socks. People with existing foot problems may also want to consult their health-care provider before doing yoga poses that put pressure on the feet.

549. If you shower in a public locker room after yoga class, be sure to wear shower sandals or slippers to protect your feet, both from foot fungus and from any objects that may have fallen onto the floor.

550. Don't be shy about letting your yoga instructor know that you have diabetes. It may be necessary, especially when you're first starting out, to check your blood sugar during class.

551. Be sure to always bring your blood glucose meter and glucose tablets with you to class; you may be surprised by how much even a gentle class may get your heart rate going from time to time, and if that happens, your blood sugar may drop.

552. Don't hesitate to stop at any time during class to check your blood sugar.

553. A general rule in yoga is that it's best not to practice on a full stomach.

554. Depending on how yoga affects your blood sugar, you may find that you need to eat some form of carbohydrate 15–30 minutes before doing yoga. If so, choose something on the lighter side, such as a

few whole wheat crackers, that will keep your blood sugar up but won't weigh you down.

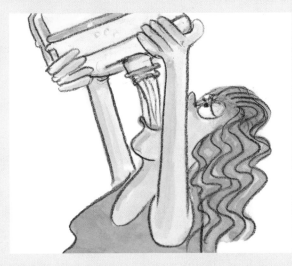

555. Be sure to drink water before and after class, and bring a bottle of water to class with you if you sweat a lot or tend to get thirsty.

556. Remember is to be gentle with yourself when you begin yoga. Don't push or strain to get into a posture.

557. When you're stiff from sitting in front of your computer all day, get up and do some simple stretches.

558. Standing in line at the grocery store, note whether you're holding any of your muscles tightly; if so, gently release them.

559. The U.S. Surgeon General recommends doing 30 minutes of moderate-intensity activity (that makes you feel warm and slightly out of breath) 5–7 days per week. The activity can be done in one bout of 30 minutes or accumulated in two 15-minute bouts or three 10-minute bouts.

560. Regular physical activity can both help manage body weight and make you healthier even if you don't lose weight.

561. If you're looking for fitness on the cheap, look no further than walking outdoors.

562. If you prefer indoor walking, check your local mall for a walking club.

563. If you're just starting a walking program, try the technique of walking for five minutes in one direction then turning around and walking five minutes back to your starting point. When your 10-minute round-trip walk starts feeling easy, increase it to six minutes out and six minutes back. Increase your distance by no more than 10% a week.

564. Try jumping rope for another cheap aerobic fitness option. Start with just 5 minutes the first few times because your calves can get very sore if you haven't jumped rope in a while.

565. Make your selection of an exercise machine based on comfort and ease of operation. Try each machine for 10–15 minutes at the store or at your gym. If it feels natural and comfortable, you're more likely to use it.

566. Choose equipment that's well built and sturdy. It shouldn't shake, rattle, or roll, or be unusually noisy. Look for in-home labor warranties (who fixes it if it breaks?) on exercise machines and ask if the warranties can be extended.

567. Make sure an exercise machine will fit into your home and won't disturb your neighbors. Treadmills have motors, so they may not be suitable for apartment living.

568. Don't let the salesperson sell you all the bells and whistles if you're looking only for the basics on an exercise machine.

569. If you're worried about motivation or would like to improve your walking, select a treadmill. They are the most popular machines, and people tend to use them at home more often than other exercise machines.

570. Select a stationary bike if you prefer to sit while you exercise; have a vascular, muscular, bone, or joint problem that prevents you from doing standing (weight-bearing) exercise; have an outdoor bike and would like to stick with riding even when the weather's bad; or simply like to bike.

571. Many rowing machines are close to the ground, so make sure you can get down to them. Rowing machines can be tough on the back; make sure your back is healthy before using one.

572. For the most effective static stretch, do a brief warm-up (3 to 5 minutes) before stretching.

573. At the gym, you might use an exercise bike or treadmill or other aerobic equipment at a light intensity to warm up your muscles before you stretch. At home, take an easy 5-minute walk to get some blood in your legs, then do your stretches.

574. Stretching helps you tune in to your body, so you pay attention to how you feel rather than pushing through pain or forcing yourself beyond your limits.

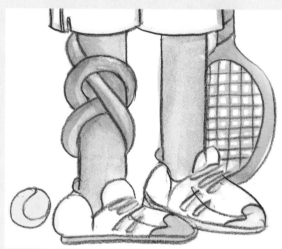

575. If tight muscles prevent you from being physically active, a stretch might be just the thing to help you get started or keep you moving.

576. If you have moderate or proliferative retinopathy, avoid stretches or exercises that place your heart lower than your waist or that cause you to hold your breath and strain, which can raise your blood pressure.

577. If you need a little instruction in stretching, there are a number of books and videos that can help. You might also ask an athletic trainer for suggestions if you belong to a gym or a physical therapist if you see one. Or you could take a stretching or yoga class.

578. As you stretch, remember that it isn't supposed to hurt. Stretch until you feel mild tension, then hold that position. As your muscles relax, you may be able to stretch a little bit more, but don't overstretch.

579. Respect your limits, and don't compare yourself to others in a stretch or yoga class.

580. Even if you regularly do some other type of aerobic exercise, vary your routine with an occasional bike ride to challenge yourself physically and stimulate yourself mentally.

581. If you're in the market for a new bike, you may want to think first about where you intend to bike—on trails or on roads—before buying one. If you intend to ride on roads, you will want either a road bike with fairly thin tires and a light-weight frame or a somewhat heavier "city bike." If you prefer biking on trails, you'll probably need a mountain bike. If you think you may be riding on both roads and fairly flat trails, a hybrid bicycle might be right for you.

582. Once you have decided which type of bike you want and approximately how much you want to spend, go to your local bike shop and try some on for size.

583. Before test-riding any bike, have the sales clerk help you pick a bike with the right frame size for your body and also show you how to adjust the seat and handlebars.

584. A good-fitting helmet is essential for bicycling and should be worn at all times, even on a leisurely ride.

585. In addition to a helmet, you may want to consider bike gloves, which give your palms some padding while leaving your fingers uncovered.

586. Wearing clothing, such as a vest, made of reflective material is a good idea if you will be biking at dawn or dusk or after dark; it makes you much more visible to motorists.

587. Biking is an aerobic exercise, so you will want a way to carry some water with you to drink as you ride.

588. If your bike is muddy after riding, clean it with soap and water (preferably gentle

soap made for bikes) and dry it off right away. Dirt and mud are abrasive and can destroy your bike components.

589. Check with a bike shop for local route and trail information.

590. Participating in a group ride organized by a bike club is also a good way to discover places to ride. Bike shops are often a good way to find a club in your area.

591. Bicycling will probably lower your blood glucose level, so you may need to stop for a snack or adjust your diabetes regimen in some other way to account for bicycling's blood-glucose-lowering effect.

592. Always tell someone where you are going and when you plan on coming back, especially if you are cycling by yourself. In general, however, biking with other people is safer. If you have a cell phone, bring it with you.

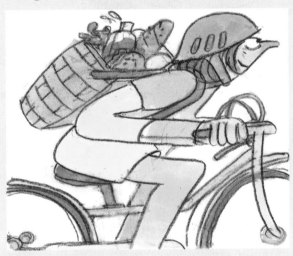

593. Always carry some food with you. On longer rides, carry your blood glucose monitoring supplies with you.

594. If you ever feel unable to control your bike—because of rain or anything else—stop and get off. You may get delayed or wetter than you otherwise would get, but you will be alive and able to take another bike ride when conditions are more favorable.

EXERCISE MYTHS AND FACTS

by Richard Weil, M.Ed., C.D.E.

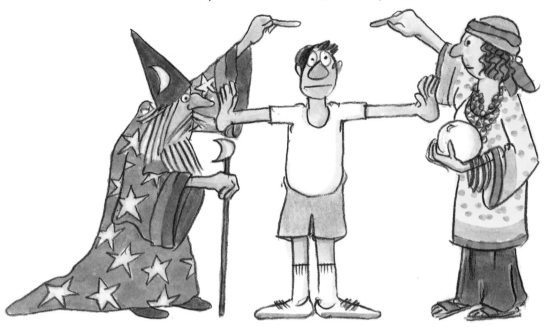

Are you confused by all the exercise advice out there? It's no wonder: With a dozen fitness magazines on the newsstand, a wealth of health and fitness news streaming into your home over the Internet, bogus ads guaranteeing an effortless 40-pound weight loss or bigger muscles in just 10 days, not to mention the free advice from well-intentioned friends, trainers, and the guy on the bench press next to you, there's a lot of conflicting information to sort through. Unfortunately, many popular fitness tips not only make exercise seem harder and more complicated than it really should be, but they can also lead to injury. To set the record straight and help you exercise safely, here are the facts—nothing but the facts—behind some of the most common exercise myths.

You don't start burning fat until 20 minutes into your workout.

This is one of the most popular myths of all time. You may have heard it from a friend or even from a fitness trainer at your gym, but the fact is, muscle burns a combination of fat and carbohydrate (glucose) simultaneously almost all of the time. It's just that you may burn a higher *percentage* of one or the other depending on the intensity of the exercise. For example, during high-intensity activities like sprinting or strenuous weight lifting, which get you out of breath, your muscles are burning a

higher percentage of carbohydrate than fat (perhaps as much as 80% to 90% carbohydrate and 10% fat). At rest and during light-intensity physical activity (such as moderate-paced walking), when breathing is easier, the percentage could change to 70% fat and 30% carbohydrate. Why does this happen?

As you start to exercise, fat and carbohydrate are released from storage sites in the body as well as from the bloodstream and enter the working muscles. (Protein is not a fuel for exercise unless your body is in a starvation crisis.) Oxygen, transported from the lungs to the muscle, burns these fuels to generate energy. Fat contains more than twice the amount of energy per gram as carbohydrate (fat contains 9 calories per gram while carbohydrate has only 4). Your muscles would prefer to burn fat, because it's so energy-dense, but the catch is, you must provide adequate oxygen to the muscle to burn it. Since fat contains more calories than carbohydrate, it also takes more oxygen to burn. When you're really out of breath—during a sprint, for example—there's not enough time for oxygen to travel from the lungs to the muscles, and so your muscles, low on oxygen, have no choice but to burn the less dense fuel, carbohydrate. As a general rule, unless you are performing brief, very intense exercise, there's always enough oxygen in the muscles to burn some fat as well as carbohydrate. Which leads us to our next myth…

The "fat-burning" option on the exercise machine at the gym is better for weight loss than the "cardio" option.

This isn't only a myth; it's really bad advice. Basically, you want to burn as many calories as possible when you exercise, whether you're trying to lose weight, increase your stamina, control your diabetes, or improve your general health. Caloric expenditure during aerobic activity is directly related to the distance you travel and how hard you work. When you select the fat-burning mode on an aerobic exercise machine, you in effect minimize the number of calories you burn, because the machine— let's say a treadmill—keeps the speed slow and the elevation low. On the "cardio" option, the speed and elevation are set higher, so that for an equivalent amount of workout time, you end up traveling farther, working harder— and burning more calories.

The reason the lower level is labeled the "fat-burning" option is that, as described above, at lower intensities you breathe more comfortably, so you deliver more oxygen to the muscles and burn a higher percentage of fat than carbohydrate. This part of the equation is accurate, but the truth is that although you may burn a higher *percentage* of fat at the slower speed and intensity, you end up burning less *total* fat. For example, if you weigh 150 pounds and walk on the treadmill for 30 minutes at 3.0 miles per hour, you will burn about 150 calories in one session. If you walk for 30 minutes at 4.0 miles per hour, you will burn 200 calories. Now let's say that at the lower-intensity, 3-mile-per-hour pace you burn 70% of your total calories from fat. That would be .70 × 150 calories, or a total of 105 calories burned from fat. At the faster, 4-mile-per-hour pace, you burn only 60% of your calories from fat (again, because you are working harder, you can't get as much oxygen to the muscles to burn fat). So, .60 × 200 calories equals 120 calories from fat. As you can see, at the slower speed, not only is the number of total calories burned less (150 versus 200), but the number of fat calories burned is also less than it is at the faster speed (105 versus 120).

If this confuses you, don't sweat it. Just remember that selecting a slower speed and lower intensity to maximize fat burning is counterproductive—unless it enables you to exercise longer and burn more calories. Whenever you exercise, try to work to the point where you feel warm and slightly out of breath. If you do, then you can be sure that you're doing the best you can to burn lots of fat and glucose, increase your level of fitness, and improve your health.

Don't lift weights if you're trying to lose weight.

Some people don't want to weight train while they're on a weight-loss program because they know that building muscle might cause some weight gain. That's true, because muscle tissue is heavier than fat, but muscle is exactly what you want to gain when you're trying to lose weight. Here's why: When you restrict calories to lose weight, you always lose some muscle. In fact, up to 25% of your body-weight loss can be from muscle. (So if you lose 10 pounds, 2.5 pounds of it could be muscle.) The problem with losing muscle during weight loss is that muscle is the engine that burns calories and helps maintain your metabolic rate. If you have less muscle, you reduce your ability to burn calories, lose more weight, and, more important, maintain your weight loss. (The plateau that many people experience during weight loss can be explained partially by loss of muscle.)

In most cases, moderate weight training will not amount to more than 3–5 pounds of weight gain anyway, but even if it did, it's what you want, because each pound of muscle consumes about 35–50 calories a day. So next time someone drops by and offers you five pounds of muscle, go ahead and take it; it'll help you use up an additional 175–250 calories daily.

Muscle is also the engine that burns glucose. The more muscle you have, the more glucose you can burn, and the better your diabetes control may be. So pour on the muscle. Lift weights all you want, whenever you want.

Exercise in the morning works better than exercise at night.

Some people believe that if you go to sleep right after exercise you won't get as much benefit from the workout, because your metabolic rate slows down while you're sleeping. If you exercise in the morning, they say, you jump-start your metabolism and burn more calories throughout the day. There's no evidence that this is true.

Another reason some people believe morning exercise is superior to nighttime exercise is that exercising right before bed supposedly keeps you awake longer. Research shows that that may be true, but generally only for deconditioned people. For fit people, exercise before bedtime does not alter sleep patterns, probably because their bodies are used to and recover quickly from the effects of exercise. Some health experts suggest that regular exercise may even help improve sleep quality and sleep onset over time.

The bottom line is that the body responds to exercise whenever you do it. If exercising at night fits your schedule better, then by all means do it then. If getting a workout first thing in the morning makes you feel more energetic, all the better. The best time to exercise is the time you are most likely to do it.

Walking isn't enough.

Walking may not be as arduous as training for a marathon, but when it comes to preventing diabetes, complications of diabetes, and heart disease, it's powerful medicine. The Diabetes Prevention Program, a three-year, government- sponsored study designed to test the ability of healthy behavior changes to prevent diabetes, showed that when people under the age of 60 who had impaired glucose tolerance, or prediabetes (a condition that often precedes Type 2 diabetes), walked 150 minutes per week (that's five 30-minute walks per week) and followed a low-fat diet (enabling them to lose 5% to 7% of their body weight), they reduced their risk of diabetes by 58%. For people over 60, the risk reduction was 71%.

In another study, close to 3,000 retired men were enrolled in the Honolulu Heart Program to study the effects of walking on heart disease. The conclusion: The more they walked, the lower their risk of heart disease. Men who walked more than 2 miles per day were half as likely to get heart disease as men who walked less than 1 mile per day.

In both of these studies, subjects walked at a moderate pace of 3.0–4.0 miles per hour.

Spot-reducing exercises can trim my trouble spots.

There's no such thing as spot-reducing. It would be nice if you could walk on the treadmill and say, "OK, today I'll burn fat from my thighs." But that's not the way it works. Whether it tends to collect on your thighs or your tummy, fat on your body belongs to your entire body, and the only way to reduce it is through regular exercise and reducing your caloric intake. Here's some information about storing and burning fat that should help you understand how aerobic exercise, weight lifting or other resistance exercise, and attention to your diet can help you lose weight.

Fat is stored in cells called adipocytes, which are located all over the body. When you eat more fat or calories than your body needs, the fat cells gobble up much of the excess and expand in size. The larger the cells, the higher your percentage of body fat. Where on the body your fat cells are located, where you tend to store fat first, and how

efficient your adipocytes are at storing fat is genetically determined; you have no control over it. As a rule, men store fat in their abdomens, and women tend to store it in their buttocks, hips, and thighs. Similarly, people generally gain and lose weight in a consistent pattern. If you've lost and regained weight multiple times, you probably know where you tend to lose it from first (perhaps the face), and where it tends to stick the longest (often in the hips, thighs, and buttocks).

How does exercise help you get rid of fat? During exercise, hormones like adrenaline are released that signal the adipocytes to release fat into the bloodstream. That fat is then transported to the muscles to be burned for energy. When an adipocyte releases its stored fat, it shrinks. The cells themselves never disappear, but as long as the fat is used by the muscle and does not return to fatten up the adipocyte, you will lose overall body fat. Because you have no control over which adipocytes are stimulated to release fat, however, you cannot "spot-reduce" fat from a particular body part.

Aerobic exercise (such as biking, walking, or swimming) stimulates the release of more fat than does resistance exercise like weight lifting, leg lifts, or pushups. However, resistance exercise builds muscle, and muscle is the engine that burns fat and helps maintain metabolic rate. So if you're trying to lose weight, an exercise program that includes aerobic activity as well as some type of calisthenics or weight lifting will probably help you the most.

Incidentally, although they don't change your weight-loss pattern, exercises that work your abdomen, thighs, hips, and buttocks will indeed strengthen and tone the underlying muscles, so even if there is still that pesky layer of fat on top, your physique will be tighter and your clothes may even feel looser.

Exercise will make me hungry.

There is no compelling evidence that moderate exercise affects a person's overall appetite; it neither makes you hungry nor suppresses your appetite. Some people report that they make better food choices if they exercise regularly, but this has not been studied carefully. The only time exercise is likely to make you hungry is if it's been 3–4 hours since your last meal or snack, and you exercise on an empty stomach.

If I don't sweat during exercise I'm not getting any benefit.

Sweating is important because it's a way of cooling off muscles that heat up during exercise, but it is not necessarily an indicator of how hard you are working. Temperature, humidity, wind conditions, and even how you are dressed all affect how much you sweat on a given day. Moreover, not everyone sweats at the same rate.

Do you ever turn beet-red during exercise? That happens because blood vessels below the skin in the face are dilating; as they widen, they transport heat from the muscles to the skin to cool off the body. Chances are, if you're a person who turns bright red in the face during exercise, you may not sweat as much as a person who does not turn red; it usually has nothing to do with the amount of exercise you do or how much effort you're putting into it. Which brings us to a related myth...

The fitter I get, the less I will sweat.

There's no relationship between how fit you are and how much you sweat. Some people sweat buckets, while others don't sweat much at all, regardless of their fitness level or degree of exertion. Heavy sweating during exercise may not be pleasant, but it means that the body is cooling itself efficiently, which may enhance your performance.

The only possible physiological downside of heavy sweating is that if you don't replace the lost fluid by drinking water, you run the risk of dehydration. Dehydration is un-healthy for all people, but it can be even more of a concern for people with diabetes, because it is more likely to occur when blood glucose levels aren't under control.

It's relatively easy to dehydrate if you sweat a lot; on a hot, humid day, you can lose more than 5% of your body weight from sweat during a workout. Athletic performance can be adversely affected by as little as a 1% drop in body weight, and when fluid loss exceeds 3% of body weight, endurance can diminish by as much as 20% to 30%. Weight loss from sweat should never exceed 2% of body weight. (For a 150-pound person, 2% of body weight is 3 pounds.)

Thirst is not a good indicator of hydration status, because by the time you feel thirsty, you may already be dehydrated. Proper hydration, or fluid replacement, should begin before you exercise and continue during and after the activity. The amount of water you drink should approximately equal the amount of fluid lost in sweat and urine. To get a sense of how much fluid you need, weigh yourself nude before and after exercise and drink 2 cups of water for every pound lost. Some people can lose ½ to 2 liters of fluid per hour (1 liter of water weighs 2.25 pounds). A more general guideline for maintaining proper hydration is as follows:
■ Drink 17 to 20 ounces of water (about 2–2½ cups) 2 to 3 hours before exercise.
■ Drink 7 to 10 ounces of water (about 1–1½ cups) 10 to 20 minutes before exercise.
■ Drink 7 to 10 ounces of water every 10 to 20 minutes during activity.

If you sweat heavily, you may need to drink more.

If I'm not sore after my workout, I'm not getting any benefit.

This myth may hail back to that old "no pain, no gain" adage that's simply not true. Muscle soreness is not a prerequisite for muscle growth. When just starting an exercise program or a new activity, it's common to feel stiff or sore for a day or more afterward. Once the body adapts to a particular exercise, however, you won't feel as sore every time you work out, though clearly you are getting stronger. You can minimize muscle pain by beginning with small amounts of activity and only gradually increasing the intensity and duration of your workout.

If you're already used to exercise, you know that you are capable of various degrees of intensity when working out. You don't need to push to the limit at each workout to realize gains in performance (in fact, overdoing it can cause burnout or injury), but if you feel you've hit a plateau in your routine, and you consider a little soreness to be "good pain," kicking your effort up a notch or two can help you reach your next fitness goal. Try lifting weights more slowly, particularly on the lowering portion of the lift, which tends to cause more soreness. You could also ask a spotter to help you with the final few repetitions once you're fatigued and cannot complete a full repetition. You begin the lift on your own, and when you cannot lift any further, the spotter helps you finish the lift; you then lower the weight on your own. This is called assisted negative training, and it will help you build muscle.

To increase the intensity of aerobic workouts, try interval training once or twice a week. Interval training involves setting up a work-to-active-recovery ratio, in which you alternate more intense periods of activity with less intense, "active recovery" periods. For example, if you usually walk on the treadmill for 30 minutes at a steady, 3.5-mile-per-hour pace, here's what a 30-minute interval training session might look like: Walk for 10 minutes at your usual pace (so you're good and warmed up), then increase the speed to, say, 3.8 mph (which will get your heart thumping) for one minute. Return to your 3.5-mph pace for another 3 minutes, then pick up the pace to 3.8 mph again for one minute.

The work-to-active-recovery ratio in this workout is 1:3: The minute at 3.8 mph is the "work," and the three minutes at 3.5 mph is the "active recovery." Over time, as you get fitter, you'll be able to extend the "work" time to 1.5 minutes and spend only 2.5 minutes at the slower pace. Eventually, your regular, steady pace will be 3.8 mph, and when you interval train, your "work" pace will be even faster.

You can't build muscle after age 50.

This myth was shattered by a landmark study published in 1990, in which 10 frail nursing home residents, ages 90 to 96, lifted weights for eight weeks. After the study was completed, their strength gain averaged 174%, thigh muscle area increased 9.0%, and walking speed increased by 48%.

Other studies have shown similar results, so it seems clear that muscle loss is caused not by aging itself but by lack of activity. Not only is muscle gain possible, but it's also very beneficial for older adults: Strength training helps increase bone mass, reduce the risk of falling, and preserve greater independence. It's fair to say that it's never too late to start lifting.

Exercise always leads to weight loss.

Disappointing as it may seem, exercise is much more important for weight maintenance than it is for weight loss. In fact, in virtually all studies that compare people who exercise to lose weight with people who diet to lose weight, the dieters always lose lots of weight, and the exercisers lose very little, if any.

That's no reason to give up on exercise, though. For one thing, you gain important health benefits from exercise even if you don't lose a pound. For another, when you lose weight by restricting calories, it's very difficult to keep the weight off permanently unless you exercise to raise your metabolic rate and prevent muscle loss. Many weight-loss researchers believe that including regular exercise in a weight-loss program is the single best predictor of long-term weight-loss success. (If you cut calories but remain sedentary, there's a high likelihood that you will regain all of the weight you lose.)

This may not sound like great news, but it is. It means that you do not have to do Herculean amounts of exercise to lose weight. If you get started on weight loss by reducing your caloric intake, then gradually increase your level of physical activity while continuing to watch your calories, you will steadily lose weight. As you lose pounds, you should find it easier to move, and by the time you reach your target weight, you should be physically active enough to keep the weight off.

If you find you have gained weight after starting to exercise, there are two probable explanations:

■ You may be gaining muscle. Muscle is heavier than fat, and it's possible to gain 3–5 pounds of muscle mass in 4–8 weeks, particularly during a weight-lifting program. (You're likely to gain more muscle from lifting weights than from doing aerobic exercise.) This is not a bad thing.

■ You may have started to eat more. Some people eat more when they begin to exercise because they feel hungrier (but it's not all that common, as mentioned before), and some eat more because they think they are "allowed to" since they're exercising. The problem is that exercise may not burn as many calories as you think. If you weigh 150 pounds and run for 30 minutes at 6.0 mph, you'll burn about 300 calories. That may seem like a lot, but if you also eat an extra 500 calories throughout the day, you're going to gain weight.

If you exercise on an empty stomach, you may eat more than usual after exercise. For instance, if you exercise after work but before dinner, and you haven't eaten since lunch, by the time you finish exercising, you may not have eaten for 5 or 6 hours. When you're famished after a workout, it's very easy to eat more than you intend to at dinner, which can cause the calories to add up. To help control hunger, try having a snack 45–60 minutes before exercise if it's been more than 3–4 hours since you last ate. Half a bagel, 8 ounces of sugar-free yogurt, an energy bar, or a banana are some suggestions for a light preexercise snack.

For people who take insulin or oral medicines that lower blood glucose level, exercising without a preexercise snack can cause hypoglycemia, or low blood glucose. Developing low blood sugar during a workout can make exercise very frustrating, and if it happens on a regular basis, the extra calories you need to treat the hypoglycemia can add up. If you're unhappy about always having to eat before or during exercise to prevent or treat low blood sugar, speak to your doctor or diabetes educator about lowering your insulin doses on days you exercise. After all, if you're trying to maintain weight loss, what's the point of exercising if you have to eat every time you work out?

The truth about exercise

So there you have some crucial facts about exercise. In today's world, where information is the name of the game, it's easy to lose track of the simplicity of movement. Exercise doesn't have to be complicated: Pick an activity that you like and that gets your heart thumping a little (remember, the key is to feel warm and slightly out of breath), then do it daily or on most days, and ignore all the hype. If you do this, you have a great shot at good health and physical fitness. □

GET MOVING WITH YOGA

by Gabrielle Kaplan-Mayer

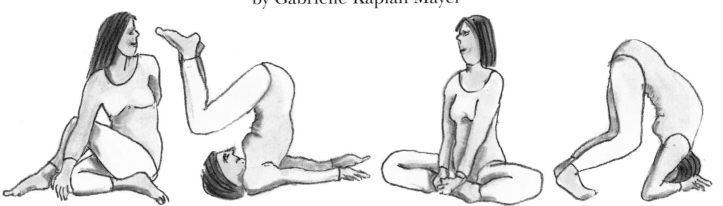

Popular images of yoga often show a sinewy person folded, pretzel-like, into a joint-defying pose, perhaps while balancing on one leg, to boot. While impressive, such images often scare people away from the very practice they are promoting or celebrating, namely yoga. That's unfortunate, because yoga has benefits for everyone, no matter how flexible or sinewy.

Yoga's benefits are not just physical, although regular practice can dramatically increase flexibility, strength, stamina, and balance. The word yoga comes from the Sanskrit word for "yoke" or "union," and the practice of yoga emphasizes the integration of physical and mental health through performing various postures (asanas), breathing exercises (pranayama), and sometimes meditation and chanting. That combination can help calm the mind, reduce mental stress, and enhance mental focus. Yoga also has a spiritual component; how much that aspect is emphasized in a yoga class depends on the instructor and the class setting.

Part of what makes yoga suitable for anyone, regardless of physical condition, is its philosophy of "being in the moment." On a physical level, that means doing the postures to the best of your ability, whatever that is. If you can stand on one foot and hold the other above your head, that's fine. If you can stand on one foot and hold the other only an inch off the ground, that's fine, too. Being in the moment also means not comparing yourself to others or even to yourself at a different time. It means doing the best you can at this moment.

On a mental level, "being in the moment" encourages you to focus on the sensations in your body—particularly the sensation of breathing—at this very minute and to allow yourself not to think about the past or the future. For many people, this isn't easy, but the benefits of practicing this type of

meditation can include feeling more relaxed and being able to deal with life stresses more effectively.

Yoga and diabetes

Any practice that enhances physical fitness and helps with stress reduction has special value for people with diabetes. Physical activity burns glucose in the short term and also builds muscle, which is the body's glucose-burning "engine." The more muscle you have, the more glucose you burn, even at rest. Regular aerobic activity (the type that gets your heart rate and breathing rate going for an extended period of time) also reduces the risk of high blood pressure and heart disease, both of which commonly occur in people who have diabetes. How much of an aerobic workout you get from doing yoga depends on the type of yoga you do and the intensity at which you practice, but the flexibility, agility, and strength you gain from doing any type of yoga will increase your ability to engage in other forms of aerobic exercise.

Stress reduction is often an unaddressed element of diabetes self-management, but uncontrolled stress can disrupt even the most diligent efforts at maintaining tight blood sugar control. Besides taking an emotional toll, stress causes a physiological response in the body, prompting the release of "fight or flight" stress hormones into the blood. Because these hormones spur the release of stored glucose or fat into the bloodstream, stress can cause elevated blood sugar if you don't have enough insulin in your system at the time. If you don't realize what is causing your blood sugar to run high, you may, in turn, feel even more stressed.

While Eastern cultures have long recognized yoga's healing benefits, Western medicine is just catching on. Some American medical schools are starting to teach yoga and meditation as a means of stress reduction, and well-known cardiologist Dean Ornish, M.D., now prescribes yoga, along with diet and exercise, as part of his plan for preventing and reversing heart disease. Studies have shown that yoga can help reduce high blood pressure (which can be partly stress-induced). It can also help reverse depression, which is more common among people with diabetes than the general population.

Exactly how yoga may relieve depression is not known, but it may work in several ways at once. According to Beryl Herrin, a yoga instructor based in Philadelphia, "Yoga gets energy moving in the body. It gives you breath awareness, which helps you to stay in the moment, rather than be consumed with worries." Exercise is known to naturally increase your brain's "feel-good" chemicals, and meditation, it seems, can have the same effect. Studies show that the increase in slower-frequency alpha and theta brain waves (both of which are associated with a state of relaxation) that occurs during and after yoga meditation corresponds with an increase in dopamine, a chemical that produces feelings of pleasure and satisfaction. And yoga may also help relieve depression simply by burning glucose, since high blood glucose itself can contribute to feelings of depression. However, yoga alone cannot treat major depression; people experiencing severe depression should seek professional help.

A style for everyone

There are many types and styles of yoga, some accentuating the physical component of yoga, others its spiritual or calming aspects. Hatha yoga is considered the "basic" yoga style and the root of most other variations. Combining physical poses and breathing exercises to increase body awareness, fitness, and flexibility, a beginner hatha yoga class is a good option for people trying yoga for the first time. Beginners and people with physical limitations might also look for classes labeled "gentle yoga," in which classical hatha postures are modified so that students can proceed comfortably at their own pace and level of ability.

For people who already have some degree of fitness, ashtanga yoga may be a good choice. Students perform a series of postures in quick succession to get a rigorous aerobic workout while increasing strength and flexibility. Sometimes called power yoga, this style is catching on in gyms and health clubs.

Another popular style is iyengar, a slower, more technique-focused method that uses props such as belts, blocks, and chairs to help students achieve precise alignment in breathing exercises and poses.

TYPES OF YOGA

Hatha yoga is the foundation of several different yoga techniques and styles. A basic hatha class is probably the best introduction to yoga, but you may find that another style suits you better. The following are types of yoga commonly taught in the United States. Within each style, a teacher may also have his own variation or focus.

Ananda. Uses gentle poses to release tension and prepare the body for meditation and increased self-awareness. Students repeat silent affirmations while holding postures.

Ashtanga. A vigorous style of yoga that uses rapid repetition of a series of postures, in order of increasing difficulty.

Bikram. Yoga practiced in sauna-like rooms heated to at least 100°F; Bikram philosophy teaches that sweating helps to release toxins in the body. People with sensitivity to extreme heat may want to avoid this style, and people who take insulin should note that insulin can be absorbed into the bloodstream more quickly in high temperatures.

Integral. A spiritual practice using gentle postures, chanting, and meditation to develop the individual as a whole.

Integrative yoga therapy. Often taught at hospitals or as part of a healthy lifestyle program, integrative yoga is usually combined with diet and exercise counseling to help people achieve better overall health or handle specific health problems.

Iyengar. Uses props such as belts, benches, and blocks to help attain greater extension and better alignment in poses and breathing exercises.

Kripalu. Aims for a state of "meditation in motion," in which the body takes over and spontaneously performs movements to release mental and bodily tension. This state is attained through gradually increasing both the intensity of meditation and the length of time poses are held.

Kundalini. This type of yoga blends postures and breathing exercises with Sanskrit chanting and meditation.

Poses are usually held much longer than in other types of yoga. The use of props allows students at all levels to progress safely and comfortably, although some people may find this style too exacting.

Kundalini yoga focuses more on the meditative side of yoga. Kundalini incorporates Sanskrit chanting, muscular contractions, meditation, and guided visualization to tap into a dormant energy force (pictured as a coiled serpent, the kundalini) at the base of the spine.

Integrative yoga therapy (not to be confused with integral yoga, which is described on page 338) is practiced in some hospitals and rehabilitation centers as a complement to standard Western medicine. Tailored to the individual, it uses yoga exercises to strengthen the mind–body connection and help people meet specific goals such as pain management, weight loss, recovery from surgery, smoking cessation, or spiritual growth.

Prenatal yoga classes allow pregnant women to move in ways that are safe and nurturing for both them and their growing babies. For women with diabetes, who are under pressure to keep blood sugar in extremely tight control to avoid birth defects in the baby and complications for themselves, the calming effects of doing yoga can be at least as important as the physical benefits. "Pregnancy was up there with the greatest challenges of my life," says Becky Rosen, 33, who has had Type 1 diabetes for 15 years. "During my first pregnancy, I was extremely exhausted and would get consumed with worries if my blood sugar went out of the really tight range. The second time around, a friend introduced me to prenatal yoga. I was so much calmer as a result. Even 10 minutes of breathing and stretching exercises in the morning helped me feel more grounded and less stressed."

These are just a few of the types of yoga classes that you may find in your area. In some areas, you may also find classes in "chair yoga" for people in wheelchairs or people who have trouble moving or working comfortably on the floor. Sometimes, there are special classes for couples or classes just for people who are overweight.

Finding the right class

To find the right yoga class for you, start by asking around for personal recommendations. Mention that you're looking for a yoga class in casual conversation; you'll probably be surprised by how many coworkers, friends, and acquaintances do or have done yoga and can either recommend or steer you away from certain classes or instructors. Beyond that, see what your community has to offer. Most metropolitan areas have a number of yoga studios. If you live in a small town or suburban area, try your local YMCA, health clubs, or community centers for yoga classes.

As you examine your options, think about what you'd like to get out of the class. Are you looking for an aerobic workout? Or would you prefer more gentle stretching and breath awareness exercises? Class brochures or listings should give some indication of the difficulty level (gentle, beginner, moderate, or advanced) and focus of the class, but if it's not clear, call and ask. You may even want to speak directly with the teacher about the style of yoga he'll be teaching and whether the class would be a good match for someone at your fitness level. A good teacher will be willing to talk about the class and to point you in the right direction, even if it means referring you to another teacher.

If you're still not ready to sign up, ask about observing a class or even taking a trial class to see if you like it. If you have never done yoga or meditation before, you may find some of the exercises new and even a little strange at first, but you shouldn't feel embarrassed or highly uncomfortable. Most classes try to welcome and encourage newcomers. However, says Beryl Herrin, "If you try a yoga class, and it doesn't feel right or the teacher isn't really inspiring, don't give up on yoga; just look for another class."

There are some other practical matters to consider before signing up for any yoga class. Cost is one of them. Some private studios charge a lot more for classes than, say, the local rec center. But you may be willing to pay a little bit more if the private studio offers smaller class sizes, meaning you'll get more individual attention, or if you want to study with a particular teacher who has an excellent reputation. You also want to find out about the length of class and how often it meets. While on average yoga classes go for about an hour, some may be longer and others shorter. Some centers allow you to drop in or pay as you go, while others require you to sign up for a given number of sessions.

If you can't find a yoga class that suits you in your area, or if you'd prefer beginning at home, yoga videos offer an excellent—and inexpensive—alternative to live instruction. You may be able to find yoga videos at your public library or local video rental store, or you can try browsing Internet yoga sites and online bookstores and reading reviews of yoga videos to find one that sounds right for you. (A couple of places to start on the Internet: www.yogajournal.com and www.yogamusicvideo.com.)

At home or in class, dress for yoga in loose or stretchy, comfortable clothing that allows you to move easily. You may want to wear some layers, such as a leotard with a light sweatshirt over it, because some parts of class may be very active and get you sweating, while others are fairly stationary, leading you to cool down quickly.

Most yoga classes require you to bring a sticky mat (available for purchase online at www.gaiam.com and www.yoga.com, among others, at some yoga centers, and at some health-food stores for about $20–$25), and a few styles of yoga, such as iyengar, may also require additional props such as special ropes and blocks. Some yoga studios have sticky mats to borrow if you forget to bring your own or haven't purchased one yet, but since most yoga exercises are done barefoot, you run the risk of picking up a foot fungus if you use the communal mats.

People who have diabetes are often admonished never to go barefoot except in the bath or in bed. However, many yoga poses are difficult to perform or hold while wearing shoes or socks. If this is a problem for you, ask your yoga teacher about alternatives such as wearing nonslip socks. People with existing foot problems may also want to consult their health-care provider before doing yoga poses that put pressure on the feet. If you shower in a public locker room after yoga class, be sure to wear shower sandals or slippers to protect your feet, both from foot fungus and from any objects that may have fallen onto the floor.

Stretch, relax…and stay safe

Don't be shy about letting your yoga instructor know that you have diabetes. It may be necessary, especially when you're first starting out, to check your blood sugar during class. Be sure to always bring your blood glucose meter and glucose tablets with you to class; you may be surprised by how much even a gentle class may get your heart rate going from time to time, and if that happens, your blood sugar may drop. Don't hesitate to stop at any time during class to check your blood sugar.

To see how yoga affects your blood sugar level, you may want to follow the example of James O'Keefe, who has Type 2 diabetes and takes insulin. When he first began yoga classes, he checked his blood sugar level before, during, and after class for several weeks to look for a pattern. "I knew how to cut back on my insulin during aerobic exercise," O'Keefe said, "but it took me some time to figure out how yoga was affecting my blood sugar. It was interesting, because my sugar wouldn't drop during class, but it would stay lower than usual for a few hours afterward."

Just like other forms of exercise, yoga may necessitate an adjustment of insulin doses, meals, or snacks. A general rule in yoga is that it's best not to practice on a full stomach. "I explain to my students that doing yoga on a full stomach just makes it harder and less comfortable to move, because the body is putting so much energy into digestion," says Beryl Herrin. Depending on how yoga affects your blood sugar, though, you may find that you need to eat some form of carbohydrate 15–30 minutes before doing yoga. If so, Herrin recommends that you choose something on the lighter side, such as a few whole wheat crackers, that will keep your blood sugar up but won't weigh you down. "If you need to bring a few crackers or a light snack along to class, go ahead. It's better to stop and eat or drink something if you need to than to not try doing yoga at all," she says.

Because your body functions best when it's well hydrated, be sure to drink water before and after class, and bring a bottle of water to class with you if you sweat a lot or tend to get thirsty.

Perhaps the most important thing—for people with or without diabetes—to remember is to be gentle with yourself when you begin. Don't push or strain to get into a posture. Yoga is about the union of *your* mind and body; it doesn't matter what the person on the mat in front of you can do. "When I first started yoga, I pushed myself a lot," James O'Keefe recalls. "Yet it was when I wasn't trying to look good—when I just focused on breathing and stretching—that I could hold the asanas [postures] much better."

You'll feel better and lower your risk of injury and soreness if you take it easy at first and gradually work your muscles up to the state of a more experienced yoga student. "Listen to your own inner teacher," recommends Beryl Herrin. "You know intuitively how much energy to use and when to go easy."

Once you get started practicing yoga, you'll discover that its benefits aren't limited only to class time. Yoga's benefits are long-lasting, and yoga techniques are accessible at any time. The next time you feel your heart racing because you're angry or anxious about something, start to take deep, gentle breaths and see how it helps to calm you down. When you're stiff from sitting in front of your computer all day, get up and do some simple stretches. Standing in line at the grocery store, note whether you're holding any of your muscles tightly; if so, gently release them. Not only will practicing these yoga techniques make you feel better, but you also may find that by reducing your stress level, they help you keep your blood sugar in better control, too. Yoga—building connections between mind and body—is a great tool for anyone trying to successfully manage his diabetes. □

THE HIGH PRICE OF INACTIVITY

by Richard M. Weil, M.Ed., C.D.E.

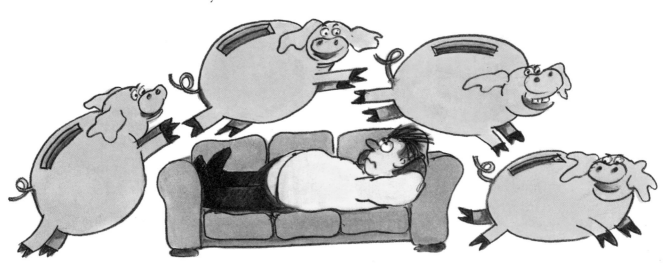

If you're like most Americans, you're concerned about the almighty dollar—how much comes in, how much goes out. If you watch every penny, you may allot very little money—or even none—to fitness. What you may not have considered, however, is how much it costs you to be sedentary. This article takes a look at both the costs of living an active lifestyle and the costs of *not* living an active lifestyle.

A nation of couch potatoes

The United States is currently experiencing an epidemic of inactivity. Less than 30% of American adults are active enough to gain any health benefits from physical activity. Another 30% are irregularly active—that is, they exercise less than 4–5 times per month—and 40% do no leisure-time physical activity at all. This trend toward inactivity in the United States has remained constant over the past 20 years, and there doesn't seem to be any indication that it's getting any better. According to the Centers for Disease Control and Prevention's National Health Interview Survey, the percentage of adults who spent most of their day sitting increased from 36.8% in 2000 to 39.9% in 2005; the percentage of adults who engaged in no leisure-time physical activity increased from 38.5% in 2000 to 40.0% in 2005; and perhaps most ominously, the percentage of adults who engaged in regular leisure-time physical activity decreased from 31.2% in 2000 to 29.7% in 2005.

America's inactivity epidemic persists in spite of widespread knowledge that an active lifestyle yields many health benefits. Regular physical activity can reduce your risk of high blood pressure and heart disease, alleviate symptoms of depression, prevent and control diabetes, and prevent some types of cancer, in addition to raising your general level of fitness.

How much does it take to keep you fit and healthy? The U.S. Surgeon General recommends doing 30 minutes of moderate-intensity activity (that makes you feel warm and slightly out of breath) 5–7 days per week. The activity can be done in one bout of 30 minutes or accumulated in two 15-minute bouts or three 10-minute bouts. The American College of Sports Medicine (ACSM) guidelines for developing and maintaining health and fitness are 3–5 days per week of continuous aerobic activity for 20–60 minutes per session. The ACSM also recommends resistance training at least two days a week that includes one set of 8–12 repetitions of 8–10 exercises that condition the major muscle groups.

The price of being sedentary

The alternative to getting regular physical activity—being sedentary—is expensive. According to research published in 1999 in the journal *Medicine and Science in Sports and Exercise*, sedentary lifestyles cost the United States an estimated $76.6 billion per year in direct medical costs (such as doctor visits, hospital stays, medication, diabetes supplies and devices, and other medical services that require direct payment of money). The $76.6 billion amount is based on the belief that physical activity reduces the incidence and helps manage the complications of certain diseases. For instance, physical activity can reduce the risk of heart attack by helping to prevent coronary heart disease, which is caused by a narrowing of the coronary arteries that feed the heart. Coronary heart disease is the number one killer of both men and women in the United States, and costs the nation $111.8 billion every year in direct and indirect medical costs. But since physically active people have a lower rate of heart disease, it is estimated that if the more than 88 million couch potatoes in the United States were active, the nation would save $8.9 billion each year on direct medical costs of coronary heart disease. Likewise, if all people with high blood pressure were active, the savings could exceed $2 billion per year.

Similarly, if all people with diabetes were active, the savings in direct medical costs would be approximately $6.4 billion. Diabetes costs the nation a staggering $132 billion per year in total medical costs, and scientists suggest that this number is an underestimate because it omits intangibles such as pain and suffering, care provided by nonpaid caregivers, and areas of healthcare where people with diabetes probably use services at higher rates than people without diabetes, (e.g., dental care, optometry care, and the use of licensed dietitians).

Although the price of inactivity for all Americans has not been updated since the original research in 1999, a study published in 2004 in the journal *American Journal of Preventive Medicine* reported that total health plan expenditures attributable to physical inactivity among members of a large health plan, Blue Cross Blue Shield of Minnesota, were 83.6 million dollars!

What all this means for your pocketbook is that you could save between $330 and $1,053 per year in direct medical costs if you were physically active. These are real numbers and may even be underestimated, according to research published in 2000 in *The Physician and Sportsmedicine*. With numbers like these, can you afford *not* to be active?

When you break down the direct medical costs of a sedentary lifestyle, one of the largest chunks is annual sales of prescription drugs, which, in the United States in 2001, exceeded $140 billion. Although no data exist on precisely how much money would be saved on drugs if all sedentary Americans were active, what is known is that doses of medicines prescribed for conditions such as diabetes, high blood pressure, and coronary heart disease can all be reduced once an individual increases his physical activity.

If you're not a believer, consider this: People with diabetes spend more than $7 billion per year on medicines. In one study published in 1999 in the journal *Diabetes Care*, researchers asked adults with diabetes to either walk or bike and do stretching exercises for 50–60 minutes per day, 4–6 days per week, for one month. At the end of the study, 16% of study participants taking insulin and 26% of participants taking diabetes pills had their treatment switched to diet and exercise therapy alone. For those who needed to remain on insulin, their total units per day were reduced by a whopping 60%, and in 22% of the people who needed to remain on pills, their doses were reduced or replaced with medicines with milder effects. Cutting back on medicines or stopping them altogether could add up to some big savings—maybe even billions of dollars each year on a national level, and certainly hundreds on an individual level.

Regular exercise can also lower the costs of another expensive problem: obesity. More than 60% of American adults are overweight or obese (approximately 80% of people with Type 2 diabetes are overweight), and the total medical costs of overweight and obesity are $99.2 billion each year. (By comparison, cigarette smoking costs only $47.6 billion.) Whether you do 20–60 minutes of vigorous exercise several days a week or accumulate 30 minutes of moderate physical activity throughout the day on most days, regular physical activity can both help manage body weight and make you healthier even if you don't lose weight.

Although there's no research to show the precise dollar amount of medical savings for overweight people who are active instead of sedentary, research published in 2005 in the journal *Preventing Chronic Disease* showed that physical inactivity, overweight, and obesity were associated with 27% of national health care charges. Since it is known that an active lifestyle reduces many of the costly complications of obesity (such as high blood pressure, heart disease, diabetes, and gallbladder disease), it stands to reason that an active lifestyle is going to put more money in your pocket.

You may be convinced now that being sedentary is pricey, but what about the price of increasing your physical activity? Doesn't that cost money too?

The price of being active

The price of physical activity is largely what you make it. You can spend a lot of money (after all, the fitness industry is a multi-billion dollar business) or you can spend very little.

If you're looking for fitness on the cheap, look no further than walking outdoors. All you need is a good pair of walking shoes—which you can find at a shoe or sporting goods store for less than

$100—and away you go. You can walk almost anywhere, the risk of injury is very low (but be sure to check your feet daily for blisters and abrasions), you already know how to do it, and it works. If you prefer indoor walking, check your local mall for a walking club.

If you're just starting a walking program, try the technique of walking for five minutes in one direction then turning around and walking five minutes back to your starting point. When your 10-minute round-trip walk starts feeling easy, increase it to six minutes out and six minutes back. Increase your distance by no more than 10% a week.

If you doubt for any reason that walking counts as "real" exercise, the Diabetes Prevention Program (DPP) has provided evidence that it does. In the DPP, men and women who walked 30 minutes per day, every day, and lost 5% to 7% of their body weight reduced their risk of developing diabetes by 58%. (If you consider that diabetes costs $132 billion dollars a year in medical costs, then a reduction of 58% comes in at over $76 billion dollars in reduced health-care costs if people walk and lose some weight). In another study, retired men who walked two or more miles per day, compared to men who walked less than one mile per day, were almost twice as likely to be alive at the end of a 12-year follow-up period.

You won't be alone if you select walking as your activity of choice. According to the National Health Interview Survey, walking is the most popular physical activity in the United States, with nearly 45% of adults reporting they walk for exercise, followed by gardening, stretching, weight lifting, biking, and jogging, most of which can also be done at little expense.

Another cheap option for aerobic fitness is a jump rope. Start with just 5 minutes the first few times because your calves can get very sore if you haven't jumped rope in a while. It's a good idea to stretch your calves before and after you jump.

Aerobic exercise machines

If you're willing to spend some money on aerobic fitness, there's plenty of exercise equipment for purchase. The most popular machines these days are treadmills, followed by stationary bikes (recumbent and upright), steppers, and ellipticals (which look like cross-country ski machines). Making a comeback are rowers and mini trampolines. Since prices vary, shop around, and keep your budget in mind. But don't forget that when you spend money on fitness, you're spending money on your health.

All the machines burn lots of calories and will improve your health and fitness (if you use them regularly, of course), so it comes down to other factors when deciding which type to purchase. Here are some tips to help you decide.

■ Make your selection based on comfort and ease of operation. Try each machine for 10–15 minutes at the store or at your gym. If it feels natural and comfortable, you're more likely to use it.

■ Equipment should be well-built and sturdy. It shouldn't shake, rattle, or roll, or be unusually noisy.

■ Warranties vary. They may cover features and components from 90 days to three years, depending on the machine's quality. Look for in-home labor warranties (who fixes it if it breaks?) and ask if the warranties can be extended.

■ Make sure the machine will fit into your home and won't disturb your neighbors. Treadmills have motors, so they may not be suitable for apartment living.

■ Don't let the salesperson sell you all the bells and whistles if you're looking only for the basics.

■ If you're worried about motivation or would like to improve your walking, select a treadmill. They are the most popular machines, and people tend to use them at home more often than other exercise machines. Prices start at around $300, although top-quality models can cost as much as $3,500 or more.

■ Select a stationary bike if you prefer to sit while you exercise; have a vascular, muscular, bone, or joint problem that prevents you from doing standing (weight-bearing) exercise; have an outdoor bike and would like to stick with riding even when the weather's bad; or simply like to bike. Choose a recumbent bike if you need back support. A recumbent bike might also be more comfortable than an upright bike if you have neuropathy in your feet. Depending on features, a stationary bike can cost you as little as $75 or as much as $2,000 or more.

■ Steppers and elliptical machines are more challenging than bikes or treadmills in terms of balance, coordination, and the difficulty of the workout—even at mild intensities, and particularly for beginners. You may like the challenge, but just be sure to try the machine for 10–15 minutes before you purchase. You can pay as little as $45 for a "mini stepper," or over $2,000 for a top professional stair-climbing machine; elliptical machines range from $90 for a bare-bones model to $3,200 and up for commercial-quality models. Convertible elliptical/stepper machines are also an option, starting in the $200–$300 range.

■ Rowers provide terrific upper-body and aerobic exercise, but using them is very challenging. Many of the machines are close to the ground, so make sure you can get down to them. They can also be tough on the back, so make sure your back is healthy before using one of these machines. Prices for rowers start around $100 and go up to over $1,000 for gym-quality models.

■ Mini trampolines are loads of fun and will work to improve your balance, coordination, and stamina. If you want a weight-bearing activity that will give you a good aerobic workout, choose a mini tramp. Prices for good-quality trampolines start at $50 and go up to $150.

Resistance exercise

Resistance exercise is good for your health (and your wallet), too. Any exercise that causes your muscles to contract against external resistance for the purpose of building strength, tone, and mass is resistance exercise. Weight machines, dumbbells, rubber tubing or bands, and calisthenics (such as push-ups) all count.

What's so great about resistance exercise? It builds muscle, and muscle is the engine in your body that burns calories and helps maintain your metabolic rate. The more muscle you have, the stronger you will be, and the better your blood sugar control may be, at any age.

In a recent study published in *Diabetes Care,* men and women from 60 to 80 years of age and with Type 2 diabetes were divided into two different groups: a weight-loss group, and a weight-loss and weight- lifting group. The idea was to see which group had a greater improvement in blood glucose control as measured by the glycosylated hemoglobin (HbA_{1c}) test. By the end of six months, the weight-lifting group had improved their HbA_{1c} three times more than the group that lost weight but did not lift weights.

That's good news, and the other good news is that it doesn't have to cost you all that much to do resistance exercise. Exercise tubes or bands are cheap, versatile, easily stored and transported, and as effective as dumbbells; if you use them regularly you'll get stronger and more toned. A complete set of exercise tubes will set you back about $20.

Feeling nostalgic for an old-fashioned calisthenics routine? Look for a copy of the out-of-print book *Royal Canadian Air Force Exercise Plans for Physical Fitness.* You can find it on the Internet at any of the Web sites of popular booksellers. It's a tough workout, but a classic.

If you feel like spending a bit of money on resistance exercise, there are plenty of opportunities to lay down some cash. Dumbbells will run you anywhere from $0.35 to over $1 per pound. A complete starter set, with a weight lifting bench, will

set you back $100 to $350 (not a king's ransom considering the health benefits). Or, if you like, you could buy a multistation weight-lifting unit, like the kind you see on TV or in sporting goods stores. Multistation machines are versatile (they have lots of exercises), and will set you back $150 to $2,500, depending on quality.

Joining a fitness center

Yet another option for exercise is joining a fitness center or health club. Among the advantages of belonging to a center are that it gets you out of the house and gives you the opportunity to meet new people (and possible exercise partners); there's a lot of equipment; there are classes and fitness trainers; and some centers even have swimming pools. A fitness center will cost you anywhere from $250 to $2,500 per year. If you're a no-frills kind of person and looking for a gym with just the basics, then a low-end center may be just right. If you want properly trained instructors, locker rooms with amenities, lots of classes, the latest equipment, and a clean, well-maintained center, then you'll probably pay more. Just keep those savings on health in mind as you get more physically active and fit!

Tennis, anyone?

Have you considered sports or outdoor activities, like hiking or riding a bike, as a way to stay fit? When's the last time you played tennis or badminton or threw a softball in the backyard? It might sound corny, but the old days when you were active may be calling to you. In fact, it might take no more than a small investment in a ball and a glove or racket to get you moving again. If you get ambitious, you might like to take a lesson to perfect your game or just get your old form back. It could cost you anywhere from less than $100 to a few hundred dollars for gear and a lesson. And when's the last time you spent an active weekend outdoors? Maybe it's time for a hike or a biking excursion. Once again, the dollar cost of pursuing active pastimes sure makes sense in light of how expensive being sedentary is.

Follow the money

Negotiating finances can be tough, but when you consider spending money on an active lifestyle, it's not just the health savings that you ought to think about. Think too about how you spend the rest of your money, and see if there isn't some way you can justify a few dollars for health and fitness. For instance, how much money do you spend on cable television each month? (While you're thinking about it, keep in mind that women who watch TV for two hours or more per day are 23% more likely to be obese than women who don't watch TV, and men who watch TV for 21–40 hours per week are 33% more likely to get diabetes than men who watch TV for 2–10 hours per week). How much do you spend on public transportation each month, and how far do you go when you ride the bus or take a cab? Could you walk those 10 blocks instead of paying for it? Have a look at your budget and see if there aren't a couple of items that could enter into the negotiation for some fitness dollars.

Remember, your health depends on it, and there may be savings you hadn't considered.

Whether you think of it as the economics of fitness or of sedentary living, it makes all the sense in the world, financially and health-wise, to become active and stay that way. There are lots of options for physical activity; some will cost you next to nothing, others will set you back a few dollars, but either way, it's worth the expense. There's no more important time than now to begin an active lifestyle, and in the end, it may even save you a few bucks. □

IMPROVING YOUR BALANCE

by Richard M. Weil, M.Ed., C.D.E.

Any physical education teacher will tell you that a fitness program has three main elements: Frequency (how often you exercise), Intensity (how hard it should feel, which is usually "warm and slightly out of breath"), and Time (how long you exercise for), otherwise known by the acronym FIT. Within FIT are the components of fit-ness—muscular strength and endurance, aerobic endurance, and flexibility—but there is more to fitness than just strength, endurance, and flexibility. Balance is a factor too, and although many people probably take it for granted, for some, poor balance can be a real obstacle to regular physical activity.

Keeping your balance

According to Webster's dictionary, balance is "an even distribution of weight ensuring stability." That sounds pretty straightforward, at least when applied to a seesaw or a stationary object such as a table or chair. But what about a human being, who not only stands but also walks, runs, skips, or dances on two legs? How does a person standing still manage not to fall over—the way a two-legged chair or table would? How does a person stay upright while walking?

The key to how human beings stand on two legs and balance so effortlessly is the brain. Think of your body as an exquisitely tuned watch that ticks with precision. Your brain is the central timekeeper with a motor and little gears that keep your body running day and night. Just as the inner workings of a watch constantly send signals to the hands of the watch to keep them moving, your brain constantly sends electrical and chemical signals to all your organs and muscles to keep them working.

But there are differences between your body and a timepiece. For one, a watch only sends signals in one direction—from the gears to the hands—to tick precisely. You send signals in two directions: Your brain sends signals to the muscles and the organs, and the muscles and organs send signals back to the brain to let it know how and what you're doing. This is called a *feedback loop*, and your body has many of them.

The feedback loops for balance use the central nervous system (CNS) as their pathway. The CNS is a complex network of nerves that start in your brain and travel down your spinal cord. At various points along your spine, the nerves exit and connect to the muscles and organs that make your body work. For instance, nerves that leave your spinal cord near your neck control your lungs and help you breathe. Nerves that leave the spinal cord in your lower back connect to muscles in your legs and help you walk.

Say you're sitting in a chair and you decide to get up and take a walk to the other side of the room. The first thing that happens is your brain thinks about what muscles need to be recruited to help you go. Once your brain thinks about it, it sends electrical signals through the nerves to the muscles that will help you rise and start walking. If all goes well, you stand up, walk smoothly to your destination, and once you get there, you stop. This sounds simple enough, until you ask the following questions: How did your brain know from moment to moment where you were in the room (your orientation) so that it could direct your muscles in the right direction? How did it know when you arrived on the other side of the room so that it could signal your muscles to stop? And how were you able to walk smoothly, in balance, without falling over?

All three questions have a similar answer: The feedback loop that your brain relies on for orientation and direction, muscle control, and balance is dependent on three very important physiological systems. They are called visual, vestibular, and somatosensory senses.

Visual senses

As it suggests, visual senses refer to your eyes and what you see. As you walk across a room, your eyes see where you want to go and feed that information to your brain. Your brain then sends signals to all the muscles necessary to keep you upright and moving in the right direction. Your brain must constantly make corrections in the muscles to keep you on course; otherwise you might wobble, drift, or simply fall down. It does that by constantly processing the feedback from the eyes.

What if you closed your eyes? Well, one thing the brain would do is rely on sound. Imagine that you got up to turn off your TV but you kept your eyes closed. You could make it to the TV because you could hear the sound, or auditory input for the brain. You might not be as steady on your feet because you've eliminated vision, which is one of the most important sensory inputs you have, but even with your eyes closed or the lights out, you could make it if you could hear the sound.

Visual and auditory input are powerful sensory inputs that help the brain make lots of decisions about where you are, how you move, and how well you balance. But what if you eliminated sight and sound?

Somatosensory senses

Even in a pitch-black room without any sound, you could, if you needed to, make it across the room. You would use your hands, your arms, your legs, your feet, your toes, your elbows, and any other body part necessary to "feel" your way across the room. You'd certainly go slowly, but you could do it. You could do it because muscles in your body have special receptors called *proprioceptors* embedded in them that continuously tell your brain the position of your joints and muscles, as well as your position in space. The complex feedback loop that allows for communication between the brain and the proprioceptors throughout the body is called *proprioception* or *somatosensory sensation*.

Proprioception is stimuli produced within the body (particularly the muscles) that provides you with a sense of position, movement, and force (or speed). Even if you didn't have anything to touch

while walking across the room in the dark, you'd be able to do it without falling down, as long as you had proprioception. An experiment you can do to test your balance and proprioception is to stand up, close your eyes, and touch your nose with one finger (but don't try this if you have balance disturbances or occasionally lose your balance). If your proprioception is good, you will "feel" how quickly your arm is moving, and you will be able to touch your finger right to the tip of your nose. You might be a bit off balance the first two or three tries because you've eliminated visual senses, but once you get used to the dark, you will be able to touch your nose and still keep good balance. Your body learns how to do this because your muscles constantly send feedback to your brain with information about where your body is in space.

Proprioception and balance for athletes, musicians, and anyone else who needs to perform at peak levels is a critical skill. Proprioception can improve with practice so that you "pattern" the communication between your brain and the muscles. For instance, a tennis player who practices thousands of serves each day gets to the point where the muscles and the brain perform seamlessly to make the ball go to the proper spot. Any deviation in the movement and the athlete will "feel" that it's not right, perhaps even before the ball lands on the other side of the net. A pianist who has practiced Beethoven hundreds of times knows precisely where his fingers should be on the keyboard because the movements have been so well practiced and coordinated between the brain and the fingers. One could even make the argument that if you made a beeline to your stationary bike every morning for your daily workout, you would pattern that movement too, so that it would get easier to do as you did more of it. Some movement experts call this "muscle memory." Proprioceptors make it happen.

Vestibular senses

Now, what if you were to keep your hands in your pockets and try to make your way across that same dark, quiet room? Without proprioceptors from your hand and arm muscles signaling your brain or visual and auditory sensation from your eyes or ears, could you still walk (or stand still for that matter), and still maintain your balance? You bet. What your brain would do is rely on the most sensitive balance mechanism of all. It's called the vestibular apparatus, and it all happens inside your head (inside your ears to be precise).

The way it works is that inside your inner ear is

STORK

The stork is one of the simplest exercises to improve balance.

1. Stand on one leg, arms at your side, shoulders relaxed.

2. Try to balance for 30 seconds. Repeat 2–3 times on each leg every day. Over the next few weeks, try to work up to 2 minutes.

3. Hint: Try not to "grab" the floor with your toes of the foot that's on the ground. Relax your muscles and you'll have more success.

4. To make the stork more challenging, try swinging your arms as if you were running. That will throw you slightly off balance and you will need to make corrections to maintain your balance. You can hold bottles of water in each hand for extra weight for even more of a challenge. Work those proprioceptors!

5. Another challenge is to try to "spell" your name with the foot in the air.

6. Yet another way to make the stork more challenging is to fold a bath towel over several times so it's four or six layers thick. Place it on the floor and stand in the center of it. It will be unstable because it's soft, but that's the idea because you want your proprioceptors to really work hard to improve your balance and strengthen your muscles.

7. For the most challenging stork of all, try any of the above with your eyes closed.

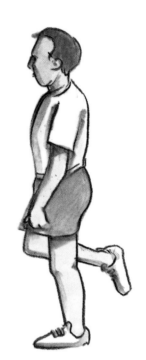

MARCHING

1. Hold on to a sturdy chair for balance and lift your right knee up toward your chest, then lower it to floor. The left knee can be bent slightly. Repeat 10–15 times with right leg, then do it with the left leg.

2. You can progress to touching the chair with one finger for balance, not holding on at all, and finally doing the exercise with your eyes closed.

3. For more of a challenge, alternate the marching between the left and right leg instead of doing a set with one leg.

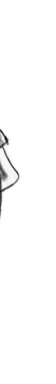

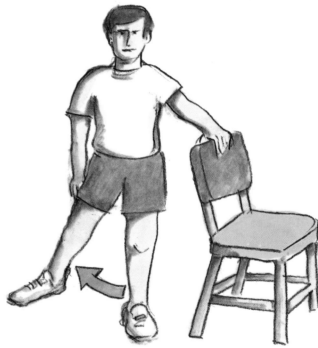

SIDE LEG RAISE

1. Hold on to a sturdy chair for balance and lift your right leg out to the side. The left knee can be bent slightly. Repeat 10–15 times with the right leg, then do the left leg.

2. You can progress to touching the chair with one finger for balance, not holding on at all, and finally doing the exercise with your eyes closed.

NOSE TOUCHER

1. Stand with your right leg approximately 24 inches in front of your left, bend your knees slightly, and try to touch your nose with one finger. The more in line your feet are with each other, the more challenging this will be. Repeat 10 times.

2. Switch your left leg to the front. Repeat 10 times.

3. Once you can do it well with either leg in front of the other, try this with your eyes closed.

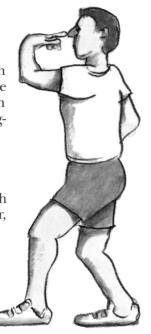

HEEL RAISES

1. Hold on to a sturdy chair for balance, rise up onto your toes, then lower your heels back to the ground. Repeat 10–15 times.

2. You can progress to touching the chair with one finger for balance, not holding on at all, and finally doing the exercise with your eyes closed.

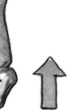

WALK A STRAIGHT LINE

1. Look for a straight line on the floor (such as a line of floor tiles) and try to walk along it. The key here is to land with one foot directly in front of the other and also to land on your heel first.

2. For variety, try walking with arms extended out and then relaxed at your sides.

3. For more of a challenge, try walking forward to one end and then backward to the other.

4. For even more challenge, try walking with your eyes closed.
Only walk with eyes closed if someone is there to assist you.

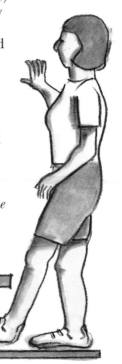

SIT-STANDS

1. Sit on the edge of a sturdy chair and try to stand up without swinging your arms forward, then sit back down slowly. Repeat 10 times.

2. If you need help, go ahead and let your arms reach forward for balance, but over time, try to stand up without the assistance of your arms.

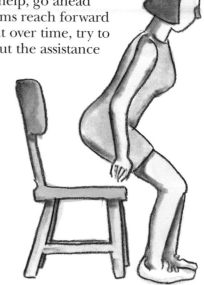

STEP-UPS

1. Stand in front of a staircase and step up with your right foot, then up with your left, then back down with your right, then back down with your left. Repeat 10 times.

2. If you need a little support, hold on gently to the railing, or better yet, just touch the wall with your fingertip and you'll be amazed at how much balance that gives you. Proprioception really works!

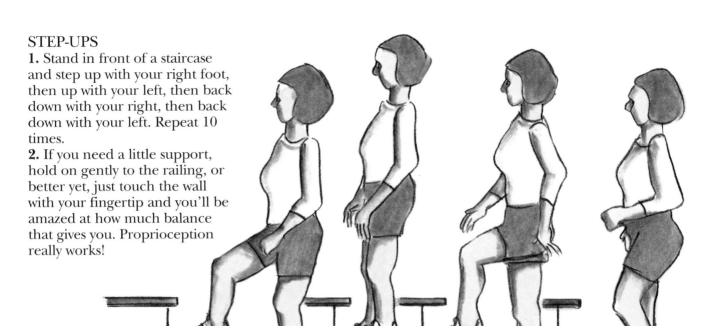

BIRDDOG

You can do this one in bed.

1. Start on your hands and knees.

2. Basic: Contract your abdominal muscles and lift one arm, then the other. Hold 2–5 seconds. Then lift one leg, then the other. Hold 2–5 seconds. Repeat each 5–10 times.

3. Advanced: Contract your abdominal muscles and lift one arm and the opposite leg simultaneously, hold 2–5 seconds, switch sides, and repeat. Repeat 5–10 times each side.

FOUR-SQUARE STEP TEST

This is an advanced exercise. *Only do this if someone is there to assist you.*

1. Lay two towels on the floor crossing each other as illustrated.

2. Stand in square number 1 facing square number 2.

3. Step forward into square 2, then sideways into square 3, backward into square 4, sideways to square 1, sideways to square 4, forward to square 3, sideways to square 2, and backward to square 1.

4. Move slowly at first until you get the hang of it. As your skill improves, you can move faster.

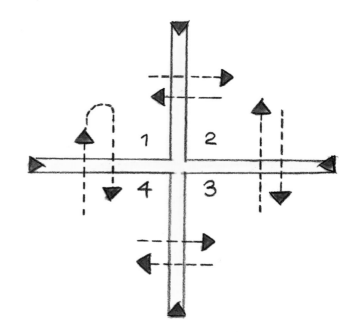

WOBBLE BOARD EXERCISES

Using a wobble board is an excellent way to help you increase your balance. The board is a wooden or plastic disk with a rise at the bottom that makes the board unstable. What you do is stand on it and try to balance.

1. Starting position: Stand with both feet on the board and either hold on to the back of a chair or touch a chair or the wall with one finger for balance if you need it.

2. Side to side. Using slow and controlled movement, rock from side to side without letting the front or back of the board to touch the floor. Keep your torso upright and your neck, shoulders, and arms relaxed. Try to do the exercise for 30–60 seconds.

3. Front to back. Same as side to side except you try for front to back.

4. Once you get the hang of it, you can try the exercises without holding on or touching the wall, and when you get really good you can try it with your eyes closed. *Do not try this with eyes closed unless you have assistance.*

5. Another challenge is to toss a ball with someone else while standing on the board.

Wobble boards can be purchased from nefitco.com; go to www.nefitco.com/balance.html to see images of wobble boards and other balance products, or call (800) 452-0980. They are also available from Orthopedic Physical Therapy Products; go to www.optp.com to view products or call (888) 819-0121.

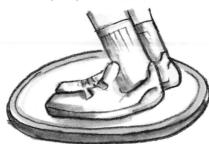

FOAM BALANCE PAD EXERCISES

Foam balance pads work like wobble boards because they are unstable surfaces, so they challenge your balance when you stand on them.

1. Starting position: Stand with both feet on the pad and either hold on to the back of a chair or touch a chair or the wall with one finger for balance if you need it.

2. Shift your weight from side to side then front to back without having feet leave the pad.

3. More advanced: March by lifting one foot then the other.

4. Try to balance on one foot and do any of the variations of the stork exercise.

5. For the most challenge of all, try this with your eyes closed. *Do not try this with your eyes closed unless you have assistance.*

Foam balance pads can be purchased from nefitco.com; go to www.nefitco.com/balance. html to see images of pads and other balance products, or call (800) 452-0980.

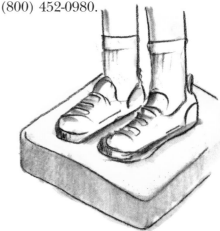

a complex system of canals and receptors. The canals are filled with special fluid, and when your head moves, the fluid shifts (like water in a drinking glass). The shifting of the fluid stimulates receptors that send signals to the brain to let it know the position of your head (upright or bent forward, backward, or to one side), the movement of the head (if you are shaking it or nodding), or if you are accelerating (for example, if you are sprinting, on a roller coaster, on an elevator, or on a ship at sea). The system is exquisitely precise and reliable and helps you keep your balance even when the other senses are diminished or absent. Of course, sometimes it is too sensitive and you get motion sickness.

Upsetting the balance

Why is it that some people, gymnasts and tightrope walkers, for instance, can balance with the greatest of ease, while others can barely walk a straight line without a wobble? It's hard to say for sure, but certainly genetics plays a part. Perhaps the prima ballerinas of the world are blessed with proprioceptors that are better tuned than the rest of us, and with hard work, they excel at balance.

On the other side of the coin, there are pathological conditions that can cause balance disturbances. Bacterial or viral infections in the inner ear can cause vestibular problems, and so can head injuries and certain drugs. Neurological conditions like Parkinson disease and dystonia are movement disorders that interfere with how the brain sends signals to the muscles, which can cause balance disturbances.

Aging is a factor, too. As we age, our strength, coordination, vision, hearing, and reflexes all start to diminish, and this can lead to problems with balance. In fact, about one-third of individuals 65 or older fall each year, and research shows that this may be due to a decrease in proprioception and somatosensory input to the brain.

Complications of diabetes can also cause balance disturbances. For instance, peripheral neuropathy in the feet can cause a loss of sensation, which will interfere with proprioception and balance. In a study of physical disability among older U.S. adults with diabetes, researchers found that diabetes in women over age 60 was associated with slower walking speed, de-creased balance, and an increased risk of falling.

Improving your balance

The good news is that balance can improve. Exercises designed to improve balance are relatively simple to do, require little or no equipment, can be done at home, and best of all, they work. In one study, researchers found that falls decreased by 11% in people given an exercise and fall-prevention program. In another study, the number of falls and fall-related injuries decreased by 35% after training.

Still other research examined the effects of placing vibrating insoles into the shoes of elderly people (with an average age of 73) then asking them to stand still for 30 seconds with their eyes closed and their hands at their sides. The researchers measured how much the subjects swayed, then compared the results to how much they swayed when they did not have the insoles in. (Measuring swaying is a standard method of measuring balance.) Interestingly, they found that there was less sway when the insoles were in than when they were not. The researchers believe the vibrations from the insoles stimulated the proprioceptors in the feet, which in turn gave the brain feedback so that the brain could make corrections in the muscles to improve balance. This is interesting research and may one day be one answer to the problem of loss of balance in people as they age.

In the meantime, the trick to improving your balance is to challenge your senses with creative exercises. Try to do balance exercises every day, because the benefits only last as long you do the exercises. If you stay consistent, you should see improvements in just a few weeks. The series of balance exercises that follow can be done in your own home, and most require no equipment or only simple household items.

Balance may not seem like it's that important, but it plays a critical role in how you move and how you function. Without balance, it's tough to move around and to pursue the active lifestyle that can improve your health and your diabetes management. Good balance, good health, and good fitness to you! □

STRETCHING

by Richard Weil, M.Ed., C.D.E.

Dogs do it. Cats do it. Even most human beings do it. Stretch, that is. You may do it every morning before you get out of bed, periodically throughout the day when you get up from a chair or get out of your car, or only when something's bothering you, like a sore back. Sometimes stretching is involuntary, like when you yawn, but most of the time it's done intentionally, to loosen up. A good stretch can help you unwind, relax, and clear your head. It will limber up your tight muscles after a tough workout or a long day at the office. And sometimes it just plain feels good.

But what do you really know about stretching? Should you do it before or after exercise? Does it prevent injuries? What's the best technique? Will it help with diabetes control? Should you do it at all? We'll stretch your mind in this article by answering all of these questions and more.

Flexibility

There are at least three main components of fitness: endurance, strength, and flexibility. In fitness terms, flexibility is the ability to move your joints through a range of motion without straining the muscles. In practical terms, it's the ability to reach up into a high cupboard without shoulder pain, scratch your back anywhere it itches, bend over and tie your shoes with ease, or walk a mile without calf tightness.

To some degree, how flexible you are is genetic; some people are just born with more flexible muscles and joints than others. Your degree of flexibility also varies naturally from joint to joint. It's possible, for example, that your hips are genetically looser than your lower back. Your flexibility in a given joint may change if, for example, an injury leads to scarring in the joint.

Your brain also has a lot to do with how flexible you are. The brain controls everything in your body, from thinking to breathing to movement, and flexibility, too. It does this via the nervous system—a complex network of nerves originating at the brain and ending, among other places, at specialized receptors in the muscles and joints called golgi tendon organs and muscle spindles. These receptors are sensitive to how much the muscles are stretched. If you stretch a muscle too quickly (for example, if you lunge for something or bend over too quickly to lift a box off the floor), the receptors sense the stress and instantly fire off a signal to the brain to tighten up the muscle to protect it against injury. Likewise, if you've got a lot of stress in your life (if you're angry about something or overworked or frustrated because your blood glucose levels aren't cooperating), your brain is stressed too, so it sends signals to the muscles to tighten up. All of this adds up to muscular tension and tightness, but it doesn't mean you can't do anything about it. Stretching can increase flexibility both through its effects on your muscles and joints and through its ability to calm the mind if done in a relaxing manner.

Stretching techniques

There are three main stretching techniques: static, ballistic, and proprioceptive neuromuscular facilitation.

Static stretching is slow, relaxed stretching. The proper technique is to stretch the muscle (or muscle group) until you feel the mildest bit of tension, hold that position until the muscle feels looser, then push just a bit further. The amount of time it takes for muscles to feel looser is different for different people, so rather than counting to 20 or 30, focus on how your muscles feel, and stretch them until they feel looser. For most people, static stretching is the most practical way to stretch. It's easy to learn, easy to do, and it works.

For the most effective static stretch, do a brief warm-up (3 to 5 minutes) before stretching. At the gym, you might use an exercise bike or treadmill or other aerobic equipment at a light intensity to warm up your muscles before you stretch. At home, take an easy 5-minute walk to get some blood in your legs, then do your stretches.

Ballistic stretching involves using repetitive bouncing motions to rapidly stretch muscles and tendons. Although some athletes are trained to stretch in this manner, most fitness professionals discourage this type of movement because of the risk of muscle strain.

Proprioceptive neuromuscular facilitation (PNF) is a stretching technique in which you push the limb against resistance—usually another person—but the person or object does not allow your limb to move. Essentially you create an isometric contraction where there is muscular tension but no movement. You hold the push for 5 seconds, then relax for 5 seconds, then start to push again.

The more times you repeat this, the more the tension in the muscles releases so that you can stretch a little further. PNF works by fooling the brain into thinking your muscles are looser than they are so that the brain releases muscular tension. It works because the isometric contraction shortens the muscle, which shortens and relaxes the muscle spindle (the specialized receptor mentioned earlier), and when that happens, the brain gets a signal from the spindle that the muscle is shorter and relaxed, so the brain decreases the tension in the muscle and you can stretch further. It's a neat little trick that has been used by movement professionals and athletes for decades.

PNF technique is considered the most effective, followed by static, and then ballistic. The drawback to PNF is that it usually requires two people and one of them has to be familiar with the technique. But it can be learned and there are resources that can help if you are interested.

Benefits of stretching

Most people agree that stretching feels good, but does it actually do any good? It's always been the mantra that you should stretch before and after exercise to prevent injury, but there's virtually no research to prove it. In fact, in a couple of special studies called meta-analyses (where large numbers of studies pertaining to a specific topic are reviewed), stretching and injury prevention was investigated and the conclusion was that stretching before exercise does not reduce the risk of injury.

In another meta-analysis, this time about stretching and prevention of muscular soreness, the research showed that stretching does not prevent muscular soreness.

Despite the lack of evidence that stretching can prevent injury or muscular soreness, I don't recommend writing it off. Feeling good may be good enough. When you're stressed or tense or your back or neck is stiff from sitting too long at the computer or helping your neighbor move furniture, a stretch may be just what the doctor ordered. Stretching also helps you tune in to your body, so you pay attention to how you feel rather than pushing through pain or forcing yourself beyond your limits. Although it's not been proven conclusively by research, many people report an improved sense of well-being and an increase in energy as the result of tuning in to their muscles. Not only that, but if tight muscles prevent you from being physically active, a stretch might be just the thing to help you get started or keep you moving.

Stretching Sampler

Stretching is most effective after a brief warm-up, but there's really no bad time to stretch.

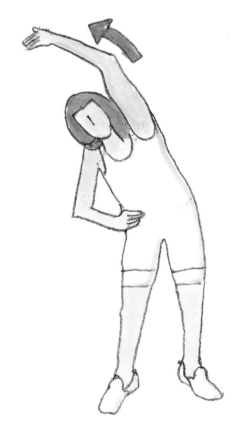

EVERYDAY STRETCHES

SIDE BEND
Stand with legs shoulder-width apart, toes pointing forward, and knees slightly bent. Place one hand on your hip and reach the other hand straight up, toward the ceiling. Slowly bend to the side, toward the hand that's on your hip. Repeat on the other side.

TORSO ROTATION

Stand 12–24 inches in front of a wall with your back to the wall. With feet shoulder-width apart and toes pointing forward, slowly turn your torso toward the wall until you can place both hands on the wall at shoulder height. Turn in one direction and then the other.

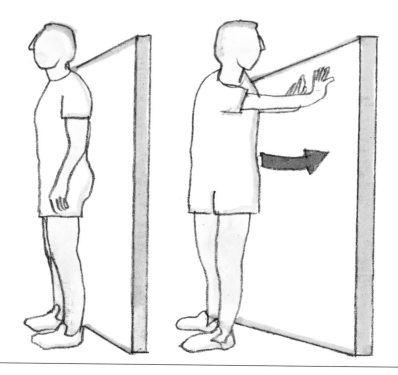

FORWARD BEND

Start in a standing position with legs shoulder-width apart and toes pointing forward. Keeping the knees slightly bent, bend forward from the hips until you feel a slight stretch in the backs of your legs. Let your head and arms hang freely, and don't bounce.

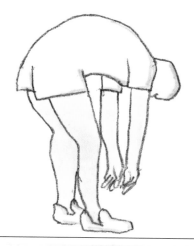

TOTAL BODY STRETCH

Lie on your back and extend your arms overhead. Reach your arms and legs in opposite directions as far as is comfortable. Hold for several seconds then relax. This stretch can also be done in a standing position.

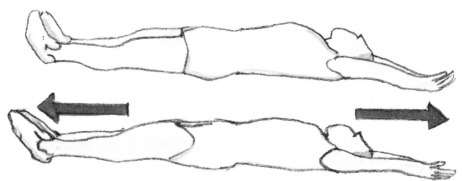

KNEES TO CHEST

Lie on your back and pull your knees into your chest with your hands for a stretch in the hip and buttock region.

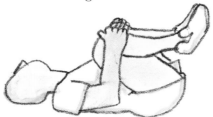

STRETCHES TO DO AT YOUR DESK
ARM AND SHOULDER STRETCH

Interlace your fingers then push your hands out in front of you, palms facing out and arms straight, with hands at about eye level.

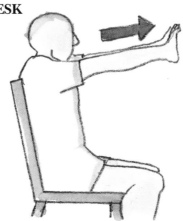

SEATED SIDE STRETCH

Extend both arms overhead, then grasp the outside of your left hand with your right hand. Lean to the right, feeling the stretch along your left side. Return to center, then grasp the outside of your right hand with your left hand and lean left.

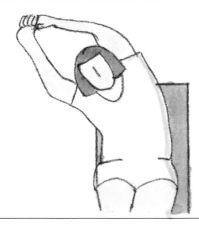

CHEST STRETCH

Interlace your hands behind your head, keeping your elbows pointed out to the sides. Imagine pulling your shoulder blades together across your back so that your elbows point even further back.

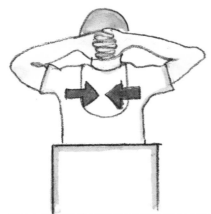

SEATED BACK STRETCH

With feet resting firmly on the floor, bend forward from your hips and rest your torso on your thighs as your arms and head hang freely.

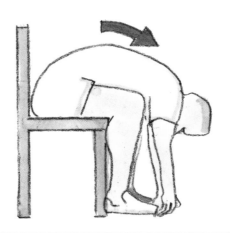

NECK STRETCHES

Keeping your back straight, slowly lean your head to the left, as if you were reaching your left ear toward your left shoulder. Repeat on your right side, reaching your right ear toward your right shoulder. Then bend your head forward, feeling the stretch in the back of your neck and upper back.

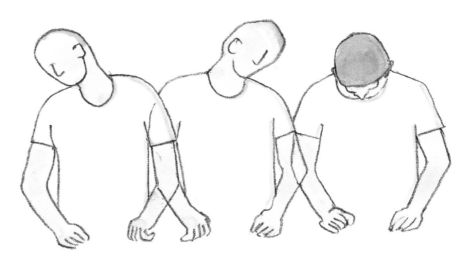

STRETCHES FOR WALKING

CALF STRETCH

Stand facing a wall or other solid support and place your forearms on the wall, head resting on hands if desired. Place one foot several inches from the wall and bend the knee of that leg. Place the other foot 12–24 inches behind you and keep that leg straight. Both heels should remain on the floor at all times, and toes should be pointing forward. Gently move your hips forward, toward the wall, keeping your back leg straight and your lower back flat. Switch legs and repeat.

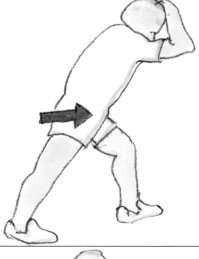

QUADRICEPS STRETCH

Position yourself between two chairs, one in front of you to hold onto for balance and one in back of you to place your foot on. Extend one leg behind you and place your foot on the chair (or table or couch). Keep the knee of the leg you're standing on slightly bent. Flex your buttocks so that the elevated thigh comes forward a bit and you feel a stretch on the front of your elevated thigh. Switch legs and repeat.

SEATED HAMSTRING STRETCH

Sit on the floor with one leg extended to the side and one leg bent so that the foot touches the inner thigh of the straight leg. Rotate your torso toward the extended leg and bend at the hips toward that leg until you feel a stretch along the back of your leg. For more of a stretch, loop a towel around the ball of your foot and gently pull your toes toward your knee.

KNEE CROSSOVER

Lie on your back and bend one knee at a 90° angle. Extend the arm on that side of your body out to the side (resting on the floor). Grasp the bent knee with the opposite hand and pull it across your body. Keeping your shoulders and head on the floor, turn your head away from the bent knee, toward the extended arm. Pull the bent knee toward the floor until you feel a stretch in your hip and lower back. Repeat on the other side.

Stretches and diabetes complications

Two conditions that commonly affect people with diabetes are neuropathy in the feet (peripheral neuropathy) and intermittent claudication. Neuropathy is a problem with the nerves, and claudication is a problem with the circulation to the calves and the feet. In both cases, some simple calf stretches may help alleviate some of the pain and muscular tightness associated with these conditions. For stretches that target the calves and legs, see the illustrations on page 356.

One note of caution for people who have moderate or proliferative retinopathy: Check with your doctor before doing any stretches or any exercise. Avoid stretches or exercises that place your heart lower than your waist or that cause you to hold your breath and strain, which can raise your blood pressure. Your doctor or diabetes educator can advise you on which activities and stretching positions are safe for you.

Getting started

You probably already know a few ways to stretch, but they may not target the muscles that feel tense or that you use for a specific activity. If you need a little instruction, there are a number of books and videos that can help. For some suggestions, see "Stretching Resources" on this page. You might also ask an athletic trainer for suggestions if you belong to a gym or a physical therapist if you see one. Or you could take a stretching or yoga class.

Doing yoga is an excellent way to increase and maintain your flexibility, as well as reduce stress and muscular tension. Yoga can also help build strength and stamina. There's even some research showing that yoga may help with blood sugar control. Certainly if it helps reduce stress, and stress makes blood sugar control more difficult, then practicing yoga might work wonders.

As you stretch, remember that it isn't supposed to hurt. Stretch until you feel mild tension, then hold that position. As your muscles relax, you may be able to stretch a little bit more, but don't overstretch. Doing so can cause your muscles to feel tighter instead of looser. Respect your limits, and don't compare yourself to others in a stretch or yoga class.

No time like the present

Unlike exercise, which often has to be planned around meals or medicines, there's almost no bad time to stretch. If you feel tension in your neck or back while sitting at your desk or on the couch,

STRETCHING RESOURCES

Need help stretching or developing a stretch routine? Look no further than the resources listed here.

STRETCHING FOR FITNESS, HEALTH & PERFORMANCE
The Complete Handbook for All Ages & Fitness Levels
Christopher A. Oswald and Stanley N. Bacso
Sterling Publishing Company, Inc.
New York, 2004
Offers stretching advice for the young, old, pregnant, and injured, as well as for specific occupations and household activities.

STRETCHING
Bob Anderson
Shelter Publications
Bolinas, California, 2000
A classic among books on stretching. Different sets of stretches are suggested for different activities.

STRETCH AND STRENGTHEN
Judith B. Alter
Mariner Books
Boston/New York, 1992
Presents both stretches and strengthening exercises with the goal of injury prevention during physical activities.

SPORT STRETCH, SECOND EDITION
Michael Alter
Human Kinetics Publishers
Champaign, Illinois, 1998
A well-illustrated book for athletes who need specific stretches.

COLLAGE VIDEO
www.CollageVideo.com
(800) 433-6769
Collage Video has three categories of stretching videos (and DVDs): yoga, tai chi, and athletic. All levels, from beginner to advanced, are available.

get up and stretch. If you've been driving for hours, take a break and stretch your legs. If you're at the gym and your legs feel stiff, give them a stretch before starting or continuing your workout, and don't forget to take a nice gentle stretch after your workout to help you cool down and relax. Stretching really is a great way to take a moment for yourself at any time of day and anywhere you happen to be.

If you've just read this entire article, it might be a good time to take a two-minute stretch break. Check pages 353 through 356 for a sampling of stretches. If you like how it feels, think about incorporating regular stretching sessions into your life. □

BIKING 101

by Marie Spano, M.S., R.D.

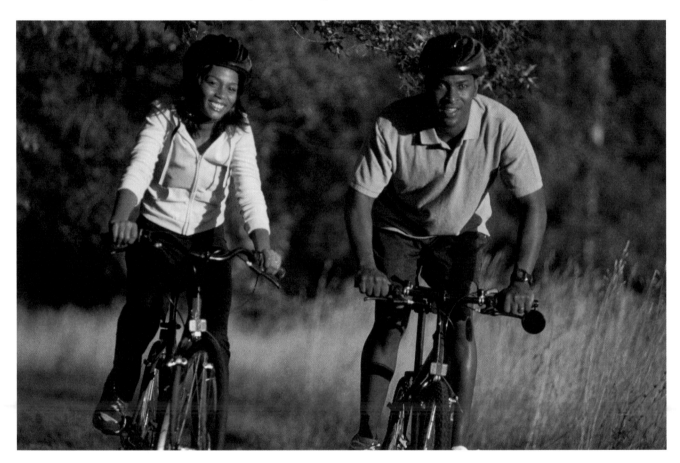

Are you tired of pedaling a stationary bike or an elliptical machine? Are you in search of a little adventure? If so, maybe you're ready to get outside and try real biking. Don't worry if several years have passed since you last rode a bike. As the saying goes, "You never forget how to ride a bicycle." However, although the fundamentals of bicycling haven't changed since you owned a ten-speed (or maybe a three-speed), many other aspects of this sport have, most of which have made it both more accessible and more enjoyable.

Technology has greatly enhanced bicycles, bicycle helmets, and even bicycling clothes. Biking clubs have sprouted up across the United States, making it easier to find others to ride with. And more communities are becoming more bike-friendly by, for example, establishing bike lanes or separate bike paths, providing bicycle parking areas, and installing bike racks on trains and buses so that bikes can be transported with their riders.

So if you haven't touched your bike in years, now's the time to get it out, dust it off, take it in to your local bike shop for a tune-up (very important), and assess whether you need any new biking accessories, such as new helmet, bike lock, or biking gloves, or even a new bike.

Why cycle?

Biking is a enjoyable activity that you can do alone or with others. It can be a good way to explore new places or to simply enjoy old favorites. There is nothing like riding down a bike path or a trail feeling the breeze on your face and the sun on your back. People who use a bike to commute to work or run errands can also have the satisfaction of knowing they're getting some exercise and not adding any pollution to the air.

Besides being a pleasant activity, biking works the muscles in your legs and arms, increases your lung capacity, and helps you maintain a healthy heart. In addition, all forms of aerobic exercise, including biking, help improve your body's response to insulin and lower blood glucose levels.

Even if you regularly do some other type of aerobic exercise, varying your routine with an occasional bike ride will challenge you physically and stimulate you mentally. Cross-training of any type works your muscles a little differently, may help prevent overuse injuries, and keeps you from getting bored with your exercise routine.

Trails or roads?

If you already have a bike and don't wish to buy a new one, the style of your bike will probably determine where you will ride it. If you're in the market for a new bike, however, you may want to think first about where you intend to bike—on trails or on roads—before buying one.

Biking on roads is convenient since you can usually just hop on outside your front door and go. However, if you have to share the road with cars, biking on roads can be scary and even dangerous. Seeking out quieter streets, back roads, and bike paths may make for more enjoyable and safer bike riding. If you intend to ride on roads, you will want either a road bike with fairly thin tires and a lightweight frame or a somewhat heavier "city bike." If you plan to commute on your bike, you might even consider getting a foldable bike for easier storage at your home and workplace.

If you prefer biking on trails, you'll probably need a mountain bike. Mountain bikes have fat, knobby tires and a thick frame, making them both sturdier and heavier than road bikes. They are also much slower on roads than road bikes. Unless you are lucky enough to live near a trailhead, mountain biking usually requires driving to your destination. (It's worth noting that not all hiking trails are open to bikes, so you will need to research where mountain biking is permitted in your area.)

If you think you may be riding on both roads and fairly flat trails, a hybrid bicycle might be right for you. A hybrid combines features from both mountain bikes and road bikes, with a mid-weight frame and tires that are thicker than those of a road bike but thinner than those of a mountain bike. Hybrid bikes cannot be used for very rugged trails.

Finding a good fit

Once you have decided which type of bike you want and approximately how much you want to spend (a used city bike may cost less than $100 [although it will almost certainly need a tune-up, which will cost a few more dollars] while a new full-suspension mountain bike can cost more than $3,000), go to your local bike shop and try some on for size. Most shops, especially those that aren't part of a national chain, are run and staffed by active cyclists who work there because of their enthusiasm for the sport and desire to help others. They are usually more than willing to help you get started and find the right equipment.

If mountain biking is in your future, you will need to choose between a full-suspension or a hardtail bike. Full-suspension bikes have both front and rear suspension, which allows for a more comfortable ride, but they're also more expensive. Hardtails have only front suspension. They are lighter and cheaper than full-suspension bikes, and they ride better on smooth terrain, but they are not as comfortable on rough terrain. Some full-suspension bikes have a "lock out" feature that lets you turn off the front and/or rear suspension when riding on flat surfaces.

Before test-riding any bike, have the sales clerk help you pick a bike with the right frame size for your body and also show you how to adjust the seat and handlebars. A properly adjusted bike will maximize both your safety and comfort. To check frame size, straddle the bike with both feet on the ground. You should have 2–4 inches of clearance between the top of the tube and your crotch for mountain bikes and hybrids and 1–2 inches of clearance for a road bike. If the bike has a sloping top tube, which is typical of women's bikes, measure your clearance from an imaginary top tube.

In addition to examining the height of the top tube, consider its length. The length of the top tube determines how far you have to bend over to reach the handlebars. You should not be stretched all the way out to reach the handlebars. Instead, your elbows should be slightly bent and your back bent from the waist at an approximately 45-degree angle (see illustration on page 361). Riding on a bike with either too much distance or too little distance between seat and handlebars will make it difficult to maneuver your bike. Bikes designed especially for women often fit them better because they take into consideration women's longer legs and shorter torsos.

Adjust the bike's seat so that when you are sitting on it with one foot on the pedal close to the lowest position, your knee is bent slightly (see illustration on page 361). With experience, you may decide to raise or lower the seat to suit your riding style. Mountain bikers, for example, typically lower the seat for greater maneuverability.

Next, adjust the handlebars to the appropriate height. You may need to ride your bike several times to find the right handlebar height for you. In general, handlebars typically range from 2–3 inches below the top of the seat to 2–3 inches above it. Your goal is to find a height that is comfortable and that allows you to easily use the brakes and shift gears.

Bike pedals come in several styles these days. Flat, "platform" pedals are best for novices or those who are doing easy riding on fairly flat surfaces. With flat pedals, you can stop your bike and immediately put your feet on the ground without any problem. Pedals with toe straps or cages secure the foot to the pedal and allow cyclists to go faster since they can use their hip flexors to apply power on the upstroke (as well as pressing down on the downstroke). "Clipless" pedals have no straps or cages but require special cycling shoes with cleats on the bottom that lock into the pedals. They, too, allow the cyclist to go faster since he can apply pressure to the pedal for its full rotation. Because clipless pedals take some getting used to, only experienced cyclists should try using them.

Other equipment

A good-fitting helmet is essential for bicycling and should be worn at all times, even on a leisurely ride. In addition to a helmet, you may want to consider bike gloves, which give your palms some padding while leaving your fingers uncovered. Although special biking clothes are not strictly necessary, many people find bike shorts with a gel pad in the seat area to be comfortable, and moisture-wicking shirts (generally made of synthetic material) can keep you drier than 100% cotton tops. Wearing clothing, such as a vest, made of reflective material is a good idea if you will be biking at dawn or dusk or after dark; it makes you much more visible to motorists.

Biking is an aerobic exercise, so you will want a way to carry some water with you to drink as you ride. If you have a bottle cage on your bike, you can carry a water bottle in it. Another alternative

is to wear a small backpack with a refillable bladder in it that has a hose with a mouthpiece that reaches over your shoulder. (Two popular brands of such bladders are Camelback and Platypus, although there are others.) The backpack can also be used to carry food, extra clothing, and other supplies.

To carry bike wrenches and extra tubes (in case of a flat tire), you may want to buy a small pouch that attaches right below your seat. Also helpful for dealing with flat tires is a small travel bike pump, which attaches to your bike. If you may be out after dark, a white headlight and a flashing red rear light are necessary to make you more visible to motorists. Reflectors on your bike will also make you more visible on city streets.

Bike maintenance

Before every ride, it is important to perform a quick inspection. Here are some things to check:
■ Check that the brakes are working properly, the tires have plenty of air and are not worn, and the wheels are secure (lift your bike so one tire is on the ground and shake the other tire in the air from side to side).
■ The rims and spokes should have no bulges, dents, or dings in them.
■ The levers on your quick-release hubs (if you have them) should be in the closed position.
■ Your chain should be well lubricated without any kinks or gunk in the links.
■ The pedals should be securely attached to the bike yet move freely.
■ The seat should be secure.

If your bike is muddy after riding, clean it with soap and water (preferably gentle soap made for bikes) and dry it off right away. Dirt and mud are abrasive and can destroy your bike components.

The Haynes Bicycle Book, by Bob Henderson, is great for basic step-by-step repair and maintenance. With nice illustrations and easy instructions, you will learn about every part of your bike, how to make easy repairs, and how to clean your bike and care for it. However, if you ride often, you should get your bike tuned up by your local bike shop at least twice a year.

Choosing a route

Bike shops are usually a good source for local route and trail information. They often have maps and books that contain detailed information such as mileage, difficulty level, and terrain.

Participating in a group ride organized by a bike club is also a good way to discover places to ride. As the sport of biking continues to increase

GETTING THE RIGHT FIT

FRAME SIZE
To see whether a bike's frame is the right size for you, straddle the bike with both feet on the ground. You should have 2–4 inches of clearance between the top of the tube and your crotch for mountain bikes and hybrids and 1–2 inches of clearance for a road bike. If the bike has a sloping top tube, measure your clearance from an imaginary top tube.

SEAT HEIGHT
Adjust your bike's seat so that when you are sitting on it with one foot on the pedal at the lowest position, your knee is bent slightly. In the pictures shown here, the leg on the top has the right amount of bend, while the leg in the middle is extended too far.

TUBE LENGTH
When sitting on your bike, you should not be stretched all the way out to reach the handlebars. Instead, your elbows should be slightly bent, and your back should be bent from the waist at an approximately 45-degree angle, as pictured here.

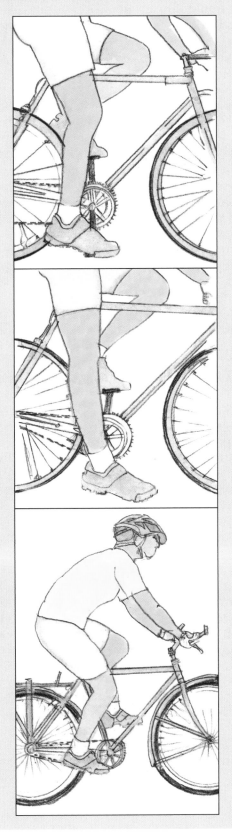

in popularity, bike clubs have sprouted up across the United States. Again, bike shops are often a good way to find a club in your area.

As you would with any new sport or physical activity, start with a route that you can cover easily, then build up your distance and difficulty gradually.

Safety first

Bicycling is great exercise and it's fun, to boot, but accidents, delays, or simply the unexpected can happen, so it's best to be prepared. In addition, bicycling will probably lower your blood glucose level, so you may need to stop for a snack or adjust your diabetes regimen in some other way to account for bicycling's blood-glucose-lowering effect. Here are some things to remember before you head out:

■ If you have a cell phone, bring it with you.

■ Always tell someone where you are going and when you plan on coming back, especially if you are cycling by yourself. In general, however, biking with other people is safer.

■ Always carry some food with you. Energy bars are easy to carry (although in warm weather, avoid bars with chocolate or yogurt coatings, which will melt in the heat). Energy gels, such as GU, Clif Shot, and PowerGel, are another option: They are essentially pure carbohydrate and can provide a quick pick-me-up when you need one.

■ On longer rides, carry your blood glucose monitoring supplies with you.

Rain can be particularly hazardous for cyclists. When it rains, the ground gets slippery, your bicycle's brakes may not work as well, and visibility—both yours and that of motorists—decreases. If you ever get caught in the rain, ride conservatively: Use your bike lights, avoid roads with heavy traffic, yield to cars at intersections, and start slowing down before you turn to avoid skidding in the turn. If you are on a low-traffic street or on a bike path, ride in the center of the lane and not on the side, where puddles and wet leaves may collect. "Dragging" your brakes, or putting a little pressure on them as you ride, can help to remove water

FOR MORE CYCLING INFORMATION

To find bike clubs in your area, good places to ride, or to book a bicycling vacation, try the following Web sites:

ADVENTURE SPORTS ONLINE
(800) 276-0770
www.adventuresportsonline.com/club/bikeclub.htm

BICYCLE CLUBS IN THE U.S.A.
www.geocities.com/Colosseum/6213

BACKROADS
(800) 462-2848
www.backroads.com
Backroads is an active travel company with bicycling trips in the United States and abroad.

LEAGUE OF AMERICAN BICYCLISTS
(202) 822-1333
www.bikeleague.org

RAILS-TO-TRAILS CONSERVANCY
(202) 331-9696
www.railtrails.org
Rail-to-Trails promotes the creation of trails from former rail lines throughout the United States.

from your tire rims, making it easier to stop with your brakes when you need to.

Last but not least, if you ever feel unable to control your bike—because of rain or anything else—stop and get off. You may get delayed (that's why you brought your cell phone) or wetter than you otherwise would get, but you will be alive and able to take another bike ride when conditions are more favorable. □

Weight Management

Tips 595–620 365

How Hunger Happens 368
The Brain's Role in Obesity

Strategies for Weight Management 373

Bariatric Surgery 376
Lifestyle Changes for Before and After

9

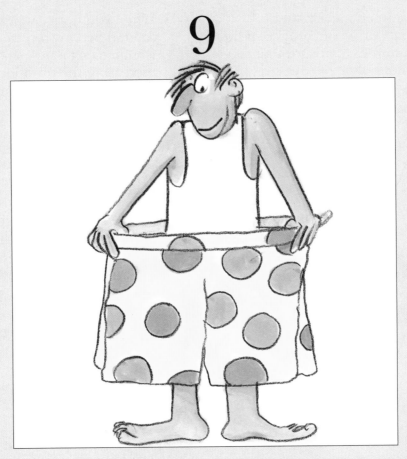

Weight Management Tips

595–620

595. Because orlistat (brand names Alli, Xenical) reduces the absorption of fat-soluble vitamins (such as vitamins A, D, E, K, and beta-carotene), people using this drug should take a daily multivitamin and mineral supplement several hours before or after taking orlistat.

596. For people who have diabetes, it's important to have blood glucose levels in a normal range before bariatric surgery.

597. Before bariatric surgery, begin taking a multivitamin, multimineral supplement every day so that it becomes part of your daily routine.

598. Start taking a calcium supplement before bariatric surgery. If you currently take calcium carbonate, switch to calcium citrate, which is more easily absorbed. Calcium citrate can be found in both powder and pill forms.

599. Before bariatric surgery, begin exercising at a level you feel comfortable with, even if it is only five minutes a day. Your goal is to establish a routine and ideally build up to 30 minutes of physical activity a day.

600. Before bariatric surgery, drink at least 48 ounces (6 cups) of water a day. Purchasing a water bottle may help you keep track of your fluid intake. Start sipping fluids throughout the day, and attempt to

drink fluids between meals. After bariatric surgery, drink one ounce of liquid every 15 minutes to ensure that you drink a minimum of 48 ounces a day.

601. After bariatric surgery, it is important to drink fluids between meals rather than at meals.

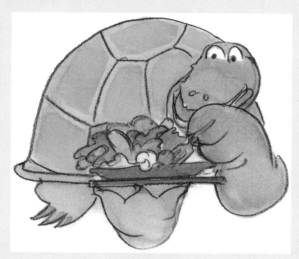

602. Get into the habit of eating slowly and chewing your food well. Eating slowly will enable you to recognize when you are full and when to stop eating. On average, a meal should last about 30 minutes.

603. Avoid concentrated sweets and beverages. Foods such as pastries, cakes, and sugar-sweetened beverages get digested rapidly and have a lot of calories.

604. When it comes to losing weight and maintaining weight loss, set small, achievable goals that can build on each other.

605. Start with any goal you are ready to tackle. For example, if you see some areas in your meal plan that you are ready to "tune up," focus on them first.

606. Be realistic about the amount of weight you wish to lose. Even a 7% to 10% weight loss has been proven to have significant health benefits, but this often strikes people as too small a goal.

607. Keep track of your progress daily. Monitoring your progress could mean maintaining a logbook to regularly record meals, exercise, and weight, or it could mean designing your own personalized system.

608. When you notice weight-loss plateaus, or a slowdown in your rate of weight loss, it is time to set a new small goal, such as increasing the duration or intensity of your exercise or making another change in your meal plan that will contribute to your progress.

609. Keep temptations out of your home and workplace to help create an environment that promotes your success.

610. Give yourself variety in your exercise and meal plans so that feelings of boredom and deprivation don't pull you off track.

611. Schedule time for exercise so that you don't feel rushed by other demands.

612. Schedule time for meal preparation so that you have nutritious foods on hand to eat when you are hungry and won't be tempted by vending machines or fast-food restaurants.

613. Be prepared to give yourself a break when life intervenes and pulls you off track.

614. Focus on your monthly weight-loss pattern to recognize the progress you're making.

615. Consider joining a club focused on an activity you enjoy, such as walking, hiking, or biking, or a support group focused on weight loss and health.

616. Reach out for exercise partners or weight-loss partners and connect to advocacy groups such as the American Diabetes Association.

617. Be on the lookout for people in your life who offer misguided help, or who take on the role of the "diabetes police" or "food police." Help them to understand what it is that you need from them through patient and assertive communication.

618. Don't forget to build in positive rewards for yourself once you meet targets along the way. Get creative in finding non-food-related rewards that are personally meaningful.

619. Remind yourself that it's not necessary to be thin to be healthy. Look for role mod-

els who aren't thin but are healthy, and aim to emulate them rather than, say, slender fashion models.

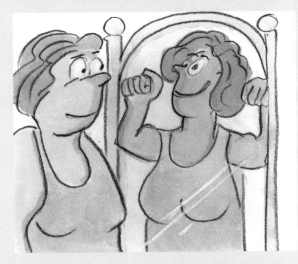

620. Decide that you and your health are worth the effort it will take to change your eating and exercise habits.

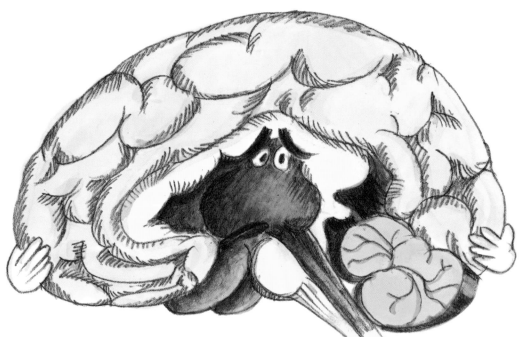

HOW HUNGER HAPPENS
The Brain's Role in Obesity

by Alisa G. Woods, Ph.D.

We have all heard reports of the obesity epidemic that is overtaking developed nations, particularly the United States. Obesity—having a body-mass index (BMI) greater than 30 kilograms per square meter—has high costs, including an increased risk of dying and the development of serious health problems, such as diabetes, cardiovascular problems, and cancer. (To determine your BMI, you can go to the Web site for the Centers for Disease Control and Prevention at www.cdc.gov/nccdphp/dnpa/bmi/calc-bmi.htm#English.) Obesity also decreases one's quality of life due to the physical limitations and social stigma associated with it.

It seems that obesity statistics become more shocking each day. For example, childhood obesity has doubled in the past 20 years, and more than 64% of people in the United States are currently estimated to be either overweight or obese according to the 1999-2000 National Health and Nutrition Examination Survey. In fact, in the United States, obesity may become the primary cause of death as a result of human behavior, even overtaking smoking. According to Robert H. Eckel, M.D., Professor of Medicine at the University of Colorado, Denver, and former president of the American Heart Association, the current obesity epidemic is "serious, and unless we become more aggressive in treating the childhood epi-

demic and/or the related complications, the worst is yet to come."

Obesity and overweight result from an energy imbalance—more energy from food is going into the body than is being used for basic body functions and physical activity—and the amount of energy going in has a lot to do with feelings of hunger and satiety (feeling full, or sated). People eat for many reasons, including but not limited to fulfilling a physical need for nutrients.

Hunger and satiety are better understood today than ever before, and major scientific findings have occurred in this field just within the past decade. Based on a new appreciation of how the brain may control hunger, the possibility of treating obesity through drugs that specifically target the nervous system is becoming more and more real.

Why hunger?

A reduced-calorie diet and exercise are the foundation of a good weight-loss plan, but if they are not enough, a physician may choose to prescribe certain medicines. Current weight-loss medicines usually achieve their effects either by reducing hunger or increasing feelings of fullness or by reducing absorption of nutrients.

Although the story of appetite seems simple—that people eat when they're hungry and stop when they're full—the complete story is actually a bit more complex. A number of hormones, metabolic processes, and neurotransmitters (signaling molecules between nerve cells) all work together to affect hunger and weight.

One way to look at how hunger and satiety work is to view them as two of the body's survival tools for protecting and maintaining itself. To prevent you from forgetting to eat (the body needs food for materials to make repairs and for keeping blood glucose levels in normal ranges), the brain signals that it's time to eat by making you feel hungry. Once the urge to eat has been obeyed, the body has little incentive to have you eat until you burst, so satiety signals are sent out that cause you to feel full. These mechanisms are critical for, say, infants, but they can cause problems in children and adults who are trying to lose weight.

Although losing weight may be in the best health interest of overweight or obese people, the body goes on carrying out its basic imperatives to maintain itself regardless. The body is not trying to be perverse; it's merely trying to prevent what could become a dangerous situation. A rapid, large amount of weight loss can throw off the delicate balance of the body's systems (and even be fatal), so the body works to prevent starvation or drastic weight loss. When a person starts trying to lose weight by giving his body a reduced-calorie diet and exercising, his body eventually intervenes to prevent the weight loss from progressing to a point that might disrupt its systems. The body's tactics in this fight are to induce hunger (to force eating and gain more calories to staunch the weight loss) and slow its metabolism, reducing the amount of energy the body burns. With the body working to increase caloric intake and reduce caloric use, you can see why people have a difficult time losing weight and maintaining the weight loss in the face of such resistance.

To overcome the body's natural tendencies to maintain weight at a set level (even if it is a level medical science considers unhealthy), researchers have looked at ways of circumventing these automatic mechanisms. Two possible approaches being examined are to block appetite-inducing signals or to increase antiappetite signals. Because a basic tenet of weight loss is to "burn more energy than you take in," some researchers are also looking at increasing metabolic rate to help people burn more calories and at blocking the absorption of some calories (see the sidebar on orlistat [brand name Xenical as a prescription medication or Alli as an over-the-counter medication] on this page).

After reading about all the hormones and neurological signaling molecules involved in hunger (and

ORLISTAT

Orlistat (brand names Xenical and Alli) is a widely used drug treatment for obesity. In February of 2007, an over-the-counter version of this medication was approved by the FDA, as a 60 mg dose. The prescription form is available at 210 mg. Unlike appetite suppressants, orlistat does not directly target the brain's hunger control system. Orlistat helps weight loss by preventing the digestion and absorption of about a third of the fat in the food a person has consumed. It has been demonstrated to cause weight loss of between 5% and 10% of the user's original body weight when taken for two years or longer. Orlistat is taken three times a day, with meals containing fat.

Orlistat is associated with several side effects including flatulence and oily stools (most last for no more than one to four weeks, although some people have experienced them for over six months). These side effects are caused by undigested fat, so people taking orlistat may start to avoid eating fat. Although this sounds positive, it can undermine the drug's weight-reducing effects (and possibly blood glucose control) if people increase their caloric intake by substituting foods rich in carbohydrate. Kidney stones or abdominal pain and other gastrointestinal problems may also occur. Because it reduces fat absorption, orlistat also reduces the absorption of fat-soluble vitamins (such as vitamins A, D, E, K, and beta-carotene). To compensate, a daily multivitamin and mineral supplement should be taken several hours before or after taking orlistat.

simply thinking about how the sight, smell, or thought of a favorite food can make a person's mouth water and his stomach rumble), it's easy to wonder if humans are mere slaves to internal chemical and metabolic processes that control hunger. However, there are also certain learned behaviors that contribute to why we eat. For example, some people eat when bored and when food is available, so simply keeping active and away from the temptations of the refrigerator or the pantry can help. People who equate food with comfort may eat when stressed and may need to find alternative ways to deal with stress. So certain behavior modifications can help some people to control their hunger and when and how much they choose to eat.

This article focuses on the approaches to weight loss that involve the metabolic, hormonal, and neurological aspects of hunger.

Hunger on the brain

The hypothalamus is a region of the brain that produces hormones that regulate functions such as sleep, mood, body temperature, thirst, and hunger. It has several divisions, including a region (the ventromedial hypothalamus) that may suppress eating and a region (the lateral hypothalamus) that seems to promote eating. Scientists identified the hunger-related function of these areas of the hypothalamus by observing that overeating and obesity developed in laboratory animals when their ventromedial hypothalamus was damaged. If an animal's lateral hypothalamus was damaged, it exhibited a severe lack of eating. Scientists also found that stimulating the ventromedial hypothalamus in animals caused them to stop eating, while stimulating the lateral hypothalamus caused the animal to eat.

Although it seems that it would be obvious to just name these sections of the hypothalamus the hunger and the satiety centers, it is not that simple. These parts of the hypothalamus do play an important part in controlling hunger, but research has identified a number of interrelating players including other parts of the brain and body and hormones from other organs. It is now widely believed that a primary role of the hypothalamus is to establish and maintain what is known as a "set point" for hunger, satiety, and weight. Different people may have different set points, which could contribute to differences in eating behavior.

Influencing the hypothalamus

The hypothalamus appears to respond to several different metabolic conditions, hormones, and neurotransmitters, including blood glucose levels. A falling blood glucose level stimulates the hypothalamus to send hunger signals that promote eating.

As you might expect, a number of hormones influencing appetite are produced by the gastrointestinal system. With its levels rising between meals and falling sharply after eating, the hormone ghrelin, from stomach cells, signals the hypothalamus to induce hunger. Other hormones, such as cholecystokinin, peptide YY, and glucagon-like peptide-1 (GLP-1), help to induce satiety after food is ingested.

Leptin, another hormone that influences the hypothalamus, is actually produced by fat tissue in the body. So what are researchers doing with this

TESTING DRUGS FOR OBESITY

It should be noted that in clinical trials examining the use of antiobesity drugs, it is currently required that people participating in these studies undergo a program of diet and exercise in addition to taking their drug. For this reason, if the clinical trial includes a placebo (sugar pill) group for comparison, these people may experience weight loss as well as the people who are taking the drug. To discover the amount of weight loss produced by the drug itself, researchers subtract the weight loss experienced by the group taking a placebo from the weight loss experienced by the group taking the drug. An additional message is also apparent: These drugs by themselves are not magic pills. When recommending a program to reduce weight, health-care providers emphasize that diet and exercise should be part of the weight-loss program in addition to medicine.

knowledge of appetite-influencing substances? Well, in several cases, clinical trials are ongoing, while in others, research has already shown that blocking a certain appetite-inducing hormone or adding a certain appetite-suppressing hormone is not effective for weight loss.

Ghrelin. Because ghrelin induces appetite, a drug that blocks ghrelin from being sensed by the hypothalamus might help to reduce appetite. The situation is complicated, though, because ghrelin stimulates the release of growth hormone as well as increasing hunger. Although its name suggests it may be of greatest concern to children and adolescents, growth hormone also affects bone density, metabolism of fat, and muscle growth in adults. (Growth hormone has also been promoted as an antiaging compound despite a lack of evidence for such cure-all properties.) Researchers have work to do before an obesity drug based on blocking ghrelin's appetite-inducing action is possible.

Cholecystokinin. Cholecystokinin was one of the first hormones to be shown to be able to inhibit appetite when injected. However, it has a short-lived effect, and volunteers who took it showed resistance to its effects over time. They ate smaller meals, but they also ended up eating more meals to compensate, so the overall energy intake was about the same.

Peptide YY. Peptide YY, released by cells in the intestines after a meal, is thought to influence the hypothalamus to induce satiety. Researchers in the United Kingdom found in 2002 that the hormone reduced food intake in humans; however, that treatment involved only a small number of volunteers, the drug had to be infused for 90 minutes, and the effects were only monitored for 24 hours. Longer-term safety and efficacy studies are needed in larger numbers of volunteers. Also, a group from the University of Cincinnati reported difficulty in replicating the British group's appetite-suppressing results in rodents in 2004.

GLP-1. GLP-1 is co-secreted with peptide YY from the intestines after a meal. It increases insulin secretion and inhibits the secretion of glucagon (a hormone that causes the liver to release stored glucose to the blood) after meals, and also seems to have some appetite-reducing effects.

Earlier this year, the U.S. Food and Drug Administration (FDA) approved a longer-lasting synthetic GLP-1–like compound called exenatide (Byetta) for use by people with Type 2 diabetes who were unable to control their diabetes with metformin and/or a sulfonylurea drug (such as glipizide, glyburide, or glimepiride). Exenatide is an injectable drug and is currently intended to be used along with metformin and/or a sulfonylurea. It has been shown to reduce glycosylated hemoglobin (HbA_{1c}, a measure of long-term blood glucose control) levels and both postmeal and fasting blood glucose levels. People also tended to lose some weight while taking the drug.

Leptin. Leptin was only recently discovered in 1994, by Jeffrey Friedman, M.D., Ph.D., of the Rockefeller University in New York and his colleagues. They were studying a specific type of mouse that becomes obese. The researchers found that these mice were lacking leptin and that the mice lost weight when they were given leptin.

It is now understood that leptin affects appetite and also increases the rate at which the body can burn fat. Most of the effects of leptin appear to be mediated by the hypothalamus. Recent studies have shown that leptin stimulates appetite-suppressing centers in the hypothalamus and inhibits parts of the hypothalamus that normally stimulate hunger. Leptin levels decrease in a person who has lost weight or who is fasting.

Despite the initial promise leptin appeared to offer as a treatment for obesity, clinical trials have not been as successful as originally expected. In obese people who do not produce their own natural leptin (a rare genetic disorder that results in obesity early in life), leptin injections do indeed help them lose weight. However, leptin deficiency only exists in a small percentage of obese people. Many obese people have actually been found to have relatively high levels of leptin, and most obese people don't respond to injected leptin by decreasing the amount of food they eat or losing weight. They are said to be resistant to leptin. So it seems that leptin may only be an effective antiobesity drug in the small number of people who fail to produce leptin and in the minority of obese people who aren't resistant to leptin.

Although the discovery of leptin did not produce a "magic-bullet" treatment for obesity, researchers have investigated modified forms of leptin that can overcome resistance and drugs that have a similar action to leptin. Scientists have found that a naturally occurring molecule known as ciliary neurotrophic factor (CNTF) may act like leptin, possibly affecting the hypothalamus and suppressing hunger.

Axokine. Axokine is a modified form of CNTF. CNTF nourishes specific types of nervous system cells, which is why axokine was originally developed to treat a neurological disease called amyotrophic lateral sclerosis (ALS), also known as Lou Gherig disease. When people with ALS were given axokine in a clinical trial, they lost weight. At that point, axokine was no longer studied as a solo treatment for ALS, but was further studied as a possible obesity treatment.

Early studies of axokine were promising and showed that people lost weight when given the drug, even people who were leptin resistant. Unfortunately, later research showed that approximately 70% of the people who take axokine develop an immune response that inactivates the drug. Axokine is therefore no longer being studied by the company that developed it.

Hoodia. The plant extract *Hoodia gordonii*, is currently very popular as an appetite suppressant and weight-loss tool. Because hoodia is a dietary supplement and not a medication, little research has been done on it. One report from researchers at Brown Medical School, published in 2004, suggested that hoodia may act in the hypothalamus by increasing the amount of ATP produced there. ATP (adenosine triphosphate) provides energy for all cells.

Signals in the brain

In addition to hormones from fat tissue and organs, neurotransmitters in the brain also affect hunger, and modifying the action of these neurotransmitters is another area of study for affecting hunger mechanisms. An approved obesity treatment and medications in late-phase clinical trials are of special interest in this category of drugs.

Sibutramine. Based on a clear connection between specific brain systems and hunger control, it would seem that directly affecting the brain would be a good mechanism of action for a drug. However, only one drug that is currently approved for use in the United States affects the brain directly. Sibutramine (Meridia) targets appetite by increasing the amount of time two neurotransmitters (noradrenaline and serotonin) have to act by preventing them from being reabsorbed by the brain cells (neurons) that produce them. Increases in serotonin caused by sibutramine may activate serotonin receptors in the hypothalamus, causing feelings of satiety. Sibutramine use has also been linked to a small increase in the user's basal metabolic rate, which could help to offset some of the body's tendency to lower its metabolic rate in people who are losing weight. Sibutramine is taken once a day.

Increases in heart rate and blood pressure can result from sibutramine use, so it's currently required that blood pressure be regularly monitored in people taking sibutramine and that people with serious cardiovascular problems not take this drug. Other side effects may include dry mouth, insomnia, loss of appetite, constipation, or headache.

Sibutramine works the same way that many antidepressants work, In fact, sibutramine was originally intended to be an antidepressant until it was noticed that it causes weight loss. Use of sibutramine has been shown to result in a 5% to 10% reduction in a person's body weight.

Lorcaserin. Lorcaserin is a medication that is currently being studied in Phase III clinical trials for the treatment of obesity. Like sibutramine, it acts on the serotonin system in the hypothalamus, but in a different way. It mimics the neurotransmitter serotonin on very specific receptors for that neurotransmitter, called $5-HT_{2C}$, once again in the hypothalamus. This may cause feelings of satiety and could also speed up metabolism.

Rimonabant. Rimonabant is a drug that acts by blocking cellular receptors in the hypothalamus for a substance called anandamide, which research is beginning to show can affect appetite, memory, and mood. When anandamide binds with its receptors, it stimulates hunger. (These are also the receptors that are triggered by the active chemical in marijuana and are thought to be responsible for marijuana's appetite-inducing effects.)

In its clinical trials, rimonabant has been linked to side effects such as nausea, depression, anxiety, and irritability. In June of 2007 the FDA con-

SHORT-TERM DRUGS

In the early 1970's, the U.S. Food and Drug Administration (FDA) declared the amphetamines and amphetamine-like drugs (also called amphetamine derivatives) effective in the treatment of obesity. Because the drugs had only ever been examined in short-term studies for weight loss and because their appetite-suppressing effects wane with time, the FDA required that use of these drugs be limited to a few weeks. However, amphetamines also cause euphoria (a false sense of well-being), which makes them likely to be abused, so few physicians prescribe them anymore as obesity treatments. On the other hand, the amphetamine-like drugs, which seem to have somewhat less potential for abuse, are still sometimes used by physicians for short-term treatment of obesity in certain people.

The amphetamine-like drugs, including phentermine (brand names Adipex-P, Ionamin, and others), mazindol (Mazanor, Sanorex), diethylpropion (Tenuate, Tenuate Dospan), and phendimetrazine (Prelu-2 and others), are thought to decrease appetite as a side effect of their stimulation of the brain. They have been linked to increases in blood pressure and heart palpitations, so they are not recommended for use in people with high blood pressure. They are also known to interact with several other drugs and may not be recommended for people who use certain asthma medicines or antidepressants.

Obesity is gaining support in medical circles as a chronic disease that may need to be managed with medicines (along with diet and exercise) for years or even a lifetime. Because of their potential for abuse and their approval for only short-term use, amphetamine-like drugs are not given much prominence in recent guidelines on the treatment of obesity from the National Heart, Lung, and Blood Institute and the American College of Physicians. Sibutramine (Meridia) and orlistat (Xenical and Alli) are currently the only drugs approved for longer-term use in the treatment of obesity.

cluded that the safety of this medication has not been demonstrated adequately, so this medication is not currently approved in the United States, although it is sold in Europe.

The fight continues

The current battle against obesity will continue to be waged with a combination of education, prevention, diet, exercise, and medical interventions. As more is understood about how the brain controls hunger, it will be interesting to see how the development of drugs that specifically target the brain and hunger-related mechanisms unfolds, and whether these treatments will indeed help halt the surging obesity epidemic. ☐

STRATEGIES FOR WEIGHT MANAGEMENT

by Ann E. Goebel-Fabbri, Ph.D.

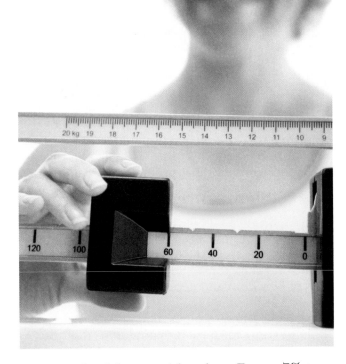

If you are overweight, you probably have had this experience more times than you care to count: being told by a health-care provider that if you could "just lose weight and keep it off," your health would improve. You may have tried numerous weight-loss programs, gym memberships, and diet books in an attempt to follow that advice. Over the years you may have lost somewhere between 50 and 100 pounds. But keeping that weight off over the long term poses its own, unique challenge.

Advice to lose weight is given routinely, yet losing weight and maintaining weight loss are very difficult goals to achieve. However, there are practical tools and strategies that can help you reach your weight-loss targets and (most important) keep that weight off over time. This article presents some of those strategies that have stood the test of time.

Set realistic goals

The most important strategy for successful weight loss—or behavioral change of any sort—is to learn how to set realistic, achievable goals for yourself. Losing weight and managing diabetes both require attention to diet and exercise. But nobody can change everything at once, so it helps to set small, achievable goals that can build on each other.

Start with any goal you are ready to tackle. For example, if you see some areas in your meal plan that you are ready to "tune up," focus on them first. On the other hand, if the weather is getting warmer and you are interested in starting a regular walking routine, go for it. Any positive lifestyle change you make that you are able to build in as a regular habit will result in improvements in your energy, mood, and motivation.

It's also important to be realistic about the amount of weight you wish to lose. Even a 7% to 10% weight loss has been proven to have significant health benefits, but this often strikes people as too small a goal. For example, someone who weighs 300 pounds and loses 30 pounds is still overweight. However, keeping this weight off over time will result in improved insulin sensitivity, lower blood glucose levels, lower blood pressure, lower blood lipids, increased mobility, and improved energy.

Setting a weight-loss goal that is too high and aiming for perfection are a recipe for burnout and make it more likely that you will give up on the overall goal of improving your health. Diabetes is a chronic disease that will be with you for your whole life, so your goals and expectations need to be maintainable and sustainable over a lifetime.

Keep track of your progress

Keeping track of your progress daily can be a powerful tool. Research shows that people who routinely monitor their progress are more likely to maintain weight loss and stick to an exercise program. Monitoring your progress could mean maintaining a logbook to regularly record meals, exercise, and weight, or it could mean designing your own personalized system. Keeping track of your weight-loss pattern will also help you decide when it is time to set a new goal. When you notice weight-loss plateaus, or a slowdown in your rate of weight loss, it is time to set a new small goal, such as increasing the duration or intensity of your exercise or making another change in your meal plan that will contribute to your progress.

Using a tracking system also helps you to increase your awareness of risky situations or foods that trigger overeating. For example, if you learn from your logbook that whenever you take home a doggie bag from a restaurant you polish it off the same night, it probably makes sense to rethink your doggie bag strategy. Keeping temptations out of your home and workplace will help you to create an environment that promotes your success.

Problem-solve ahead of time

Approach your weight-loss goals with strategic planning in mind. Since you are working on lifestyle changes for the long haul, give yourself variety in your exercise and meal plans so that feelings of boredom and deprivation don't pull you off track. Schedule time for exercise so that you don't feel rushed by other demands. Similarly, schedule time for meal preparation so that you have nutritious foods on hand to eat when you are hungry and won't be tempted by vending machines or fast-food restaurants.

By sticking to a schedule and creating a routine for your new behaviors, they will gradually become more reliable habits for you. However, it's still a good idea to devise a game plan ahead of time for how you might handle times when you are feeling bored or too stressed to exercise or cook, as well as for how you will handle changing seasons and unpredictable weather. Over time, your new habits will become your everyday approach to how you live your life. They will be just part of "what you do."

Expect setbacks

Be prepared to give yourself a break when life intervenes and pulls you off track. Slips and setbacks are a normal and expectable part of working to change longstanding habits. Accepting that

---

RESOURCES FOR WEIGHT CONTROL

The following resources can provide inspiration and guidance for people trying to lose weight and keep it off.

NATIONAL WEIGHT CONTROL REGISTRY
www.nwcr.ws
This national study tracks over 5,000 people who have lost significant weight and kept it off for long periods. The Web site is a comprehensive, noncommercial resource for reading inspiring real-life stories as well as research findings.

GREEN MOUNTAIN AT FOX RUN
www.fitwoman.com
This weight-loss retreat is exclusively for women and focuses on a lifestyle, nondiet approach. Specialized wellness programs are offered three times a year. The Web site has information on nutrition, fitness, and women's health.

JOSLIN'S WHY WAIT PROGRAM
www.joslin.org
A one-of-a-kind program created expressly to address the weight-management needs of people with Type 2 diabetes, Why WAIT is a 13-week program offered several times per year at the Joslin Clinic in Boston.

CALORIE KING
www.calorieking.com
This database provides calorie, fat, and carbohydrate information on commonly eaten foods and meals from popular restaurants across the United States. It also serves as a comprehensive guide for healthy eating approaches to weight and diabetes management.

---

you cannot anticipate every crisis before it happens will help you to bounce back from those times when you are faced with the unpredictable. This is when it becomes necessary to take a deep breath, look at the situation with fresh ideas, and try to recommit to healthier choices. Self-criticism will only pull you further off track.

You may also sometimes experience setbacks in your weight-loss progress even when you're doing everything "right." This is normal. You can expect some ups and downs along the way, but you should see a gradual downward trend over time.

Losing one or two pounds a week is considered a healthy rate of weight loss, but this is often too subtle to keep people motivated. Focusing on your monthly weight-loss pattern instead can help you recognize the progress you're making.

Get support from family and friends

Find the supports you need. This may include your spouse, other family members, friends, and coworkers. In addition, consider joining a club focused on an activity you enjoy, such as walking, hiking, or biking, or a support group focused on weight loss and health. Reach out for exercise partners or weight-loss partners and connect to advocacy groups such as the American Diabetes Association.

Be on the lookout for people in your life who offer misguided helping, or who take on the role of the "diabetes police" or "food police." These are usually people who love you and are worried about your health but simply do not know how to express their concern in a way that feels supportive to you. Help them to understand what it is that you need from them through patient and assertive communication. This involves first knowing yourself and tuning in to what it is that you need for support. For example, do you need someone to take care of your kids while you exercise? Or do you need the companionship of an exercise partner? Perhaps you need both.

It helps to assume that your family members and friends love you and are doing what they are doing out of love and concern. That does not mean that you should just put up with what they are doing. But it may make it easier to approach them and communicate your needs clearly and openly so that they can change their behavior to something that really is helpful to you.

Seek a supportive health-care team

In addition to finding supports in your social and family life, take the time to build a supportive medical team. This ideally will include a primary-care doctor and an endocrinologist and may also include a nutritionist, nurse educator, exercise physiologist, and mental health practitioner. Look for team members who are willing to help you define specific and clearly achievable goals together as a collaborative process. If you're not sure which targets to prioritize, ask your team members for advice. For example, should you focus first on improving your blood glucose levels or your blood pressure? Or should you focus on establishing a maintainable exercise routine? Keep in mind, however, that your input is important because you are the one who will be carrying out the steps to reach your health goals.

Make health a priority

Decide that you and your health are worth the effort it will take to change your eating and exercise habits. This can be the most challenging part of the process for some people because of feelings of low self-worth or because of the feeling that it's impossible to achieve an "ideal" thin body size.

How to overcome these feelings? One way is to note how much better you feel when you are actively engaged in the process of improving your health and well-being. Another is to remind yourself that it's not necessary to be thin to be healthy. Look for role models who aren't thin but are healthy, and aim to emulate them rather than, say, slender fashion models.

Reward yourself

Nobody can deny that the possible complications of diabetes are real and can be frightening; this is truly a "high stakes" disease. However, fear and self-criticism are not good motivators for behavior change. In fact, they often make people feel powerless and stuck. Rather than focusing exclusively on avoiding complications in the future, determine what the "here and now" positive rewards for your behavior changes (and their short-term results) will be. When setting goals for behavior change, don't forget to build in positive rewards for yourself once you meet targets along the way. Get creative in finding non-food-related rewards that are personally meaningful.

By using these weight management strategies, you will soon notice changes in your blood glucose levels, and you may need to cut back on your insulin doses or doses of other diabetes medicines. (See your health-care provider for help in making these medication changes.) Make a point to also take time to register the subtler, "real life" rewards that come from feeling healthier: Notice whether you have improved energy and stamina, feel stronger, have better concentration and improved mood, and feel more self-confident. These are meaningful changes that will influence your overall quality of life. ☐

BARIATRIC SURGERY
Lifestyle Changes for Before and After

by Laurie Block, M.S., R.D., C.D.E.

The American public spends nearly $35 billion annually on weight-loss products and services. However, whether the money is spent on assistance with behavior modification, fitness programs, medicines, or diet books, traditional methods of weight loss often prove unsuccessful. In fact, 90% of overweight people who try to reduce their weight do not sustain significant weight loss. So it should come as no surprise that alternative methods of weight loss are on the rise. One of these methods is weight-loss surgery, often called bariatric surgery, which has been increasing in popularity since it was introduced in the United States in 1969. According to the American Society for Bariatric Surgery, more than 175,000 such surgeries were performed in the United States in 2006, and more than one million surgeries have been performed since its introduction.

The World Health Organization now states that bariatric surgery is the most effective way of reducing and maintaining weight in severely and morbidly obese people. Clinical studies from the United States report that people who have the surgery lose approximately 60% of their excess weight in 12 months and continue to lose weight 18–24 months after surgery. Studies also show that people who have had this surgery maintain a loss of between 35% and 75% of their excess weight 10–15 years after surgery.

Besides bringing about weight loss, bariatric surgery can lead to reductions in blood pressure, blood glucose levels, and symptoms of sleep apnea. However, this surgery is not an easy road to weight loss. It requires significant lifestyle changes both before surgery and for the rest of a person's life.

Gastric bypass procedure

Bariatric surgery is considered an option for people who are severely obese and have at least one substantial obesity-related condition and for people who are morbidly obese. Severe obesity is defined as having a body-mass index (BMI) greater than 35. Obesity-related conditions include diabetes, high blood pressure, sleep apnea, and arthritis. Morbid obesity is defined as being more than 100 pounds above an ideal body weight or having a BMI greater than 40.

The most common form of bariatric surgery performed in the United States is the Roux-en-Y gastric bypass procedure. Considered the gold standard in weight-loss surgery, it restricts both the amount of food that can be eaten at any one time and the amount that is absorbed by the body. It is believed to offer the best balance of effectiveness versus risk.

In the procedure, the stomach is divided into two parts: an upper part and a lower part. The upper part becomes a small pouch about the size of an egg and is able to hold 5% of its original capacity. This small pouch is then connected to the jejunum (the middle section of the small intestine). The procedure essentially reroutes food, bypassing the upper half of the intestine known as the duodenum.

With the upper part of the intestine bypassed and essentially 95% of the stomach unavailable for digestion, many changes occur that are believed to be helpful for weight reduction. The first obvious change is a smaller upper stomach pouch, which allows for a quicker feeling of fullness. Second, without the upper half of the intestine available, fewer nutrients are absorbed.

In addition, gastric bypass surgery causes changes in the amount of *ghrelin* a person produces. Ghrelin is a hormone normally released in the stomach and upper part of the small intestine that stimulates hunger. In lean individuals, blood levels of ghrelin tend to be high before meals and much lower after meals. Some studies suggest that in obese individuals, ghrelin levels don't fall as much after meals, possibly causing continued feelings of hunger even though food has been eaten. After gastric bypass surgery, however, ghrelin levels have been found to be barely measurable, which may promote a feeling of fullness and decrease the desire to eat.

Preparing for surgery

Bariatric centers vary in their presurgical recommendations, but most aim to prepare you and your support system for the psychological, dietary, and lifestyle changes necessary after surgery. Nutrient requirements and preventing complications are the major focuses of the presurgical discussion. Losing some weight before surgery is recommended to help decrease the size of the liver and allow for an easier operation. For people who have diabetes, it's important to have blood glucose levels in a normal range before surgery.

Your presurgical consultation with a registered dietitian will likely include a review of portion sizes; advice on getting enough fluids and protein in your diet; a discussion of "dumping syndrome" and how to prevent it, including choosing unsweetened beverages over sweetened ones; and a discussion of the potential for food intolerances, such as lactose intolerance, to develop after surgery. Your dietitian may also recommend meal schedules and exercise, as well as appropriate protein bars or shakes and vitamin supplements.

It has become increasingly common for medical centers to start those scheduled for bypass surgery on a liquid diet as much as 10 days before surgery in an attempt to deplete liver glycogen stores. Depleting glycogen stores reduces the size of the liver by as much as 40% and decreases abdominal size, making it easier for the surgeon to perform the operation.

Even before the 10-day countdown to surgery, however, it helps to have made some lifestyle changes that will prepare you for life—and proper nutrition—after surgery. Here are some steps to take once you have been approved for gastric bypass surgery:

Start a meal schedule. In preparation for surgery, start a consistent meal schedule. Get into the habit of having three meals a day, including breakfast, and have some protein at each meal. Both of these habits are important for getting adequate nutrients, and having protein in a meal promotes a feeling of fullness after the meal.

Take a multivitamin supplement. Begin taking a multivitamin, multimineral supplement every day so that it becomes part of your daily routine. Discuss with your surgical team when (at what hour of day) you should take your supplements. Often, multivitamins are taken in the morning and evening, and calcium and iron are taken two hours apart to maximize absorption. Ask your team to recommend a multivitamin that you are likely to be able to tolerate after surgery, and purchase a daily pill dispenser if that will make it easier for you to remember to take your supplements.

Take a calcium supplement. Start taking a calcium supplement. If you currently take calcium carbonate, switch to calcium citrate, which is more easily absorbed. Calcium citrate can be found in both powder and pill forms.

Exercise. Begin exercising at a level you feel comfortable with, even if it is only five minutes a day. If you are unable to walk, try upper-body exercises and seated leg exercises to promote better blood circulation. Your goal is to establish a routine and ideally build up to 30 minutes of physical activity a day. Daily exercises to strengthen and build muscles will help you maintain muscle mass, aid in healing, and assure good circulation. Remember that performing strenuous exercise or lifting more than 15 pounds during the six weeks after your surgery is discouraged. Arrange for any heavy lifting that needs to be done before your surgery date.

Increase fluids. Drink at least 48 ounces (6 cups) of water a day. Ideally, 64 ounces of water daily is recommended. Purchasing a water bottle may help you keep track of your fluid intake. Start sipping fluids throughout the day, and attempt to drink fluids between meals. After surgery, it is important to drink fluids between meals rather than at meals. If you prefer beverages other than water, start purchasing noncarbonated, sugar-free, caffeine-free beverages.

Practice portion control. One of the most common complications of surgery is dumping syndrome, or rapid emptying of stomach contents into the small intestine. This typically causes symptoms such as light-headedness and sweating. Dumping syndrome tends to occur when too much fatty food or when sugar-sweetened liquids are consumed. Reviewing portion sizes with measuring cups and spoons or a food scale may help you to avoid eating or drinking too much at one time and experiencing dumping syndrome after surgery.

Limit snacking. Snacks may be necessary to control hunger, but try to limit them to once or twice a day. Snacks should contain no more than 100–150 calories and should contain some protein. Protein bars or shakes with at least 14 grams of protein but no more than 150 calories are good choices for snacks. High-fiber fruits and vegetables are also good snack choices before surgery.

Chew your foods. Get into the habit of eating slowly and chewing your food well. Eating slowly will enable you to recognize when you are full and when to stop eating. After surgery, it can also help to prevent vomiting. On average, a meal should last about 30 minutes.

Practice deep breathing exercises. Deep breathing exercises enhance lung capacity in preparation for general anesthesia. Before surgery, you can build lung strength by blowing up balloons. After surgery, you may be instructed to use an *incentive spirometer* to help perform deep breathing and keep your lungs clear. You may want to ask your surgeon to show you an incentive spirometer before surgery. You may use the incentive spirometer for up to four weeks after discharge from the hospital.

Avoid smoking. Some medical centers simply will not operate on smokers. If you are giving up smoking to have this surgery, you may want to purchase some acetaminophen (Tylenol) to combat any headaches associated with quitting smoking.

Stock your kitchen. After surgery you will have to follow a liquid then a soft diet for a period of time. You can plan ahead by stocking up on sugar-free clear liquids, gelatins, Popsicles, broths, teas, and soft foods. Sugar-free products sweetened with sorbitol may be used both before and after surgery, but be aware than most people can tolerate no more than 10–15 grams a day. More than that may cause gastrointestinal symptoms.

Discuss medicines. Ask your surgeon whether to discontinue any medicines you currently take before surgery. You will also need a game plan for restarting all or some of the medicines you take after surgery. In addition, you may want to purchase a pain reliever such as acetaminophen, because after surgery you will need to avoid aspirin and nonsteroidal anti-inflammatory drugs such as ibuprofen (Advil, Motrin) and naproxen (Aleve).

After surgery

Immediately after surgery, hydration is a priority, and a clear liquid diet is recommended. People recovering from surgery are generally offered 1–3 ounces of clear, noncarbonated, caffeine-free liquid to sip slowly. Sugar-free beverages or gelatin, water, bouillon, caffeine-free herbal tea, or uncarbonated beverages are usually well-tolerated. Flat diet soft drinks or artificially sweetened drinks such as Crystal Light may also be used. Ideally, you should drink one ounce of liquid every 15 minutes to ensure that you drink a minimum of 48 ounces a day. Drinking from a medicine cup, which holds about an ounce of liquid, can help you keep track of how much you're drinking. Using a straw, however, is discouraged because people tend to suck up air along with the liquid, making it more difficult to assess how much has been drunk.

One to two weeks after surgery most people are ready to start on a "full liquid" diet, which can include milk-based products such as nonfat or low-fat milk, no-sugar-added Carnation Instant Breakfast, low-fat pudding and yogurt, and commercially prepared protein drinks. Your surgical center may be able to recommend a particular protein shake. Use lactose-free products if you are unable to tolerate milk.

Pureed foods can generally be added to the diet two to four weeks after surgery. Using a food processor or blender and adding a small amount of liquid will help to get the right consistency. High-protein foods such as tofu, baked fish, eggs, cottage cheese, and ground dark turkey or chicken meat are often tolerated. During this phase, it is important to begin separating meals and fluids. Drink water or noncaloric beverages 30 minutes before meals and 90 minutes after meals. Eating solid foods with little or no fluid slows digestion and helps you to feel full longer.

At four to six weeks after surgery, solid foods can usually be reintroduced one at a time. Focus on adding high-protein foods such as soy products, quinoa, eggs, milk, low-fat soups, moist ground lean meats, flaked fish, ground beef, tuna, and salmon. Begin your meals by eating protein, then add soft cooked vegetables and unsweetened cooked, canned, or fresh fruit. Pay close attention to your bodily sensations and stop eating at the earliest sign of fullness.

Avoid tough dry cuts of meat such as steak. You will also need to avoid fibrous foods such as asparagus, popcorn, peanuts, celery, and rhubarb. Fibrous foods may get stuck in the small opening of the stomach pouch.

The need for hydration will continue to be important, and high-protein drinks may be continued.

Lifetime habits

Once you've had gastric bypass surgery, your gastrointestinal tract is permanently changed, and you need to take special steps to ensure proper nutrition.

Vitamins. You will need to continue taking a multivitamin that contains thiamine to supplement your diet. There is a lifelong need for vitamins since your total calorie intake will be low, and because the surgery bypasses the duodenum, where many nutrients are normally absorbed. People who develop food intolerances may also have trouble getting all the vitamins they need. You may initially take a chewable multivitamin, then progress to a tablet or capsule when you can tolerate it.

In addition to a multivitamin, you will need to start taking vitamin B_{12} (cyanocobalamin) supplements. A daily dose of 500 micrograms is usually enough to prevent deficiencies. Supplementation can be taken as tablets, in a nasal spray such as Nascobal, or as monthly intramuscular injections. The importance of vitamin B_{12} should not be underestimated. Lifelong use is necessary to prevent anemia and neurological damage.

Protein. Consuming adequate amounts of protein is one of the most important issues for people who have had bariatric surgery. Protein is needed to maintain body tissues and help in the healing process. The recommendation is to consume approximately 1 gram of protein per kilogram ideal body weight per day. Most men require a minimum of 56 grams of protein per day, and most women, a minimum of 46 grams. However, many bariatric centers recommend consuming 60 grams of protein per day. One ounce of meat or other foods derived from animals has approximately 7 grams of protein. Most meal plans contain 6–7 ounces of high-protein foods daily.

Fluids. It is important to keep hydrated, but it is also important not to drink and eat at the same time. The usual advice is to drink fluids 30 minutes before meals and 90 minutes after meals. Separating fluids from meals will help you feel fuller longer. In addition, drinking and eating together can distend the gastric pouch, which can result in discomfort, vomiting, or light-headedness associated with dumping syndrome.

Caffeine recommendations vary. Because caffeine may irritate the stomach, and other components of coffee and tea may inhibit iron absorption, some programs recommend avoiding caffeinated drinks entirely. If you wish to drink coffee or tea, ask your medical team for individualized advice.

Sweets. Avoid concentrated sweets and beverages. Foods such as pastries, cakes, and sugar-sweetened beverages get digested rapidly, have a lot of calories, and contribute to dumping syndrome. Replacing sweetened beverages with low-sugar beverages will help prevent nausea and vomiting.

Portions. As the stomach pouch heals and the pouch expands, the stomach will have a capacity of about one cup. Being able to recognize when you're full and keeping portion sizes controlled will be a significant part of keeping weight off and preventing dumping syndrome. Eating too much, as well as eating too fast and not chewing foods well, are all associated with vomiting and nausea.

Iron. Even with a diet high in animal proteins, which contain easily absorbed iron, people who have had bariatric surgery—particularly premenopausal women—can develop iron deficiency anemia, with the accompanying symptoms of extreme fatigue and weakness. To prevent anemia, iron supplementation may be necessary. Ferrous sulfate is commonly recommended and likely to be absorbed. Feosol, Slow FE, and Niferex are common iron supplements. Ask your physician to evaluate your total iron levels and hemoglobin levels. If constipation occurs when you take iron supplements, try to include more high-fiber foods such as well-chewed apples, berries, and whole grains in your diet. A product called Benefiber can also be added to liquids to alleviate constipation.

Calcium. Calcium citrate with vitamin D is required after surgery to prevent deficiencies. Most surgical centers recommend taking between 1200 and 1500 milligrams of calcium daily to prevent fractures and maintain good bone health. Vitamin D is typically included in both calcium supplements and multivitamin supplements; a total of approximately 800 IU a day is recommended.

Including low-fat cheeses and milk in the diet also boosts calcium intake. Even people who are lactose intolerant can often tolerate as much as 4 ounces of milk, or as much as 6 grams of lactose (milk sugar) per meal. Those who must avoid lactose because of symptoms such as cramping or diarrhea may want to try low-lactose milk or calcium-fortified soy or rice milk.

Alcohol. Recommendations for alcohol vary. Many programs do not recommend drinking alcohol until six months after surgery. People who have had bariatric surgery produce limited amounts of the enzymes needed to metabolize alcohol, so they often feel the effects of alcohol quicker and are also more sensitive to its effects. In addition, alcoholic drinks are caloric, so they may interfere with weight loss. However, some people choose to and can tolerate one to two drinks—with a drink equaling 12 ounces of beer, 4 ounces of wine, or 1 ounce of a distilled spirit—six months after surgery.

Exercise. Immediately after surgery you will be encouraged to walk. Upon discharge, walking for 15 minutes four times a day is recommended. Walking should be gradually increased for the first 6–8 weeks. A one- to two-mile walk per day is a reasonable goal. If you have degenerative joint problems, water aerobics is a good option. Exercise helps prevent formation of blood clots and stimulates muscle growth and strength. Weight training and muscle strengthening will help improve appearance and maintain metabolic rate.

However, exercise does not eliminate the excess skin that may become apparent with quick weight loss. Support garments may be helpful, and additional surgical procedures can remove excess skin.

Follow-up care. Staying in touch with your medical team and joining a support group will help you stick to your postsurgery guidelines. For the first year, it is recommended that you meet with your doctor as recommended, usually no less than every three months. After the first year, annual exams are suggested, especially to check for any nutrient deficiencies.

WHAT'S OVERWEIGHT?

This graph shows what is considered a normal weight
and what is considered overweight or obese for people of different heights.

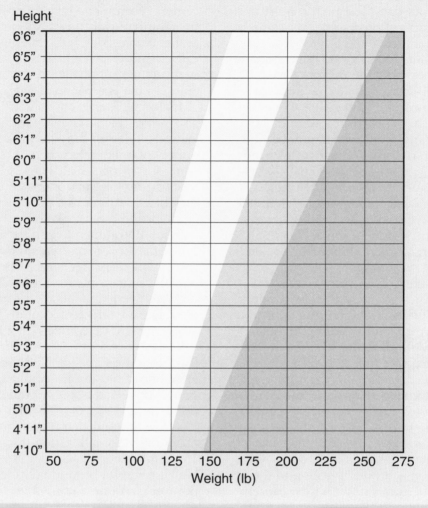

Height

Weight (lb)

Normal Weight   Overweight   Obese

At about 18–24 months after surgery, most people stop losing weight and need to start a weight-maintenance plan that includes both an appropriate meal plan and support from others. If a support group is not available in your area, try an online group such as www.obesityhelp.com or groups.msn.com/GastricBypassSupportGroup.

Learning more

Gastric bypass surgery is not without risks, and it requires major lifestyle changes for those who have it done. In spite of the potential complica-

tions, however, bypass surgery has improved the health and quality of life of many people.

For more information on bariatric surgery and other obesity treatments, as well as opportunities for advocacy, look through the Web sites of the American Society for Bariatric Surgery, www.asbs.org, or the American Obesity Association, www.obesity.org. You can also call the American Society for Bariatric Surgery, at (352) 331-4900, and the American Obesity Association, at (202) 776-7711. □

Nutrition and Meal Planning

Tips 621–679 383

Are You Label-Able? 388

Sizing Up Your Servings 396

Vegetarian and Vegan Meal Planning 400

Trans Fat begone! 412

Extreme Makeover—Recipe Edition 416

10

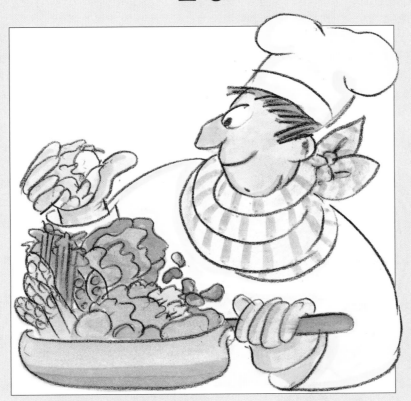

Nutrition and Meal Planning Tips

621–679

621. Find nutrition information on the Nutrition Facts label, where manufacturers provide serving size information, quantities of specific nutrients, and percent Daily Values (%DV). Nutrient information required on all food labels includes total calories, calories from fat, total fat, saturated fat, *trans* fat, cholesterol, sodium, total carbohydrate, dietary fiber, sugars, protein, vitamin A, vitamin C, calcium, and iron.

622. Don't assume that the nutrition information listed on the label is for the entire package of food. To find out how many portions of food a package contains, look at the "Servings Per Container."

623. Do not use the number of grams of "Sugars" listed on the food label to consider when evaluating how a food will affect your blood glucose level. "Total Carbohydrate" will give you a more accurate picture of how a serving of a particular food will affect your blood glucose level since it takes into account all of the carbohydrates that will affect blood glucose.

624. To increase your fiber intake, try to choose breads, grains, and snack foods that provide at least 3 grams of fiber per serving and cereals and entrées that provide 5 or more grams of fiber per serving.

625. If you are eating a food with more than 5 grams of dietary fiber per serving, you can subtract half the grams of "Dietary Fiber" from the grams of "Total Carbohydrate" before you calculate the number of carbohydrate choices in your meal.

626. If a food contains more than 5 grams of sugar alcohols or more per serving, you can subtract half the grams of "Sugar Alcohols" from the "Total Carbohydrate" value before calculating the carbohydrate choices in your meal or snack.

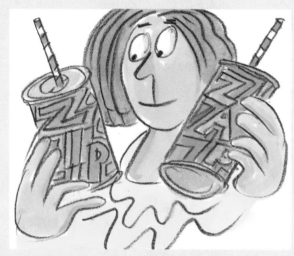

627. Reading the ingredients list can be helpful when comparing two products with similar names.

628. People who follow a vegan diet may need to take extra care to meet their nutrition needs. Some vegans (and vegetarians) may need to supplement their meal plan with a multivitamin or calcium.

629. Combining grains or seeds with legumes or beans will provide a complete protein. It's not necessary to eat these combinations at the same meal, but they should be eaten the same day.

630. Get calcium from calcium-fortified foods such as soy milk, rice milk, orange juice, and calcium-processed tofu. Legumes, almonds, peanuts, walnuts, and dark, leafy greens such as broccoli, collards, kale, mustard greens, and spinach are also rich in calcium.

631. Get vitamin D by getting 5–15 minutes of sun exposure every day, if possible (but protect yourself with sunscreen for prolonged exposure). If your sun exposure is limited, be sure to eat vitamin-D-fortified foods.

632. Look for products low in fat and sodium, and if you are a vegan, examine food labels closely for ingredients such as casein and whey, which are milk derivatives found in some soy cheeses, margarine, and processed foods.

633. To keep your saturated fat intake down, try to avoid products that contain palm oil, palm kernel oil, or coconut oil, which are high in saturated fat.

634. If you're trying to cut back on fat, try using vegetable or fruit juice, vegetable or mushroom broth, or wine as a cooking liquid.

635. Vegetable oil sprays are also helpful because they allow you to use less; you can make your own by pouring oil into a spray bottle.

636. Discard dried herbs and spices that have lost their zing; even when stored in a cool, dry place in an airtight container, most dried herbs and spices lose their flavor after about a year.

637. Pasta and rice come in all sorts of colors, shapes, and flavors. Trying a different variety can liven up your basic meals.

638. Instead of dried pasta, look for fresh pasta in the refrigerated section of the supermarket. (If you won't eat an entire package of fresh pasta in a day or two, cook what you'll eat and freeze the rest for later.)

639. If cold cereal is a morning mainstay, read labels carefully; one may have more B vitamins while another has more iron.

640. Store cereal in airtight containers or food bags so they don't go stale.

641. Consider precut or bagged salads, precut vegetables or fruit, and other ready-to-use items. While they can be more costly, convenience ingredients may be worth the expense if they mean preparing a decent meal for yourself.

642. If you're experiencing green salad burnout, bagged salad mixes can offer other interesting meal possibilities.

643. It's perfectly OK to use ready-to-eat foods, but they usually taste better and have greater nutritional value if you jazz them up.

644. When you go to a restaurant in an ethnic area, take some time to check out the neighborhood groceries for new ingredients to incorporate into your own cooking.

645. Work with a health-care provider or registered dietitian to ensure that your eating plan is balanced and will help you maintain blood glucose control.

646. Keeping careful food and blood-glucose-monitoring records can make it easier to resolve any fluctuations in blood glucose levels as you try new foods and eating habits.

647. Becoming more familiar with standard serving sizes can help you figure out how much you are eating and whether you are meeting or exceeding guidelines for a healthy diet.

648. If you have trouble controlling your portion sizes, using packaged foods such as frozen meals can help remove the temptation to overeat.

649. Use the food label or ask your dietitian to help you figure out how to fit preportioned foods into your meal plan.

650. When eating out, request small portions (such as "kid size" or "lunch size" portions), resist the urge to super-size, try an appetizer and a salad as a meal, or share a meal (and the calories) with a friend.

651. If you order a full portion, ask for half of it to be wrapped in a doggy bag before it is served to remove the temptation to eat it all. For food safety reasons, be sure your doggy bag gets to your refrigerator within two hours of the beginning of your meal.

652. Because heart disease and stroke are the main causes of death among people with diabetes, focus a discerning eye on the type and amount of fat in the diet as well as the type and amount of carbohydrate.

653. Manmade *trans* fat should be avoided entirely if possible. Identify foods containing *trans* fat by reading the ingredients list and looking for any type of hydrogenated vegetable oil in the list. Any partially hydrogenated vegetable oil contains *trans* fat.

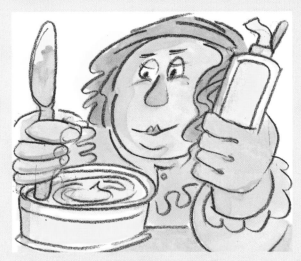

654. If you have no choice but to buy margarine that contains partially hydrogenated oil, choose the tub or squeeze-bottle variety rather than stick margarine.

655. Until there are more widespread regulations on *trans* fats, most diners will need to be aware of which restaurant foods commonly have them and avoid those foods.

656. If you frequent a particular restaurant chain, research your favorite foods and find alternatives on the menu if you find they contain *trans* fat.

657. In cooking, oil almost always can be substituted for butter or margarine with similar results.

658. In baking, consider using butter instead of margarine or shortening. If the amount of fat in the recipe is important to the quality, you may also use half oil and half butter, or substitute completely with oil. It is a good idea to test this method on a small recipe since using oil may change the result.

659. One quick trick for eating more healthfully while still enjoying favorite foods is to simply decrease your portion size when eating high-fat, high-sugar, or high-sodium foods.

660. Eliminating "optional" ingredients such as salt in the cooking water or high-fat, high-calorie sauces on vegetables can help you achieve healthy eating goals.

661. To improve the health benefits of a favorite recipe, look over the list of ingredients, consider the role each plays in the recipe, and modify only one at a time. This gives you an opportunity to judge the success of your single change.

662. While yeast breads require salt to control the rising of the dough, in other recipes, salt can be cut in half or totally eliminated without compromising the final results.

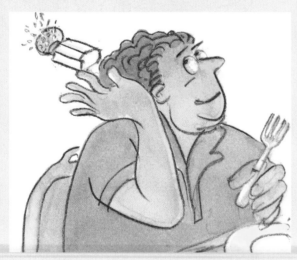

663. Tasting foods before salting them and removing the saltshaker from the table are two great starts to healthier eating.

664. Adding fiber adds to the health benefits of a dish, and adding herbs, spices, and other low-calorie but flavorful ingredients makes nutritious dishes more appealing to eat.

665. Lighten up packaged mixes by trying lower-fat options in preparation. For example, use half of the oil called for in packaged pasta salad mixes, or try using low-fat or skim milk when making instant pudding.

666. Make soup or stew ahead of time, then refrigerate and skim off the hardened fat on top before reheating to serve.

667. Reduce the fat content in homemade baked goods by substituting unsweetened applesauce, pureed prunes, or another pureed fruit for part of the oil, shortening, margarine, or butter.

668. Fortify the taste of low-fat dishes with fat-free seasonings, spices, and herbs.

669. Use artificial sweeteners in recipes when sugar is used only for its sweet taste, not to add body or texture to a dish.

670. For baked items, a special baking version of an artificial sweetener may be necessary. For foods that will be heated, consult the sweetener manufacturer's directions to determine whether a particular product can be used.

671. Low-salt or low-sodium versions of canned vegetables, soy sauce, broth, and seasoning mixes substitute nicely for the full-salt versions.

672. Limit the use of high-sodium foods in your recipes. Cured foods such as bacon and ham, foods packed in salty brine such as pickles, olives, and sauerkraut, and condiments such as mustard, ketchup, and barbecue sauce can be significant sources of sodium in your recipes.

673. Whole wheat flour can replace from one-quarter to half of the all-purpose flour in most recipes.

674. Use whole-grain pasta or brown rice in recipes to boost their fiber content.

675. Add beans to enhance the fiber content and flavor of a recipe. However, don't forget to count the carbohydrate content of added beans: 15 grams of carbohydrate per one-third cup of cooked beans.

676. For the best flavor, buy the freshest ingredients you can find. Buy locally grown fruits and vegetables in season, when possible, or purchase frozen fruits and vegetables, which are generally frozen immediately after picking, so they retain a fresh taste and maximum nutrients.

Nutrition and Meal Planning

677. If you want to substitute fresh herbs for dry in a recipe, use one tablespoon of fresh herb for each teaspoon of dried.

678. Add seasonings to chilled foods, such as salad dressings and dips, several hours before serving to allow time for their flavors to blend.

679. If you're making a hot dish such as soup or stew, add herbs toward the end of the cooking time so their flavor won't disappear.

ARE YOU LABEL-ABLE?

by Belinda O'Connell,
M.S., R.D., C.D.E.,
and Laura Hieronymus,
M.S.Ed., A.P.R.N., B.C.-A.D.M., C.D.E.

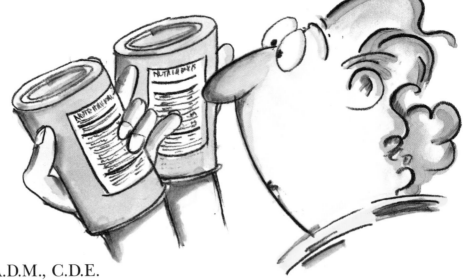

Eating healthfully and following a meal plan are key components of good diabetes care whether you use oral or injectable medicines or diet and exercise to manage your diabetes. Knowing how to read a food label can help you choose healthful foods, figure out portion sizes, count carbohydrates, limit sodium or fat, and keep track of calories. Understanding how to use the information found on food labels can also help you to choose foods that meet your vitamin and mineral requirements. In short, being "label-able" can take the guesswork out of healthy eating.

Label legalities

A majority of the prepared foods you find in your local grocery store are required to have a nutrition label. Nutrition labeling of most foods is regulated by the Food and Drug Administration (FDA), under the Nutrition Labeling and Education Act of 1990, which identifies the nutrients that must be listed on food labels, other nutrients that may be listed, allowed health claims, and standard portion sizes. The Act also defines terminology commonly used on labels such as "light," "reduced-fat," and "sodium free."

Raw, unprocessed fruits and vegetables, meat, fish, and poultry are not required to have nutrition labels, though voluntary labeling is strongly encouraged, and many U.S. food stores provide this information, either by posting it near fresh food displays or by labeling foods such as meats that are packaged in the store. Other foods that are not required to bear nutrition labels include food prepared for immediate consumption such as restaurant, cafeteria, and airplane food; ready-to-eat food prepared primarily on-site, such as bakery store items; foods prepared by some small businesses; and medical foods (special foods prescribed by a physician to manage a disease or health condition). Restaurants that make health claims for certain foods on their menus or in advertising are required to provide nutrition information for those foods.

Nutritional and herbal supplements have Nutrition Facts labels similar to those on packaged foods, but they are regulated by the FDA under a different set of guidelines, the Dietary Supplement Health and Education Act of 1994. Under this act, supplement manufacturers are responsible for making sure dietary supplements are safe before they are marketed and that label information is truthful and not misleading. The FDA has strict guidelines that regulate the types of information and health or nutrition claims allowed on supplement labels.

Nutrition information on food labels can be found in several locations. These include the Nutrition Facts label, the ingredients list, and other areas of the label where health claims may be displayed.

The Nutrition Facts label

Your best source of nutrition information is the Nutrition Facts label, where manufacturers provide serving size information, quantities of specific nutrients, and percent Daily Values (%DV). Nutrient information required on all food labels includes total calories, calories from fat, total fat, saturated fat, *trans* fat, cholesterol, sodium, total carbohydrate, dietary fiber, sugars, protein, vitamin A, vitamin C, calcium, and iron.

SAMPLE FOOD LABELS

These Nutrition Facts labels from two different types of pizza show how standard labeling practices make it easier to compare two similar food items.

INDIVIDUAL GOURMET VEGETARIAN PIZZA
made with whole wheat flour

LARGE MEAT LOVERS SUPREME DEEP DISH PIZZA

Nutrition Facts

Serving Size: 1 pizza (170 g)
Servings Per Container: 1

Amount Per Serving
Calories 329   Calories from Fat 81

	% Daily Value*
Total Fat 9 g	**14%**
Saturated Fat 3 g	**16%**
Trans Fat 3 g	
Cholesterol 15 mg	**5%**
Sodium 360 mg	**15%**
Total Carbohydrate 47 g	**16%**
Dietary Fiber 6 g	**24%**
Sugars 4 g	
Protein 15 g	

Vitamin A 8%	Vitamin C 10%
Calcium 15%	Iron 8%

*Percent Daily Values are based on a 2,000 calorie diet. Your daily values may be higher or lower depending on your calorie needs.

Nutrition Facts

Serving Size: ¼ pizza, 2 slices (154 g)
Servings Per Container: 4

Amount Per Serving
Calories 510   Calories from Fat 235

	% Daily Value*
Total Fat 26 g	**40%**
Saturated Fat 12 g	**62%**
Trans Fat 3 g	
Cholesterol 55 mg	**18%**
Sodium 890 mg	**37%**
Total Carbohydrate 43 g	**14%**
Dietary Fiber 3 g	**12%**
Sugars 6 g	
Protein 26 g	

Vitamin A 0%	Vitamin C 0%
Calcium 4%	Iron 17%

*Percent Daily Values are based on a 2,000 calorie diet. Your daily values may be higher or lower depending on your calorie needs.

Nutrient information allowed but not required on nutrition labels includes calories from saturated fat, polyunsaturated fat, monounsaturated fat, potassium, soluble fiber, insoluble fiber, sugar alcohols and other carbohydrates, percent of vitamin A present as beta-carotene (a nutrient found in plant foods that is converted to vitamin A in the body), and other essential vitamins and minerals (those the body cannot make at all or in sufficient quantities to meet its daily needs). If a health claim is made anywhere on the food package about a nutrient that is allowed but not required, that nutrient must be included in the Nutrition Facts panel.

No nutrients other than those specifically required or allowed are permitted on the Nutrition Facts label.

Serving size. The serving size is the portion size for which all of the nutrition information on the food label is based. In the past, serving sizes on labels were determined by individual manufacturers, and they varied a great deal. Today, serving sizes are standardized, and all manufacturers are required to use the same standard portion sizes. Standard serving sizes are based on amounts people typically eat in a single sitting, and they must be provided in both familiar measures, such as cups, tablespoons, or slices, and in metric measure, such as weight in grams (g) or volume in milliliters (ml).

If you look at the sample food labels for pizza on this page, you can see that the serving size for the vegetarian pizza is 1 pizza (170 g), while the serving size for the meat pizza is 2 slices (154 g).

PERSONALIZING THE PERCENT DAILY VALUE

The Percent Daily Values (%DV) on food labels are based on a 2,000-calorie diet, which may or may not be appropriate for you. To individualize these values according to the number of calories you eat daily, follow the steps below.

STEP 1: Determine your approximate daily calorie needs:

WOMEN		MEN	
Weight Loss..............	1,500 calories	Weight Loss..............	1,800–2,000 calories
Weight Maintenance	1,800–2,200 calories	Weight Maintenance	2,200–2,500 calories
Active..................	2,200+	Active..................	2,500+

STEP 2: Use this chart to find your personal Percent Daily Values. Keep in mind, however, that even though these values have been adjusted according to calorie intake, they are still based on average adult needs. Individuals may need more or less of these nutrients depending on their age, sex, and overall health.

	1,500 CALORIES	1,800 CALORIES	2,000 CALORIES	2,200 CALORIES	2,500 CALORIES	3,000 CALORIES
Total Fat (grams)	Less than 50 g	Less than 60 g	Less than 65 g	Less than 73 g	Less than 80 g	Less than 99 g
Saturated Fat (grams) (includes *trans* fat)	Less than 15 g	Less than 18 g	Less than 20 g	Less than 24 g	Less than 25 g	Less than 30 g
Cholesterol (milligrams)	Less than 300 mg	Less than 300 mg	Less than 300 mg	Less than 300 mg	Less than 300 mg	Less than 300 mg
Sodium (milligrams)	Less than 2,400 mg	Less than 2,400 mg	Less than 2,400 mg	Less than 2,400 mg	Less than 2,400 mg	Less than 2,400 mg
Dietary Fiber (grams)	At least 20 g	At least 20 g	At least 25 g	At least 25 g	At least 30 g	At least 35 g

Even though the pizzas themselves are different sizes, because the nutrition values are calculated for a similar amount of pizza, you can easily compare the fat, calories, carbohydrate, and other nutrients in the two products.

Not all foods fit neatly into standard serving size categories, however, so the FDA allows manufacturers to adjust serving sizes and to round off values based on specific guidelines. This means that if you need very precise nutrition information about foods, it is most accurate to weigh foods on a food scale yourself.

A common mistake people make when reading food labels is to confuse the weight of the entire serving of food for the amount of carbohydrate in the food. For example, the total weight of the vegetarian pizza is listed as 170 grams, but only 47 grams are carbohydrate. If you want to know how much carbohydrate is in a serving of a food, be sure to look for "Total Carbohydrate" on the label.

Another common mistake is to assume that the nutrition information listed on the label is for the entire package of food. Sometimes, it is, but often, it is not. For example, one 24-ounce soda is actually three servings, and therefore, three times the calories and carbohydrate if you drink the whole bottle. To find out how many portions of food a package contains, look at the "Servings Per Container." If this number is 1, the nutrition information provided is for the whole package, but if this number is greater than 1 and you intend to eat the entire package, you must multiply the amount of calories, fat, carbohydrate, etc., by the number of servings per container to find out how much of these nutrients you will be consuming.

For example, the "Serving Size" for the meat pizza on page 389 is ¼ pizza, 2 slices (154 g). If you were going to eat the whole pizza, you would be eating four servings, so to figure out the amount of nutrients in your actual serving, you would multiply the nutrition information provided by 4. In this case, one serving has 510 calories and 43 grams of carbohydrate. If you were to eat the entire package, you would be consuming 2,040 calories (4×510) and 172 grams of carbohydrate (4×43 grams).

Percent Daily Value (%DV). Major nutrients on food labels, such as fat, cholesterol, sodium, carbohydrate, and protein, must be listed as a quantity, in grams or milligrams, and as a percent Daily Value. Percent Daily Values are reference values designed to help people see how a food fits into their overall diet. Generally, a %DV of 5% or less means the food is a low source of the nutrient, while a %DV of 20% or more means the food is a high source of the nutrient. For example, the amount of fat in one serving of the vegetarian pizza is 9 grams, and the %DV is 14%. This means that one serving of this food provides about 14% or one-seventh of a typical person's recommended maximum daily fat intake, and, therefore, seven servings would provide 100%. One serving of the meat pizza has 26 grams of fat and provides 40% of a typical person's daily fat intake, so just 2½ servings would supply an entire day's recommended maximum fat intake.

The percent Daily Value also provides context for interpreting the quantities of nutrients in a food. For example, you could mistakenly think the meat pizza is a low-fat food, because 26 grams is a relatively small number, but when you look at the %DV, you see that it is actually a high-fat food, since one serving provides 40% of your day's fat intake. Alternatively, you might think that the vegetarian pizza is a high-sodium food because it has 360 milligrams of sodium, a fairly large number, but when you look at the %DV, you see that one serving provides only 15% of the average person's recommended daily maximum.

Most of the percent Daily Values on food labels are calculated for someone who needs 2,000 calories a day. (Exceptions are cholesterol, sodium, and vitamin and mineral values, which are the same for all healthy adults, no matter how many calories they eat.) Since you may have higher or lower calorie needs, the percent Daily Values on food labels may not be exactly correct for you. You can still use them to compare foods and to quickly determine the general nutritional quality of a food, but to find your personal nutrient values see "Personalizing the Percent Daily Value" on page 390.

Calories. The "Calorie" information tells you the number of calories in one standard serving of the food. (The standard serving size is listed on the label under Serving Size.) Remember, the number of calories in your serving of food will depend on the portion size you actually eat, which may or may not be the same as the standard serving size. To determine the number of calories in your serving of food, measure how much you are eating and compare this to the standard serving size from the food label. If your portion is larger than the standard serving from the food label, you will need to adjust the calories from the food label up to account for your larger portion. If your portion of food is smaller than that listed on the label, you will need to adjust the calories down to account for your smaller portion.

Fat and cholesterol. This section tells you the amount of total fat, saturated fat, *trans* fat, and cholesterol provided by one standard serving of food. (Again, if your portion is larger or smaller, you will need to adjust these values accordingly.) On some products, polyunsaturated fat and monounsaturated fat are listed as well. The Dietary Reference Intake recommends limiting fat intake to 20–35% of calories. The American Diabetes Association (ADA) recommends that people with diabetes limit their saturated fat intake to less than 7% of calories and minimize intake of trans fats.

To figure out how much fat and saturated fat is OK for you, see "Personalizing the Percent Daily Value" on page 390.

Sodium. This tells you the amount of sodium in one standard serving of a food. The ADA recommends that people with diabetes keep their daily total sodium intake under 2300 milligrams per day, and, conveniently, the percent Daily Value for sodium is based on 2400 milligrams per day, so it can help you see if a food is a high-sodium or low-sodium food and how easily it will fit into your diet. For example, ½ cup of regular chicken noodle soup may have up to 940 mg of sodium, which uses up 39% of your daily sodium intake. Reduced-sodium chicken noodle soup, however, may have only 450 mg of sodium, or 19% of your daily recommended maximum intake, so it is a healthier choice.

Carbohydrate. Understanding how to use carbohydrate information from food labels is particularly important for people with diabetes. The most important number for you to look at in this section is "Total Carbohydrate." It is listed in bold letters and tells you the amount of carbohydrate, in grams, found in one standard serving of a food. If you count carbohydrates, "Total Carbohydrate" is the number you should use to calculate carbohydrate choices. This is because research shows that most forms of carbohydrate (including starches, processed sugars, sugar from fruit, and sugars in milk) increase blood glucose levels similarly when they are eaten in equal portions. (The exceptions are dietary fiber, "resistant" starches, and sugar alcohols, which have less of an effect on blood glucose than other carbohydrates.) For more on using food labels to determine carbohydrate choices, see "Calculating Carbohydrate Choices" on this page.

Listed under "Total Carbohydrate" are the amounts of the different types of carbohydrate present in the food. These may include Dietary Fiber, Sugars, Sugar Alcohols, and Other Carbohydrates.

Many people are concerned about the amount of sugar they are getting. The amount of "Sugars" on a food label can give you important clues about how generally healthy a food is: Foods that contain a great deal of sugar are generally not good sources of fiber, vitamins, or minerals and may be high in total fat or saturated fat as well. Nonetheless, the number of grams of "Sugars" listed on the food label is not the most important factor to consider when evaluating how a food will affect your blood glucose level. "Total Carbohydrate" will give you a more accurate picture of how a serving of a particular food will affect your blood glucose level since it takes into account all of the carbohydrates that will affect blood glucose.

The "Dietary Fiber" listing on food labels can be used to identify healthier entrées, breads, grains, cereals, sweets, and snack foods. The percent Daily Value for fiber is 25 grams for a 2,000-calorie diet, but most Americans do not get that much fiber on a daily basis. To increase your fiber intake, try to choose breads, grains, and snack foods that provide at least 3 grams of fiber per serving and cereals and entrées that provide 5 or more grams of fiber per serving.

If you are eating a food with more than 5 grams of dietary fiber per serving, you can subtract half the grams of "Dietary Fiber" from the grams of "Total Carbohydrate" before you calculate the number of carbohydrate choices in your meal. This is done because dietary fiber is not digested and does not increase blood glucose levels.

Many sweets marketed to people with diabetes contain sugar alcohols, such as xylitol, mannitol, and sorbitol. Sugar alcohols have a lower caloric value and raise blood glucose levels less than other forms of carbohydrate, but foods made with sugar alcohols are not necessarily "healthier" or even lower in carbohydrate than foods sweetened with sugar. To determine how a food fits into your meal plan, look at the number of calories and amounts of "Total Carbohydrate," "Total Fat," and "Satu-

CALCULATING CARBOHYDRATE CHOICES

Use the pizza labels on page 389 and the steps below to learn how to calculate the amount of carbohydrate choices in the foods you eat.

STEP 1: Figure out how much carbohydrate is in your portion of food.
■ Find the standard Serving Size from the label.
■ Find the amount of Total Carbohydrate on the label for one standard serving.
■ Measure the portion of food you are actually going to eat.
■ Compare that portion of food to the standard Serving Size from the food label.
■ If your portion of food is larger or smaller than the standard Serving Size, increase or decrease the Total Carbohydrate content accordingly. One way to do this is to divide your portion (in cups, tablespoons, slices, etc.) by the standard Serving Size (using the same unit as before).

STEP 2: Once you know the amount of carbohydrate in your portion of food, you can calculate the number of carbohydrate choices in your portion of food.
■ One carbohydrate choice has 15 grams of carbohydrate.
■ Divide the Total Carbohydrate in your portion of food by 15 grams per carbohydrate choice. Less than 5 grams does not count as a carbohydrate choice; 5–10 grams equals ? carbohydrate choice, and more than 10 and up to 20 grams equals 1 carbohydrate choice.

EXAMPLE:
MEAT LOVERS SUPREME PIZZA
Standard Serving Size: 2 slices
Total Carbohydrate: 43 grams
Portion eaten: 3 slices
Comparison of portion eaten to Serving Size:
  3 ÷ 2 = 1½ servings
Total carbohydrate eaten:
  65 grams (43 grams × 1½ servings)
Number of carbohydrate choices: 4½
(65 grams of carbohydrate eaten ÷ 15 grams of carbohydrate per carbohydrate choice)

rated Fat" the food contains. If the food has fewer calories and less carbohydrate and fat than other, similar products, it is probably a better choice, but in many cases, the amounts of "Total Carbohydrate," "Total Fat," or other nutrients are not significantly different for foods containing sugar alcohols than for other, similar foods. For example, if you compare the nutrition information for Murray Sugar-Free Fudge Dipped Shortbread Cookies made with sugar alcohols and a grocery store brand of Regular Fudge Dipped Shortbread Cookies made with sugar, you can see the sugar-free version is not necessarily a better choice.

MURRAY SUGAR-FREE FUDGE DIPPED SHORTBREAD COOKIES
(Made with sorbitol)
  Serving Size: 5 cookies (29 g)
  Calories: 130
  Total Fat: 7 g
  Total Carbohydrate: 20 g
  Sugars: 0 g
  Sugar Alcohol: 9 g
  Number of Carbohydrate Choices: 1

REGULAR FUDGE DIPPED SHORTBREAD COOKIES
(Made with sugar)
  Serving Size: 2 cookies (25 g)
  Calories: 120
  Total Fat: 6 g
  Total Carbohydrate: 17 g
  Sugars: 8 g
  Sugar Alcohol: 0 g
  Number of Carbohydrate Choices: 1

Since sugar alcohols have a lower caloric value (2–3 calories per gram versus 4 calories per gram for other carbohydrates) and cause a somewhat lower blood glucose response, they are counted somewhat differently from other carbohydrates. If a food contains 5 grams of sugar alcohols or more per serving, you can subtract half the grams of "Sugar Alcohols" from the "Total Carbohydrate" value before calculating the carbohydrate choices in your meal or snack.

Protein. The amount of protein you need is based on your size, calorie needs, and stage of life. The ADA recommends that adults with diabetes eat about the same amount of protein as the general population. The Dietary Reference Intake for protein recommends getting 10-35% of total daily calories from protein. Most labels do not list a percent Daily Value for protein because most Americans get adequate amounts of protein and it is not considered a nutritional concern, so it does not need to be highlighted on the food label. In gen-

eral, men need about 60 grams of protein per day, and women need about 45–50 grams of protein per day.

Vitamins and minerals. Labels are required to list vitamin A, vitamin C, calcium, and iron and are allowed to list information about other essential vitamins and minerals. This information is provided only as a percent Daily Value and is the same for all healthy adults. This information can help you make sure you meet the guidelines for intake of these important nutrients. For example, when choosing fruit juice, you can use the percent Daily Values to help you choose the juice that provides the greatest amounts of vitamins and minerals if you don't get enough of these nutrients elsewhere in your diet. If you look at the two apple juice labels below you can see that Apple Juice A is regular apple juice and has no calcium or vitamin C, but Apple Juice B has been fortified with these nutrients, and one 4-ounce serving provides 100% of the daily vitamin C requirement and 20% of the daily calcium requirement.

APPLE JUICE A
  NUTRITION FACTS
    Serving Size: 8 fl oz (240 ml)
    Servings Per Container: 8
    Calories 120
    Total Fat 0 g
    Sodium 25 mg
    Total Carbohydrate 29 g
    Sugars 26 g
    Protein 0 g
    % Daily Value*
    Vitamin A 0%
    Vitamin C 0%
    Calcium 0%
    Iron 2%
* Percent Daily Values are based on a 2,000 calorie diet.

APPLE JUICE B
  NUTRITION FACTS
    Serving Size: 8 fl oz (240 ml)
    Servings Per Container: 8
    Calories 120
    Total Fat 0 g
    Sodium 40 mg
    Total Carbohydrate 30 g
    Sugars 26 g
    Protein 0 g
    % Daily Value*
    Vitamin A 0%
    Vitamin C 100%
    Calcium 20%
    Iron 0%
  * Percent Daily Values are based on a 2,000 calorie diet.

LABEL TERMS

The FDA regulates the descriptive terms food manufacturers may use on labels and the way in which they may use them, so that "low fat" on one label means the same thing as "low fat" on another. The following list spells out the official meanings of some of the most common label terms.

LABEL TERM	DEFINITION
Free	Means one serving of a food contains no or insignificantly low amounts of a nutrient such as fat, cholesterol, or sodium.
Calorie Free	Less than 5 calories per serving.
Sugar Free	Less than 0.5 grams of sugar per serving.
Sodium Free	Less than 5 milligrams of sodium per serving.
Fat Free	Less than 0.5 grams of fat per serving.
Low Fat	3 grams of fat or less per serving or per 50 grams of the food if the serving size is 2 tablespoons or less or 30 grams or less.
Low Saturated Fat	1 gram of saturated fat or less per serving and 15% or less of calories from saturated fat.
Low Sodium	140 milligrams of sodium or less per serving or per 50 grams of the food if the serving size is 2 tablespoons or less or 30 grams or less.
Very Low Sodium	35 milligrams of sodium or less per serving or per 50 grams of the food if the serving size is 2 tablespoons or less or 30 grams or less.
Low Cholesterol	20 milligrams of cholesterol or less and 2 grams of saturated fat or less per serving or per 50 grams of the food if the serving size is 2 tablespoons or less or 30 grams or less.
Low Calorie	40 calories or less per serving or per 50 grams of the food if the serving size is 2 tablespoons or less or 30 grams or less.
Lean (meats, poultry, fish)	4.5 grams of saturated fat or less, less than 10 grams of fat total, and less than 95 milligrams of cholesterol per serving (of about 3 ounces).
Extra Lean	Less than 2 grams of saturated fat, less than 5 grams of fat total, and less than 95 milligrams of cholesterol per serving (of about 3 ounces).
High	Can be used if the food contains 20% or more of the Daily Value for protein, vitamins, minerals, dietary fiber, or potassium in one serving.
High Fiber	5 grams of fiber or more per serving.
Good Source of	Means one serving of a food contains 10% to 19% of the Daily Value for a nutrient.
Reduced or Less	Means the food contains at least 25% less of a nutrient or of calories than the regular or average representative product.
Light or Lite	For foods deriving less than 50% of calories from fat, means the food is reduced in calories by at least one-third or reduced in fat by at least 50%. For foods deriving more than 50% of calories from fat, the product is reduced in fat by at least 50%. For foods with modified sodium content, the product is reduced in sodium by at least 50%.

HEALTH CLAIMS

UNQUALIFIED HEALTH CLAIMS

The FDA has guidelines for how and when manufacturers may assert that their product may prevent a certain disease or benefit health beyond providing basic nutrition. The FDA has approved 12 "unqualified" nutrient–disease label claims, listed below. Because these statements are sufficiently supported by scientific evidence, they do not need a disclaimer or other qualification to temper the claims being made.

NUTRIENT	DISEASE
(high) Calcium	Osteoporosis
(low) Fat	Certain cancers
(low) Saturated fat and cholesterol	Heart disease
Fiber-containing grain products, fruits, and vegetables	Certain cancers
Fiber (particularly soluble)-containing grain products, fruits, and vegetables	Heart disease
(low) Sodium	High blood pressure
Fruits and vegetables	Certain cancers
Folate	Neural tube defects
Dietary sugar alcohols	Dental cavities
Soluble fiber from certain foods (such as whole oats and psyllium seed husk)	Heart disease
Soy protein	Heart disease
Plant sterol/stanol esters	Heart disease

QUALIFIED HEALTH CLAIMS

In addition to the well-supported health- or disease-related claims listed above, the FDA now allows "qualified" health claims, which apply to nutrients and foods that appear to have beneficial effects but have less supporting evidence. These must have a disclaimer indicating the limited nature of the evidence to ensure that the beneficial effects of the nutrient or food are not misrepresented.

Ingredients lists

Additional information about a packaged food can be gleaned from its ingredients list. Ingredients are listed in order of predominance by weight, so the ingredient that makes up the greatest proportion of the food is listed first, and other ingredients are listed in descending order. Reading the ingredients list can be helpful when comparing two products with similar names. For example, you can't tell from the names of the following two breads which is healthier, but when you look at the ingredients lists, you can see Bread A has whole wheat flour as the first ingredient, and Bread B has wheat flour as the first ingredi-

ent. Wheat flour is simply another term for refined white flour, which contains very little fiber. Whole-grain flours, such as whole wheat, are a better choice because they are higher in fiber.

BREAD A: *Whole Wheat Bread*
Ingredients: 100% stone ground whole wheat flour, water, brown sugar, wheat bran…

BREAD B: *Hearty Classic Health Nut Bread*
Ingredients: Enriched wheat flour, water, high fructose corn syrup, walnuts, whole wheat flour…

Ingredients lists are particularly useful for people with food allergies. Common allergens such as wheat, milk products, nuts, and eggs are now highlighted in food ingredients lists or noted in a separate statement to simplify identification for consumers.

Label terms and claims

The Nutrition Facts label provides information on the quantity of nutrients in foods, such as calories, fat, carbohydrate, and fiber, that play a role in major health concerns in the United States. Food manufacturers often attempt to draw consumers' attention to the amount of fat, sodium, or other nutrients in a food with prominent wording declaring, for example, "Reduced fat!" To protect consumers from misleading claims, the FDA regulates the way terms such as "low calorie" or "fat free" can be used on labels. These terms have specific definitions to ensure that all manufacturers use them in the same manner. (See "Label Terms" on page 394 for a list of these terms and their official definitions.)

The FDA also regulates the use of health- or disease-related claims on food labels. A health claim is a statement about the role of a specific nutrient in maintaining health or preventing disease. Since these statements are commonly used by consumers to help them select more healthful foods, only health claims approved by the FDA are allowed on food labels. Foods that carry a health-related claim are required to contain specified levels of nutrients believed to be adequate to bring about the health result described in the claim. (See "Health Claims" on page 395 for a list of these claims.)

You be the judge

By regulating what and how information is presented on food labels, the FDA has made following a balanced, healthy diet a much more manageable feat. Although individual dietary needs also have to be taken into account, the information on food labels can serve as a valuable tool in helping to determine what to eat and how much of it to eat at a time. So the next time you're at the grocery store, just remember—you can judge a food by its label. □

SIZING UP YOUR SERVINGS

by Belinda O'Connell, M.S., R.D., C.D.E.,
and Laura Hieronymus, M.S.Ed., A.P.R.N., B.C.-A.D.M., C.D.E.

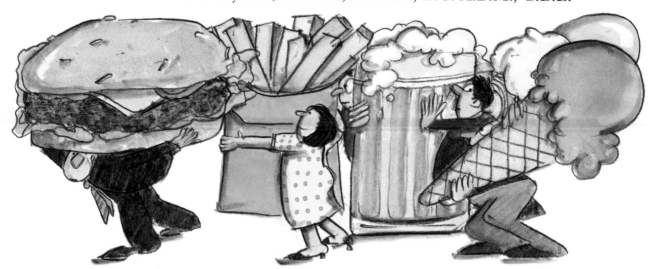

In the food service industry, "smalls" have become "talls," "mediums" have become "grandes," and "larges" are now "super supremes." In many cases, the new, larger sizes are actually cheaper per ounce of food or drink than their smaller predecessors. But while getting more for your money may seem like a good thing on the surface, when you look more closely at the costs in terms of health, portion size inflation is too much of a good thing.

Why portions matter

Increased portions of food mean increased calorie, carbohydrate, and fat intake and in many cases, weight gain or high blood glucose levels. The percent of Americans who are struggling with extra weight continues to increase dramatically, with nearly 66% of adults, 17% of children, and a majority of adults with Type 2 diabetes overweight or obese. Researchers have found that food portion sizes in the marketplace are consistently larger than in the past and that these increases mirror changes in the weight of Americans. Others have found that larger portion sizes are linked to higher calorie intakes in both adults and children.

Being aware of super-sized food portions is particularly important for people with diabetes because gaining weight can make diabetes—as well as high blood pressure and high blood choles-terol— more difficult to control. Eating large portions of carbohydrate-containing foods can also affect blood glucose control if not adequately covered by diabetes medicines or insulin.

Portion size increases

The trend toward increasing portion sizes began in the 1970's and 1980's. Prior to that time, a "family size" soft drink container was 26 ounces; today a "single serve" soft drink weighs in at a hefty 24 ounces. Researchers have found that portion sizes of many other commonly consumed foods, including bread, crackers, cookies, ready-to-

SUPER-SIZE SURPRISE

Here's how basic fast-food items compare to their "super-size" brethren. Keep in mind that an extra 100 calories per day can add up to about 10 pounds of weight gain per year. One extra carbohydrate choice at a meal can increase blood glucose by 30 to 50 "points," depending on the individual. For information on foods not listed here or specific restaurant brands, see the Web site www.calorieking.com.

FOOD ITEM	CALORIES	CARBOHYDRATE (g)	FAT (g)	SODIUM (mg)	ADDITIONAL CALORIES AND CARBOHYDRATE CHOICES
Hamburger	250	31	9	520	
Quarter Pounder with cheese	510	40	26	1,190	260 calories, ½ more carbohydrate choices
Junior roast beef sandwich	272	34	10	740	
Super roast beef sandwich	398	40	19	1,060	126 calories, ½ carbohydrate choice
6 chicken nuggets	252	16	14	672	
10 chicken nuggets	420	26	24	1,120	168 calories, 1 carbohydrate choice
Single slice of cheese pan pizza (medium, 12″ pizza; ⅛ pizza)	270	27	13	570	
Personal cheese pan pizza (about 6″ across)	620	69	26	1,370	350 calories, 3 carbohydrate choices
Small order of French fries	248	31	13	144	
Super-size order of French fries	570	70	30	330	322 calories, 2½ carbohydrate choices
Small vanilla ice cream cone (5 oz)	240	38	8	115	
Large vanilla ice cream cone (10 oz)	480	76	15	230	240 calories, 2½ carbohydrate choices

eat cereals, pasta, French fries, beer, wine, juice, and other soft drinks have also gotten larger over the past five years. The average soft drink portion increased by 2 ounces (containing approximately 25 calories) as did fruit drink portions (for an increase of approximately 30 calories).

At first glance, these changes may seem small, but when considered cumulatively, they add up to potentially large health problems. For example, an additional 100 calories a day will cause a weight gain of about ten pounds a year unless more physical activity is done to burn off the added calories.

As Americans' portions have increased, so have the sizes of the dishes and cups we use. In the past, people drank juice from 4-ounce juice glasses. Today, we use 10- to 16-ounce tumblers for juice. In the past, we ate ice cream in ½-cup dessert dishes (remember the pudding dishes your grandmother used?). Today, we eat ice cream in cereal bowls that hold two cups or in special ice cream bowls the size of small mixing bowls. We also make muffins in extra-large muffin tins and eat on oversized, "restaurant-style" plates. Because a normal-size portion looks small on a large plate or in a large bowl, using oversized plates, bowls, cups, and mugs can all lead to oversized portions.

Meal "deals"

Portion size increases are most obvious with "super-size" fast-food meal deals, where the trend is more food for less money. These deals may be tempting until you consider the hidden costs of that extra food. A regular size hamburger (250 calories, 31 grams carbohydrate) and small order of French fries (248 calories, 31 grams carbohydrate) has about 500 calories and 62 grams of carbohydrate (4 carbohydrate choices). Switching to a Quarter Pounder with cheese [510 calories, 40 grams carbohydrate) and a super-size order of French fries (570 calories, 70 grams carbohydrate) adds up to 1,080 calories and 110 grams of carbohydrate (about 7 carbohydrate choices). Make this switch even once a week and you could be gaining close to 10 pounds a year—probably not the deal you were looking for. (A carbohydrate choice is an amount of food containing roughly 15 grams of carbohydrate.)

Because meal deals are more cost-effective, many people choose them, some figuring they just won't eat it all, but surveys show that the majority of people eat all the food they are served in a restaurant all or most of the time. (See "Super-Size Surprise" on page 397 to see how calories, carbohydrate, and sodium amounts differ with different portion sizes.)

Standard serving sizes

While portion sizes have increased, the standard "serving sizes" found on food labels—and used by dietitians when designing diabetes meal plans—have not. For example, most people who eat corn-flakes eat a portion of about 1½ cups, but a standard serving and 1 carbohydrate choice is ¾ cup. If a person assumes that his usual portion is one standard serving (which many people do), he may be unwittingly eating twice as many carbohydrate choices as intended. Doing this frequently can lead to high blood glucose.

Becoming more familiar with standard serving sizes can help you to figure out how much you are eating and whether you are meeting or exceeding guidelines for a healthy diet.

Tips to help control portions

Measuring foods, reading labels, and using a meal-planning system such as carbohydrate counting can help you to manage portion sizes and improve your blood glucose control.

Measuring. If you really want to know how much you are eating, you need to measure it. You can use measuring cups and measuring spoons or a food scale that measures food in grams. Most people are surprised to see how much larger the portions they eat are than standard serving sizes on food labels . Pour out your usual portion of cereal, juice, or pasta, guess the portion size, then measure it. How close did you get? Next measure out a standard serving or the portion specified in your meal plan of foods you typically eat; note how much of your plate, bowl, or glass this portion fills.

Estimating. Measuring the food you eat is the most accurate way to figure out what you are eating, but there are times when this is simply not practical. In those instances use the following rules of thumb to help you estimate portion sizes when eating out or other times when measuring is not possible:

- Thumb tip = 1 teaspoon
- Full thumb = 1 tablespoon or 1 ounce
- Palm of hand or deck of cards = 3 ounces meat
- 4 stacked dice = 1 ounce cheese
- Tennis ball = small fruit
- Closed fist = 1 cup
- Inside of slightly cupped hand or racquetball = ½ cup
- Golf ball = ⅓ cup

Reading labels. Reading labels can help you determine portion sizes, calories, carbohydrate, fat, and sodium in the packaged foods you eat. When reading labels, first find the "standard serving size" on the Nutrition Facts panel. This is the portion of

USING MYPYRAMID

MyPyramid (www.mypyramid.gov) shows a range of recommended servings for each food group. The number of servings that are right for you depends on the number of calories you need based on whether you are male or female, your age, your size, and how active you are. Use the guidelines below to determine the number of servings you need from each food group.

	SEDENTARY WOMEN AND SOME OLDER ADULTS	MOST SCHOOL-AGE CHILDREN, TEENAGE GIRLS, ACTIVE WOMEN, AND MANY SEDENTARY MEN	TEENAGE BOYS AND ACTIVE MEN
Calories per day	1600	2200	2800
Grains per day	5 oz	7 oz	10 oz
Vegetables per day	2 cups	3 cups	3½ cups
Fruit per day	1½ cups	2 cups	2½ cups
Milk per day	3 cups	3 cups	3 cups
Meat & Beans per day	5 ounces	6 ounces	7 ounces

food that the nutrition information is calculated for. If you are eating a larger portion than the standard serving, you will need to adjust calories, carbohydrate, and other nutrients upward. Conversely, if you are eating a smaller portion, you should decrease these values accordingly.

Keeping records. Keeping food and blood glucose records can help you to see the effects of the foods you eat on your blood glucose level. This information can also be used to adjust your medicine or insulin doses to better match your lifestyle and allow you greater flexibility. Try to keep track of what you eat and how much as well as your blood glucose levels before and after meals for at least 3–5 days before you see your diabetes care provider.

Your diabetes-care provider should go over your blood glucose and food logs with you to help analyze how your food choices are affecting your blood glucose and to suggest ways to improve your diabetes control. However, your diabetes-care provider can make individualized recommendations that are tailored to your lifestyle only if your logs reflect how you really eat and live.

Meal plans. Following a meal plan will help you to keep portions in line. Many people use either carbohydrate counting or food exchanges (or a combination) to plan what they eat. Others find the "plate method" of meal planning easier and more intuitive. This method uses a plate (ideally a 9-inch to 10-inch dinner plate) to demonstrate a healthy meal plan. Most standard menus recommend ¼ of the plate as starch choices, preferably whole grain (1–2 carbohydrate choices), ½ of the plate as non-starchy vegetables (0–1 carbohydrate choices), and ¼ of the plate as meat or meat substitutes, plus a glass of milk and a serving of fruit (each providing 1 carbohydrate choice). If milk is not included at the meal, another starch or fruit can be added.

Preportioned foods. If you have trouble controlling your portion sizes, using packaged foods such as frozen meals can help remove the temptation to overeat. In addition, they make carbohydrate counting a breeze since you can easily locate the carbohydrate content on the Nutrition Facts label. It may also help you to visualize standard food servings when you eat out or prepare food yourself. Use the food label or ask your dietitian to help you figure out how to fit preportioned foods into your meal plan.

Share a meal. When eating out, request small portions (such as "kid size" or "lunch size" portions), resist the urge to super-size, try an appetizer and a salad as a meal, or share a meal (and the calories) with a friend. If you order a full portion, ask for half of it to be wrapped in a doggy bag before it is served to remove the temptation to eat it all. (For food safety reasons, be sure your doggy bag gets to your refrigerator within two hours of the beginning of your meal.)

Fighting the tide of ever-increasing portion sizes takes some thought initially, but once you become more aware of your portions and where large portions may be causing you to eat excess calories or carbohydrate, taking steps to reverse the trend is a relatively simple way to tune up your eating habits and your health. □

VEGETARIAN AND VEGAN MEAL PLANNING

by Nancy Berkoff, R.D., Ed.D., C.C.E.

A few decades ago, many Americans considered vegetarianism a fringe fad, a practice for hippies and health nuts. Over the past several years, however, vegetarian diets have gone increasingly mainstream. Baby Boomers value the health benefits and "exotic" appeal of ethnically influenced vegetarian meals, high school students think vegetarianism is "in," and others associate it with environmental and animal protection.

Age group and philosophy aside, one of the best reasons for trying meatless eating these days is taste. Appetizing vegetarian recipes, ready-made entrées, and even restaurant dishes are now easier to find than ever. In fact, according to a National Restaurant Association survey, more customers requested vegetarian options while dining out in 2000 than in any previous year.

For people with diabetes, who are at higher risk than the general public for cardiovascular disease and other diet-related health conditions, vegetarian eating is worth considering. Cutting out (or cutting back on) meat, and choosing flavorful vegetarian meals that are low in cholesterol and saturated fat and high in fiber, vitamins, and calcium and other minerals can help reduce blood pressure, LDL "bad" cholesterol, and body weight and possibly help stabilize blood glucose levels.

Vegetarian nutrition 101

What exactly is a vegetarian diet? It depends who you ask. Many vegetarians avoid meat, fish, and poultry, but do eat milk, other dairy products, and eggs; they are called lacto-ovo vegetarians. Pescans are lacto-ovo vegetarians who also include fish and seafood in their diet. Vegans do not eat meat, fish, poultry, or dairy foods, and most avoid honey, wool, and any other product made from animals. Fruitarians eat only uncooked fruits, seeds, and nuts. (Vegetables are considered off-limits because the entire plant must be "killed" to consume them. Apples, for example, can be picked without killing the tree, but harvesting carrots or onions destroys the entire plant.)

Special health concerns for vegetarians depend on what foods they eliminate and how much variety they get in their diet. Vegetarian diets that include dairy products and eggs can easily meet nutrition requirements and don't greatly restrict food choices. In fact, many people who cut back on their meat intake for health reasons become vegetarians without even noticing it. A meatless menu can be very healthful, as long as you choose low-fat or nonfat dairy foods, limit consumption of egg yolks, and stick to low-fat cooking techniques.

For some, the temptation when making the switch to a vegetarian diet is to load a baked potato with full-fat sour cream or cheese because "I'm not having the prime rib, after all," or to sauté vegetables in puddles of butter since they're not getting cholesterol from bacon or chicken skin anymore. This approach can quickly undermine the health benefits of cutting out meat. Using nonfat or low-fat cheeses in sandwiches, garnishes, and soups; nonfat and low-fat yogurt in salad dressings; reduced-fat cottage or ricotta cheese on salads or in casseroles; and low-fat egg substitute at breakfast or in baked goods are simple modifications that can help keep the fat content of your vegetarian diet low.

Vegan diets, which exclude all animal products, tend to be high in fiber and nutrients and can help reduce the risk of major chronic diseases. Because they restrict more categories of food, though, people who follow a vegan diet may need to take extra care to meet their nutrition needs. Some vegans (and vegetarians) may need to supplement their meal plan with a multivitamin or calcium. However, the key to a nutritionally sound vegan diet, as for any balanced diet, is choosing a wide variety of healthful foods.

Some people who are interested in vegan eating are concerned that they would not be getting enough protein. Not to worry. Soy foods are a convenient source of complete protein; like eggs, dairy products, and meat, soybeans contain all nine of the essential amino acids (the building blocks of protein) that the body needs but can't make on its own. It's also possible to get adequate protein by eating a diversity of whole grains, seeds, nuts, and legumes throughout the day. Usually, combining grains or seeds with legumes or beans will provide a complete protein. It's not necessary to eat these combinations at the same meal, but they should be eaten the same day. Vegan menu items that are high in protein include bean soup with crackers, lentil soup with potato salad, stir-fried tofu and almonds with rice, a veggie burger on a bun, three-bean chili with pasta or barley, peanut butter and bread, and pasta with nondairy pesto, to name just a few.

While protein is not usually a problem, getting enough calcium, iron, zinc, vitamin B_{12}, and vitamin D can be a concern for people who no longer obtain these nutrients from dairy foods or meat. To help prevent nutrient deficiencies, try to eat daily servings of plant foods rich in these important vitamins and minerals. Here are a few good sources:

Calcium. Calcium-fortified foods such as soy milk, rice milk, orange juice, and calcium-processed tofu. Legumes, almonds, peanuts, walnuts, and dark, leafy greens such as broccoli, collards, kale, mustard greens, and spinach are also rich in calcium.

Iron. Enriched and fortified cereals, whole-grain breads and whole grains, lentils, black-eyed peas, kidney beans, seeds, dark, leafy greens, dried fruit, cashews, wheat germ, and sea vegetables (seaweed). You can enhance your iron intake by eating iron-rich foods together with foods containing vitamin C, which helps the body absorb iron. Try adding orange sections to a fresh spinach salad, serving a tomato and green pepper sauce (both vegetables are high in vitamin C) with steamed kale, or having a glass of grapefruit juice with a bowl of iron-enriched cereal.

Zinc. Whole-grain breads and cereals, adzuki beans, chickpeas, lentils, nuts, sea vegetables, tofu, and wheat germ contain zinc.

Vitamin B_{12}. Fortified cereals, soy foods and meat analogs such as vegetarian burgers, and nutritional yeast are good sources of vitamin B_{12}. Nutritional yeast can be sprinkled on hot cereal, soy yogurt, frozen desserts made from soy or rice milk, salads, cooked vegetables, and pasta. It can also be used to make homemade, nondairy, "fake" cheese. If you are a vegan, read the label before purchasing nutritional yeast to be sure that it does not contain whey, which is derived from milk. Red Star Vegetarian Support Formula is a nondairy yeast.

Vitamin D. Exposure to ultraviolet rays from the sun enables the body to make vitamin D, so try to get in 5–15 minutes of sun exposure every day, if possible (but protect yourself with sunscreen for prolonged exposure). This method may not be effective in the winter, when sun intensity is low, or for older adults, who are less able to make vitamin D in the skin. If your sun exposure is limited, be sure to eat vitamin-D-fortified foods such as soy or rice milk, breakfast cereals, and soy meat analogs.

Food pyramid planning

A food pyramid diagram illustrating what foods to emphasize and which to eat less of can be a useful tool for planning a nutrient-rich diet. One guide that may help potential vegetarians and vegans is the Oldways Traditional Healthy Vegetarian Diet Pyramid, which can be viewed on the Internet at www.oldwayspt.org (click on Traditional Diet Pyramids). The base of this pyramid places equal emphasis on fruits and vegetables, whole grains, and legumes and beans, which should be eaten at every meal. The middle level is made up of nuts and seeds, egg whites, soy milk and other soy products, plant oils, and dairy. These items provide protein, calcium, and fat and should be eaten daily. Foods at the top level, including whole eggs and sweets, should be eaten only once or twice a week. The Oldways guide does not suggest serving sizes but gives a general idea of how to balance your daily food choices. The Web site describes a variety of foods from each pyramid category, some of which may be new to you.

For those who prefer a more precise meal-planning pyramid, here is an outline of a daily meal plan based on the Food Guide for Vegetarian Meal Planning. The number of servings you choose from each group depends on your total caloric needs:

Grains group. (6–10 servings per day) Examples of 1 serving: 1 slice bread, ½ bagel or English muffin, ½ pita, 1 6-inch tortilla, 1 ounce ready-to-eat cereal, 3 small crackers, ½ cup cooked pasta, rice, or cereal, 2 bread sticks, 2 cups popped popcorn, 3 tablespoons wheat germ. Remember, at least half of your grains should be whole.

Vegetable group. (5–8 servings per day) Examples of 1 serving: ½ cup raw or cooked vegetables, 1 cup raw leafy vegetables, ½ medium potato, or ¾ cup vegetable juice.

Fruit group. (3–5 servings per day) Examples of 1 serving: 1 medium piece of fresh fruit, ½ cup frozen or canned fruit, ½ cup juice, ¼ cup dried fruit.

Dry beans, nuts, seeds, eggs, and meat substitutes group. (2–4 servings per day) Examples of 1 serving: ½ cup cooked dried peas, beans, or lentils, 2 tablespoons nuts or seeds, 2 tablespoons peanut butter, 4 ounces tofu or tempeh, 1 cup soy milk, 1 ½ ounces soy cheese, 1 egg or 2 egg whites, 3 ounces meat substitute (such as a veggie burger).

Milk group. (0–3 servings per day) Examples of 1 serving: 1 cup milk, 1 cup yogurt, 1½ ounces part-skim cheese. (Vegans should select calcium-rich plant foods or dairy substitutes.)

Fats and sweets. (Use sparingly) Butter, stick margarine, shortening, soft drinks, candy, syrups, jelly, and jam. Liquid plant and fish oils are not part of this group; 5–8 teaspoons of these should be consumed daily, either as part of the dry beans, nuts, seeds, eggs, and meat substitutes group, or separately. To see how much of these healthy oils are in various foods, visit www.mypyramid.gov/pyramid/oils_count.html.

Menu planning

So now you know the building blocks of healthy eating, but you still can't picture a vegetarian menu. Won't your meals be monotonous or your food choices limited? They certainly don't have to be.

Your breakfasts might include poached egg whites with salsa, an egg-white omelet with mushrooms and tomatoes, scrambled egg substitute with soy "bacon" strips or breakfast links, a nonfat yogurt parfait with fresh or frozen fruit and whole-grain cold cereal, low-fat cottage cheese with fresh melon and whole wheat toast, or whole-grain cold

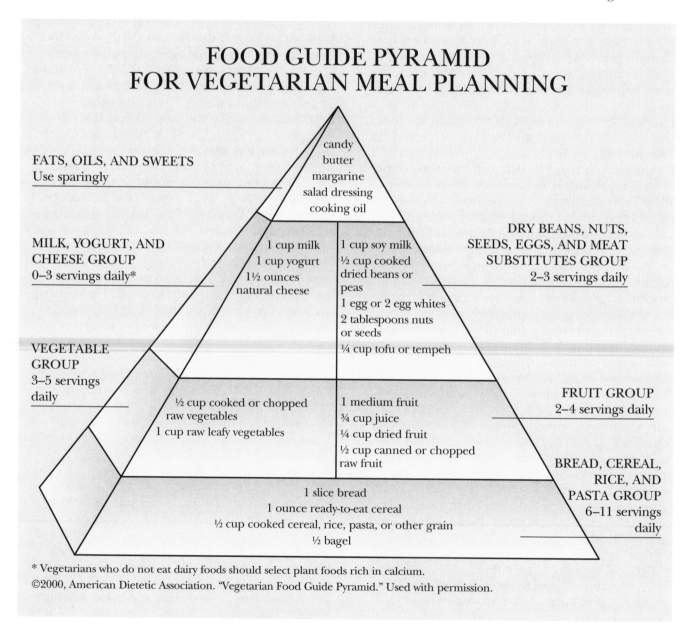

FOOD GUIDE PYRAMID FOR VEGETARIAN MEAL PLANNING

FATS, OILS, AND SWEETS
Use sparingly

candy
butter
margarine
salad dressing
cooking oil

MILK, YOGURT, AND CHEESE GROUP
0–3 servings daily*

1 cup milk
1 cup yogurt
1½ ounces natural cheese

1 cup soy milk
½ cup cooked dried beans or peas
1 egg or 2 egg whites
2 tablespoons nuts or seeds
¼ cup tofu or tempeh

DRY BEANS, NUTS, SEEDS, EGGS, AND MEAT SUBSTITUTES GROUP
2–3 servings daily

VEGETABLE GROUP
3–5 servings daily

½ cup cooked or chopped raw vegetables
1 cup raw leafy vegetables

1 medium fruit
¾ cup juice
¼ cup dried fruit
½ cup canned or chopped raw fruit

FRUIT GROUP
2–4 servings daily

1 slice bread
1 ounce ready-to-eat cereal
½ cup cooked cereal, rice, pasta, or other grain
½ bagel

BREAD, CEREAL, RICE, AND PASTA GROUP
6–11 servings daily

* Vegetarians who do not eat dairy foods should select plant foods rich in calcium.
©2000, American Dietetic Association. "Vegetarian Food Guide Pyramid." Used with permission.

or cooked cereal with skim milk and fresh, frozen, or dried fruit.

Easy, low-fat, vegetarian lunch or supper entrées could include a fresh spinach or vegetable salad with walnuts and shredded skim milk mozzarella, a Greek salad with low-fat Feta or goat cheese, vegetable lasagna or macaroni and cheese made with low-fat ricotta or cottage cheese, veggie burgers with nonfat shredded cheese and sliced vegetables, a sandwich stuffed with a little cheese and lots of grilled vegetables, or cheese strata, a baked, layered cheese sandwich made by alternating slices of bread with sliced tomatoes or tomato sauce and low-fat cheese. When you don't have time to cook, there are many frozen vegetarian entrées and side dishes to choose from in most grocery stores. (Look for products low in fat and sodium.)

Vegan menus may seem to present more of a problem in menu planning, but many of the foods you eat are "naturally" vegan or can easily be prepared without animal products. With simple foods like fruits and fruit salad, applesauce, breads, raw and cooked vegetables (without butter), pasta (made without eggs), cooked or cold cereals, potatoes, rice, hearty vegetarian salads (such as three-bean salad or marinated mushroom salad), vegetable and bean soups (made with vegetable stock), and steamed or baked grains, you can construct many a mouthwatering meal. To see how this is done, take a look at three days' worth of enjoyable menus, all made with basic vegan ingredients.

Whether you "go vegan" all at once or simply work in a few vegetarian meals a week, perhaps the easiest way to make the transition is to convert some of the items you are used to serving. Leave off the cheese and sausage and load up a prepared pizza crust with marinara sauce, chopped onions, peppers, garlic, mushrooms, and tomatoes. Prepare vegan mashed potatoes with vegetable stock and a dab of margarine instead of milk and butter. When you light up the barbecue, try soy or veggie burgers or vegetable kebabs, and throw some sliced portobello mushrooms, tomatoes, and onions on the grill to use in a grilled vegetable sandwich the next day. Leave out the meat and add another variety or two of beans to create a two-, three-, or four-bean chili. Skipping the meat leaves more room for savory, fiber-rich beans, jalapeños, chopped vegetables, and salsa in

BREAKFAST 1
Oatmeal or kasha with raisins, chopped dates, sliced banana, and enriched soy milk
Whole grain toast with peanut butter
Orange juice

LUNCH 1
Spinach, potato, and black-eyed pea stew
Sautéed corn with tomato sauce
Baked apple with chopped dried apricots

DINNER 1
Steamed tofu with Asian vegetables
Brown rice with peas and almonds
Baked cinnamon pear

BREAKFAST 2
Toasted bagel with soy cream cheese
Fruit smoothie (made with orange juice, nutritional yeast, frozen berries, and rice milk or soy milk)

LUNCH 2
Falafel (fried, ground chickpeas) on a pita with shredded romaine lettuce, carrots, and tomato wedges
Tomato, onion, and parsley salad
Fresh grapes

DINNER 2
Creamy carrot soup
Pasta-lentil salad
Corn muffin (from a vegan baking mix)
Sliced melon

BREAKFAST 3
Soy yogurt with fresh or frozen berries and slivered almonds
Orange-raisin muffin with vegan margarine and preserves
Cranberry juice

LUNCH 3
Veggie burger on a whole wheat bun with sliced tomato and cucumber, shredded lettuce and carrot, sliced onion, ketchup, mustard, and relish
Vegan peanut butter cookie
Chocolate soy or rice milk

DINNER 3
Tomato stuffed with seasoned brown rice and mushrooms
Kale or spinach braised in vegetable stock
Dinner roll with vegan margarine
Butterscotch pudding (made with soy milk), topped with banana

vegan tacos or burritos. In fact, replacing meat with extra vegetables and/or beans works well in most casseroles, stews, stir-fries, soups, and pasta dishes.

Traditional vegan ingredients

Preparing vegetarian (and especially vegan) meals may also encourage you to experiment with new recipes and new foods, from dairy and meat substitutes to less familiar ingredients from traditionally vegetarian societies. If you're ready for something new, give some of these "traditional" vegetarian foods a try:

Tofu. Tofu is made by curdling soy milk with a coagulating agent (either calcium sulfate or magnesium chloride). Unless it is aseptically packaged (in packages resembling juice boxes), tofu is packed in water and should be kept refrigerated. Some people rinse their tofu before cooking; if using only a part of a block at a time, store the remainder in fresh water.

There are several varieties of tofu, each suitable for different types of dishes. Firm and extra-firm tofu hold up well to chopping and slicing and keep their shape when grilled, simmered, stewed, baked, or stir-fried. Soft tofu is better for blending and using in recipes where a creamy ingredient is needed, such as salad dressings, dips, thick beverages, and sauces. Silken tofu is custardlike and has a faint, nutty flavor. It goes well in puddings, "cream" pies, casseroles, soups, and sauces. In addition, there are low-fat versions as well as smoked and meat-flavored varieties of tofu.

Plain tofu has a neutral flavor and texture, so you must give it inspiration by marinating or seasoning it prior to or during cooking. Try marinating tofu in dried basil, oregano, and black pepper with a drop of vinegar to give it an Italian flavor; in red pepper flakes, lime juice, and chopped fresh jalapeños for a Southwestern spin; or in soy sauce, chopped fresh garlic, and green onions for an Asian flair. To satisfy a sweet tooth, add a couple of drops of almond extract to some reduced-sugar maple syrup and let tofu marinate in it for several hours. Then slice it and serve it on top of sliced fresh oranges.

A half-cup serving of tofu contains approximately 94 calories, 2 grams of carbohydrate, 10 grams of protein, and 6 grams of fat.

Seitan. Sometimes called the "meat of the wheat," seitan is a compressed extract of gluten (the protein found in flour). Seitan is sold in strips or chunks and can be frozen until you're ready to use it. It can be stir-fried, roasted, poached, or baked; seitan "steaks" can be marinated and grilled for a

fast entrée. Seitan adds a chewy texture to dishes and can be used as a substitute for meat in just about any recipe.

A 4-ounce serving of seitan contains approximately 77 calories, 12 grams of carbohydrate, 7 grams of protein, and less than 1 gram of fat.

Tempeh. Tempeh is made from cooked, fermented soybeans (sometimes mixed with sea vegetables or a grain such as rice or barley) that are formed into a cake. You may see some black spots

---

VEGAN MENU SUGGESTIONS

As you can see from the menus below, vegan meals can suit any mood, schedule, or celebration. Diversity in color, texture, and seasoning is the antidote to a bland and boring meal.

GRAB-AND-GO BREAKFAST
Enriched cold cereal with chopped dried fruit, nuts, and soy milk
Orange sections
Fruit smoothie with calcium-processed soft tofu or soy yogurt blended with a banana, fresh berries, and wheat germ

CRUNCHY BOXED LUNCH
Carrot sticks, raw green beans, or pea pods with tomato salsa
Pita pocket with shredded romaine lettuce, shredded carrots, and tofu cheese slices
Vegan peanut butter raisin cookie
Calcium- and vitamin-D-fortified chocolate rice milk

DELECTABLE DINNER PARTY
Vichyssoise (cold potato and leek soup) with tomato-thyme whole-grain bread
Carrot and spinach pâté en croute (in pastry)
Herbed orzo with fresh basil
Tossed baby greens with walnuts and lime vinaigrette
Apple-Calvados sorbet (Calvados is an apple liqueur)

SIMPLE SUPPER
Tomato-vegetable soup with rosemary breadsticks
Lentil and potato ragout
Glazed baby carrots
Four-bean salad
Baked apple with lemon sauce

Nutrition and Meal Planning

FITTING IN NEW FOODS

When planning your meals, keep in mind that 15 grams of carbohydrate counts as one carbohydrate choice or carbohydrate exchange, even if the food is considered a "meat substitute." This table may make it easier to see how to fit some common vegetarian foods into your meal plan.

FOOD	SERVING SIZE	CARBOHYDRATE (g)	EXCHANGES
Boca Burger, original	2½-ounce patty	6	½ starch, 2 very lean meat
Cooked dried beans, peas, lentils	½ cup	20*	1 starch, 1 very lean meat
Gardenburger Original	2½-ounce patty	14	1 starch, 1 lean meat
House Original Tofu Steak	5 ounces	0	2½ medium-fat meat
Minestrone soup, canned, ready-to-serve	1 cup	20	1 starch, 1 lean meat
Morningstar Farms Grillers	2½-ounce patty	5	2 lean meat
Nasoya Extra Firm Tofu	3 ounces	2	1 medium-fat meat
Nasoya Lite Firm Tofu	3 ounces	1	1 very lean meat
Nutritional yeast	3 tablespoons	11*	1 starch, 2 very lean meat
Rice Dream Chocolate Enriched Rice Milk	1 cup	34	2½ starch, ½ fat
Rice Dream Original Enriched Rice Milk	1 cup	23	1½ starch, ½ fat
Seitan	4 ounces	12	1 starch, 3 very lean meat
Silk Chocolate Soy Milk	1 cup	23	1½ starch, 1 medium-fat meat
Silk Unsweetened Soy Milk	1 cup	4	1 medium-fat meat
Silk Vanilla Soy Milk	1 cup	10	1 starch, 1 medium-fat meat
Soy Delicious nondairy frozen dessert	3-fluid-ounce sandwich	28	2 starch, ½ fat
Soy nuts (roasted soybeans)	1 ounce	10	½ starch, 1 high-fat meat
Tempeh	4 ounces	14	1 starch, 2 lean meat
Tofurky Deli Slices, original	1½ ounces	5	1½ very lean meat
Tofutti Cutie vanilla (frozen dessert)	1½-fluid-ounce sandwich	17	1 starch, 1 fat
Yves meatless hot dog	1 ½-ounce dog	2	1 very lean meat
Yves meatless chicken skewer	3-ounce skewer	7	½ starch, 2 very lean meat
Wheat germ	¼ cup	15	1 starch, 1 lean meat

* Contains more than 5 grams of fiber per serving.

on the surface of the tempeh—this is the bacterium still working (similar to the active cultures in yogurt and other fermented dairy products) and is not a sign that the product is spoiled. Tempeh should be refrigerated (it lasts about ten days) and can be frozen for several months. Be sure to thaw it in the refrigerator.

Tempeh has a chewy texture and a smoky taste and is a good stand-in for meat. When made with soy only, it has the distinctive, nutty flavor of soybeans. Tempeh can be cut into small pieces and added to soups, stews, stir-fries, or casseroles, or it can be grilled and served in a sandwich. Tempeh is higher in fiber (containing 2.5 grams per serving) and carbohydrate and slightly higher in fat than tofu. A half-cup serving contains 160 calories, 14 grams of carbohydrate, 16 grams of protein, and 9 grams of fat.

Soy and rice milk. Soy milk is made by boiling soybeans in water, grinding them, and pressing out the liquid. Rice milk is a liquid drained from cooked rice. Both beverages are available in plain, vanilla, and chocolate flavors, low-fat and nonfat varieties, and regular or calcium- and vitamin-D-fortified versions. If sold in aseptic packages, they can be stored at room temperature, but once opened, soy and rice milks are perishable and must be kept refrigerated. Soy milk or rice milk can be substituted for cow's milk in recipes. Calorie, carbohydrate, and fat content depend on the brand and variety of milk. Generally, soy milk is lower in carbohydrate and higher in protein than rice milk.

"Fake" meats and dairy products. Soy yogurt, cheeses, mayonnaise, sour cream, and ice cream are a boon to vegans, because most can be used interchangeably with dairy products. (Soy cheeses, however, do not melt as easily as dairy cheese.) For those who miss the taste of meat, there are refrigerated or frozen soy-based hot dogs, burgers, sausage, bacon, and other meats. Depending on where you live and the stores in your area, you may find meat-substitute products that range from jerky to "sloppy joe" mixture, to stuffed "turkey," to sliceable "roasts." Not all products are vegan and not all are meant to imitate the taste of meat; you may need to try several brands to find products you like. Look for products low in fat and sodium, and if you are a vegan, examine food labels closely for ingredients such as cassein and whey, which are milk derivatives found in some soy cheeses, margarine, and processed foods.

Soybeans. Fresh, whole soybeans (edamame) can be found at farmers' markets, Asian food stores, and some supermarkets. You may also find soybeans frozen, either in the pod or shelled, or canned. Steamed fresh or frozen soybeans in the pod make a good appetizer or garnish (the inedible pods are fuzzy and the beans green). Canned soybeans go well in soups and stews and can be used as a garnish for salads. One half-cup serving of cooked soybeans offers 19 grams of "complete" protein.

Shopping and meal-planning suggestions

There's nothing easier than grilling up a veggie burger for dinner when you're in a rush, but variety and preparation are the secrets to a satisfying vegetarian diet. This doesn't mean having hundreds of ingredients on hand or spending hours on complex recipes, but it does mean careful shopping and creative use of some staples. Here, for instance, are some versatile vegetarian ingredients that may figure on your new shopping list:

Canned beans and vegetables. You may not have the time or inclination to shop for and prepare fresh vegetables and dried beans every day, but when the ingredients are only a can opener away, it's easy to prepare a hearty stew, soup, salad, or casserole using kidney, black, white, lima, or butter beans (baby limas), as well as garbanzos, soybeans, and lentils, to name just a few. Yes, fresh vegetables may be tastier, but you can't beat low-sodium canned vegetables for easy-to-use add-ins. Keep a range of colors on hand for greater nutrient variety, including canned corn, green beans, yellow wax beans, sliced or julienned beets, sliced carrots, sauerkraut, pickled red cabbage, sliced or whole mushrooms, and chopped tomatoes.

Dried fruit and vegetables. Dried fruits are high in carbohydrate and calorie-dense, but even a small portion is chock-full of nutrients and texture. Dried dates, apricots, figs, raisins, prunes, apples, peaches, nectarines, cranberries, cherries, and blueberries are just some of the delicious dried fruits that you can toss into cereal, pancakes, smoothies, and salads, or just eat out of hand. Sun-dried red and yellow tomatoes, dried vegetable soup mixes, dried mushrooms, and dried chilies make excellent additions to soups, salads, pastas, and combination dishes.

Nuts and seeds. Nuts, seeds, and nut butters can add an interesting kick to many meals. Plain old oatmeal gets more exciting with a walnut or pecan crunch, while stir-fries, salads, and soups go well with a garnish of toasted almonds or sesame seeds. If peanut butter sounds dull, try soy, hazelnut, almond, or macadamia nut butter. They are

Oven-poached pears

4 tablespoons apricot or raspberry jam or preserves
4 ripe Bartlett or Bosc pears (apples, fresh peaches, or nectarines also work well in this recipe)
4 tablespoons chopped almonds or hazelnuts
4 teaspoons margarine
4 teaspoons apple juice concentrate
2 teaspoons ground ginger
2 teaspoons grated lemon or orange zest
Raspberries or strawberries (optional)

Preheat oven to 375°F. Cut four pieces of foil that are about 2½ times the size of the pears. Fold each piece in half and place one tablespoon of jam in the crease of the fold. Cut pears lengthwise through the stem, about halfway down, so that you create four wedges that are still held together at the base of the pear. Place pears in the center of foil on top of the jam (it's OK if the wedges separate a bit), and fill them with 1 tablespoon nuts, 1 teaspoon margarine, 1 teaspoon apple juice concentrate, ½ teaspoon ground ginger, and ½ teaspoon citrus zest. Set the pears upright and wrap them in a loose but well-sealed foil envelope. Place pears on a baking sheet or in a baking dish and bake for about 10–20 minutes or until the pears are soft and heated through. Test with a fork for doneness. Unwrap the pears and serve them on a pink palette of puréed raspberries or strawberries, if desired.

Note: The pears can be assembled the night before and stored in the refrigerator until ready to cook. Once cooked, do not leave pears in foil; store them in a covered plastic or glass dish.

Preparation time: 15 minutes

Yield: 4 pears

Per serving:
    Calories: 182
    Carbohydrate: 30 g
    Protein: 2 g
    Fat: 7 g
    Saturated fat: 1 g
    Sodium: 54 mg
    Calcium: 30 mg
    Fiber: 5 g

Serving size: 1 pear

Exchanges per serving:
    ½ starch, 1½ fruit,
    1 fat
Carbohydrate choices: 2

Graham pudding parfaits

1 package instant pudding mix
1½ cups low-fat rice milk or soy milk
1 cup coarsely crumbled graham cracker pieces
1 cup mixed berries (fresh or frozen and thawed)
3 tablespoons shredded coconut

Prepare pudding according to package directions. Place a thin layer of graham cracker crumbs in the bottom of three parfait cups or small bowls and cover with a thin layer of berries then a layer of pudding. Complete parfaits by layering graham crackers, pudding, and berries until all ingredients are used. Garnish with coconut and chill for one hour before serving.

Note: This dessert freezes well. For variation, use sliced bananas and peaches in addition to berries, or try fruit-flavored soy yogurt in place of pudding.

Preparation time: 15 minutes

Yield: 3 parfaits

Serving size: 1 parfait
    (¾ cup)

Per serving (prepared with soy milk):
    Calories: 371
    Carbohydrate: 70 g
    Protein: 7 g
    Fat: 8 g
    Saturated fat: 2 g
    Sodium: 734 mg
    Calcium: 27 mg
    Fiber: 5 g

Exchanges per serving:
    2 starch, 1 fruit,
    1 low-fat milk, 1 fat
Carbohydrate choices:
    4½

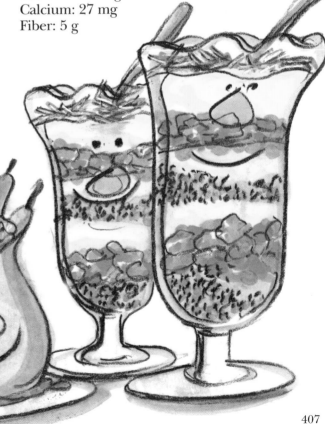

Corn and potato chowder

Vegetable oil spray
½ cup chopped onions
2 cloves garlic, minced
⅛ cup chopped fresh parsley
1½ cups frozen corn, thawed (or corn kernels
  from 4 ears of corn)
3 cups water
4 boiling potatoes, cubed
1 teaspoon dried dill
2 cups soy milk
1 cup drained and mashed silken tofu
1 teaspoon thyme
½ teaspoon black pepper

Spray a large pot with vegetable oil and heat. Add onions, garlic, parsley, and corn; cover and simmer over low heat for 20 minutes, stirring frequently. Add water and bring to boil. Add potatoes and simmer uncovered for 30 minutes, or until potatoes are tender. Stir in dill, soy milk, tofu, thyme, and pepper, and simmer for 15 minutes or until very hot.

Preparation time: 15 minutes

Yield: 4½ cups

Serving size: 1½ cups

Per serving:
  Calories: 310
  Carbohydrate: 53 g
  Protein: 15 g
  Fat: 7 g
  Saturated fat: 1 g
  Sodium: 39 mg
  Calcium: 75 mg
  Fiber: 8 g

Exchanges per serving:
  1½ starch, 3 medium-
  fat meat
Carbohydrate choices:
  3½

Asian noodle bowl

1½ cups cooked noodles, chilled (start with
  ½ cup uncooked noodles)
½ cup shredded green cabbage
⅛ cup sliced radishes
½ cup chunked firm tofu or meat substitute
2 teaspoons minced fresh garlic
1 teaspoon minced fresh ginger
3 teaspoons vegetable oil
1 teaspoon soy sauce
2 tablespoons cashews or peanuts

In a large serving bowl, toss noodles, cabbage, radishes, tofu, garlic, and ginger until combined. Mix together oil and soy sauce and add to noodles. Stir to combine and garnish with nuts.

Preparation time: 15 minutes

Yield: 2 servings

Serving size: ½ recipe

Per serving (using
tofu and peanuts):
  Calories: 400
  Carbohydrate: 37 g
  Protein: 23 g
  Fat: 20 g
  Saturated fat: 5 g
  Sodium: 180 mg
  Calcium: 187 mg
  Fiber: 6 g

Exchanges per serving:
  2 starch, 3 medium-fat
  meat, 2 fat
Carbohydrate choices:
  2½

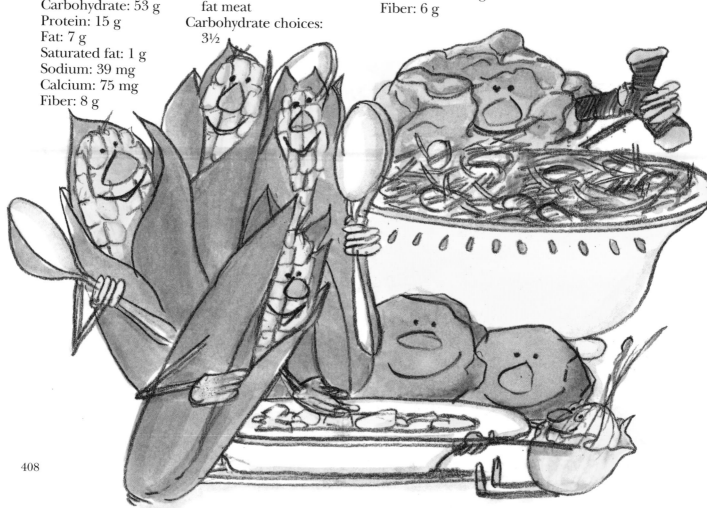

good—and good for you (eaten in moderation, of course).

Root veggies. Root vegetables can be stored for a long time, so select your favorites (from white potatoes to purple potatoes, Yukon golds, sweet potatoes, carrots, rutabagas, parsnips, beets, and turnips), give them a dark, cool home, then roast, microwave, bake, or steam them. Make a meal of a white baked potato served with canned lentils and salsa or a sweet potato topped with crushed pineapple, mashed tofu, dried cranberries, and canned mandarin oranges.

Many root vegetables can be grated for a crunchy salad topping, mashed with margarine or vegetable stock for a side dish, or puréed to use as the base for soups. Looking for a healthful snack food? Thinly slice fresh beets, purple potatoes, Yukon Gold potatoes, carrots and taro (if you've got it), arrange the slices on an oil-sprayed baking sheet, and bake at 425°F until they are crispy for fresh, hot chips.

Oils. Limiting the fats in your meal plan is a good idea, but oil is still an important ingredient. Olive oil is flavorful and contains a high percentage of monounsaturated fat (one of the good guys). Sesame seed and hazelnut oils are specialty oils that give unique flavors to dishes. If you're selecting unflavored oils, go for canola, corn, safflower, or sunflower oils, which are lower in saturated fat.

Margarine often contains whey and may not be vegan, so read labels carefully if you choose to use it. In addition, health experts advise limiting your consumption of *trans*-fatty acids; these can be found in solid stick margarines (soft tub margarine is a better choice) and in products such as cookies or snack bars containing hydrogenated or partially hydrogenated fats. To keep your saturated fat intake down, try to avoid products that contain palm oil, palm kernel oil, or coconut oil, which are high in saturated fat.

Remember, a little fat in the diet is necessary, but if you're trying to cut back on fat, try using vegetable or fruit juice, vegetable or mushroom broth, or wine as a cooking liquid. Four ounces of fruit juice contains about 50 calories, the same as 2 teaspoons of most oils. Vegetable oil sprays are also helpful because they allow you to use less; you can make your own by pouring oil into a spray bottle.

Herbs. Always have on hand the sweet staples (cinnamon, nutmeg, orange zest, ground ginger, cloves), the savory staples (granulated garlic, black and white pepper, onion powder, dried basil, oregano, thyme, red pepper flakes, curry powder, dried parsley), and any other herbs and spice blends (such as lemon-pepper or Cajun spices) that you use often. Discard dried herbs and spices that have lost their zing; even when stored in a cool, dry place in an airtight container, most dried herbs and spices lose their flavor after about a year.

The following simple strategies can help you keep your meals lively, healthful, and quick to prepare:

Vary your staples. Every time you go to the store, you grab four boxes of spaghetti, an economy-size bag of white rice, and your favorite brand of cold cereal. Sure, it's easy to remember, but it can get a bit boring. Pasta and rice come in all sorts of colors, shapes, and flavors. Trying a different variety can liven up your basic meals. Instead of dried pasta, look for fresh pasta in the refrigerated section of the supermarket. (If you won't eat an entire package of fresh pasta in a day or two, cook what you'll eat and freeze the rest for later.) Try brown, wild, or even black rice, and pasta made with whole wheat, spinach, carrots, tomatoes, mushrooms, chilis, or lemon-basil seasoning. If you're feeling more adventurous, try replacing rice or pasta with a less familiar grain, such as quinoa, bulgur, or kasha.

If cold cereal is a morning mainstay, read labels carefully; one may have more B vitamins while another has more iron. Select several different kinds, so that you're getting a variety of nutrients, then combine the cereals or alternate them daily. (Store cereal in airtight containers or food bags so they don't go stale.)

Take shortcuts. Consider precut or bagged salads, precut vegetables or fruit, and other ready-to-use items. While they can be more costly, convenience ingredients may be worth the expense if they mean the difference between preparing a decent meal for yourself and opting for yet another bowl of cereal at mealtime. If you're experiencing green salad burnout, bagged salad mixes can offer other interesting meal possibilities. For instance, take a prepared cole slaw mix (usually shredded green cabbage and carrots) or bagged, shredded red cabbage and sauté it with a little bit of oil and a lot of cracked pepper. Mix the sautéed cabbage with cooked broad noodles and you have a fast, colorful supper.

Mix and match a meal. A can of tomato soup for lunch? Yawn. A can of tomato soup with fresh tomatoes, some chunked tofu, a few canned garbanzo beans, and some leftover baked potato—now that's a meal! It's perfectly OK to use ready-to-eat foods, but they usually taste better and have greater nutritional value if you jazz them up.

RESOURCES

Whether you're vegetarian, vegan, or just curious, the resources below provide a wealth of new recipes and information on healthy vegetarian eating. To learn more about available meat and dairy alternatives, visit the food manufacturers' Web sites or call their consumer information lines.

FOOD MANUFACTURERS

BOCA FOODS COMPANY
www.bocaburger.com
Boca produces meatless Boca Burgers, lasagna, sausage, chicken patties and nuggets, and ground "beef" for use in tacos, "meat" sauce, and "meat" balls, and chili. Some of their products are vegan. The Web site lists stores and restaurants that sell Boca foods.

FIELD ROAST GRAIN MEAT COMPANY
www.fieldroast.com
(800) 311-9497
Field Roast Grain Meats are vegan wheat-gluten products that can be used in place of roast meat, cutlets, burgers, sandwich meats, or ground meat. Recipes for using various Field Roast products and locations of stores that carry them can be viewed on the Web site.

LIGHTLIFE FOODS
www.lightlife.com
(800) SOY EASY (769-3279)
Lightlife makes meatless burgers and hot dogs, sliced turkey-, chicken-, and beef-style deli slices, ground "beef," chicken-style patties, tempeh, and seitan. Most products are soy-based and vegan. Nutrition facts, menu ideas, and information on where to purchase these products are on the Web site.

MORNINGSTAR FARMS
www.morningstarfarms.com
Morningstar Farms makes vegetarian breakfast patties, burgers, sausages, egg substitute, meatless crumbles, and more. A collection of recipes using Morningstar Farms products is available online.

TURTLE ISLAND FOODS
www.tofurky.com
(800) 508-8100
Maker of the famous Tofurky Vegetarian Roast, this company also sells several varieties of tempeh, soy and tempeh burgers, vegan stuffing, and more. The Web site offers recipes, menu-planning suggestions, and complete nutrition information for these products.

YVES VEGGIE CUISINE
www.yvesveggie.com
(800) 434-4246
With headquarters in Canada and facilities in several U.S. states, Yves makes vegan Canadian bacon, pepperoni, burgers, hot dogs, deli slices, vegan cheeses, chicken-style skewers, and soy-based prepared entrées such as chili and stew. The Web site provides nutrition information for all products.

BOOKS
The following two books can be found in many online and local bookstores.

THE VEGETARIAN MEAT AND POTATOES COOKBOOK
Robin Robertson
Harvard Common Press
Boston, 2002

THE NEW VEGETARIAN GRILL, REVISED EDITION
250 Flame-Kissed Recipes for Fresh, Inspired Meals
Andrea Chesman
Harvard Common Press
Boston, 2008

Add nuts and dried fruit to pancake or waffle mix; frozen and fresh berries to muffin mixes; canned mushrooms, frozen vegetables, or dried chilies to an instant soup cup; or granola and nuts to an instant pudding snack.

Think ethnic. Borrowing from different ethnic cuisines is a great way to spice up your supper. Just picture it: You unceremoniously dump a can of white beans into a bowl. Big deal. Now you toss in some salsa. Hmmm, getting better. If you're a fire-eater, you add some pickled jalapeños and hot sauce. Throw your feast into the microwave until it's hot and now you've got something!

When you go to a restaurant in an ethnic area, take some time to check out the neighborhood groceries for new vegetarian or vegan ingredients

AMERICAN DIABETES ASSOCIATION
www.diabetes.org
(800) 342-2383
Visit this Web site to review the Diabetes Food Pyramid and get diabetes-care and meal-planning advice.

AMERICAN DIETETIC ASSOCIATION
www.eatright.org
(800) 877-1600
The American Dietetic Association Web site offers a number of vegetarian fact sheets and references. While they do not specifically address a vegetarian diet for people with diabetes, they offer excellent advice on healthy meal planning.

OLDWAYS PRESERVATION AND EXCHANGE TRUST
www.oldwayspt.org
(617) 421-5500
Oldways Preservation and Exchange Trust is a nonprofit group that promotes the healthful eating patterns of traditional societies to combat obesity and other health problems in developed countries. The Web site offers three culturally specific food pyramids, as well as the Traditional Healthy Vegetarian Diet Pyramid and a fact sheet on vegetarian eating.

THE VEGETARIAN RESOURCE GROUP
www.vrg.org
(410) 366-8343
The Vegetarian Resource Group compiles information on vegan and vegetarian diets, health and nutrition tips, consumer product information, recipes, shopping tips, and links to additional vegetarian Web sites and resources. For a registration fee of $25, members receive *Vegetarian Journal,* a bimonthly magazine with recipes, product reviews, and answers to reader questions.

to incorporate into your own cooking. Prowl Indian stores for curry pastes and powders, aromatic sauce mixes, tandoori rubs (great for seasoning vegetables and tofu), pickled vegetables, chutneys, long-grained rice, and interesting breads and crackers.

Visit Middle Eastern stores for spices, hummus, tahini, harisa (a fiery chili paste), pomegranate molasses (makes a wonderful addition to salad dressings and cold beverages), nut and seed blends, and pita breads.

Look in Asian markets for different varieties of tofu, soy beverages and soy nuts, various spices, sauces, canned fruits and vegetables, long- and short-grained rice, and different types of produce.

Carbohydrate concerns

Making the switch to a vegetarian or vegan diet may require reworking your meal plan and possibly adjusting insulin or diabetes medicine doses. When trying new recipes or adapting old ones, you can calculate the carbohydrate content by adding up the grams of carbohydrate in each ingredient and dividing the total by the number of servings the recipe makes. Replacing meat or eggs with beans, grains, or soy substitutes probably means you'll be consuming more carbohydrate overall. However, a vegetarian diet may also be higher in fiber, which does not immediately affect blood glucose level. (Over the long term, a vegetarian diet high in soluble fiber—the kind in oats, fruits, and legumes—may eventually lower blood glucose levels and possibly insulin needs.) If a food contains more than 5 grams of fiber per serving, you can subtract the grams of fiber from the carbohydrate grams.

Working with a health-care provider or registered dietitian can ensure that your eating plan is balanced and will help you maintain blood glucose control; keeping careful food and blood-glucose-monitoring records will make it easier to resolve any fluctuations in blood glucose levels as you try new foods and eating habits. □

TRANS FAT BEGONE!

by Julie Lichty Balay, M.S., R.D.

If you've read a newspaper in the past 40 years, you're probably already aware that not all fat is created equal. There are three major categories of fat in the diet: unsaturated, saturated, and *trans* fat. Unsaturated fats are considered "good" fats because small amounts of these in the diet can improve blood cholesterol levels and slow hardening of the arteries (atherosclerosis) that contributes to high blood pressure and cardiovascular disease.

Saturated fat is considered "bad" fat because it has the opposite effect: It raises low-density lipoprotein (LDL, or "bad") cholesterol levels and promotes atherosclerosis.

Trans fat is the new bully on the block. It has been shown not only to raise LDL cholesterol levels but also to lower high-density lipoprotein (HDL, or "good") cholesterol. Both of these effects increase the risk for heart disease, stroke, and high blood pressure. Because heart disease and stroke are the main causes of death among people with diabetes, it is especially important for those with diabetes to focus a discerning eye on the type and amount of fat in the diet as well as the type and amount of carbohydrate.

What is *trans* fat?

Trans fat is produced when liquid oils are solidified into margarine or vegetable shortening by a process called *partial hydrogenation*. The term *trans* fat is a chemist's way of describing the straight chain of particles that make up this unhealthy fat molecule. (For an illustration, see page 414.) Believe it or not, the difference between straight-chained fats and bent-chained fats is the difference between healthy and unhealthy fats. Saturated fat likewise has a straight chain, which is

why both saturated and *trans* fats do similar damage in the arteries and are both categorized as "bad" fats. However, as an oil derivative, *trans* fat is technically still an unsaturated fat, but because it is now shaped differently, it has vastly different properties than the naturally occurring unsaturated fats found in liquid oils, nuts, seeds, and fish.

Partial hydrogenation of any type of oil will result in *trans* fat formation. (Full hydrogenation of oil does not result in the creation of *trans* fat, but the end result should be considered a saturated fat.) Common food sources of *trans* fat are fast foods (such as French fries, chicken nuggets, and fish fillets), prepared foods (such as burritos, pizza, and croutons), snack foods (such as crackers, microwave popcorn, chips, and granola bars), and baked goods (such as hamburger buns, doughnuts, cookies, cakes, and pies). Using margarine or vegetable shortening will add *trans* fat to home-cooked foods.

If *trans* fat is like saturated fat, does it matter which one you eat as long as you do not eat too much of either? It may. At the very least, *trans* fat is as harmful as saturated fat, but many recent studies have shown that it is even more so. An article published in April 2006 in *The New England Journal of Medicine* reviewed many studies in which diets containing saturated fat were compared with diets containing an equal amount of *trans* fat. The people whose diets had the *trans* fat had higher levels of LDL cholesterol, lower levels of HDL cholesterol, and higher levels of triglycerides (which are lipids, or fats, circulating in the blood). Each of these is a well-known risk factor in the development of cardiovascular disease. Other findings in the *trans* fat groups included elevated levels of Lp(a) lipoprotein and smaller

LDL particles, both of which also translate into a higher risk of heart disease.

Interestingly, when the researchers compared the incidence of cardiovascular disease between the two groups, rates were even higher in the *trans* fat group than the changes in cholesterol and other blood lipids suggested they should be. The NEJM article concluded from several major studies involving 140,000 subjects that an increase of *trans* fat by just 2% of total energy intake (about 4 grams of *trans* fat per day, based on the average 2000-calorie-per-day diet) raises the risk of cardiovascular disease by 23%.

The review article also cited studies linking *trans* fat intake with increased risk of dying from a heart attack or stroke and increased systemic inflammation. It is this chronic inflammation, caused by long-term exposure to things like smoking, pollution, and bad fats that is thought to be at the root of many chronic diseases, including diabetes.

In another study, which followed almost 85,000 female nurses for 16 years, *trans* fat intake was shown to increase the risk of diabetes by up to 39% in the nurses who consumed the most *trans* fat.

Trans fat has also been hypothesized to affect insulin sensitivity and blood glucose levels, which means it may have a very direct effect on day-to-day diabetes management. An article published in *Diabetes Care* studied 16 obese people with Type 2 diabetes who were placed on three different diets over the course of six weeks. One diet was high in unsaturated fat, the second high in saturated fat, and the third high in *trans* fat. Although the researchers observed no significant difference in blood glucose levels, the subjects were found to have hyperinsulinemia (overproduction of insulin by the pancreas) after meals on both the high-saturated-fat and high-*trans*-fat diets. Hyperinsulinemia is linked to insulin resistance, the hallmark of Type 2 diabetes. Other research on glucose and insulin sensitivity has been less conclusive, but it has also not used subjects with diabetes. More research is therefore needed to know what effect the ingestion of *trans* fat might have on diabetes control.

Why hydrogenate fat?

The hydrogenation process was developed in the early 1900's and became particularly popular in the years since the 1960's. In the 1960's and 1970's, when it was recognized that saturated fat had unhealthy effects on the body, food companies marketed plant-based margarines and vegetable shortenings as healthier alternatives to butter and lard in home cooking and baking and as "good" fats in packaged food products. However, there

AMOUNT OF *TRANS* FAT IN TYPICAL SERVINGS

PREPARED AND FAST FOODS

French fries	4.7–6.1 grams
Chicken nuggets	5.0 grams
Pizza	1.1 grams

PACKAGED SNACKS

Tortilla chips	1.6 grams
Microwave popcorn	1.2 grams
Granola bar	1.0 gram

BAKERY PRODUCTS

Doughnut	2.7 grams
Cookie	1.8 grams
Danish	3.3 grams

MARGARINES

Vegetable shortening	2.7 grams
Stick margarine	0.9–2.5 grams
Tub margarine	0.3–1.4 grams

These numbers were adapted from the article *Trans fatty acids and cardiovascular disease*, published in the April 13, 2006, issue of *The New England Journal of Medicine*, pages 1601–1613.

DETECTING *TRANS* FAT

Even if a product lists no *trans* fat in the Nutrition Facts panel, check the ingredients list for hydrogenated oils. Any oil that has been partially hydrogenated will contain *trans* fat.

INGREDIENTS: PEANUTS, SUGAR, PARTIALLY HYDROGENATED VEGETABLE OILS (RAPESEED, COTTONSEED AND SOYBEAN) TO PREVENT SEPARATION were also practical reasons hydrogenated fats were already being widely used before this time.

For one thing, vegetable oils and hydrogenation are inexpensive. Corn and soybeans are staple crops in the United States, and it is much cheaper to produce oils from these crops than to raise the cattle and swine needed to make butter and lard. In addition, hydrogenated oils do not spoil easily, so packaged goods made with hydrogenated oils have much longer shelf lives than their natural-fat counterparts.

A benefit of partially hydrogenated oils for the consumer is that they spread more easily than animal fats. Have you ever tried to spread cold butter on a piece of toast and watched your toast tear to shreds? Try it with a cold stick of margarine and see how much easier the job becomes. (Full hydrogenation, in contrast, yields a hard, waxlike product.) Not only do partially hydrogenated oils increase spreadability, but they help maintain the emulsion in foods like peanut butter, which means the oil from the peanuts will not separate and rise to the top of the jar. Partially hydrogenated oils also have a very high smoking point, which means they are ideal for frying.

So food manufacturers have had good reasons to use partially hydrogenated oils, but the negative effects they have on health give consumers even better reason to avoid them.

Avoiding *trans* fats

The average American consumes approximately 5–8 grams of *trans* fat per day, or 45–72 calories' worth, accounting for about 2% to 3% of total calories consumed per day. Most dietary *trans* fat is manmade through the hydrogenation process. However, small amounts of *trans* fat are produced naturally by the bacteria found in the stomachs of ruminant animals such as cows and sheep, so there are trace amounts of *trans* fat found in dairy products, beef, and lamb. However, natural *trans* fat makes up only about 0.5% of the calories in the average American diet, and natural *trans* fat is bound to other important nutrients such calcium and iron. Avoiding the manmade variety, therefore, will likely have a greater positive effect on health.

There remains the question as to how much, if any, *trans* fat is safe to eat. The current consensus among the experts is that manmade *trans* fat should be avoided entirely if possible.

Avoiding *trans* fat got easier as of January 1, 2006, when rules took effect requiring food manufacturers to list *trans* fat separately on the Nutrition Facts panel required on the label of all packaged

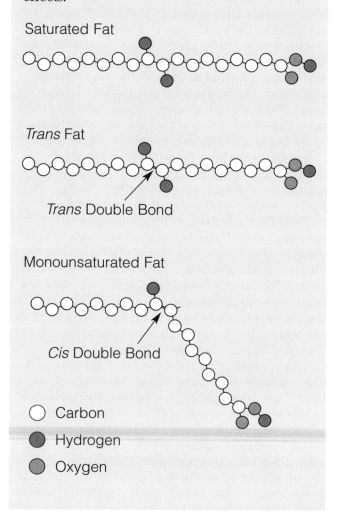

CHEMICAL STRUCTURE OF FAT

The structure of a fat molecule changes how it behaves in the body. Straight-chained fats such as saturated fat and *trans* fat have unhealthy effects in the body, while bent-chained fats such as monounsaturated fat have healthful effects.

Saturated Fat

Trans Fat

Trans Double Bond

Monounsaturated Fat

Cis Double Bond

○ Carbon

● Hydrogen

● Oxygen

goods. However, just reading the Nutrition Facts panel may not be good enough to get all the *trans* fat out of your diet. If the amount of *trans* fat in one serving of food is 0.5 grams or less, the manufacturer is allowed to state on the label that it contains 0 grams of *trans* fat. You might think that 0.5 grams is too scant an amount to do any harm, but if more than one serving of the food is consumed over the course of the day, or if several foods containing small amounts of *trans* fat are eaten, it's easy to consume several grams of *trans* fat in a day, and, as mentioned earlier, it only takes a few grams a day to have negative health effects.

There is another way to identify foods containing *trans* fat and that's to read the ingredients list and look for any type of hydrogenated vegetable oil in the list. Any partially hydrogenated vegetable oil contains *trans* fat.

As you read labels, you will probably find that some of your favorite foods contain *trans* fat. Most varieties of peanut butter, for example, are labeled as having 0 grams of *trans* fat, but they also list partially hydrogenated vegetable oil in the ingredients list. This can be a disappointing experience, but fortunately, due to the new labeling laws and public awareness about *trans* fat, many manufacturers have either reformulated many of their products or developed new "*trans*-fat–free" ones. So you should be able to find substitutes for the packaged goods you enjoy. Margarines are a very common source of dietary *trans* fat, but there are now margarines made without partially hydrogenated oils that are widely available. They are more expensive than regular margarine, but they are worth it if you use such spreads regularly. If you have no choice but to buy margarine that contains partially hydrogenated oil, choose the tub or squeeze-bottle variety rather than stick margarine. The softer the margarine, the less *trans* fat it has. (Hydrogenation makes oils harder, so softer products have undergone less hydrogenation.)

Eating out is tricky when it comes to *trans* fat. Unless you specifically ask what type of oil is used for frying (and get an accurate answer), you cannot be sure of the presence of *trans* fat. Hopefully, there will be a similar trend for restaurants to remove the hydrogenated oil from their recipes the way manufacturers of packaged food have begun to do. In New York City, the Board of Health has taken matters into its own hands, requiring restaurants to eliminate all artificial *trans* fats from their menus by July 2008. (Using them in most frying oils has already been banned in the city.) However, until there are more widespread regulations on *trans* fats (as in some European countries), most diners will need to be aware of which restaurant foods commonly have them and avoid those foods.

Restaurant and fast-food chains have the nutrient values of their menus available in the restaurant or online, so if you frequent a particular restaurant chain, it would be advisable to research your favorite foods and find alternatives on the menu if you find they contain *trans* fat. It should be pointed out that all fried foods should be eaten sparingly because of their high fat content; steering away from them in general will limit both *trans* fat and total fat in the diet.

In cooking, oil almost always can be substituted for butter or margarine with similar results. In baking, consider using butter instead of margarine or shortening: The flavor is superior and because of this you may feel satisfied with less of the food. Because butter contains a lot of saturated fat (and trace amounts of naturally occurring *trans* fat), consider using less butter than the recipe calls for (most recipes come out just fine with 50% to 75% of the fat listed). If the amount of fat in the recipe is important to the quality, you may also use half oil and half butter, or substitute completely with oil. It is a good idea to test this method on a small recipe since using oil may change the result.

Keep in mind that all fats have the same amount of calories (9 calories per gram), and eating a lot of any fat can contribute to overweight. That means olive oil can make you gain as much weight as butter or as margarine made with hydrogenated oil.

Most major health organizations recommend keeping fat intake to about 30% of daily calories, which works out to about 65 grams of fat per day for a person who consumes 2,000 calories per day. Most also say that saturated and *trans* fat intake combined should account for no more than 10% of daily calories, or about 20 grams of fat. However, the American Heart Association released new guidelines in June 2006 advising Americans to limit their *trans* fat intake to less than 1% of total calories, or about 2 grams.

Since it is really not yet known if any amount is safe, to be on the safe side, read the labels on packaged foods, and don't buy any that contain either *trans* fat or that list partially hydrogenated oils in the ingredients list. Your arteries will thank you for your efforts. □

EXTREME MAKEOVER— RECIPE EDITION

by Patti Geil, M.S., R.D., C.D.E.,
and Laura Hieronymus, M.S.Ed., A.P.R.N.,
B.C.-A.D.M., C.D.E.

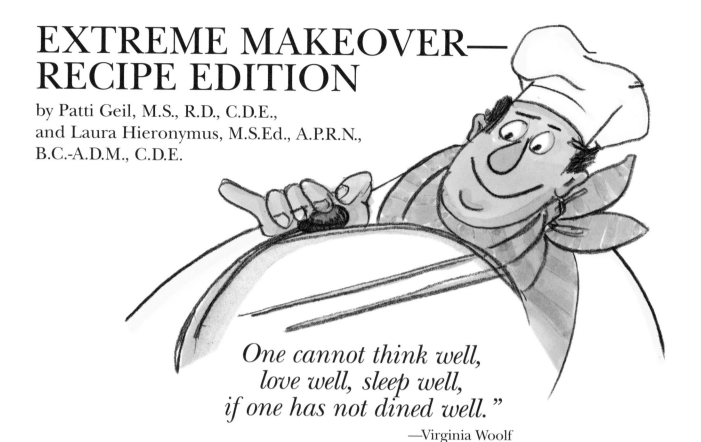

*One cannot think well,
love well, sleep well,
if one has not dined well. "*

—Virginia Woolf

Man does not live by bread alone… or by tasteless but healthful "diabetic recipes." There is no denying that smart food choices have a positive effect on your blood glucose levels, but food has to taste good for anyone to want to eat it. Often, people newly diagnosed with diabetes become overwhelmed with information about meal planning and feel they need to count the nutrients in each morsel of food. Because many old favorite family recipes tend to be high in fat, sugar, and salt, enjoying them may seem to be a thing of the past.

As you become more comfortable living with diabetes, however, you'll find that it's not necessary to give up all of your favorite foods to achieve good blood glucose control. There is a place in your meal plan for treats as well as tradition. Creative cooking techniques can help you modify recipes to fit your meal plan while retaining the flavors you enjoy.

Healthy eating: not hocus-pocus

The principles of healthy eating for diabetes are not magical mysteries. In fact, people with diabetes can eat the same food the rest of the family enjoys. Eating healthfully benefits everyone and reduces the risk for many chronic conditions such as heart disease.

The American Diabetes Association as well as the new U.S. Department of Agriculture "MyPyramid Plan" (www.mypyramid.gov) describe a healthy meal plan as one that emphasizes fruits, vegetables, whole grains, and fat-free or low-fat milk and milk products, lean meats, poultry, fish, beans, eggs, and nuts, and is low in saturated fats, *trans* fats, cholesterol, salt (sodium), and added sugars. People with diabetes also need to pay special attention to carbohydrate (sugars and starches) and portion sizes.

The first published cookbooks describe the kitchen as a household "laboratory," which is an apt description of the room in which you should freely experiment with creating healthier versions of your favorite recipes. As you attempt new approaches to your tried-and-true recipes, make notes to yourself directly on the recipe or in the cookbook so you'll know which changes worked well and which did not.

Tricks of the trade

One quick trick for eating more healthfully while still enjoying favorite foods is to simply decrease your portion size when eating high-fat, high-sugar, or high-sodium foods. For example, serve salad dressing on the side, and measure out 1 or 2 tablespoons for your portion. Use 1 tablespoon of sour cream rather than 2 on a baked potato. Sprinkle foods with herbs and spices, or add steamed, chopped vegetables to your dishes to punch up the flavor and fiber. Reduce the amount of oil you use to sauté foods, or use flavored cooking spray instead of oil. Eliminating "optional" ingredients such as salt in the cooking water or high-fat, high-calorie sauces on vegetables also helps you achieve your healthy eating goals.

To improve the health benefits of a favorite recipe, look over the list of ingredients, consider the role each plays in the recipe, and modify only one at a time. This gives you an opportunity to judge the success of your single change. Surprisingly, even one or two seemingly small recipe adjustments can greatly improve the nutrient profile.

Knowing the role each ingredient plays in a recipe will help you determine the amount needed to ensure a tasty product before you make sweeping changes.

Fat. Fat is a key ingredient in cooking for a number of reasons. In baked goods, fat tenderizes, adds moisture, and affects the shape of the finished product. Fat also carries, blends, and stabilizes flavors. It adds a creamy texture to sauces and dips, and it makes you feel full. Because of the varied roles that fat plays in cooking, it can be difficult to make great-tasting low-fat and fat-free foods without careful substitutions. In addition, a small amount of fat is necessary in the diet to absorb fat-soluble vitamins and other nutrients.

Sugar. Sugar provides texture, color, and bulk to a variety of foods. In yeast breads, sugar helps the bread rise; it also gives the light-brown color and crisp mouth-feel found in many baked goods. It is often possible to cut back on added sugar in a recipe by one-quarter to one-third without making a difference in quality, but eliminating it entirely or using a sugar substitute in its place will not yield a satisfactory product in many cases.

Salt. Salt or sodium occurs naturally in many foods, but a significant amount of the salt we eat comes from food preparation and processing or adding salt at the table. While yeast breads require salt to control the rising of the dough, in other recipes, salt can be cut in half or totally eliminated without compromising the final results. Tasting foods before salting them and removing the salt-shaker from the table are two great starts to healthier eating.

Modifying recipes is not always about subtracting. Adding fiber adds to the health benefits of a dish, and adding herbs, spices, and other low-calorie but flavorful ingredients makes nutritious dishes more appealing to eat.

RECIPE RESOURCES

Having the right recipes can make following a healthy meal plan much easier. However, with almost 17,000 cookbooks on the market, you may find it challenging to determine which ones meet your needs. Here are a few tips for finding recipes you can use with confidence:

■ Glance through a cookbook before buying it to be sure nutrition information and serving sizes for recipes are provided. Having diabetes exchange information for each recipe is an added bonus.

■ Cookbooks published by Rapaport Publishing, Inc., including *Diabetes Self-Management's Meals & Menus for 1 or 2* and *Healthy & Hearty Diabetic Cooking*, provide detailed nutrition facts for each recipe, as do recipes that appear in *Diabetes Self-Management* magazine.

To order cookbooks, call (800) 664-9269 or log on to www.DiabetesSelfManagement.com.

■ Cookbooks published by the American Diabetes Association (ADA) and the ADA membership magazine *Diabetes Forecast* also provide detailed nutrition facts for recipes.

To order cookbooks, call (800) 232-6733 or log on to http://store.diabetes.org.

■ Registered dietitians, county extension agents, and public health departments often have created special diabetes cookbooks and recipes available to you at no cost.

■ Check out interesting cookbooks from the public library for a "test drive" before purchasing one for home.

■ The Internet can be a wonderful source of information. One popular recipe program for those with Type 1, Type 2, or prediabetes is GlucoMenu (located at www.glucomenu.com), which is under the direction of a registered dietitian and certified diabetes educator. The GlucoMenu program provides complete menus, recipes, and grocery lists with nutrition facts for diabetes, based on your specified calories. Other services include an online diabetes progress tracking chart, food substitution list, and full access to professional articles about diabetes. Cost begins at $49 for a month of menus and additional services, with discounts for longer periods of time.

■ Magazines such as Diabetic Cooking (www.diabeticcooking.com) and Diabetes Health (www.diabeteshealth.com) also publish recipes with nutrition information.

Fiber. Because most Americans, with or without diabetes, don't eat near the amount of fiber recommended each day, they aren't enjoying the health benefits it can provide. Increasing the fiber in your diet contributes to better digestion and a lower risk for heart disease and cancer. Fiber, particularly the soluble variety found in oats and beans, slows the release of glucose into the bloodstream after a meal and improves blood fat levels.

Flavor. Preparing the healthiest recipes in the world won't make a bit of difference if they aren't consumed. After all, food is more than just something to eat. We prefer certain foods for social, emotional, and physical reasons. Consumer research shows that when we purchase a certain food, taste tops nutrition as the number one reason we buy one food over another. Because reducing fat, sugar, and salt may remove certain flavors, it's often necessary to boost the taste in other ways. Also, the senses of taste and smell diminish with age, making it even more important to create flavorful dishes.

To reduce fat

One easy way to reduce the fat in the meals you prepare at home is to use specially modified low-fat or reduced-fat ingredients. For example, fat-free sour cream or yogurt can easily replace full-fat sour cream in a chilled dip without a change in quality. However, using fat-free margarine to sauté vegetables does not work well. Follow manufacturers' directions for modified ingredients to obtain the best results. Here are some other tips:

■ Lighten up packaged mixes by trying lower-fat options in preparation. For example, use half of the oil called for in packaged pasta salad mixes, or try using low-fat or skim milk when making instant pudding.

■ Make soup or stew ahead of time, then refrigerate and skim off the hardened fat on top before reheating to serve. For each tablespoon you remove, you skim off more than 100 calories!

■ Reduce the fat content in homemade baked goods by substituting unsweetened applesauce, pureed prunes, or another pureed fruit for part of the oil, shortening, margarine, or butter. In a banana bread recipe, for example, you can substitute an equal amount of applesauce for at least half of the fat.

■ Fortify the taste of low-fat dishes with fat-free seasonings, spices, and herbs. A simple pepper-garlic herb rub made from garlic powder, cracked black pepper, and cayenne pepper can be gently pressed onto the surface of meat, poultry, or fish prior to grilling for extra snap.

To reduce sugar

Buying products that contain no added sugar or that are artificially sweetened can reduce the amount of table sugar in your diet. However, the words "sugar-free" or "no added sugar" on the food label don't necessarily mean a food or ingredient is calorie- or carbohydrate-free. Sweeteners such as sugar alcohols and polyols may provide fewer calories per gram but should be counted as part of your day's carbohydrate allowance for the best blood glucose control. Similarly, naturally occurring sugars must be counted as well. Here are some ways to trim the sugar in your diet:

■ When fruit is called for, use fresh fruits, unsweetened frozen fruits, or fruits canned in their own juices, or rinse the syrup off canned fruits to cut the sugar and calories.

■ Use artificial sweeteners in recipes when sugar is used only for its sweet taste, not to add body or texture to a dish. For example, in most cases, sugar-free gelatin can be substituted for the full-sugar version. For baked items, a special baking version of an artificial sweetener may be necessary. For foods that will be heated, consult the sweetener manufacturer's directions to determine whether a particular product can be used.

■ Vanilla or peppermint extracts enhance the sweetness of foods. Spices such as allspice, cardamom, cinnamon, coriander, ginger, mace, and nutmeg also increase the perception of sweetness.

To reduce salt

Cutting back on sodium can help many people prevent or control high blood pressure. Here are some tips for doing that:

■ Use herbs and spices in place of salt. Basil, bay leaves, dill, marjoram, mint, parsley, rosemary, sage, savory, tarragon, and thyme are particularly good herbs for replacing salt in recipes.

■ Low-salt or low-sodium versions of canned vegetables, soy sauce, broth, and seasoning mixes substitute nicely for the full-salt versions.

■ Limit the use of high-sodium foods in your recipes. Cured foods such as bacon and ham, foods packed in salty brine such as pickles, olives, and sauerkraut, and condiments such as mustard, ketchup, and barbecue sauce can be significant sources of sodium in your recipes.

To increase fiber

For best results, increase your fiber intake gradually. Here are some ways to add high-fiber ingredients to the foods you prepare:

■ Whole wheat flour can replace from one-quarter

SLIMMED DOWN MACARONI AND CHEESE

A classic comfort food, macaroni and cheese can be modified to taste good yet still be good for you. Several approaches were used to cut over 380 calories and 42 grams of fat per serving from this recipe, while maintaining a rich, cheesy flavor. The main strategy was ingredient substitution: reduced-fat rather than full-fat cheese, reduced-calorie stick margarine rather than butter, and skim milk rather than whole milk. Fat, cholesterol, and calories could be slashed even further by using egg substitute in place of the egg and by making the topping with crumbs from fat-free croutons rather than dry breadcrumbs stirred into melted, reduced-calorie margarine. Using whole-wheat macaroni would increase the fiber content to about 3 grams per serving. Experiment to find your ideal balance of good taste and good health.

Original Momma's Macaroni and Cheese

5 cups cooked macaroni (approximately 3 cups uncooked)
5 tablespoons butter
2 eggs
½ teaspoon salt
½ teaspoon pepper
3 cups whole milk
2 cups shredded mozzarella cheese
4 cups shredded Cheddar cheese

Yield: 6 servings   Serving size: 1 cup

Per serving:
    Calories: 737
    Carbohydrate: 27 g
    Protein: 38 g
    Fat: 53 g
    Saturated fat: 33 g
    Sodium: 1,037 mg
    Fiber: 1 g

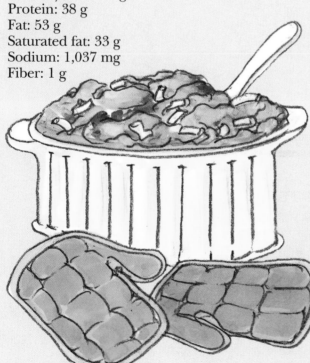

Momma's Slimmed-Down Macaroni and Cheese

4 cups cooked elbow macaroni (about 2 cups uncooked)
2 cups (8 ounces) shredded, reduced-fat sharp Cheddar cheese
1 cup 1% low-fat cottage cheese
¾ cup nonfat sour cream
½ cup skim milk
2 tablespoons grated fresh onion
1½ teaspoons reduced-calorie stick margarine, melted
¼ teaspoon salt
¼ teaspoon pepper
1 egg, lightly beaten
Vegetable cooking spray
¼ cup dry breadcrumbs
1 tablespoon reduced-calorie stick margarine, melted
¼ teaspoon paprika
Fresh oregano sprigs

Combine first 10 ingredients; stir well and spoon into a 2-quart casserole coated with cooking spray. Combine breadcrumbs, 1 tablespoon melted margarine, and paprika; stir well. Sprinkle over casserole. Cover and bake at 350°F for 30 minutes. Uncover; bake 5 minutes or until set. Garnish with oregano.

Yield: 6 servings   Serving size: 1 cup

Per serving:
    Calories: 356
    Carbohydrate: 38 g
    Protein: 25 g
    Fat: 11 g
    Saturated fat: 5 g
    Sodium: 627 mg
    Fiber: 1 g

to half of the all-purpose flour in most recipes.
■ Use whole-grain pasta or brown rice in recipes to boost their fiber count.
■ Add extra vegetables to casseroles, soups, and pasta or rice dishes. Pasta primavera provides an excellent opportunity to add fiber in the form of vegetables such as artichokes, asparagus, broccoli, cauliflower, mushrooms, peas, peppers, tomatoes, and zucchini.
■ Beans can enhance the fiber content and flavor of a recipe. Add kidney beans to chunky vegetable soup or pinto beans to the meat filling for tacos or burritos. However, don't forget to count the carbohydrate content of added beans: 15 grams of carbohydrate per one-third cup of cooked beans.

To increase flavor

For the best flavor, buy the freshest ingredients you can find. Buy locally grown fruits and vegetables in season, when possible, or purchase frozen fruits and vegetables, which are generally frozen immediately after picking, so they retain a fresh taste and maximum nutrients. Adding herbs and spices to recipes can also make food tastier. Here are a few things to keep in mind when doing so:
■ Keep in mind that dry herbs are stronger than fresh and that powdered herbs are stronger than crumbled. If you want to substitute fresh herbs for

dry in a recipe, use one tablespoon of fresh herb for each teaspoon of dried.
■ When using herbs to increase flavor in your recipes, timing is everything. Add seasonings to chilled foods, such as salad dressings and dips, several hours before serving to allow time for their flavors to blend. If you're making a hot dish such as soup or stew, add herbs toward the end of cooking time so their flavor won't disappear.
■ Spices that hold up well if added early in the cooking time include allspice, coriander, cumin, ginger, and nutmeg.

Enjoying your food— and good health

It's no longer necessary to choose either favorite recipes or good blood glucose control. They can coexist when you stick to small portions or make a few recipe alterations. For an example of how it can be done, see "Slimmed-Down Macaroni and Cheese" on page 419.

The French writer and gastronome Maurice Edmond Sailland once said, "Cuisine is when things taste like themselves." That thought surely describes the ideal way of cooking for diabetes: choosing quality ingredients to create good-for-you foods that taste good too! □

Preventive Health

Tips 680–772 423

Lower Cholesterol to Lower Heart Risk 429

Lifestyle Habits for a Healthy Heart 433

The Benefits of Tight Control 437
No End in Sight

Avoiding Eye Complictions. 440

Boning Up on Bone Health 445

Emergency Preparedness 450
Just In Case

Getting the Sleep You Need 454

Diabetes and Your Skin. 460
Protecting Your Outermost Layer

How to Avoid Errors in Diabetes Care. 465

11

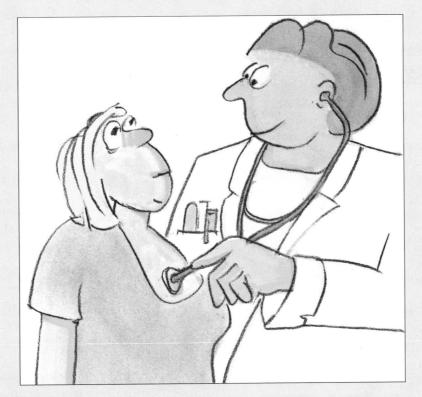

Preventive Health Tips

680–772

680. To help yourself sleep, reduce caffeine, limit alcohol, and stop smoking.

681. Get in the habit of using your bed only for sleep and sex.

682. Don't read, eat, talk on the phone, or watch television in bed.

683. Get up at the same time every morning, whether you've slept or not.

684. Be patient, as it can take at least two weeks to learn new sleep behaviors.

685. Sex can also be a good sleep-inducer for some people.

686. Exercise during the day to promote sleep at night.

687. Maintain the best possible blood glucose control to improve sleep.

688. Lose excess weight to make it easier to sleep.

689. Get some sun exposure during the day to improve sleep at night.

690. Use a "white noise generator," a fan, or a tape of nature sounds to block unwanted noise when trying to sleep.

691. Thinner pillows may give better posture and more comfortable sleep to people who sleep on their backs, while people who sleep on their sides may need thicker pillows for more neck support.

692. Try a pillow or bolster behind you when you sleep on your side, or a pillow under your feet or between your knees to reduce back strain.

693. Set your thermostat appropriately for a comfortable sleeping temperature.

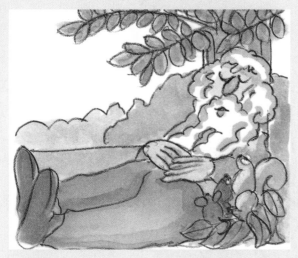

694. Avoid long naps if you have insomnia.

695. Keep a sleep diary to figure out what's keeping you up or what works best to help you sleep. In your sleep diary each morning, write down when you went to bed, about how long it took to go to sleep, about how many times you recall waking up, when you got up, and how rested you feel. Record any naps you took the day before. Also rate your energy level and alertness during the day on a scale of 1 to 10. If this doesn't work, you may want to consult a sleep specialist.

696. Tell your doctor about any prescription or over-the-counter drugs you are taking. Bring a list of all of your medicines to your appointments, or bring the drugs themselves (in their original containers).

697. Fill all of your prescriptions at one pharmacy, if possible.

698. Keep an up-to-date list of your medicines in your wallet or purse.

699. Talk to your doctor before starting any dietary or herbal supplements.

700. When you refill your prescriptions, note whether your pills (or insulin) look different from those you normally take. If they do, check it out with your pharmacist.

701. Don't stop taking a prescribed medicine because you feel better.

702. To learn more about the medicines you take, read the information sheets given out with prescriptions by your pharmacist, or talk to your doctor, nurse, or diabetes educator about your medicines.

703. If your doctor has not adjusted your medicines or doses recently, ask him to review your medicines with a view to keeping you in good control.

704. Review generic drugs with your doctor or pharmacist with a view to lowering costs, and consider using combination tablets that contain more than one drug to reduce your co-pays and the number of pills you take each day.

705. Keep in mind that, often, it is both cheaper and safer to use older, proven medicines than to use brand-new ones.

706. Have a sick-day plan that you have discussed with your doctor and diabetes educator. It should specify how to maintain blood glucose control while you are ill and also when to call your health-care provider for advice.

707. If you think your blood glucose level is low, address the problem promptly. Stop what you're doing, check your blood glucose level with your meter, and have a snack if necessary, even if you have to stop your car or interrupt a conversation to do it. If you don't have your meter with you or can't use it for any reason, go ahead and treat your symptoms of hypoglycemia without checking your blood glucose level first.

708. To treat hypoglycemia, chew and swallow four glucose tablets (containing about 4 grams of carbohydrate each) or drink about 5 ounces of orange juice or a regular (not diet) soft drink.

709. It is a good idea for anyone with diabetes to wear a medical identification bracelet indicating that he has diabetes, just in case he is ever unable to speak for himself.

710. Participate in your in-hospital diabetes care by knowing what your readings are

and by making sure your meals are designed to accommodate your diabetes control plan.

711. Before you enter the hospital, talk to your doctor about which medicines to continue taking and which to stop (and when).

712. If you are having surgery, it's a good idea to ask who will be in charge of your diabetes control while you are having surgery and recuperating from it.

713. Before you leave the hospital, make sure you have in writing what your medicines and doses should be when you arrive home.If some of the medicines you were taking before hospitalization are not on the list of medicines to take after, ask why. Also, ask your usual pharmacist to check your new combination of medicines for potential drug interactions or anything that you may be allergic to.

714. If you are not sure how to carry out parts of your diabetes regimen or are not getting the results you expect from your efforts, speak to your doctor or diabetes educator.

715. If you have any doubt about the safety of foods, particularly meat or dairy foods, which spoil quickly, throw them out.

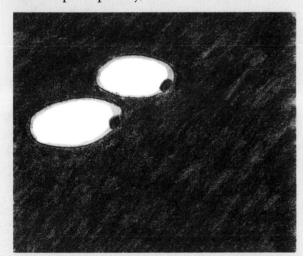

716. Plan ahead for power outages or other disasters by keeping at least a three-day supply of nonperishable food—and a manual can opener—in your home. Pick foods that require no cooking or preparation in case you cannot heat foods.

717. To maintain blood glucose control in an emergency, do your best to eat meals and snacks on your usual schedule, and continue to monitor your blood glucose on schedule as well.

718. Find a place to store a gallon of water, some glucose tablets, and some shelf-stable snacks at your office in case you get stuck there overnight.

719. If you typically wear dress shoes at work, keep an old pair of sneakers there in case you have to evacuate the building.

720. In your car, it's a good idea to keep a flashlight (with working batteries), a small first aid kit, a plastic bottle of water, glucose tablets, some nonperishable snacks, and a pair of sneakers (in case you have to get out and walk) just in case.

721. In cold weather, you may also want to keep some extra clothes and a blanket in your car.

722. Do not plan on keeping a blood glucose meter and strips or insulin in your car; car temperatures can get very hot (and very cold), which will make strips inaccurate and insulin ineffective.

723. Even if you're just going for a walk or a bike ride, pop a small bottle of water, a snack, some money, and your basic diabetes supplies into a fanny pack.

724. Choose a friend or family member who lives out of state to serve as a contact person in case local phone lines are down or in case not all evacuating family members are equipped with cell phones.

725. Your emergency bag should be stored near your front or back door. If it's a bright color, it will be that much easier to find when you're in a rush, and it should be marked with your name.

726. The American Diabetes Association recommends starting diet and exercise changes if one's LDL cholesterol level is over 100 mg/dl and adding drug therapy if it exceeds 130 mg/dl

727. For people with diabetes who already have cardiovascular disease, drug therapy should be started along with lifestyle

changes if their LDL levels are above 100 mg/dl.

728. To reduce your risk of coronary heart disease, reduce your intake of saturated fat and cholesterol. Saturated fat should be less than 7% of your total calories per day and dietary cholesterol should be less than 200 mg per day.

729. If you do not know your recommended calorie intake, ask your physician for a referral to a registered dietitian. A registered dietitian can calculate your calorie goals and give you personalized recommendations for how to achieve your saturated fat intake goal and other diet modification goals using foods that you like and enjoy.

730. Saturated fat and *trans* fats should be replaced with monounsaturated fats (up to 20% of calories) and polyunsaturated fats (up to 10% of total calories).

731. To further lower LDL cholesterol, try adding plant stanols or sterols to your diet.

732. If you are at a healthy weight, work with your physician to prevent weight gain. Develop strategies for weight maintenance and anticipate high-risk occasions for possible weight gain (for example, times of significant stress).

733. If you are overweight, start with a weight-loss goal of 10% through dietary change, portion control, and daily physical activity.

734. Once you get the OK to exercise, try 30 minutes of moderate-intensity activity on most, if not all, days of the week—even if you are not overweight.

735. To lower triglyceride levels, reduce your intake of refined or processed carbohydrates, such as candy, table sugar, white flour, and baked goods made with white flour.

736. Eat foods rich in monounsaturated and polyunsaturated fats instead of those that contain refined sugar.

737. Substituting fish rich in omega-3 fatty acids (found in fatty fish such as salmon, sardines, and tuna) may also lower triglycerides.

738. Discuss the risks and benefits of taking fish oil with your physician.

739. If triglycerides are a problem for you, it would be a good idea to cut down on alcohol as much as possible.

740. People meeting their diabetes treatment goals should have an HbA_{1c} test at least twice a year, and those whose therapy has changed or who are not meeting their goals should be tested four times a year.

741. It is important to keep skin well moisturized. The best way to moisturize is to apply lotion or cream right after showering and patting the skin dry.

742. Help skin lesions heal faster with the use of antibiotic washes and creams.

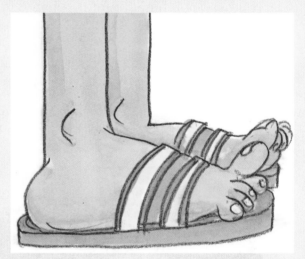

743. To help prevent athlete's foot, it is always a good idea to wear slippers or shoes of some sort in public areas such as locker rooms or showers.

744. Get immediate attention and treatment for foot ulcers. Treatment may include oral or intravenous antibiotics to control the infection, as well as dressings and salves with lubricating, protective, antibiotic, or cleansing properties.

745. To protect your skin and help prevent skin ailments from developing, observe good hygiene. Bathe regularly and wash your hands often.

746. People who live in hot, humid areas should change their clothing once it becomes wet from perspiration.

747. Keep an eye out for skin reactions that arise as a result of allergies to medicines.

748. Injuries to the skin should be kept covered and inspected on a regular basis to make sure they are not worsening.

749. Inspect your hands and feet daily for the presence of cuts or scrapes, since these parts of the body may have decreased sensation due to neuropathy, and wounds may therefore go unnoticed.

750. A large part of keeping your skin healthy involves maintaining practices that are good for your whole body, such as eating a balanced diet, drinking plenty of water, managing stress, and controlling your blood glucose level.

751. To prevent eye disease, keep your blood glucose levels as close to the normal range as possible.

752. Tight control is best achieved with close consultation with members of your diabetes care team, careful attention to diet (especially portion control), regular exercise, medicine if necessary, and blood glucose monitoring on a regular basis.

753. Keep your blood pressure well controlled through diet, regular physical activity, and medicine, if needed, to avoid eye complications.

754. Keeping your blood pressure at or below 115/75 mm Hg will greatly reduce the risk of losing vision to diabetes.

755. Check, know, and improve your blood lipid levels through diet, regular physical activity, and medicine, if necessary, to lower risk of retinopathy and other eye diseases.

756. Make sure you get a dilated eye examination every year by an optometrist or ophthalmologist knowledgeable about and experienced with diabetes and diabetic eye disease.

757. Insist that your eye doctor send timely reports to your other doctors and health advisors, and ask them to send reports to your eye doctor.

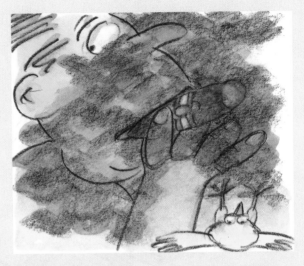

758. If you have diabetes, quitting smoking is arguably the single best thing you can do for your eyes (as well as your heart, lungs, kidneys, dental health, etc.).

759. Adequate levels of many nutrients, including calcium, vitamin D, magnesium, and vitamin K, are necessary to build healthy bones. The most important of these are calcium and vitamin D.

760. Exercise, particularly weight-bearing activities where your body is working against gravity, can help keep bones strong. Weight-bearing activities include walking, dancing, climbing stairs, and weight training.

761. Balance exercises are useful to prevent falls that could lead to fractures.

762. If you drink alcohol, keep your regular intake to no more than one to two servings per day.

763. Have your risk for osteoporosis evaluated now, before problems occur, then do your part to lower your risk by taking steps such as increasing your activity level and consuming enough calcium and vitamin D to prevent it early.

764. Leave a light on in the hall or bathroom at night so you are not stumbling in the dark if you need to go to the bathroom.

765. Keep floors, hallways, stairways, and outdoor walkways free of clutter.

766. Use rubber bath mats in the tub and shower. Consider using a shower chair if your balance is poor.

767. Avoid walking on rough or uneven surfaces if your balance is poor. Watch your step at curbs, and look for misaligned areas when walking on sidewalks. Consider using a cane or walker.

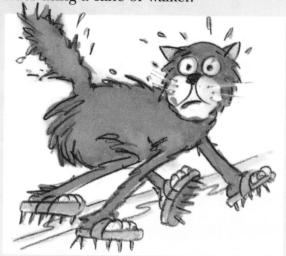

768. If it's icy outside, carry a small bag of sand, salt, or kitty litter to sprinkle on slippery sidewalks and steps or wear lightweight crampons.

769. To meet your calcium needs, try to eat at least 2 to 3 servings of low-fat dairy products or other calcium-rich foods each day.

770. If you need a calcium supplement to meet your calcium requirements, choose one that contains calcium citrate, calcium lactate, or calcium carbonate.

771. Choose supplements that have the USP (United States Pharmacopeia) seal, showing they meet government guidelines for production and dissolution.

772. Avoid "natural" calcium supplements that contain calcium from coral, oyster shells, dolomite, or bone meal, because these sources are more likely to be contaminated with lead and other dangerous substances.

LOWER CHOLESTEROL TO LOWER HEART RISK

by Wayne L. Clark

The news out of the United Kingdom in June 2003 was a call to action for people with diabetes and their physicians. Investigators in the Heart Protection Study had reported a year earlier that the drug simvastatin had lowered cholesterol levels in study subjects and reduced the risk of heart attack and stroke by 25%. The researchers then looked at the subgroup of subjects who had diabetes, and published their findings in June 2003.

They found that lowering levels of low-density lipoprotein (LDL) cholesterol (often referred to as "bad" cholesterol) by 39 mg/dl resulted in a 22% reduction in the likelihood of a first heart attack or stroke in people with diabetes. Significant cardiac benefits were found even in people who entered the study with no signs of arterial hardening and those whose LDL levels were within ranges that don't automatically suggest the need for LDL-lowering drugs. These results led the researchers to conclude their report with a declaration that "statin therapy should now be considered routinely for all diabetic patients at sufficiently high risk of major vascular events, irrespective of their initial cholesterol concentrations."

The relationship between heart disease and the various forms of lipids (blood fats such as cholesterol and triglycerides) was described as early as the 1930's and confirmed in the Framingham Heart Study in the 1970's and by many other studies since then. Cholesterol is a key contributor to atherosclerosis, the "hardening of the arteries" that leads to heart disease, stroke, and peripheral vascular disease.

This is particularly important to people with diabetes, in whom atherosclerosis is much more prevalent. Three-quarters of people with diabetes will die of complications that arise from atherosclerosis. They have a 2–4 times higher risk of heart attack and stroke and are more likely to die in the hospital undergoing a cardiac procedure. They also do less well following a heart attack or surgery. Atherosclerosis in the peripheral circulation, primarily in the arteries of the legs, is 2–4

times more likely in people with diabetes. This can lead to dangerous clots, pain, and amputation.

People with diabetes, in particular Type 2 diabetes, have a characteristic dyslipidemia (lipid disorder) that puts them at higher risk of atherosclerosis. They tend to have high blood levels of triglycerides and low levels of high-density lipoprotein (HDL) cholesterol. HDL cholesterol is often referred to as "good" cholesterol, because it appears to protect against atherosclerosis. Although people with diabetes tend to have levels of LDL cholesterol that are the same (or only slightly elevated) as people who don't have diabetes, their LDL particles are of a different and more dangerous kind.

The LDL particles in people with diabetes are different because they contain more triglycerides. "When you increase the concentration of triglycerides in LDL cholesterol, its structure changes and it becomes a smaller, denser particle," says Leonard M. Keilson, M.D., M.P.H., a lipids specialist practicing in Portland, Maine. "These dense LDL particles are particularly dangerous, because they can more easily cross the endothelium—the lining of the arteries—and enter the wall of the vessels." Fatty deposits in arterial walls lead to atherosclerosis.

Diet modification and exercise can help with this dyslipidemia, although Dr. Keilson cautions that they are most effective in people who have metabolic syndrome (a group of problems including cholesterol abnormalities, abdominal obesity, high blood pressure, and insulin resistance that increase the risk of diabetes, heart disease, and stroke) as opposed to full-blown Type 2 diabetes.

"You can 'convert' a person with metabolic syndrome to what is essentially a nondiabetic state with diet modification and exercise," Dr. Keilson says. "In true diabetes, though, the risk of heart disease is profound, and many physicians will go directly to pharmaceutical therapy to give their patients maximum protection."

Even with the known benefits of diet and exercise and the existence of a variety of medicines, however, many people with diabetes are still at increased risk. At least half of the people with diabetes in the United States have total cholesterol levels above 200 mg/dl, which is the upper limit of the desirable range.

This disturbing report comes from a January 2004 review of data in the National Health and Nutrition Examination Survey 1999–2000. The review found that 51.8% of the people with diabetes in the survey had total cholesterol levels above 200 mg/dl. This was improved from a similar survey conducted between 1988 and 1994, but it means that millions are still above current cholesterol-lowering treatment goals.

Treating dyslipidemia

The primary focus of dyslipidemia treatment in all people, with diabetes or not, is LDL cholesterol. Overwhelming evidence from clinical trials, experimental animals, laboratory research, and epidemiology points to LDL cholesterol as the form of cholesterol most likely to cause atherosclerosis.

There are two ways to lower LDL levels: lifestyle changes and drug therapy. The American Diabetes Association (ADA) recommends starting diet and exercise changes if one's LDL level is over 100 mg/dl and adding drug therapy if it exceeds 130 mg/dl. For people with diabetes who already have cardiovascular disease, however, drug therapy should be started along with lifestyle changes if their LDL levels are above 100 mg/dl.

Current guidelines notwithstanding, recent studies have shown that intensive treatment of LDL, lowering levels to the 60's and 70's, may dramatically decrease cardiovascular events. The largest of them, the Treating to New Targets (TNT) study, reported a 22% reduction in events with aggressively lowered LDL levels.

Therapy still begins with diet and exercise, however. Observational studies have concluded that people who adopt healthier diets and get more exercise have fewer heart attacks and other such cardiac events. Both diet modification and exercise have been shown to improve the dyslipidemia of diabetes, so by extension they are considered the best first-line treatment.

The ADA calls diet modification "medical nutrition therapy," or MNT, and the American Heart Association includes it with exercise in what it calls "therapeutic lifestyle changes," or TLC. Both recommendations call for reducing saturated fat in the diet and replacing it with an increased intake of carbohydrate or monounsaturated fat. Intensively following such a diet has been shown to result in a 15–25 mg/dl reduction in LDL levels.

"Diet and exercise can be expected to reduce

LDL levels by no more than about 10%," Dr. Keilson says. "Appropriate drug therapy, on the other hand, can bring about a 30% to 50% decrease. Exercise and diet are still important, for a variety of reasons, but the risk of heart disease is so high in people with diabetes that most should probably have drug therapy as well."

Drugs for lowering LDL cholesterol

The first drug of choice to lower LDL cholesterol levels is usually an HMG CoA reductase inhibitor, or "statin." These drugs, including pravastatin (brand name Pravachol), simvastatin (Zocor), lovastatin (Mevacor), fluvastatin (Lescol), rosuvastatin (Crestor), and atorvastatin (Lipitor), are well tolerated with few short-term or long-term side effects. The Heart Protection Study used simvastatin and reduced cardiovascular events by 25% in people with diabetes. (The authors of the study note that the 25% reduction was observed in people who didn't always take their statin properly; taking simvastatin as prescribed 100% of the time, they predict, could reduce cardiac events by 33%.) Trials of the other statins have had similarly convincing results, with mean reductions in cholesterol of 20%, average reductions in the incidence of coronary artery disease of 30%, and average reductions in mortality of 29%. Statins also have the bonus effect of lowering triglycerides as much as 35% and raising HDL levels 10%. The newest statin, rosuvastatin, appears to be the most powerful of all, with significantly greater effect on all the lipids than other members of the family.

Safety concerns about statins have been largely laid to rest. After rare reports of muscle weakness and aches in people taking statins, a national review in 2006 found little reason for concern so long as regular blood tests are used to catch problems early in those few people who would develop them.

"Given a one-in-five chance of heart disease in diabetes," Dr. Keilson says, "the one-in-10,000 chance of serious side effects from the statins shouldn't keep anyone from reaping the benefits of the therapy."

A five-year study funded by the National Institutes of Health comparing the side effects of simvastatin and pravastatin against placebo is due to be completed this year. The $5 million study is investigating issues such as muscle pains and anecdotal reports of cognitive dysfunction in people taking statins.

Alternative LDL-lowering drugs include the bile acid sequestrants, such as cholestyramine (Questran, Questran Light) and colestipol (Colestid). These drugs lower LDL cholesterol and have few serious side effects, though they have been associated with bothersome gastrointestinal side effects. Some may also find cholestyramine and some forms of colestipol unpalatable because they are powders or granules that must be mixed with water. (A tablet form of colestipol is available.) A newer drug in this class, colesevelam (WelChol), comes in tablet form and may be better tolerated and as effective as its predecessors.

The bile acid sequestrants can raise triglyceride levels, so in a person with high triglycerides, nicotinic acid, or niacin, is sometimes used instead because it has been shown to decrease levels of LDL cholesterol and triglycerides and to raise levels of HDL cholesterol. The Coronary Drug Project examined the benefits of niacin in people who had had heart attacks and found an 11% lower mortality after 15 years. The side effects of therapeutic niacin treatment include flushing, gastrointestinal upset, and liver damage. Flushing can be reduced by using extended-release (Niaspan) or sustained-release formulations of niacin, but risks of liver damage increase with use of sustained-release (but not extended-release) niacin.

Niacin can also cause high blood glucose levels in some people, so there has been concern about using it in people with diabetes. However, a study published in 2000 concluded that niacin could be safely used in people with diabetes, increasing HDL levels by 29% while lowering LDL levels by 8% and triglycerides by 23%. Current guidelines for people with diabetes allow for its use with mindfulness of the potential side effects.

Ezetimibe (Zetia) is the first in a new class of drugs called cholesterol absorption inhibitors. In clinical trials, it significantly lowered LDL levels and moderately lowered triglyceride levels and raised HDL levels. Ezetimibe is much better tolerated than the bile acid sequestrants and may ultimately replace them in routine therapy.

Lowering triglycerides

Once LDL levels are brought under control, the next step is to address elevated triglyceride levels. The drugs of choice for this therapy are the fibrates: gemfibrozil (Lopid), clofibrate, and fenofibrate (Lofibra, Tricor). In addition to lowering triglycerides, they also moderately lower LDL cholesterol and can change the size of LDL particles from the small, dense type that is more likely to cause atherosclerosis to a larger type. The most common side effects of the fibrates are primarily gastrointestinal symptoms.

The Helsinki Heart Study of gemfibrozil demonstrated a 10% drop in total cholesterol, an 11% drop in LDL, a 35% drop in triglycerides, and an 11% increase in HDL. The Diabetes Atherosclerosis Intervention Study (DAIS) used fenofibrate therapy and measured the progress of atherosclerosis using angiography, documenting a 40% reduction in the progress of the disease.

Other triglyceride-lowering agents include fish oils that have high levels of omega-3 fatty acids. In addition to lowering triglycerides, omega-3 fatty acids also help reduce blood clotting and improve other facets of heart function. Flaxseed oil is also rich in omega-3 fatty acids and has the advantage of not having a fishy taste.

The role of diabetes drugs

There are a number of drugs that are often prescribed for people with diabetes for other purposes but which have some positive effect on lipids as well. Since people with diabetes may be taking these medicines anyway, Dr. Keilson feels they can be an important part of the management of dyslipidemia.

The thiazolidinediones (TZDs), rosiglitazone (Avandia) and pioglitazone (Actos), are used primarily to reduce the insulin resistance common in Type 2 diabetes. In people taking a TZD, the size of LDL particles increases, and HDL levels rise. Pioglitazone also lowers triglyceride levels, but rosiglitazone raises LDL levels.

The primary side effects of the TZDs are weight gain and fluid retention. The American Heart Association and the ADA have long recommended caution in using them in people with congestive heart failure or risk factors for it and additionally recommended that they not be used in people with advanced congestive heart failure. There are new concerns about the TZDs, which have been linked to as much as a 43% increased risk for heart attack and a 64% increased risk for cardiovascular death. There is still controversy about the findings, but the FDA has ordered a "black box" warning on the labels.

At higher doses, metformin (Glucophage, Glucophage XR) is able to reduce total cholesterol levels. Metformin is also linked to some weight loss, which can have a beneficial effect on lipids.

Acarbose (Precose) is used primarily to slow the absorption of complex starches in the intestine, helping to reduce high blood glucose levels after a meal. It also appears to lower LDL levels and raise HDL levels in the process. The evidence for lipid benefits from miglitol (Glyset), which is in the same drug class as acarbose, is inconclusive.

METABOLIC SYNDROME AND LIPID GOALS

The metabolic syndrome is a collection of risk factors that increases a person's chances of developing diabetes, heart disease, or stroke. People are diagnosed with metabolic syndrome when they have three or more of the risk factors at the levels listed in the table. Also included in the table are the corresponding lipid goal thresholds that the American Diabetes Association currently advises people with diabetes to aim for.

RISK FACTOR	DEFINING LEVEL FOR METABOLIC SYNDROME	GOAL FOR PEOPLE WITH DIABETES
Abdominal obesity (Waist circumference)		
Men	Greater than 40 inches	—
Women	Greater than 35 inches	—
LDL cholesterol	—	Less than 100 mg/dl
Triglycerides	150 mg/dl or higher	Less than 150 mg/dl
HDL cholesterol		
Men	Less than 40 mg/dl	Greater than 40 mg/dl
Women	Less than 50 mg/dl	Greater than 50 mg/dl
Blood pressure	130/85 mm Hg or higher	Below 130/80 mm Hg
Fasting glucose	Greater than 100 mg/dl* (and less than 126 mg/dl)	—

The defining levels of metabolic syndrome were taken from the Third Report of the Expert Panel on Detection, Evaluation, and Treatment of High Blood Cholesterol in Adults (Adult Treatment Panel III).

* The 2002 ATP III report originally listed a fasting plasma glucose level greater than 110 mg/dl as being diagnostic of metabolic syndrome, but in 2004, the American Diabetes Association lowered the definition threshold for impaired fasting glucose to 100 mg/dl.

The anti-obesity drugs orlistat (Xenical) and sibutramine (Meridia) are primarily used for weight loss but may have positive effects on blood lipids as well. Orlistat blocks the enzymes that break down fat in food, preventing as much as 30% of the fat from being absorbed. Treatment with orlistat has produced statistically significant lowering of total cholesterol, LDL cholesterol, and triglycerides in a clinical trial.

Sibutramine works through the central nervous system to suppress appetite. The Sibutramine Trial of Obesity Reduction and Maintenance (STORM) found that in addition to its weight-loss benefits, sibutramine lowered levels of triglycerides and increased levels of HDL cholesterol.

Combination therapy

The complex dyslipidemia of diabetes often calls for a combination of drugs to achieve target levels of cholesterol. Most common are combinations of statins, which are effective for lowering LDL levels, with other drugs that address high triglycerides and low HDL levels.

"If you have a person with a low LDL level but who has high triglycerides and a low HDL level," Dr. Keilson says, "you need to treat him differently than a person with high LDL levels. You can attempt to control his problem with more intensive blood sugar control, which will lower triglycerides, and with dietary modifications that reduce carbohydrates. After that, the next step would be to add a fibrate, fish oil or flaxseed oil, or niacin. The addition of ezetimibe to statin therapy may be especially helpful in raising HDL levels."

In one study that added ezetimibe to statin therapy, for instance, LDL levels were reduced, HDL levels were increased, and triglyceride levels were lowered compared to statin plus placebo therapy.

Combination therapy also can have an additive effect on lowering LDL levels. The addition of the bile acid sequestrant colesevelam to statin therapy has been shown to result in an 8% to 12% greater reduction in LDL levels than statin therapy alone.

Niacin is also used with statin therapy, because the two drugs have complementary effects. A combination drug that contained both extended-release niacin and lovastatin (Advicor) was put to the test against atorvastatin and simvastatin in the Advicor Versus Other Cholesterol-modulating Agents Trial Evaluation (ADVOCATE). The combination drug lowered LDL levels, increased HDL levels, and decreased triglyceride levels better than atorvastatin or simvastatin alone.

Niacin plus statin combination therapy was also explored in the HDL-Atherosclerosis Treatment Study (HATS). Subjects who had already had coronary artery disease were given either placebo or niacin and simvastatin, with or without antioxidant vitamins. The group on niacin and simvastatin that did not receive antioxidants achieved a 42% reduction in LDL levels, a 36% decrease in triglycerides, a 26% increase in HDL levels, and a 90% reduction in coronary events. (The group taking antioxidants with niacin and simvastatin had slightly lesser improvements in cholesterol, but more important, the reduction in cardiovascular events disappeared.) LDL levels in the placebo groups were unchanged.

The goal of lipid therapy in diabetes is to return the levels of all lipids to as close to normal as possible. It is achievable in nearly every person, and the arsenal of drugs that can add to the benefits of diet and exercise is growing steadily. ☐

LIFESTYLE HABITS FOR A HEALTHY HEART

by Heidi Mochari, M.P.H., R.D.

It is no secret that abnormal levels of fats and cholesterol in the blood are associated with an increased risk of coronary heart disease. These fats and cholesterol are called blood lipids, and the good news is that there is a lot of information about how to manage them. In fact, dramatic improvements in lipid levels can be achieved through simple lifestyle changes.

The National Institutes of Health National Cholesterol Education Program (NCEP) has come up with some therapeutic lifestyle changes for reducing the risk of coronary heart disease. These modifications are designed primarily to reduce low-density lipoprotein (LDL, or "bad") cholesterol to a desirable level and to manage factors associated with the *metabolic syndrome*. This is a cluster of risk factors associated with cardiovascular disease and diabetes and includes the following: abdominal obesity, high blood pressure, abnormally low high-density lipoprotein (HDL, or "good") cholesterol, a high level of triglycerides (the chemical form in which most fat exists in the body), and high blood glucose. National guidelines have established an LDL cholesterol of less than 100 milligrams per deciliter (mg/dl) as ideal and have recently given physicians the option to lower LDL cholesterol to less than 70 mg/dl in people considered to be at very high risk (such as those with established coronary heart disease and/or diabetes). A fasting triglyceride level of less than 150 mg/dl is considered normal for both men and women. An HDL cholesterol value of at least 40 mg/dl is recommended for men and a value of at least 50 mg/dl is recommended for women.

LDL-lowering strategies

The first change recommended by the NCEP is to reduce your intake of saturated fat and cholesterol. Saturated fat should be less than 7% of your total calories per day and dietary cholesterol should be less than 200 mg per day.

Saturated fats are found mostly in foods that come from animals: meat, poultry fat, lard, butter, cheese, and other dairy products. They are also found in foods from tropical plants such as coconut oil, palm oil, and cocoa butter. Saturated fats are solid at room temperature. If you can see solid fat in your food—such as the fatty strips in bacon or the fat found under chicken skin—chances are that there is a significant amount of saturated fat present.

Saturated fat grams can add up quickly. For example, a grilled cheese sandwich made with two pieces of bread, two slices of American cheese, and one pat of butter contains 11 grams of saturated fat. If additional butter is used to cook the sandwich, or if it is served with French fries, the meal has even more saturated fat. So what many might consider a simple lunch contains more than the daily upper limits for saturated fat intake. If you do not know your recommended calorie intake, ask your physician for a referral to a registered dietitian. A registered dietitian can calculate your calorie goals and give you personalized recommendations for how to achieve your saturated fat intake goal and other diet modification goals using foods that you like and enjoy.

Dietary cholesterol can also add up quickly. Cholesterol is only found in foods that come from animals, such as meat, poultry, egg yolks, butter, and cheese, and is usually found in the same places as saturated fat. When you reduce your intake of saturated fat to your target goal, you will probably meet your dietary cholesterol goals as well. Many people wonder if they should avoid foods such as eggs and shellfish altogether because one serving of them may exceed daily recommendations. Although these foods are higher in cholesterol than others, they are lower in saturated fat than other sources of animal protein. Consequently, they can become part of a sensible meal plan if consumed in small portions. For example, by choosing one small or medium egg, with 157 mg and 187 mg of cholesterol respectively, you can stay within daily upper intake limits, but remember to balance the dietary cholesterol in that egg with the other foods that you eat. For example, don't use butter to cook the egg (use a nonstick spray, or have it boiled or poached) and have vegetarian meals for lunch and dinner. Alternatively, you could have just the egg whites for protein and avoid any cholesterol whatsoever.

Trans fats are another issue to pay attention to. *Trans* fats are generally produced by hydrogenation of vegetable oils, though some are found naturally in animal fats. Hydrogenation increases the shelf life and flavor stability of many processed foods—for instance, shortening, some margarines, and fried foods. Other major sources of *trans* fats include foods made with partially hydrogenated oils such as certain crackers, cookies, doughnuts, and fast foods. The problem with *trans* fats is that they can raise LDL cholesterol and lower HDL cholesterol levels. As of January 1, 2006, the Food and Drug Administration requires that the amount of *trans* fat in a serving be listed on a separate line under saturated fat on the Nutrition Facts panel. You should check this information and try to keep your *trans* fat intake as low as possible. If you can't find *trans* fat on the Nutrition Facts label, it's probably because you're looking at an older label.

Reducing the saturated fat, *trans* fats, and choles-

SATURATED FAT GOALS

One way to lower your LDL ("bad") cholesterol level is to make sure your intake of saturated fat accounts for less than 7% of your total calorie intake.

Calorie level	Grams of saturated fat equal to less than 7% of total calories
1,200	9
1,400	10
1,600	12
1,800	13
2,000	15
2,200	17
2,400	18

terol in your diet does not mean that you should follow an extremely low-fat diet. On the contrary, for persons with the metabolic syndrome, lipid disorders, and/or diabetes, total fat should make up 30% to 35% of total calories. Saturated fat and *trans* fats should be replaced with monounsaturated fats (up to 20% of calories) and polyunsaturated fats (up to 10% of total calories). Evidence suggests that replacing saturated fat with unsaturated fat is more effective in lowering the risk of coronary heart disease than reducing total fat consumption.

The two types of unsaturated fats in the diet—monounsaturated and polyunsaturated—are found in a variety of foods. Monounsaturated fats are found in avocados, almonds, olives, peanuts, and olive, peanut, and canola oils. Polyunsaturated fats can be divided into two groups: omega-6 polyunsaturated fats, which are found mainly in seeds and vegetable oils such as corn and soy oils, and omega-3 polyunsaturated fats, which are found in fish, flaxseed, and walnuts. Consuming omega-3 fatty acids from fish and plant sources may lower your risk of coronary heart disease.

Substituting saturated fat for monounsaturated or polyunsaturated fats can be as simple as putting avocado on your sandwich instead of cheese, having nuts for a snack instead of chips or baked goods, or using salad dressing made with olive oil or canola oil instead of using a creamy salad dressing.

Going even lower

If reducing your intake of saturated fat, cholesterol, and *trans* fats does not get you to your LDL goal, you might try two additional strategies.

First, try adding plant stanols or sterols to your diet. These are derived from natural plant components such as soy. They reduce the absorption of cholesterol in the digestive tract, resulting in lower total and LDL cholesterol levels. They can be found in some soft margarine products and also in supplement form. If you choose to use one of the margarine products, be sure to adjust your calorie level to account for the calories contained in the product. Plant stanol or sterol intakes of 2–3 grams per day have been found to lower LDL cholesterol by 6% to 15%.

A second strategy is to try adding more soluble fiber to your diet. See "Sources of Soluble Fiber" on page 436 for a list of foods that contain soluble fiber. A total fiber intake of 20–30 grams per day is part of the diet recommended by the NCEP. By increasing their soluble fiber intake by only 5 to 10 grams per day, most people can reduce their LDL cholesterol by about 5%.

Weight management and physical activity are also fundamental components of the NCEP-recommended changes. If you are at a healthy weight, work with your physician to prevent weight gain. Develop strategies for weight maintenance and anticipate high-risk occasions for possible weight gain (for example times of significant stress). If you are overweight, start with a weight-loss goal of 10% through dietary change, portion control, and daily physical activity. You should also consider regular visits with your physician to follow up and examine your progress. Any increase in physical activity should be based on your cardiac status, your age, and your physician's assessment of your limitations and goals. Once you get the OK to exercise, try 30 minutes of moderate-intensity activity on most, if not all, days of the week—even if you are not overweight.

Triglycerides

Triglycerides in the blood come from the foods we eat. Calories that are not immediately used by the body are converted into triglycerides and transported to the fat cells to be stored. Like LDL cholesterol, excess triglycerides in the blood are linked to increased risk for coronary artery disease.

If triglycerides remain elevated once LDL cholesterol is reduced to your goal, losing weight and engaging in regular physical activity should become your primary focus. Overweight and lack of physical activity are strong contributors to high triglyceride levels, so working with your health-care provider to start a program of weight loss and daily exercise could lead to an improved triglyceride level.

In addition to reducing your calorie intake and exercising, there are some other changes that can reduce triglyceride levels. First, reduce your intake of refined or processed carbohydrates, such as candy, table sugar, white flour, and baked goods made with white flour. These foods can promote an increase in triglyceride levels. Excessive intake of these foods may also increase blood glucose levels, and it is very common to see high blood triglycerides when diabetes is not well controlled.

Eat foods rich in monounsaturated and polyunsaturated fats instead of those that contain refined sugar. Substituting fish rich in omega-3 fatty acids (found in fatty fish such as salmon, sardines, and tuna) may also lower triglycerides. Omega-3 fish oil capsules may be therapeutic in some cases, but over-the-counter fish oil supplements have been found to contain varying amounts of fish oil, so only prescription supplements are recommended at this time. Discuss the risks and benefits of taking fish oil with your physician. High doses can cause excessive bleeding in some people.

Even small amounts of alcohol can increase triglycerides. So if triglycerides are a problem for you, it would be a good idea to cut down as much as possible.

HDL cholesterol

HDL cholesterol is called "good" cholesterol because higher levels protect against coronary heart disease by carrying cholesterol away from the arteries and back to the liver where it is disposed of. A low level of HDL cholesterol is associated with an increased risk for coronary heart disease.

When triglyceride levels are elevated, HDL cholesterol levels begin to fall. So when you make changes to improve your triglycerides, this may also lead to improved HDL cholesterol levels. However, low HDL cholesterol may also be present in the absence of high triglycerides. This is called *isolated low HDL cholesterol* and is attributed to many of the same factors that may promote high triglycerides, including overweight and obesity, physical inactivity, cigarette smoking, very high carbohydrate intake (more than 60% of calories), Type 2 diabetes, and genetic factors.

All the lifestyle changes covered in this article are essential components in HDL cholesterol management. In particular, losing weight or maintaining a healthy weight, being physically active on most, if not all, days of the week, and not smoking can improve your HDL cholesterol. Additionally, maintaining a low intake of saturated fat and *trans* fat, avoiding processed carbohydrates, and consuming an adequate amount of monounsaturated

SOURCES OF SOLUBLE FIBER

A total fiber intake of 20–30 grams per day is recommended as part of the TLC diet. Increasing soluble fiber intake by 5 to 10 grams a day has been found to reduce LDL cholesterol by 5% on average. The foods listed here are good sources of soluble fiber.

FOOD	SERVING SIZE	SOLUBLE FIBER (grams)	TOTAL FIBER (grams)
Apples	1	1	4
Barley	½ cup cooked	1	4
Beans	½ cup cooked	1.5–3.5	5.5–7
Broccoli	½ cup cooked	1	1.5
Brussels sprouts	½ cup cooked	3	4.5
Chickpeas	½ cup cooked	1	6
Lentils	½ cup cooked	1	8
Oat bran	½ cup cooked	1	3
Oatmeal	½ cup cooked	1	2
Pears	1	2	4
Psyllium supplement	1 teaspoon	2	3

Adapted from Third Report of the National Cholesterol Education Program (NCEP) Expert Panel on Detection, Evaluation, and Treatment of High Cholesterol in Adults (Adult Treatment Panel III).

and polyunsaturated fats are all associated with promoting a healthy level of HDL cholesterol.

Special considerations for diabetes

The combination of high triglycerides and low HDL cholesterol is common among people with diabetes (especially Type 2 diabetes) and is often referred to as *diabetic dyslipidemia* or *atherogenic dyslipidemia*. Abnormalities in blood lipids, high blood pressure, high blood glucose, insulin resistance, and other factors also contribute to the increased risk for coronary heart disease among people with diabetes.

Just having diabetes is considered a coronary heart disease "risk equivalent." This means that the lipid management goals for people with diabetes are the same as for people who have established coronary heart disease. A change in lifestyle is always the first thing to do to lower lipid levels, but physicians may also use lipid-lowering drugs to further reduce the risk—even if lipid goals are met through lifestyle changes alone. To keep track of your lipid levels, annual cholesterol testing is recommended, with follow-up and management by your physician. And because nutrition issues can be complex, it is also recommended that people

with diabetes meet with a registered dietitian to assess their calorie needs and to discuss personal diet strategies for meeting their dietary goals.

The payoff

Improvement in lipid levels is not always easy to accomplish and may take time, but significant change *is* possible. An estimated LDL cholesterol reduction of 8% to 10% can be achieved by cutting your intake of saturated fat to less than 7% of calories. An additional reduction of 3% to 5% can be achieved by cutting your cholesterol intake to less than 200 mg per day. A 10-pound weight loss could mean as much as a 5% to 8% decrease in LDL cholesterol. The addition of plant sterol and stanol esters to the diet could reduce LDL cholesterol even further, by up to 15%. And adding soluble fiber can reduce it up to 5% more. This adds up to a possible 36% to 43% reduction in LDL cholesterol through lifestyle changes alone.

These lifestyle modifications may not only improve lipids—they may have a ripple effect. Blood glucose control and blood pressure may also improve. The best way to start is to talk with your physician. Review your lipid profile with him, set lifestyle change goals, and set a date to follow up and track your progress. ☐

THE BENEFITS OF TIGHT CONTROL

No End in Sight

by Wayne Clark

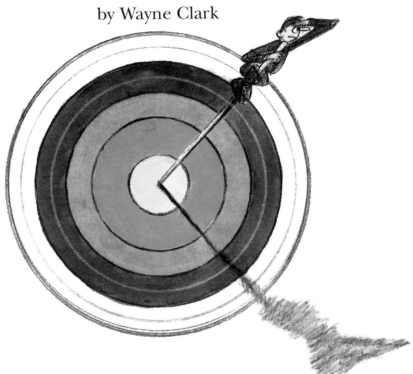

The results of the landmark Diabetes Control and Complications Trial (DCCT) were published in 1993. Despite its continuing legacy of proof that maintaining blood glucose levels as close to normal as possible reduces the risk of diabetes complications, today less than half of people with diabetes are reaching target blood glucose levels, according to most estimates. Health-care providers and researchers continue to struggle with how to improve those numbers.

Recalling the DCCT

Researchers began recruiting participants for the DCCT in 1983. They signed up 1,441 people with Type 1 diabetes, roughly half within five years of their diagnoses and the rest within 15 years of diagnosis. The subjects were randomly assigned to either conventional insulin treatment or intensive treatment. Those on intensive treatment took three or more insulin injections each day or used an insulin pump and monitored their blood glucose levels three or four times a day. The goal for the intensive treatment group was to keep their glycosolated hemoglobin, or HbA_{1c} levels (a meas-

ure of blood glucose control over two to three months) at or below the top of the normal range: 6.05%. In actuality they achieved a median HbA_{1c} of 7.2%. The study's subjects were followed for six and a half years, and the publication of the results in late 1993 changed the standards of Type 1 diabetes management forever.

The research team had hoped to be able to demonstrate a 30% to 40% reduction in complications among those on intensive treatment. What they actually saw was so significant that they ended the study early and advised the subjects on conventional treatment to switch to intensive treatment.

Those who were within five years of diagnosis and had been assigned to intensive treatment experienced a 76% reduction in the risk of diabetic retinopathy, or eye disease, a 34% reduction in the risk of microalbuminuria (an early stage of diabetic nephropathy, or kidney disease), and a 69% reduction in the risk of diabetic neuropathy, or nerve disease. Results for those within 15 years of diagnosis and on intensive treatment were less dramatic but still significant: a risk reduction of 54% for retinopathy, 43% for microalbuminuria, and 57% for neuropathy. In both groups there was a 41% reduction in the risk of cardiovascular disease.

The drawbacks for the intensive treatment group were a three-times higher incidence of severe hypoglycemia (very low blood glucose levels), and an average weight gain of 4.6 kilograms (about 10 pounds).

The study also answered the question of whether or not there is a point below which a lower HbA$_{1c}$ does not yield additional benefit. The answer was that there is no "glycemic threshold": The closer to normal the better.

The DCCT ended in 1993, but more than 1,370 of its subjects were then enrolled in a long-term follow-up study called Epidemiology of Diabetes Interventions and Complications (EDIC). The news from EDIC in the past few years has been almost too good to be true: The benefit of intensive blood glucose management continues even after treatment becomes less monitored and less rigorous.

A report from the EDIC group in 2002 found that the people from the intensive treatment arm of the DCCT still had a 62% reduction in the risk of retinopathy seven years after the end of the DCCT. Long-term results for nephropathy were published in 2003, covering eight years of follow-up, and members of the intensive treatment group still enjoyed a 59% reduction in the risk of microalbuminuria. More striking still, that group saw an 84% reduction in the risk of developing clinical albuminuria, a more advanced stage of kidney disease. The latest data for neuropathy were published in 2006, and showed that eight years after the DCCT ended, the participants who had been on intensive treatment experienced a 64% reduction in the risk of neuropathy.

The DCCT studied Type 1 diabetes, but the vast majority of cases of diabetes are Type 2. However, the value of intensive therapy was demonstrated for Type 2 diabetes by the United Kingdom Prospective Diabetes Study (UKPDS), published in 1998. The UKPDS covered a 20-year period and included more than 5,100 people with Type 2 diabetes in England, Northern Ireland, and Scotland.

The UKPDS showed that intensive treatment of Type 2 diabetes, using sulfonylurea drugs (oral medicines that increase the secretion of insulin by the pancreas) or insulin, reduced microvascular complications (primarily retinopathy and nephropathy) by 25%. Another group of people in the study who were overweight and received intensive treatment with metformin (an oral medicine that suppresses glucose production by the liver and enhances the body's sensitivity to insulin) saw a 32% decrease in diabetes complications.

Where are we now?

Despite the overwhelming evidence of the importance of "tight" blood glucose control in people with Type 1 and Type 2 diabetes, it is still far from the norm. In a study published in the January/February 2006 issue of *Annals of Family Medicine*, Dr. Stephen J. Spann and his colleagues reported on a review of charts of people with Type 2 diabetes from four large primary-care-based research networks. They found that only 40.5% of these people had HbA$_{1c}$ values below 7%. Moreover, 31.3% of HbA$_{1c}$ values were above 8%.

These findings echo those of the National Health and Nutrition Examination Survey (NHANES) from 1999–2000, in which only 37% of participants were found to have achieved the target goal of an HbA$_{1c}$ level less than 7%. Another 37.2% of the participants had an HbA$_{1c}$ above 8%. It is notable that these percentages did not change significantly from the earlier NHANES covering 1988–1994.

Not even a majority of people who get their diabetes care in specialized clinics at academic medical centers are reaching target HbA$_{1c}$ values. A 2002 review from 30 academic medical centers in the United States found that while nearly all patients with Type 1 or Type 2 diabetes had received an HbA$_{1c}$ test within the previous year, only 34% were at 7% or less.

"The reason we did our study," said Dr. Spann, who is Chairman of Family and Community Medicine at Baylor College of Medicine in Houston, Texas, "is that while we understand that improved glycemic control is better, we struggle with how to make it happen in primary care. We wondered what we could learn about elements that might predict good glycemic control.

"We didn't really find anything that was absolutely predictive of good control," he said. "We did learn that the level of complexity rises as you start adding the other important treatment targets, such as blood pressure and cholesterol. It's hard enough to hit one target, and even harder to achieve targets simultaneously for multiple risk factors."

Barriers to tight control

There are many reasons tight blood glucose control is not more widespread, despite its clear benefits. "Some people have access problems," Dr. Spann says, "such as insurance that doesn't cover extensive treatment. It also is difficult to get many people to a point where they're willing and able to make lifestyle changes to improve their control."

Since diabetes is a progressive condition, it can become increasingly difficult to achieve treatment targets. Several studies have noted that the percentage of people achieving targets diminishes with duration of diabetes.

What's more, the "system" of medical care may be a problem in itself, according to Dr. Spann and others. The way primary care is organized and reimbursed by insurance companies probably serves as a barrier to achieving optimal blood glucose control for many people. Dr. Spann points to the "Chronic Care Model" developed by Dr. Ed H. Wagner at Improving Chronic Illness Care (ICIC), a national program of the Robert Wood Johnson Foundation based in Seattle, as a way to change the system.

"I think that the proponents of the Chronic Care Model are right on," Dr. Spann says. "There have been a number of studies that have shown that practices that have most of the elements of the model in place do better in getting more of their patients to treatment targets." Those elements include electronic registries that track and report important patient information, multidisciplinary treatment teams, and care management. "The doctor can't do it all," Dr. Spann says. "We know that nurses and diabetes educators probably do better health education than we do."

One health system that has adopted the Chronic Care Model and applied it to diabetes is MaineHealth in Portland, Maine. In conjunction with its physician–hospital organization, the MMC PHO, MaineHealth has developed an Internet-based Clinical Improvement Registry for primary-care doctors. The doctors enter information about their patients, and the system provides current clinical data at each visit, including the latest laboratory results, status of key tests (for example, HbA$_{1c}$ and blood pressure), and problems to be addressed. The system can also be used to generate notices for patients and doctors, to remind them of overdue examinations or laboratory tests. Data may be viewed for each patient or for a doctor's overall practice.

The MMC PHO also employs 14 Chronic Illness Care Managers, who are embedded in primary-care practices as part of the patient care team (they manage not just diabetes, but asthma and heart failure). These nurse specialists provide patients with intensive education and motivational support, even paying home visits if that will help.

The most recent data from the program covers the experience of 15 primary-care practices over a period from the program's inception to the end of its first year. Before the program existed, 80% of people with diabetes had received an HbA$_{1c}$ test within the past year. After a year, 93% of people had received one. The percentage of people with HbA$_{1c}$ values less than 7% rose from 41% to 49%—a 20% increase. The percentage of people with HbA$_{1c}$ values above 8% decreased from 31% to 24%, and the percentage of people with HbA$_{1c}$ values above 9.5% decreased from 13% to 9%. There were similar results in measures of LDL (or "bad") cholesterol and blood pressure.

"This is not a question of bad doctors or bad patients," says Larry Anderson, M.D., Senior Director for Quality Improvement and Medical Affairs at the MMC PHO. "It is a question of a care model that is focused on illness instead of prevention, and systems that have been created that don't accommodate a change in focus. We're changing the focus, including offering financial incentives for physicians whose patients do better."

What does it mean to you?

The HbA$_{1c}$ test is considered the gold standard for the evaluation of blood glucose control. While the test has been in use for nearly 30 years, widely accepted target levels are a relatively recent development.

Before the DCCT, the American Diabetes Association's (ADA) Standards of Medical Care (which is considered the primary source of recommendations for effective treatment), did not recommend a target HbA$_{1c}$ level. In response to the DCCT, the ADA in 1995 set a target of less than 7%, and set 8% as the "action" limit, above which additional intervention should be undertaken. The action limit was removed in the 2003 recommendations, effectively indicating that any level above 7% was cause for action.

The trend toward recommending lower blood glucose levels continued in 2004, when the ADA stated that "more stringent" targets could be considered for individuals. This year, that position was clarified further to indicate that while the HbA$_{1c}$ goal for people in general is less than 7%, the goal for an individual should be as close to normal (less than 6%) as possible without significant hypoglycemia.

"There's no doubt, lower is better," Dr. Spann says. "Is a 6% HbA$_{1c}$ achievable for every patient? Probably not. There are tradeoffs, such as the risk of hypoglycemia when striving for very tight control. The new ADA guidelines recognize that targets should be tailored to individuals."

The ADA recommends that people meeting their treatment goals have an HbA$_{1c}$ test at least twice a year, and that those whose therapy has changed or who are not meeting their goals be tested four times a year.

It's important not just to have the test, but to understand and be familiar with the results. A pair of recent studies found that only about a quarter of people with diabetes knew their most recent HbA$_{1c}$ value.

There is a growing recognition that the approach to diabetes management needs an over-haul to reflect the condition's many challenges. An international task force called the Global Partner-ship for Effective Diabetes Management recently published a series of recommendations for Type 2 diabetes that includes aggressive interventions for any HbA$_{1c}$ level that stays above 6.5% for a six-month period. Combinations of oral diabetes drugs and the addition of insulin should be prescribed sooner, according to the group. Moreover, the group recommends pursuing cholesterol and blood pressure targets with equal aggressiveness, and implementing a multidisciplinary team approach to help people take control of their diabetes.

Meanwhile, the good news about tight blood glucose control keeps coming in. A DCCT/EDIC study published in December 2005 demonstrated that the risk of cardiovascular events was reduced by 42% in people who had been in the intensive treatment arm of the DCCT—even a dozen years after the study ended. The findings extended ear-lier observations that the intensive control group had slower progression of carotid intima–media thickness and coronary artery calcification, both signs of developing atherosclerosis (hardening of the arteries).

We will know in 2010 if the beneficial cardiovas-cular effect of intensive control extends to Type 2 diabetes. The Action to Control Cardiovascular Risk in Diabetes (ACCORD) trial is following 10,000 people with Type 2 diabetes across the United States and Canada for eight years, to deter-mine the impact of intensive control (and also of cholesterol and blood pressure treatment) on the development of cardiovascular disease.

"The bottom line is that this is very difficult," Dr. Spann says. "As our study and others have shown, even with good practices with good physi-cians, and even with motivated patients, it's so hard that only 40% of people hit the targets. But there's really solid evidence that hitting those tar-gets prevents blindness, amputations, and kidney disease. That's a significant payoff— and a reason to keep trying." □

AVOIDING EYE COMPLICATIONS

by A. Paul Chous, M.A., O.D.

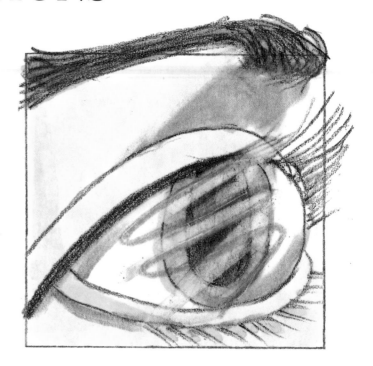

When it comes to diabetes-related eye complications, the good news is that most cases of severe vision loss due to diabetes are preventable. The bad news is that tens of thousands of people still lose vision to diabetes each year, despite all that is known about prevention and treatment.

Diabetes is the leading cause of new blindness for American adults between the ages of 20 and 74. The American Diabetes Association (ADA) estimates that 12,000–24,000 people in the United States lose their vision to diabetic retinopathy each year, and studies have shown that people with dia-betes have a fivefold to twenty-fivefold increased risk of blindness in their lifetimes.

However, these numbers very likely underesti-mate the true incidence of vision loss and blind-ness, because diabetes can cause a variety of eye diseases other than retinopathy, several of which can cause severe visual impairment (see "Eye Diseases Associated With Diabetes" on this page). Moreover, these statistics ignore vision loss less severe than "legal blindness" (defined as vision on the eye chart worse than 20/200 with the use of prescription lenses or severe loss of peripheral vision to within 20 degrees of central vision). But even less severe vision loss can and does substantially affect quality of life for thousands of people with diabetes.

Prevention strategies

Why do so many people continue to lose their sight to diabetes when so much is known about preventing and treating these complications? This question has dogged eye doctors, diabetes specialists, and public health experts for years, and the consensus answer boils down to four critical and interrelated elements: the epidemic of new diabetes cases, lack of patient education, lack of patient motivation and support, and lack of access to excellent diabetes care.

I do not pretend that these issues are easily solved, but I believe the tools are at hand to greatly reduce all the dreaded complications of diabetes—including blindness—as well as the human suffering they entail. I believe that a collaborative effort among people who have diabetes, health-care providers, and policy makers is the surest and fastest route to that end.

With that goal in mind, here is some of what I have learned in my 36 years of living with diabetes and my 15 years as a doctor of optometry specializing in diabetes care and education. Most of these strategies, in addition to minimizing the risk of eye complications, will go a long way toward preventing all diabetes complications. This is not all that surprising since eye problems caused by diabetes often go hand in hand with nerve, kidney, and cardiovascular disease.

Blood glucose control

Keep your blood glucose levels as close to the normal range as possible. High blood glucose levels are directly or indirectly responsible for all forms of diabetic eye disease. The landmark Diabetes Complications and Control Trial, published in 1993, showed that in people with Type 1 diabetes, each 10% reduction in average blood glucose levels, as reflected by a person's glycosylated hemoglobin (HbA_{1c}) level, lowers the risk of developing diabetic retinopathy by roughly 60% and lowers the risk of preexisting diabetic retinopathy getting worse by 43%.

This means, for example, that if your HbA_{1c}

EYE DISEASES ASSOCIATED WITH DIABETES

Having diabetes raises the risk of developing a number of eye problems, including the following:

DIABETIC RETINOPATHY. Damage to the smallest blood vessels serving the light-sensitive retina of the eye. Retinopathy results in bleeding, leakage of serum and other blood components, a decreased oxygen supply, and the possible development of new but abnormal blood vessels that bleed profusely and cause fibrovascular scar tissue that detaches the retina, causing severe loss of vision.

CATARACT. A clouding of the eye's internal lens that results in loss of vision.

GLAUCOMA. Damage to the optic nerve associated with increased internal eye pressure, leading to permanent loss of vision. It typically causes few or no symptoms until late in the disease.

ANTERIOR ISCHEMIC OPTIC NEUROPATHY. A sudden loss of blood supply to the optic nerve, resulting in severe vision loss. It can be thought of as a stroke of the optic nerve.

KERATOPATHY. Chronic damage to the cornea (the clear "windshield" at the front of the eye), causing irritation, redness, dry eye, reflex watering of the eyes, and sometimes impaired vision.

EYE MUSCLE PALSY. A loss of blood supply to the nerves responsible for controlling the coordinated movements of both eyes, resulting in double vision.

RETINAL VASCULAR OCCLUSION. A sudden blockage of the arteries or veins serving the retina, sometimes resulting in severe vision loss.

level is typically 7.0% (equivalent to an average blood glucose level of 172 mg/dl) and you bring your HbA_{1c} down to 6.3% (equivalent to an average blood glucose level of 147 mg/dl), you have dramatically reduced your chances of developing retinopathy. If you already have some degree of retinopathy and you lower your HbA_{1c} level by this amount, you have substantially lowered the chances of your retinopathy getting worse. These risk-reduction statistics hold true until HbA_{1c} levels are below 5.0% (which is equivalent to an average blood glucose level of 101 mg/dl), at which point the risks of retinopathy development and progression are minimal.

The landmark United Kingdom Prospective Diabetes Study showed similar results for people with Type 2 diabetes. If you can keep your HbA_{1c} results around or under 6.0%, you will greatly lower the odds of having serious eye complications from diabetes.

Why and how does high blood glucose damage the eyes? The "stock" answer given by medical professionals is that high blood glucose levels damage the smallest, most fragile blood vessels throughout the body, and the eyes have lots of small blood vessels. While this explanation is not incorrect, it is somewhat simplistic. The fuller answer is quite a bit more complex. Essentially, high blood glucose has two harmful effects in the eyes:

■ It impairs the ability of small blood vessels to precisely control the volume of blood traveling through them. The result is excessive blood flow that mechanically injures those vessels, making them leaky. To visualize this, imagine a garden hose trying to accommodate the water flow from a fully opened fire hydrant.

■ The breakdown (metabolism) of excess glucose by the body leads to an increase in the formation of harmful biochemicals (called *glucose metabolites*). These biochemicals make blood vessels in the retina leaky, promote the formation of abnormal, new blood vessels, and bind ("stick") to the proteins that make up body tissues (including parts of the eyes), causing those proteins to function abnormally. Some of the harmful by-products of glucose metabolism include *advanced glycosylation endproducts* and *protein kinase C.*

Of course, the clear benefits of "tight" blood glucose control have to be balanced against the risks of severe hypoglycemia (low blood glucose). Tight control is best achieved with close consultation with members of your diabetes care team, careful attention to diet (especially portion control), regular exercise, medicine if necessary, and blood glucose monitoring on a regular basis.

Living with diabetes is admittedly often like walking a tightrope between high and low blood glucose levels. There is great variability in each person's response to specific foods, activities, and treatments. The point is that the better you can learn to recognize and react to your unique blood glucose patterns, the closer to normal you can keep your blood glucose levels, and the healthier your eyes will be.

Blood pressure control

Keep your blood pressure well controlled through diet, regular physical activity, and medicine, if needed. The United Kingdom Prospective Diabetes Study showed that for Type 2 diabetes, controlling high blood pressure lowers the risk of retinopathy and worsening of existing retinopathy even more than tight blood glucose control. A 10/5 mm Hg reduction in blood pressure (for example, from 150/90 mm Hg to 140/85 mm Hg) reduced the risk of severe vision loss by nearly 50%. (In addition, this same blood pressure reduction lowered stroke risk by 44% and death by 32%!)

Elevated blood pressure in-creases blood flow into the eye, accelerating diabetic retinopathy. It also increases the turbulence of blood flow to the retina and optic nerve, which increases the risk of abnormal blood clotting (as happens in *ischemic optic neuropathy* and *retinal vascular occlusion*).

Recent research on the dynamics of blood flow to the eyes (called *ocular hemodynamics*) has given new insight into the importance of blood pressure control. The results of this work can help eye doctors gauge the risk of severe vision loss from diabetic retinopathy for individual patients. Research has demonstrated (using a technique called *laser Doppler velocimetry*) that at the onset of retinopathy, the volume of blood flow into the retina increases dramatically. As mentioned earlier, this is believed to be caused by high blood glucose, which impairs the ability of retinal vessels to constrict and precisely regulate blood flow. The pressure generated by this blood flow, known as *retinal perfusion pressure* (RPP), injures the walls of the smallest blood vessels (making them leaky) and redirects blood away from the smallest vessels (capillaries) into larger vessels. This results in destruction of the capillaries and inadequate blood circulation within retinal tissues (a phenomenon known as *capillary nonperfusion*). This destruction, in turn, leads to the release of biochemical messengers that promote the growth of new but abnormal blood vessels that bleed profusely and can lead to retinal detachment (as happens in *proliferative diabetic retinopathy*).

Retinal perfusion pressure (RPP) is highly dependent on the average pressure inside the blood vessels (known as the *mean arterial pressure,* or MAP) and somewhat dependent on the internal eye pressure (*intraocular pressure,* or IOP). Together, these pressures predict the risk of vision loss from diabetes. Both MAP and RPP can be calculated quite simply by knowing your blood pressure and your internal eye pressure, the latter of which is routinely measured at the eye doctor's office. The formula is as follows:

$$RPP = \frac{2}{3} \times MAP - IOP$$

where MAP = Mean Arterial Pressure = (systolic blood pressure – diastolic blood pressure) ÷ 3 + diastolic blood pressure.

For example, if your blood pressure averages 150/90 mm Hg and your intraocular pressure is 15 mm Hg, your MAP = (150 – 90) ÷ 3 + 90 = 110 mm Hg, and your RPP = ⅔ × 110 – 15 = 58.3 mm Hg.

If your blood pressure averages 110/80 mm Hg and your intraocular pressure is 15 mm Hg, your MAP = (110 – 80) ÷ 3 + 80 = 90 mm Hg, and your RPP = ⅔ × 90 – 15 = 45 mm Hg.

This may look like a lot of math, but it's worth doing it if it helps you to gauge your personal risk of developing severe retinopathy that threatens your vision. Considerable research has shown that RPP and MAP strongly predict the risk of developing severe, sight-threatening retinopathy in Type 1 and Type 2 diabetes, respectively.

Specifically, the risk of severe retinopathy increases by fourfold to sixfold (400% to 600% increased risk) when RPP is higher than 50.1 mm Hg (in Type 1 diabetes) and MAP is higher than 97.1 mm Hg (in Type 2 diabetes).

Amazingly, in one large study, RPP and MAP predicted the development of severe diabetic retinopathy as well as or better than HbA$_{1c}$ and duration of diabetes. My advice is to know your blood pressure, know your intraocular pressure, calculate your MAP and RPP, and discuss these numbers and their implications with both your eye doctor and your diabetes physician. Since IOP is almost always above 10 mm Hg (the normal range is between 10 mm Hg and 21 mm Hg), keeping your blood pressure at or below 115/75 mm Hg (a level at which MAP = 88.3 mm Hg and RPP is less than 48.9 mm Hg) will greatly reduce the risk of losing vision to diabetes.

Blood lipid control

Check, know, and improve your blood lipid levels through diet, regular physical activity, and medicine, if necessary. Diabetic retinopathy is often more severe in people with abnormal blood lipids, especially elevated low-density lipoprotein (LDL, or "bad") cholesterol and triglycerides. The risk of ischemic optic neuropathy, retinal vascular occlusion, and cataract is also higher in these people.

Ideally, LDL cholesterol should be below 100 mg/dl, triglycerides should be below 150 mg/dl, and HDL ("good") cholesterol should be above 45 mg/dl in men and above 55 mg/dl in women.

There is some evidence that the cholesterol-lowering statin drugs may reduce the risk of diabetic eye disease (and strong evidence that they reduce the occurrence of stroke and heart attack) even in people with normal blood lipid levels. Reduced consumption of saturated fats, *trans* fats, and hydrogenated fats, and increased consumption of foods high in monounsaturated fats (such as olive oil and avocados), omega-3 fats (such as flaxseed or flaxseed oil, cold-water fish, and fish oil supplements), and dietary fiber appear to improve blood lipid levels. So does regular physical activity, such as walking 30 minutes each day. Increased physical activity can also improve blood glucose control which, in and of itself, improves your blood lipid levels.

Smoking

If you smoke, quit. Smoking constricts blood vessels, thereby raising blood pressure and increasing the risk of diabetic eye disease. Nicotine, the primary addictive ingredient in cigarettes, reduces the ability of red blood cells to carry oxygen, resulting in *retinal hypoxia* (oxygen starvation) that further damages the eye. Smoking also generates *free radicals,* chemical compounds that damage cells. This is why smokers are much more likely to develop cataracts at a younger age than nonsmokers and much more likely to develop *macular degeneration,* the leading cause of vision loss in people over 50 in the Western world. We all know that smoking is bad for health. If you have diabetes, quitting smoking is arguably the single best thing you can do for your eyes (as well as your heart, lungs, kidneys, dental health, etc.).

Regular dilated eye exams

Make sure you get a dilated eye examination every year by an optometrist or ophthalmologist knowledgeable about and experienced with diabetes and diabetic eye disease. It is estimated that 40% to 50% of people with diabetes do not get annual dilated exams. This is tragic, because most cases of severe vision loss from diabetes are preventable with early diagnosis and timely treatment. For example, laser therapy for severe, vision-threatening cases of diabetic retinopathy has been shown to decrease the risk of severe vision loss by 50% to 75%, and vision loss from glaucoma can be largely prevented with drugs, laser treatment, and/or surgery. Unfortunately, by the time people have symptoms of diabetic eye disease, very often, irreversible eye damage has already occurred, and the prognosis for successful treatment is poorer. This is why it is so critical for people with diabetes to have their eyes examined on a regular basis. Remember that all people with diabetes, whether they have Type 1 or Type 2 diabetes and whether or not they use insulin, are at increased risk for losing vision.

Why is dilation of the eyes so important? Dilating, or enlarging, your pupils allows the eye doctor to see more of the inside of your eye, view it more easily, and view it in stereo (in 3-D), factors that greatly improve the chances of early diagnosis. Remember that good vision (on an eye chart test or in the real world) does not mean there is no diabetic eye disease. Many people with diabetic retinopathy and glaucoma, two potentially blinding eye diseases, have 20/20 or better vision and absolutely no symptoms at the time they are diagnosed. If you have diabetes and wait for symptoms of eye disease, it may very well be too late. However, if you follow the guidelines described here, your annual visits to the eye doctor are more likely to end with the words, "Everything looks normal and healthy. Keep doing what you're doing and we'll see you next year!"

Round up a diabetes team

Seek out health-care professionals who are knowledgeable, communicate effectively, and serve as your advocates. Knowledge is power, and you want a health-care team with plenty of both. Members of your diabetes team should explain their findings and recommendations in understandable language and should encourage you to ask questions and actively participate in the management of your diabetes. You, the person with diabetes, must also strive to become knowledgeable. This will empower you to make educated health-care decisions, to ask better questions, and to get better care.

Effective communication also means that members of your health-care team should communicate well and often with each other, because diagnoses and treatments given by one specialist often affect the treatments and recommendations offered by others. In short, you want your team members to be on the "same page." Insist that your eye doctor send timely reports to your other doctors and health advisors, and ask them to send reports to your eye doctor. Because good diabetes care requires frequent visits to members of your health-care team, it is very important that each one encourages you, advocates for you, and works with you and the other team members in your best interest. Put simply, this is what good health-care professionals do, and if you've got diabetes, you cannot settle for anything less.

Stopping diabetes and its complications

Even as science discovers more about the causes and complications of diabetes, and even as more effective treatments become available, the epidemic of diabetes and its complications continues to grow. Perhaps the most effective way to stop diabetes complications, including blindness, is to prevent diabetes in the first place.

The groundbreaking Diabetes Prevention Program, a study that examined what might prevent diabetes, has shown that simply walking 30 minutes each day, five days per week, reduces the diagnosis of Type 2 diabetes in at-risk people by nearly 60%. But for those of us who have already been diagnosed, the risk of severe eye complications can be reduced by as much as 95% if we can work together to educate, motivate, and support ourselves, our health-care providers, and our policy makers to take every action possible in turning the tide. Hopefully, this article will serve as another springboard toward that end. □

BONING UP ON BONE HEALTH

by Belinda O'Connell, M.S., R.D., C.D.E.

What are your plans for retirement? Are you saving for your financial future with an IRA or a work retirement account? Are you watching your fat and cholesterol intake to keep your heart healthy? Are you taking steps to prevent osteoporosis and ensure the health of your bones?

Most of us do not think about the health of our bones very often. We tend to take their supporting presence for granted. But perhaps we shouldn't. Without strong bones, many daily activities such as grocery shopping, house cleaning, and walking can become increasingly difficult to do.

Osteoporosis, a disease that causes bones to weaken and fracture, can have surprisingly broad effects on the quality and length of your life. Your risk of developing osteoporosis is influenced by your genetic back- ground, your lifestyle, and even your diabetes. Because most people are not aware that they have osteoporosis until bone loss is serious, it is important to take steps to prevent or slow bone loss early, before significant problems occur.

Bone growth and loss

Most people think of their bones as hard, unchanging structures, but this could not be further from the truth. Bone is a living, growing tissue that is continually being broken down and rebuilt. In child- hood and adolescence, bone tissue is built more quickly than it is broken down, and there is a net increase in bone mass. Your body builds bone tissue efficiently until about the age of 30, when peak bone mass is reached. Peak bone mass refers to the point when bone mass is at its greatest and bones are at their strongest. After age 30, your body's ability to build new bone decreases, and your bones begin to break down faster than new bone can be made. This results in a gradual, age-related loss in total bone mass. In women, loss of bone mass is accelerated by menopause, when the ovaries stop producing estrogen, a hormone that prevents bone loss. But men develop osteoporosis, too.

Although some loss of bone mass is a natural part of aging, when bone tissue is lost too quickly, or rebuilding of bone is too slow, osteoporosis can develop. Osteoporosis is more likely to occur in people who do not reach their maximum potential bone mass when they are young. Reasons for not reaching maximum potential bone mass include poor nutrition (particularly inadequate calcium and vitamin D intake), chronic or prolonged illness, and drug side effects.

Osteoporosis can affect any bone, but fractures of the wrist, hip, and spine are most common. One in two women and one in four men over age 50 will have an osteoporosis-related fracture in their lifetime. Hip fractures usually require surgery and hospitalization to repair, and they can permanently reduce mobility. In fact, 85% of people who have had a hip fracture cannot walk unaided across a room six months later. Degradation or collapse of spinal bone tissue can also decrease mobility and is often very painful. Since many fractures occur when a person falls, taking steps to prevent falls can reduce the risk of bone fractures. (See "Preventing Falls and Fractures" on page 446 for tips on staying upright.)

Risk factors for osteoporosis

Approximately 10 million Americans currently have osteoporosis and another 34 million are at high risk for developing the disease because they have decreased bone mass. Factors that affect risk of osteoporosis include the following:

Genetics. Your genes influence your peak bone mass and your rate of bone loss as you age. Genetics may also influence how likely you are to experience a bone fracture. If your parents or grandparents had osteoporosis, you are at high risk of developing it too. You can't change your genes, but you can control other risk factors for osteoporosis.

Sex. Women are four times more likely than men to develop osteoporosis. This is because women tend to have smaller bones than men and because hormonal changes in menopause dramatically increase the rate of bone loss. Women can lose up to 20% of their bone mass in the five to seven years following menopause.

Age. Because the ability of the body to build bone decreases as you age, the older you are, the greater your risk of osteoporosis. People who reach a higher peak bone mass when they are young are better protected against age-related bone loss.

Ethnicity. People of Latino and African-American heritage have a lower risk for osteoporosis than people of Caucasian and Asian ethnicity. But this does not mean that osteoporosis is not a concern for Latinos and African-Americans; it is, and they also need to control the risk factors that they can.

Body size. The size of your bones influences your risk of developing osteoporosis. People with small bones and a thin body build are at greater risk than people who have large, dense bones. People who weigh more often have stronger bones because bone is stimulated to grow and make new tissue by weight-bearing activity. Women who weigh more may also produce greater amounts of estrogen. Eating disorders like anorexia can cause severe loss of bone tissue and greatly increase the risk of having osteoporosis at a young age.

Hormone levels. The sex hormones, estrogen in women and testosterone in men, protect against bone loss. When hormone levels are low, the rate of bone loss increases. Hormone levels are decreased in amenorrhea (the abnormal loss of menstrual periods in young women) and menopause. Medroxyprogesterone (brand name Depo-Provera), an injectable contraceptive, may also cause bone loss.

Nutrition. Adequate levels of many nutrients, including calcium, vitamin D, magnesium, and vitamin K, are necessary to build healthy bones. The most important of these are calcium and vitamin D. Bones and teeth hold more than 99% of the body's calcium stores. If your dietary calcium intake is low, the body pulls calcium from bone stores to perform other necessary functions in the body. Chronic low calcium intakes cause calcium loss from bones, weakening them. Vitamin D is necessary for absorption and use of calcium in the body, and low levels are also associated with increased osteoporosis and fractures. (To read more about calcium, see "The Calcium Connection" on page 448.)

Conditions such as food allergies, Crohn disease, and intestinal surgery that limit food intake

PREVENTING FALLS AND FRACTURES

Falls increase the chances of fracturing a bone that has been weakened by osteoporosis. Falls can be caused by unsafe surroundings, poor vision, poor balance, drugs that increase dizziness or confusion, and medical conditions that affect gait, vision, or mental function. People with diabetes are at increased risk for falls if their diabetes has changed their vision or neuropathy has affected their balance or gait. Hypoglycemia (low blood sugar) can also increase the chances of a serious fall.

Here are some tips to lower your risk of falling:

■ Make sure rooms, hallways, and stairways in your home are well lit, and keep a flashlight in your car and by your bed.

■ Leave a light on in the hall or bathroom at night so you are not stumbling in the dark if you need to go to the bathroom.

■ Keep floors, hallways, stairways, and outdoor walkways free of clutter.

■ Wear rubber-soled shoes and slippers. Do not walk in socks or stockings on smooth or slippery surfaces. Avoid shoes with high heels.

■ Use rubber bath mats in the tub and shower. Consider using a shower chair if your balance is poor.

■ Have handrails installed in stairwells and grab bars in the bathroom.

■ Use nonslip carpet pads or tack down area rugs in your home. If you use throw rugs, choose ones with a nonslip backing.

■ If you have mobility problems, consider carrying a cordless phone on your person, or use an answering machine so you are not tempted to run to answer the phone when it rings.

■ Keep your blood glucose meter and something to treat low blood glucose (such as glucose tablets) nearby when you are napping or sleeping.

■ Avoid walking on rough or uneven surfaces if your balance is poor. Watch your step at curbs, and look for misaligned areas when walking on sidewalks. Consider using a cane or walker.

■ If it's icy outside, carry a small bag of sand, salt, or kitty litter to sprinkle on slippery sidewalks and steps or wear lightweight crampons.

or decrease absorption of nutrients can also increase risk of osteoporosis. In addition, excessive intake of retinol, a form of vitamin A, has been shown to interfere with normal bone metabolism and to increase the risk of fractures. The upper intake limit for retinol is 600 micrograms for children up to 3 years, 900 micrograms for children 4–8 years, 1700 micrograms for children 9–13 years, 2800 micrograms for teens 14–18 years, and 3,000 micrograms for people 19 and older. The upper intake level does not include beta-carotene, a nutrient found in plant foods that is converted to vitamin A in the body. Retinol is found in animal products; vitamin supplements; fortified foods such as milk, cereals, and energy bars; and skin preparations.

Activity level. A low physical activity level is a risk factor for osteoporosis. Exercise, particularly weight-bearing activities where your body is working against gravity, can help keep bones strong. Weight-bearing activities include walking, dancing, climbing stairs, and weight training. Balance exercises are also useful to prevent falls that could lead to fractures.

Smoking. Smoking can decrease estrogen levels and may promote early menopause in women. Smoking-related bone loss is a major risk factor for osteoporosis.

Alcohol intake. Regular consumption of more than one to two servings of alcohol a day can be toxic to bone cells and can prevent bone from growing and rebuilding itself. Alcohol use can also decrease absorption of nutrients from food, change calcium and vitamin D metabolism, and in-crease risk of falls and incidence of fractures.

Medicines. Some drugs can in-crease the risk of osteoporosis by decreasing the ability of bone cells to make new bone or increasing the breakdown of bone, decreasing calcium absorption and metabolism, or changing hormone levels. Drugs can also increase the risk of having a fall-related fracture if they cause dizziness. Common drugs that can lead to osteoporosis include glucocorticoids, such as prednisone, some anticonvulsants, such as phenytoin (Dilantin), hormones used to treat endometriosis, and too much thyroid medicine. Excessive use of aluminum-containing antacids can decrease calcium absorption.

Diabetes and bones

In the past, it was thought that risk of osteoporosis was increased in people with Type 1 diabetes but not in those with Type 2 diabetes. More recent research suggests this may not always be the case. The reasons for changes in bone metab-

---

RECOMMENDED CALCIUM INTAKES

Children
1–3 years	500 mg/day
4–8 years	800 mg/day

Boys and men
9–18 years	1300 mg/day
19–50 years	1000 mg/day
50 and older*	1200 mg/day

Girls and women
9–18 years	1300 mg/day
19–50 years	1000 mg/day
50 and older*	1200 mg/day

Upper intake limit.....2500 mg/day

* Some experts believe calcium intakes for men and women over 65 should be as high as 1500 mg/day.

---

olism in diabetes are not completely clear, but they likely include lack of insulin, high blood glucose levels, and changes in vitamin D and calcium metabolism.

People who develop Type 1 diabetes in childhood or adolescence tend to have decreased bone mass as adults and are more likely to develop osteoporosis and experience fractures than people who don't have diabetes. It is thought that lack of insulin, which is a growth factor for bone, causes poor bone growth and lower peak bone mass in adolescents with Type 1 diabetes. High blood glucose levels may also cause poor bone growth, though studies of blood glucose control and bone mineral density have not always shown a link between the two.

People with Type 1 diabetes have also been shown to have reduced levels of vitamin D on diagnosis and abnormal seasonal changes in vitamin D levels, which could contribute to poor bone growth. Other conditions that can increase risk of osteoporosis, such as gluten intolerance (also called celiac disease) and thyroid disorders, are also more common in Type 1 diabetes.

Research studies of people with Type 2 diabetes have found in-creases, decreases, and no change in bone mineral density associated with diabetes. It is true that people with higher body weights tend to be protected against bone loss, and many people with Type 2 diabetes are overweight, but several studies have found that people with Type 2 diabetes experienced a greater number of fractures than people without diabetes, while others

THE CALCIUM CONNECTION

Calcium is a nutrient that is needed for the proper growth and development of bones. It is also required for heart contraction, nerve function, and many other cell reactions. If dietary calcium intake is too low, the body takes calcium from bones to meet other needs. Over time, this can cause calcium depletion and bone weakening.

Your body's calcium level is a function of more than just what you eat. Calcium balance is determined by how much calcium you get in your diet, how much of that calcium your body absorbs, and how much calcium your body loses each day, mostly through urine.

Intake. Research shows that low calcium intakes decrease bone mass and increase bone loss and fractures. This is a serious concern since many Americans get less than half the calcium they need to keep their bones healthy. Those people who need calcium the most—teen-age girls, young women, and adults over 65—tend to have the lowest intakes.

Current recommendations for calcium intake vary by age and sex. To meet your calcium needs, try to eat at least 2 to 3 servings of low-fat dairy products or other calcium-rich foods each day. People who do not meet this goal and people with potentially higher requirements, such as older women, may need a supplement to reach their recommended daily intake for calcium.

Good sources of calcium include low-fat milk, yogurt, and cheese; dark green, leafy vegetables such as broccoli, collard greens, bok choy, and spinach; fish with edible bones such as canned sardines and salmon; calcium-fortified tofu and soy milk; almonds; and foods fortified with calcium such as orange juice, cereals, nutrition bars, breads, and rice.

If you need a calcium supplement to meet your calcium requirements, choose one that contains calcium citrate, calcium lactate, or calcium carbonate. Choose supplements that have the USP (United States Pharmacopeia) seal, showing they meet government guidelines for production and dissolution. Avoid "natural" calcium supplements that contain calcium from coral, oyster shells, dolomite, or bone meal, because these sources are more likely to be contaminated with lead and other dangerous substances. Calcium supplements are better absorbed when taken with meals and in moderate doses. If you need to take more than 300–500 milligrams as a supplement

have found significant bone loss in people with Type 2 diabetes compared to age- and sex-matched control subjects. Other studies have found low serum vitamin D levels in post-menopausal women with Type 2 diabetes.

No matter what type of diabetes a person has, diabetes-related complications such as hypoglycemia, retinopathy and vision loss, and changes in balance caused by neuropathy, can increase the risk of falls and fractures.

Diagnosing osteoporosis

Osteoporosis can be diagnosed with a test called a bone mineral density test. The most accurate form of bone mineral density testing is called dual energy x-ray absorptiometry, or DXA (formerly called DEXA). This test uses a very small amount of radiation, less than a common x-ray, to measure the amount of calcium and tissue that you have in your bones. It is painless and takes about 10 to 15 minutes to perform. Many health clinics and physician's offices offer bone mineral testing right in their office, and Medicare will pay for these tests for beneficiaries who are at risk for developing osteoporosis. The U.S. Preventive Services Task Force has issued recommendations that all women 65 and older be screened for osteoporosis, as well as those 60 to 65 who are at risk of osteoporosis.

After you get your bone mineral density tested, your physician will compare your results against a "normal" standard. One standard, the T-score, compares your bone mineral density to an average, healthy 30-year-old's bone density. The other standard, the Z-score, compares your bone mineral density to that of a typical healthy person of your age and body size. Because most people lose bone as they age, the age-matched Z-score is less useful in determining risk.

T-scores and Z-scores are measured as a *standard deviation,* or how different your measurement is from normal. Bone mineral density values that are one standard deviation or less from normal are considered healthy. T-scores that are more than one standard deviation below normal but less than 2.5 standard deviations below normal indicate each day, divide your dose and have part in the morning and part in the evening with meals. Some people may need a supplement that also contains vitamin D.

Absorption. Calcium absorption is a function of how much calcium you eat and how available the calcium from that food is. Not all sources of calcium are absorbed equally. Calcium from dairy products and fortified foods is absorbed better than calcium from vegetables or supplements, though some research suggests that other nutrients in fruits and vegetables may enhance bone density.

Calcium absorption and normal bone development also depend on adequate levels of vitamin D. The primary source of vitamin D is sunshine, which the body uses to make vitamin D in the skin. Summer sun exposure of at least 15 minutes per day without sunscreen is believed to meet requirements. Sun exposure in the winter, in northern latitudes, and in polluted areas may not be as efficient. Older people and people with kidney disease do not make vitamin D well. The best food source of vitamin D is fortified milk; most other dairy products are not fortified.

Recommended intakes of vitamin D are 5 micrograms per day (200 International Units [IU]) for children and adults up to age 50; 10 micrograms per day (400 IU) for adults 50–70 years; and 15 micrograms (600 IU) for adults over 70. Studies suggest that many older people have significantly depleted levels of vitamin D and that supplements containing up to 800 IU of vitamin D and 1200 milligrams of calcium protect against fractures when taken daily. However, vitamin D can be toxic in high doses. The safe upper intake level for vitamin D is 50 micrograms per day (2,000 IU).

Other nutrients in foods can also affect calcium balance but play a smaller role than either calcium or vitamin D. High-protein and high-sodium diets can cause increased urinary calcium loss, which can negatively affect calcium balance in those with low calcium intakes. Caffeine, oxalates in vegetables like spinach, and phytates in wheat bran can bind to calcium in the intestine, decreasing its absorption, as can phosphorus from soft drinks and other foods. Too much retinol, a form of vitamin A, can interfere with calcium absorption and normal bone metabolism. Soy isoflavones, because of their similarities to estrogen, may be bone protective.

osteopenia, or low bone mass. Scores that are more than 2.5 standard deviations below normal indicate osteoporosis.

Prevention and treatment

Although osteoporosis can be treated, it cannot be cured, so the best treatment is to take steps to prevent it from developing in the first place. The best protection against osteoporosis is to build as much bone as possible while you are young. Bones are a bit like a bank savings account. If you "deposit" a lot of bone tissue when you are young, you have more to "withdraw" as you age without hitting critically low levels. For children and younger adults, this means being physically active and getting enough calcium and vitamin D. Research indicates that adequate calcium intakes early in life may reduce incidence of hip fractures by 50% later.

Even if you have passed the time period when bone is built most efficiently (from preadolescence until about 30), there is still a great deal you can do to preserve the bone you have. To avoid osteoporosis, or to slow bone mass loss if you already have osteoporosis, take the following steps to control your risk factors:

■ Begin to participate in weight-bearing activities such as walking, dancing, or weight lifting. Ask your health-care team to recommend back-strengthening exercises. Try an activity like tai chi or yoga that improves balance.

■ If you smoke, ask your physician to help you find a smoking cessation program or to prescribe a medicine to help you control your desire for cigarettes as you quit.

■ If you drink alcohol, keep your regular intake to no more than one to two servings per day.

■ Make sure that your diet includes the right amount of nutrients like calcium and vitamin D to keep your bones strong.

There are also several different types of medicines that may help slow bone loss or strengthen bone in those diagnosed with osteoporosis. These include the following:

■ Bisphosphonates, which include alendronate (Fosamax), ibandronate (Boniva), and risedronate

(Actonel), decrease bone loss, increase bone density, and decrease the risk of fractures in the spine, hip, and other sites. These drugs are used to treat and prevent osteoporosis in men and women as well as bone loss due to steroid therapy. Bisphosphonates must be taken on an empty stomach, and food must be delayed for 30 to 60 minutes after taking the medicine.

■ Calcitonin is a hormone that helps the body regulate calcium and bone metabolism. A synthetic version, sold as Miacalcin, is available as a nasal spray or an injection. It can decrease bone loss, increase bone density of the spine, and lower risk of spinal fractures. It may also help control pain associated with spinal fractures. It is FDA-approved to treat osteoporosis only in postmenopausal women, but it may be prescribed off-label to men as well.

■ Parathyroid hormone helps to regulate bone and calcium metabolism. A genetically engineered version of parathyroid hormone is available as an injection, called teriparatide (Forteo). Teriparatide promotes the growth of new bone and can decrease hip and spine fractures. It is approved for use in men and postmenopausal women as a treatment for osteoporosis.

■ Selective estrogen receptor modulators (called SERMs) are drugs that mimic some of the positive effects of estrogen without the same risk of negative side effects. One that is approved for treatment of osteoporosis is raloxifene (Evista). It has been shown to increase bone mass and decrease bone breakdown and the incidence of fractures.

No time like the present

Too often, the first sign of osteoporosis is a bone fracture, which is not only painful but can seriously affect a person's quality of life. Don't let yourself be surprised by osteoporosis. Have your risk for osteoporosis evaluated now, before problems occur, then do your part to lower your risk by taking steps such as increasing your activity level and consuming enough calcium and vitamin D to prevent it early. Talk with your health-care team about your risk factors for osteoporosis today, before frail bones and possibly fractures slow you down. □

EMERGENCY PREPAREDNESS
Just In Case

by Judith Jones Ambrosini and Laura Laria

Where were you when the lights went out? That was the question many Americans asked each other in August 2003, when large sections of the Midwest, Northeast, and parts of Canada lost electrical power. While some lucky people got their power back within hours, others were without electricity for several days. While they waited for the lights to come back on, any food in their refrigerators—and any insulin—slowly warmed up.

Two years later, in August 2005, Hurricane Katrina struck the Gulf Coast of the United States, forcing hundreds of thousands to abandon their homes and flee to shelters and temporary housing. Many were eventually able to return home, often after waiting for months, but some were not. In the meantime, all were separated from most of their possessions, including, for some, their diabetes supplies.

Both of these incidents serve as reminders that disasters and emergencies can and do happen, suddenly wiping out conveniences such as refrigerators, air conditioning, fresh food, and even running tap water. This makes life more difficult for everyone, and it can particularly complicate managing one's diabetes. Still, there are ways to plan ahead so you don't get caught unprepared and empty-handed when normal life is suddenly disrupted.

Power outage

The August 2003 power outage prompted a run on flashlights, batteries, and bottled water, so it's better to stock up on these items before you need them. Be sure you have enough batteries to use your flashlights and a battery-operated radio or television, as well as extras to replace those in use. It's not a bad idea to have some candles and matches in your home as well, but remember that candles present a fire hazard and should not be left unattended. Matches can also come in handy for lighting a gas stove with an electric ignition.

The American Red Cross recommends storing one gallon of water per household member per day (don't forget pets!), and keeping at least a three-day supply of water per person in your home. The average person needs to drink at least two quarts of water a day, but hot weather or intense physical activity—as well as breast-feeding or illness—will increase those needs. Water should be stored in plastic containers such as soft drink bottles, which should be emptied and refilled every six months. While you're refilling your water bottles, you may want to check your supply of other seasonal items such as extra blankets or sleeping bags, which could be useful if your heat went out along with your power in the winter.

What about food in the refrigerator or freezer? If the refrigerator door is kept shut, foods can last for 4–6 hours. In addition, many fruits and vegetables can keep for several days without refrigeration. Frozen foods can stay frozen for three days if the freezer is full and well insulated and the door is kept shut. As long as frozen foods still have ice crystals in their centers, they should be safe to eat. To extend your food supply as long as possible, eat refrigerated foods first, frozen foods next, and shelf-stable foods last. However, if you have any doubt about the safety of foods, par-ticularly meat or dairy foods, which spoil quickly, throw them out. Don't risk food poisoning.

To avoid running out of food completely, plan ahead for power outages or other disasters by keeping at least a three-day supply of nonperishable food—and a manual can opener—in your home. Pick foods that require no cooking or prepara-tion in case you cannot heat foods. Some examples of foods to keep on hand include canned meats, fish, pasta dishes, beans, vegetables, fruits, and fruit juices; shelf-stable boxes of milk, soy

milk, and fruit juice; powdered milk; crackers, energy bars, hard candy, peanut butter, jelly, canned nuts, and dried fruit. While these foods have a long shelf life, they will not keep forever, so it's nec-essary to keep an eye on "use by" dates and rotate your stock.

For people who use insulin, lack of refrigeration brings up another concern: How long will insulin remain usable? In general, a vial of opened, unrefrigerated insulin lasts for 28 days at room tempera-ture, with many pens and pen cartridges good for 7, 10, or 14 days. Unless your power is out for an extended period, therefore, the insulin in the vial or pen you are currently using should remain usable for the duration. However, if your indoor air temperature is over 86°F—which could easily be the case if your power goes out in August—you will need to devise a way to keep your insulin cooler than room temperature (but not frozen). One way to do this is to place insulin in water that is cooled with ice or refreezable ice packs. Another is to place your insulin in water-activated cold packs (such as Frio brand products), which stay cold for many hours after being saturated with water.

Once your power comes back on, ask your health-care provider about the safety of any unopened insulin that you had stored in the refrigerator. Depending on how long the power was out, it may be safer to discard it and buy new.

Although other diabetes sup-plies do not generally require refrigeration, getting more sup-plies could be a problem if the traffic lights in your commu-nity are not working or nearby drugstores are closed. (Hospitals, however, have backup generators, so in an emergency you can still go to the hospital.) This is where having a sick-day box with some

FOR MORE INFORMATION

If you would like to learn more about how to respond to specific
types of disasters and emergencies, use the resources listed below.

AMERICAN RED CROSS
www.redcross.org
Find out how to take a class in first aid or CPR
or click on "Publications" to find "Community
Disaster Education Materials," which include
videos and brochures. To order these materials,
contact your local chapter of the Red Cross.
(Look under "A" in your phone book for "American Red Cross.") Click on "Disaster Services"
then "After a Disaster" to find lists of things
you'll need to think about after a disaster has
struck, from food safety and first aid to financial
recovery and evacuation. Sign up for their
"1 Minute Update" e-mail newsletter for tips,
news, and disaster updates.

EMERGENCY PREPAREDNESS AND RESPONSE
www.bt.cdc.gov
(800) CDC-INFO (232-4636)
(888) 232-6348 (TTY)
Developed by the Centers for Disease Control
and Prevention, this Web site has information
on responding to radiation exposure, bioterror-
ism, and chemical agents as well as natural disasters. A version of this site is available in Spanish.

FEDERAL EMERGENCY MANAGEMENT AGENCY
www.fema.gov
(800) 621-FEMA (3362)
(800) 462-7585 (TTY)
At FEMA's Web site, you can get news and
updates on emergencies and disasters across the
United States. Click on the "Plan Ahead" tab for
guidance on preparing for emergency scenarios,
or on "Publications & Forms" under "Quick
Links" to look for information on a more specific topic. For regional information or to contact a regional office, click on "Regional Offices"
under "About FEMA."

PREPARE.ORG
www.prepare.org
In 14 different languages, this site is sponsored
by groups such as the American Red Cross and
has information on disaster preparedness for
seniors and their caregivers, pet owners, people
with disabilities, and children. People with
screen readers or slow Internet connections will
appreciate the text-only version of the site
(www.prepare.org/text/indexTX.htm).

READY CAMPAIGN
www.ready.gov
(202) 282-8000
(202) 447-3543 (TTY)
This site, from the Department of Homeland
Security, has three subsites on emergency management for businesses, kids, and the general
public. It contains instructional videos that can
be viewed online, including ones about precautions for senior citizens, people with disabilities,
and pets. It also has numerous publications that
can be either downloaded from the site or
ordered by calling (800) BE-READY (237-3239).

---

extra supplies can come in handy. (For more on
assembling a sick-day box, see "Sick-Day Supplies"
on page 33.) Just be sure to replace any sick-day
supplies you use once the power comes back on
and you can travel freely.

The tools and techniques that can get you
through a power outage—flashlights, batteries,
battery-operated radio, stored water, nonperishable foods, extra diabetes supplies—will also come
in handy if you are stuck in your home for several
days because of a snowstorm, ice storm, or similar
weather-related situation. To maintain blood glucose control under these circumstances, do your
best to eat meals and snacks on your usual schedule, and continue to monitor your blood glucose
on schedule as well.

When you're away from home

What if you're stranded away from your home—
and your carefully assembled emergency supplies—for hours or even days? Clearly, you can't
carry around three days' worth of food and water
at all times, but you can put some safeguards in
place at your workplace, in your car, and even in
your backpack or briefcase to prevent being
caught with no supplies.

At work, for example, you can probably find a
place to store a gallon of water, some glucose

Preventive Health

tablets, and some shelf-stable snacks in case you get stuck there overnight. You may also want to keep a flashlight, batteries, and a battery-operated radio at work, particularly if you work in a remote location. If you typically wear dress shoes at work, keeping an old pair of sneakers there is a good idea in case you have to evacuate the building.

In your car, it's also a good idea to keep a flashlight (with working batteries), a small first aid kit, a plastic bottle of water, glucose tablets, some non-perishable snacks, and a pair of sneakers (in case you have to get out and walk) just in case. In cold weather, you may also want to keep some extra clothes and a blanket in your car. Do not plan on keeping a blood glucose meter and strips or insulin in your car; car temperatures can get very hot (and very cold), which will make strips inaccurate and insulin ineffective.

Carrying a small bottle of water, a snack, some money (including change for pay phones), and your basic diabetes supplies with you whenever you leave your home may seem like a chore, but you really never know what can happen between your front door and your destination. So even if you're just going for a walk or a bike ride, pop these items into a fanny pack. That way, if a sudden rainstorm comes up and you're stuck across town for several hours, you can worry about whether you left your windows open, but you won't have to worry about your diabetes control.

Leaving in a hurry

In some situations you may be stuck in your home; in others, you may have to leave in a hurry. If your life is in danger because, for example, your house is on fire, you will have no time to grab your diabetes supplies or anything else, and you shouldn't try to. Your priority in these cases is to get away from danger.

Because sudden evacuations can be confusing, make a plan for reuniting with your family before disaster strikes. Select two emergency meeting places, one right outside your house or apartment building, and another outside your neighborhood

in case the problem is widespread. In addition, choose a friend or family member who lives out of state to serve as a contact person in case local phone lines are down or in case not all evacuating family members are equipped with cell phones.

If you have a little more time to leave your home—which could be the case if, say, a hurricane is on the way—it's a good idea to pack a bag with some essentials to ride out the next few days. In fact, many experts recommend packing an emergency bag long before there's any emergency on the horizon so you can grab it and go if needed.

What should you have in your bag? Here are some ideas:
- Shelf-stable diabetes supplies such as an extra meter, lancets, syringes, pump infusion supplies, alcohol wipes, hand cleanser, and glucose tablets.
- Perishable diabetes supplies such as test strips and insulin—but keep in mind that these items will have to be replaced at regular intervals and that your health insurance may not cover them.
- First-aid supplies such as Band-Aids and small bandages.
- Flashlight with working batteries.
- Medical identification wallet card.
- List of telephone contact numbers, including close relatives and health-care providers.
- List of all the medicines you take.
- Bottle of water.
- Snacks such as energy bars or candy.
- Money, both small bills and change for pay phones.
- Some items of clothing, such as a T-shirt, underwear, and socks.
- Some toiletries such as soap, toothbrushes, and toothpaste.

To be useful, your emergency bag should be stored near your front or back door. If it's a bright color, it will be that much easier to find when you're in a rush, and it should be marked with your name.

We hope you never have to use your emergency kit, but if you do, you won't regret taking the time and making the effort to assemble it. □

GETTING THE SLEEP YOU NEED

by David Spero, R.N.

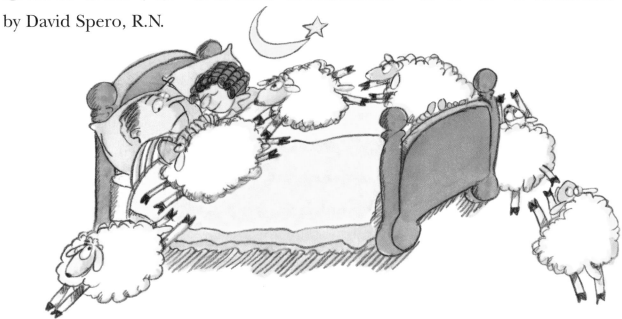

Sleep that knits up the ravell'd sleeve of care,
The death of each day's life, sore labour's bath,
Balm of hurt minds, great nature's second course,
Chief nourisher in life's feast.

—William Shakespeare, *Macbeth*

You don't need to be a great poet to describe the healing value of sleep. Nearly everyone knows the dragged-out feeling that comes with a sleepless night and how much better we feel after a restful one. What many people may not realize, however, is that sleep is not just "pleasant" or "refreshing" but necessary for good health.

Sleep gives the body time to relax and repair and is now also understood to play a role in learning. Insomnia, however, is one of the most common complaints in America, and it also has a link to diabetes: Sleep deprivation can make diabetes worse, and diabetes symptoms can make it harder to sleep.

The good news is that sleep problems are nearly always treatable. Usually, you don't need any medicines or surgery to get to sleep, just some simple behavior changes. This article gives the basic concepts that sleep specialists use to help people get to sleep, stay asleep, and wake up rested. You will also learn what sleep conditions benefit from a doctor's care.

What is insomnia?

Insomnia isn't just an occasional rough night or sleeping less than you think you should. The key question to determine if you have insomnia is "how rested do I feel?" If you have all the energy and alertness you want, you don't have insomnia, no matter how little sleep you get. On the other hand, if you're tired and drowsy all day, you may have insomnia, even if you're in bed 12 hours a night. The quality of sleep is as important as the quantity. For example, if you're struggling for breath all night or your body can't relax because of stress and tension, you may not feel rested no matter how much you sleep.

There are at least three kinds of insomnia: problems getting to sleep, problems staying asleep, and waking up too early and not being able to go back to sleep. Problems getting to sleep (sleep-onset insomnia) are often due to stress, too much activity or anxiety at bedtime, or bad sleep habits.

Problems staying asleep (sleep-maintenance insomnia) are often due to medical problems described later in this article such as sleep apnea or an enlarged prostate. We all wake up 12–15 times a night, but we usually get right back to sleep without ever realizing or remembering we've been awake. It's insomnia if you can't get back to sleep easily.

Problems with waking up too early are often a sign of depression, or they may be caused by noise and light in the bedroom.

Insomnia and health

Our fast-paced society takes its toll on sleep. The average American sleeps about 7–7½ hours a night. A century ago, the average was 9 hours.

Francis Buda, M.D., cofounder of the Atlanta Center for Sleep Disorders, says, "The American population as a whole is chronically sleep deprived."

Until recently, though, it was thought that lack of sleep had few long-term health effects. The main concern has been accidents and mistakes due to poor concentration and fatigue. But recent studies at institutions such as the University of Chicago and Pennsylvania State University have shown that sleep deprivation (getting at least two hours less than you want) leads to insulin resistance, increases in appetite, and higher levels of stress hormones in the blood—conditions that can contribute to the development of diabetes. Some researchers believe there may also be a connection between sleep disorders and heart disease.

While sleeplessness can promote diabetes, symptoms associated with high blood glucose, low blood glucose (hypoglycemia), and some diabetes complications can also interfere with sleep. If your blood glucose level is high, you may be in the bathroom urinating every few hours during the night. Hypoglycemia can cause nightmares, night sweats, or headache; hunger that wakes you up to get food; or symptoms associated with daytime hypoglycemia such as rapid heartbeat, dizziness, or shaking. Tracy Kuo, Ph.D., insomnia specialist and clinical psychologist at the Stanford Sleep Disorders Clinic, says that a vicious circle can occur with diabetes and insomnia because "diabetic neuropathy can cause restless legs and pain. Fatigue from a poor night's sleep may keep some people with diabetes from getting enough daytime activity, which in turn makes it harder to sleep the following night."

Things that keep us awake

As many as 36% of Americans have some type of sleep disorder. That's a huge number. Why is sleeping so difficult? Sleep specialists have identified the following reasons, among others.

Substances. Sleep specialist Peter Hauri, Ph.D., Co-Director of the Mayo Clinic Sleep Disorders Center, says, "There are three things that have an excellent chance of helping you sleep, no matter what other factors are involved. These things are reducing caffeine, limiting alcohol, and stopping smoking."

Although coffee and soft drinks are the most commonly recognized sources of caffeine, chocolate, some teas, and some medicines also contain caffeine. Even one cup of tea or a chocolate bar in the afternoon can keep some people up after midnight. Dr. Hauri suggests cutting all caffeine out of your diet. Once you get some normal sleep going, you can try slowly adding the caffeine back. If you

smoke, nicotine cravings don't stop at night, and they can wake you up. The only way out of this trap is to stop smoking completely. Of course, smoking and diabetes are a horrible combination anyway, so if getting a good night's sleep encourages you to quit, it's a win–win proposition.

People used to think an alcoholic drink was a good sleep aid, hence the term "nightcap." But Dr. Hauri says, "Drinking alcohol late in the evening produces troubled and fragmented sleep. The person does not sleep soundly but wakes up several times and does not get back to sleep promptly. By morning, there invariably is less sleep than without alcohol." Some foods, especially spicy foods, also cause insomnia in some people.

Sleeping pills. Almost all sleep specialists now try to avoid prescribing sleeping pills for people with chronic sleep problems. Although they can be useful for treating some short-term sleep disturbances, hypnotics (sleeping pills) are not usually given to people with chronic insomnia because they can become habit-forming, and people may even experience a rebound effect of more pronounced insomnia when the drugs are stopped. People also rapidly build up a tolerance to many sleep medicines, needing more and more over time to get to sleep. In addition, with some drugs, you can wake up in the morning feeling as tired as if you hadn't slept at all. You're also in danger of falling if you wake up in the night to go to the bathroom with sedatives in your system. This is a major cause of broken hips and other injuries for older people, especially people in nursing homes. Over-the-counter sleep medicines are just as bad, according to Dr. Buda.

Depression. Both insomnia and "hypersomnia" (sleeping too much) are classic symptoms of depression. If you lie in bed having thoughts of hopelessness or worthlessness, especially in the early morning, you may be depressed. Because depression is a risk factor for other problems and because it is treatable, you should seek professional help.

Sleep apnea. A number of medical conditions interfere with sleep. One is sleep apnea, where the person experiences interruptions of breathing during the night. Sleep apnea normally happens to heavy snorers, who are usually, but not always, overweight. Sleep apnea is typically observed when loud snoring is interrupted by about 10 seconds or more of silence as breathing stops and then starts again— often with a loud snort or gasp—which may wake you. (Some people think they woke to go to the bathroom, when actually it was sleep apnea.) This pattern may repeat many times an hour throughout the night. If you have a bed partner, he or she would probably notice the signs of sleep apnea first. You could also spend a night in a sleep lab for an official diagnosis. It's worth checking out, because sleep apnea is associated with serious health problems, including diabetes and heart disease.

Other medical conditions. Gastroesophageal reflux disease (GERD) is commonly known as heartburn. When people with GERD lie down, acid from the stomach can leak back into the esophagus, causing pain and, sometimes, severe damage. Other people have periodic limb movements or restless legs syndrome, in which jumping of the legs makes sleep difficult. (Sometimes it's even more difficult for the bed partner!) Older men may develop a benign enlargement of the prostate, which can cause more frequent urges to urinate, waking them several times a night. These conditions are treatable and should be checked out by a physician.

Many other diseases, including heart, kidney, liver, nerve, and thyroid problems, can cause insomnia. Many prescription and over-the-counter drugs can cause insomnia in some people. Check the labels on the drugs you take or ask your pharmacist if you suspect a drug may be causing or contributing to your sleep difficulties.

Pain, whether from neuropathy, headache, arthritis, or some other source, can make it hard to get to sleep.

Stress and anxiety. What's happening in your life—money problems, job hassles, family stress, worrying about the world situation, or whatever— can leave you too worked up to relax and sleep. "Emotional arousal, frustration, and worry are incompatible with sleep," says Dr. Kuo. "Relaxation, not distress, is a necessary condition for sleep." Even if the cause of the stress is long-term, relaxation techniques could help you to calm down enough at night to sleep.

If you lie there at bedtime with a rapid heartbeat, worrying about bad things that could happen, or have trouble falling or staying asleep, you may have an anxiety disorder. Anxiety disorders are highly treatable.

Conditioned insomnia. Another big cause of sleep problems is trying to sleep when conditions aren't right for it. Some people spend too much time in bed; others don't get enough activity during the day. Some think they should sleep more than their bodies really want. Dr. Buda says, "You can't get more sleep than you need each night. When your body is rested, it just won't sleep."

Once people get into a pattern of struggling to sleep, they can have insomnia for years, just out of

habit. The key is to start applying good sleep practices like the ones outlined later in this article. To determine whether you might have conditioned insomnia, ask yourself if you sleep better away from home. If you do, you could be conditioned to associate your own bed with insomnia.

Eliminating the struggle

Nothing bad happens when you miss one or two nights of sleep, as long as you're careful about driving the next day. It's chronic insomnia that causes problems. So if you regularly have problems falling asleep, don't lie in bed tossing and turning. Sleep specialist Richard Bootzin, Ph.D., Professor of Psychology and Psychiatry at the University of Arizona, says that if you're not asleep in 10 minutes, you should get up and go to another room. Dr. Kuo says it's not the length of time that matters but that you should get up if you feel it's taking too long to get to sleep or you're getting frustrated. Then do something relaxing or soothing for at least 10 minutes, preferably out of bed. Don't go back to bed until you're really tired. If you still can't sleep as quickly as you'd like, get up and try relaxing again. But if you're comfortably relaxed in bed, Dr. Kuo says it's OK to stay there, even if you're not asleep. The idea is to associate your bed with relaxation, comfort, and getting to sleep easily, not with frustration and wakefulness.

To help your body and mind connect your bed with relaxation, get in the habit of using your bed only for sleep and sex. Don't read, eat, talk on the phone, or watch television in bed. Once you've established sound sleep, you may be able to loosen up a bit.

Whatever you do, don't *try* to go to sleep. Dr. Hauri says, "The harder you try to stay awake, the easier you will fall asleep. The harder you try to sleep, the longer you will stay awake."

In Dr. Bootzin's plan, it's also crucial to get up at the same time every morning, whether you've slept or not. You're trying to form a new habit of easy and regular sleep, and a couple of days of tiredness may be a small price to pay.

Be patient. Dr. Kuo says it takes at least two weeks to learn new sleep behaviors. "Changing long-time sleep patterns is a process. It's not something you can change all at once. If you've had insomnia for a long time, it may take at least six to eight weeks to establish improvement. And many people benefit from the help of a sleep specialist."

Routine, routine, routine

Sleep doctors recommend having a bedtime ritual, or a set of habits you can form that promote sleep.

SLEEP LOG

Because your daily activities can affect your sleep, keeping track of them can help you to figure out which promotes or hinders sleep for you.

NAME_____   DATE _____

	Sunday	Monday	Tuesday	Wednesday	Thursday	Friday	Saturday
Time to bed last night?							
Approximate time needed to fall asleep?							
About how many times did you wake up? For about how long?							
Approximate time you woke for the last time?							
When did you get up for the last time?							
How rested did you feel in the morning? (1–10)							
How rested did you feel in the evening? (1–10)							
Rate your energy level for today. (1–10)							
How many naps today? How long?							
What else happened? (Exercise, sleep ritual, arguments, caffeine, anything you want to investigate?)							

After sitting at a computer or watching TV, talking or doing physical exercise, many people find it hard to go right to sleep. You need to wind down first. You should faithfully go through your ritual every evening, if possible. Rituals vary from person to person. Whatever works for you is OK. Here are some ideas:

- Dim the lights 20 minutes or so before bedtime (to simulate sunset).
- Take a warm bath.
- Have a snack. Most bedtime snacks will work, but avoid spicy food. Warm milk, herbal tea, and turkey are especially good for many people.
- Pray or meditate.

- Do some gentle stretching, but not vigorous exercise.
- Taking acetaminophen or aspirin at bedtime helps some people stay asleep by lowering body temperature, which triggers sleep-inducing signals in the brain.
- Repeat an affirmation such as, "I have done all I needed to do today."
- Listen to restful music or nature sounds or a relaxation tape.
- Put on socks or down booties so that cold feet don't keep you awake.
- Sex can also be a good sleep-inducer for some people.

Some of these things can also help you get back to sleep after waking up in the middle of the night.

Sleep-promoting lifestyles

What you do during the day makes a big difference in how you sleep at night.

Exercise. Bodies need to move. If you don't move all day, your body won't want to stay still at night. Of course, exercise also helps blood glucose control. Exercising too close to bedtime could keep you awake, though, so it may be good to avoid vigorous exercises three to six hours before you go to bed.

Stress. Anything that makes your life less stressful helps you sleep, and vice versa. Relaxation and self-soothing skills are crucial and are taught at most sleep clinics. If worries keep you awake, Dr. Hauri suggests spending 10–30 minutes a day (not in the evening) in a "worry session," thinking of all your worries and writing some ideas on "worry cards." You know they'll be there in the morning, so you don't have to worry at night.

Blood glucose control. Maintain the best possible blood glucose control.

Excess weight. Overweight makes it harder to sleep and can cause sleep apnea. Another reason to get in shape.

Sunlight. Get some sun exposure during the day. Without sunlight, your brain is not properly cued to produce melatonin, the body's natural sleep aid. Being unable to see sunlight is why most blind people have problems with insomnia.

Get comfortable

Some people can sleep anywhere. Most of us need a quiet, safe, dark room. If you can't get such a room, a blindfold and/or ear plugs might help. A "white noise generator," a fan, or a tape of nature sounds can block unwanted noise. Use curtains or shades to block outdoor lights and morning light if it wakes you.

Get a comfortable mattress. Most people can sleep on any decent mattress. You probably don't need to toss out your current one and spend tons of money on the most expensive model, but mattresses were not designed to last a lifetime, so you will need to replace them every so often. Pillows should also be comfortable. Thinner pillows may give better posture and more comfortable sleep to people who sleep on their backs, while people who sleep on their sides may need thicker pillows for more neck support. Some people like a pillow or bolster behind them when they sleep on their sides, or a pillow under their feet or between their knees to reduce back strain.

Temperature can also be a factor. An overactive radiator could have you waking up in a sweat, so be sure to set your thermostat appropriately.

The pros and cons of naps

Napping may leave you less tired at bedtime, setting the stage for insomnia. Some experts, including Dr. Bootzin, have a strict rule: No naps! Others are more flexible, but the National Sleep Foundation suggests limiting a nap to no more than 20–30 minutes, while the American Academy of Sleep Medicine says a nap should be less than an hour and no later than 3 PM. Long naps should be avoided if you have insomnia.

Studies on the health effects of naps have given conflicting results. But for some, napping can be a healing break from the stresses of the day. In a review of the medical literature, Masaya Takahasi, D.M.Sc., of Japan's National Institute of Industrial Health, found several studies that indicate that short naps (less than 20 minutes) may be linked to a reduction in the risk of heart disease.

Keep a sleep diary

Since so many things can hinder or promote sleep, many people find it helpful to keep a sleep diary to figure out what's keeping them up or what works best to help them sleep. (The sample "Sleep Log" on page 457 gives one format for keeping such a diary.) Each morning, write down when you went to bed, about how long it took to go to sleep (but don't watch the clock for an exact time; clock-watching can keep you up), about how many times you recall waking up, when you got up, and how rested you feel. Record any naps you took the day before. Also rate your energy level and alertness during the day on a scale of 1 to 10.

Finally, write down what else happened. You won't be able to record everything, so focus on three or four issues at a time. (Some people keep a separate "day log" for this.) Perhaps start with

SLEEP RESOURCES

To learn more about sleep disorders and their treatments,
check out some of the following resources.

Books

HOLISTIC SLEEP
Beating Insomnia with Commonsense,
Medical, and New Age Techniques
Francis B. Buda, M.D.
Citadel Press
New York, 2000

NO MORE SLEEPLESS NIGHTS
Peter Hauri, Ph.D., and Shirley Linde, Ph.D.
John Wiley & Sons
New York, 1996

SAY GOOD NIGHT TO INSOMNIA
A Drug-Free Program Developed at
Harvard Medical School
Gregg D. Jacobs, Ph.D.
Owl Books
New York, 1999

Organizations

AMERICAN ACADEMY OF SLEEP MEDICINE
www.aasmnet.org
(708) 492-0930
This association's Web site features less consumer-oriented information than the others listed here, but the site is still useful for people interested in locating an accredited sleep study center near them. Click on "Find a Sleep Center" under "Patients & Public."

AMERICAN SLEEP APNEA ASSOCIATION
www.sleepapnea.org
(202) 293-3650
The ASAA provides information on sleep apnea and also organizes a national network of support groups.

NATIONAL SLEEP FOUNDATION
www.sleepfoundation.org
An organization that offers information on sleep disorders and funds sleep research. A number of brochures and fact sheets with helpful hints for better sleep can be viewed on its Web site.

RESTLESS LEGS SYNDROME FOUNDATION
www.rls.org
(507) 287-6465
The foundation's Web site has information on restless legs syndrome, a directory of providers who specialize in its treatment, and a list of support groups. To receive a free booklet on dealing with restless legs syndrome, call (877) INFO-RLS (463-6757).

SLEEPNET.COM
www.sleepnet.com
This site offers information and links on sleep disorders, discussion forums, and an e-mail newsletter.

---

caffeine, nicotine, alcohol intake, and medicines. Record your bedtime ritual. Other possible issues to monitor: watching TV, exercise, family or work hassles, or anything else that may bother you. Over a couple of weeks, you might discover what helps you sleep and what gets in the way.

When to see a doctor

If none of this works, if you keep waking up all night, or if you have trouble waking up in the morning or staying alert during the day, you may want to consult a sleep specialist. You may have a treatable medical condition such as sleep apnea, or you may need help overcoming years of bad habits. Learning how to get a good night's sleep can make a difference in your blood glucose control and your quality of life. As Dr. Buda says, "Sleeping better means living better." And it's not that hard to learn. Get started, and sweet dreams! □

DIABETES AND YOUR SKIN
PROTECTING YOUR OUTERMOST LAYER

by May Leveriza-Oh, M.D.

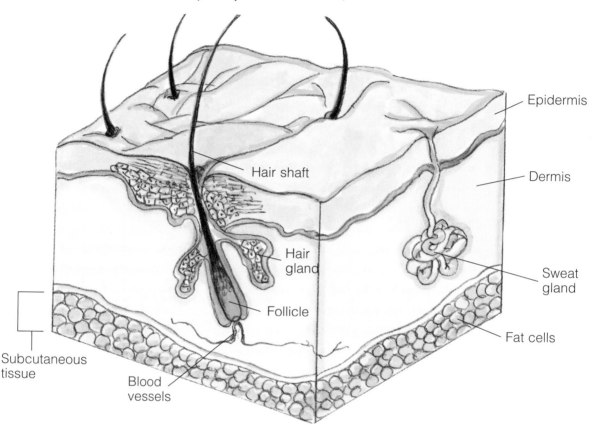

Epidermis

Dermis

Hair shaft

Hair gland

Sweat gland

Follicle

Fat cells

Subcutaneous tissue

Blood vessels

T he phrase "feeling comfortable in your own skin" is usually used figuratively to describe a level of self-confidence or self-acceptance. But when your skin itches, hurts, flakes, breaks out, changes color, or just doesn't look or feel the way you'd like it to, the phrase can take on a new, very literal meaning.

Diabetes can affect the skin in a number of ways that can make a person feel less than comfortable. In fact, as many as a third of people with diabetes will have a skin condition at some point in their lifetime. While some conditions may appear uniquely in people with diabetes, others are simply more common in people with diabetes. The good news is that a fair number of these conditions are treatable or can be prevented by maintaining blood glucose control and taking good daily care of your skin.

Dry, itchy skin

Dry skin can occur as a result of high blood glucose. When the blood glucose level is high, the body attempts to remove excess glucose from the blood by increasing urination. This loss of fluid from the body causes the skin to become dry. Dry skin can also be caused by neuropathy (damage to the nerves) by affecting the nerves that control the sweat glands. In these cases, neuropathy causes a decrease or absence of sweating that may lead to dry, cracked skin. Cold, dry air and bathing in hot water can aggravate dry skin.

Dryness commonly leads to other skin problems such as itching (and often scratching), cracking, and peeling. Any small breaks in the skin leave it more exposed to injury and infection. It is therefore important to keep skin well moisturized. The best way to moisturize is to apply lotion or cream right after showering and patting the skin dry. This will seal in droplets of water that are present on the skin from the shower. Skin that is severely dry may require application of heavy-duty emollients 2–3 times a day.

Itchy skin is usually related to dryness, but it can

460

also be related to poor circulation, especially in the legs and feet. This is typically due to atherosclerosis, a disease in which fatty plaques are deposited in the arteries. Fungal infections, which can be more common when a person has high blood glucose, can also be very itchy.

Bacterial infections

When blood glucose levels are high, a person with diabetes is more susceptible to infection. This is believed to be why there's a higher incidence of certain bacterial infections among people with diabetes and why these infections tend to be more serious than in the general population. The following are some of the more common bacterial infections in people who have diabetes.

Impetigo and ecthyma. Impetigo is a common, contagious, superficial skin infection that starts out as fluid- or pus-filled blisters or pimples that rupture to form erosions on the skin. These erosions are then covered by crusts. Minor breaks in the skin may lead to an impetigo infection, or it may arise as the result of an existing skin problem, such as atopic dermatitis, contact dermatitis, psoriasis, ulcers, traumatic wounds, burns, or insect bites. This infection most often arises on the face, arms, legs, buttocks, hands, and skin folds such as the underarms and groin.

Ecthyma has many features similar to those of impetigo and can in fact result from untreated impetigo. The main difference is that ecthyma goes into the deeper layers of the skin, forming ulcerations, which then become covered with thick crusts. This condition most commonly occurs on the legs and sometimes the buttocks. Poor hygiene increases the risk of ecthyma.

Impetigo may improve on its own, or it may become chronic and widespread. The use of oral antibiotic medicine, coupled with topical antibiotics such as bacitracin, antibacterial soaps, and good hygiene, is typically sufficient to clear the infection within a week. Ecthyma is usually treated the same way but for a longer period of time; generally, antibiotics are taken for 10–14 days. Since lesions (areas of damaged tissue) are deeper in ecthyma, they usually take a longer time to close, and they may heal with some degree of scarring.

Folliculitis, furunculosis, and carbuncles. Folliculitis, furunculosis, and carbuncles are all infections that arise in the hair follicles. Sweat and other conditions that cause moisture on the skin (such as high temperatures and humid weather), the shaving of hairy regions such as the underarms and legs, and the blockage of hairy areas by clothing, bandages, or casts or by lying or sitting in one spot for a long period of time can all increase the risk of an infection in the hair follicles.

Folliculitis is inflammation of the hair follicle that is characterized by the formation of a pustule (a small pimple or blister containing pus) or a group of pustules. Furunculosis is distinguished by the development of furuncles—deep, red, hot, tender nodules—that may develop from the pustules found in folliculitis. The nodules usually enlarge, become painful, and rupture after several days, forming abscesses (swollen areas containing pus). Furuncles generally occur on the neck, face, underarms, and buttocks. A carbuncle is a larger, painful, more serious lesion with a deeper base, generally occurring at the nape of the neck, on the back, or on the thighs. The area is red, swollen, and covered in pustules. Fever and a feeling of illness may also occur with a carbuncle.

The chances of getting folliculitis may be lessened by using clean or new razors to shave, exposing areas of the skin that are typically covered, such as the back, to the air, and wearing loose, cool clothing. Lesions usually improve on their own, but they heal faster with the use of antibiotic washes and creams. Simple furunculosis is treated by the local application of antibiotic creams and warm, moist compresses, which relieve discomfort and promote drainage. A carbuncle or furuncle with a significant amount of redness or swelling or an associated fever should be treated with a systemic antibiotic (one that affects the entire body), since one of the risks of these lesions is an infection of the bloodstream. This can spread bacterial infection to many of the body's organs, including the heart, brain, and kidneys.

When the lesions are large, painful, and fluctuant (they can be shifted and compressed), draining them via surgery is usually the best option. In these cases, the person should receive antibiotics until all evidence of inflammation has disappeared. After the lesion is drained, the area should be covered with a thin layer of antibiotic ointment and a sterile dressing.

Cellulitis and gangrene. Two of the more serious and complicated bacterial infections that occur in people with diabetes include cellulitis and infectious gangrene. Cellulitis is an infection that spreads through the deeper layers of the skin as well as the fat layer directly underneath the skin. People who develop cellulitis usually have an open wound that acts as an entry point for bacteria, although occasionally, the skin infection originates from a bacterial infection of the blood. Areas infected by cellulitis are typically red, warm, painful, and swollen. The lesions feel hard to the touch, and there is no clear line between skin that is infected and skin that isn't infected. This condition usually affects the face and extremities, and sometimes it also occurs on the trunk. The legs are affected three times more often than the arms.

Cellulitis requires prompt medical care. It is important that the health-care provider take a culture to determine what organism is causing the infection so that the right antibiotic is used. Once oral or intravenous antibiotics are started, the average time for healing is 12 days, with a range of 5–25 days.

Infectious gangrene is a serious condition that usually develops on the hands or feet at the site of an injury such as a laceration, needle puncture, or surgical incision. It can also occur in surgical incisions on the abdomen. The condition generally begins as cellulitis, which is followed by fever and other generalized symptoms as the infection rapidly spreads. The area then becomes dusky blue in color, and blisters appear and rupture, forming areas of black skin.

Since the mortality rate (death rate) for infectious gangrene is high, it is important that it is diagnosed early and treated aggressively.

Fungal infections

High blood glucose levels can also predispose people with diabetes to developing common fungal skin infections from organisms such as *Tinea* and *Candida*.

Fungal infections can occur just about anywhere, including the feet (*Tinea pedis*), the hands (*Tinea manuum*), the body (*Tinea corporis*), and the groin (*Tinea cruris*). *Tinea pedis,* or athlete's foot, usually occurs in the web spaces between the toes or on the soles of the feet. Lesions are itchy and may develop vesicles (sacs filled with air or fluid) or may simply be red and scaly. It is usually contracted by walking barefoot on a contaminated floor. To help prevent athlete's foot, it is always a good idea to wear slippers or shoes of some sort in public areas such as locker rooms. *Tinea manuum* is characterized by papules (small, raised pimples or swellings), vesicles, or scaling, typically on the dominant hand, and is associated with touching athlete's foot lesions. *Tinea corporis,* or ringworm, presents as multiple red or pinkish circular lesions with a distinct, scaly border. In severe cases, the lesions may merge, forming large, discolored areas on the body. *Tinea cruris,* or jock itch, results in red to brownish, scaly, itchy lesions that cover the groin and sometimes extend to the pubic region and upper thighs.

Candidiasis of the skin tends to occur in folds of skin such as the underarms, groin, under the breasts, and between the buttocks. This condition begins with pustules on a red base that eventually result in softened, thickened areas of skin.

All of these superficial fungal infections are treated in more or less the same way. Applying antifungal creams two to three times daily for approximately two to four weeks should clear the infection. Keeping the affected areas dry, and using medicated powders in skin folds to reduce friction and moisture are also helpful measures. Infections that don't respond to topical treatment may be treated with oral antifungal medicines.

Skin conditions associated with diabetes

The following skin conditions are strongly associated with having diabetes, but they can occur in people who don't have diabetes as well.

Acanthosis nigricans. This condition is characterized by the formation of velvety, brownish, thickened areas of skin in the groin, underarms, under the breasts, and in the creases of the neck. The affected skin may become leathery or warty or develop tiny skin tags. Acanthosis nigricans is common in people who are obese, but it may also be associated with certain forms of cancer as well as endocrine disorders such as polycystic ovarian syndrome (PCOS), acromegaly, Cushing syndrome, and diabetes.

There is no cure for this condition, but it may improve with weight loss, topical bleaches, or a class of drugs known as keratolytics.

Vitiligo. Vitiligo is a skin disorder that causes white spots or large areas of depigmentation to occur on various areas of the body. About 30% of people with vitiligo have a family history of the condition, and it is more common in people with Type 1 diabetes than Type 2 diabetes. Vitiligo progresses slowly over the years, commonly affecting the backs of the hands, the face, and body folds such as the underarms and groin.

Treatment of vitiligo is necessary only in people who have severe cases or who are considerably distressed by the condition. Treatment involves the use of steroids or chemical agents called psoralens that are either placed directly on the skin or taken orally. The most popular treatment, known as PUVA, uses oral psoralens in combination with phototherapy sessions, in which the person is exposed to ultraviolet light, specifically ultraviolet A.

Granuloma annulare. A common skin disorder of unknown cause, granuloma annulare manifests as skin-colored or pinkish groups of bumps, or papules, that may be arranged in rings. There are several subtypes of granuloma annulare; the one associated with diabetes is called disseminated, or generalized, granuloma annulare, in which lesions are widespread over the body. The use of steroid creams or ointments or steroid injections is sometimes used to treat lesions. Most, however, disappear on their own within two years.

Diabetes-related skin conditions

The following skin conditions occur almost exclusively in people who have diabetes.

Diabetic dermopathy. This common skin condition is characterized by depressed, irregularly round or oval, light brown, shallow lesions. Lesions may vary in number from few to many and are usually found on both legs but are not symmetrically distributed. Because these lesions do not itch, hurt, or open up, they are often overlooked and not reported to the health-care provider.

Diabetic blisters (bullosis diabeticorum). This is an uncommon condition in which blisters occur on the hands and feet and sometimes also the legs and forearms. The blisters are unrelated to trauma or infection; they develop spontaneously and may become quite large. However, they are usually not painful and typically heal without scarring in several weeks.

Foot ulcers. Foot ulcers are a serious problem that can ultimately lead to amputation if left untreated. Each year, about 2% to 3% of people with diabetes develop a foot ulcer. Approximately 15% of people with diabetes develop a foot ulcer at some point in their lifetime.

Foot ulcers are erosions on the skin of the feet. Some affect just the outermost layers of skin, while others extend to deeper tissues. Ulcers often begin as a result of minor trauma, such as irritation from ill-fitting shoes that goes unnoticed or untreated. The most common locations for ulcers to develop are the weight-bearing areas of the foot such as the heel and the ball of the foot and sites subject to pressure such as the toes or ankles.

A number of factors make people with diabetes more likely to develop foot ulcers than those without diabetes. Neuropathy is one risk factor. Almost all people with diabetes who develop typical foot ulcers have neuropathy that affects their motor, sensory, or autonomic nerves. Neuropathy in the motor nerves causes weakness, thinning, and limitation in the movement of certain muscles in the foot, leading to deformities in the normal foot shape such as atypically high arches, claw toes (all toes except the big toe bend toward the floor) and

hammer toes (the longest toe bends toward the floor at the middle toe joint). Neuropathy of the sensory nerves results in loss of protective sensation to pain, pressure, and heat. People with sensory neuropathy may therefore not be aware of cuts, abrasions, and calluses that can lead to ulcers. Depending on the amount of sensory neuropathy, people may even be unaware of major traumas to their feet, such as occur from stepping on pins, glass, and other sharp objects. Neuropathy of the autonomic nerves can lead to warm, excessively dry feet that are prone to skin damage.

Peripheral vascular disease is another factor that can contribute to the formation of foot ulcers in people with diabetes. Because of the decreased blood circulation to the feet in this condition, there is an impaired delivery of oxygen, nutrients, and antibiotics. Therefore, wounds tend not to heal well and to become infected.

Foot ulcers warrant immediate attention and treatment. The physician will need to determine how deep and infected the ulcer is. He may take an x-ray of the foot to check whether infection has spread to the bone. Treatment for a foot ulcer may include oral or intravenous antibiotics to control the infection, as well as dressings and salves with lubricating, protective, antibiotic, or cleansing properties. Taking care of the ulcer and following up with health-care providers is very important for preventing complications that could eventually lead to an amputation.

Necrobiosis lipoidica diabeticorum. This condition occurs in about 0.3% of people with diabetes and is three times more common in women than in men. Lesions tend to form on the fronts and sides of the lower legs, although they may also occur on the face, arms, and trunk. The typical lesion begins as a tiny, dusky red, elevated nodule with a defined border. It gradually enlarges, becoming irregular in shape. It may then become de-pressed and turn a brownish-yellow color, except for the border, which remains red. Affected areas may lack sensation because of the destruction of some nerves and nerve endings.

The course of this condition is usually chronic and recurrent. Although topical steroids may halt progression of active lesions, it is very difficult to completely cure the affected areas. Untreated lesions can readily deteriorate to form shallow, painful ulcers. Unfortunately, not even the normalization of blood glucose levels is sufficient to control this skin condition in many cases.

Digital sclerosis and scleredema adultorum. Digital sclerosis is a condition in which the skin on the hands becomes thickened and waxy and may develop multiple, pebble-like growths. Scleredema adultorum is a similar condition that affects the back and sides of the neck, with the possibility of painless swelling spreading to the face, shoulders, and upper torso.

Although there is no effective treatment for these conditions, they generally resolve on their own within six months to two years.

Saving your skin

To protect your skin and help prevent skin ailments from developing, observe good hygiene. Bathe regularly and wash your hands often. Keep areas of the skin that are susceptible to infections, such as the underarms, groin, area under the breasts, neck, web spaces of the feet and hands, and inner thighs clean and dry. If necessary, use antichafing powders or creams and choose proper clothing that allows air to circulate. After bathing, dry these areas well to prevent infections from beginning. People who live in hot, humid areas should change their clothing once it becomes wet from perspiration.

Be sure to use mild or hypoallergenic varieties of products that come in contact with the skin, such as soaps, lotions, washes, and creams. Products with additives such as fragrances or coloring can irritate the skin or cause an allergic reaction.

Also keep an eye out for skin reactions that arise as a result of allergies to medicines. Reactions to oral drugs may take the form of itching, rashes, or wheals, while reactions to insulin may appear as bumps, rashes, or depressions in the areas where insulin is injected. If you suspect you are allergic to one of your diabetes drugs, inform your health-care provider.

Wounds should be treated promptly. Since people with diabetes may not heal as well as others, it is important to give immediate attention even to cuts and wounds that seem minor. Injuries to the skin should be kept covered and inspected on a regular basis to make sure they are not worsening. The hands and feet should be inspected daily for the presence of cuts or scrapes, since these parts of the body may have decreased sensation due to neuropathy, and wounds may therefore go unnoticed. Dryness and itching can be self-treated, but more serious conditions should be brought to the attention of a doctor.

Preventing foot ulcers

Proper foot care is a vital part of preventing minor wounds from developing into ulcers. This means the feet should be inspected daily for cuts, sores,

or other forms of irritation. The toenails should be cut straight across. (If a person cannot see or reach his feet, a health-care provider should cut his toenails.) The feet should be washed daily in warm water and carefully dried, especially between the toes. A moisturizing lotion should then be applied, but not between the toes.

A health-care provider should examine the feet at least once a year. People with risk factors for developing a foot ulcer, such as neuropathy, foot deformities, calluses, or a history of foot ulcers, should have their feet inspected by a doctor more often, preferably every one to six months. If a person notices a blister, cut, scratch, sore or other form of irritation, he should be sure to notify his health-care provider immediately.

People with diabetes should avoid walking barefoot, even when indoors. Socks or stockings should also be worn to reduce friction between the foot and the shoe. If possible, choose seamless socks and stockings. Socks with lumpy seams can be worn inside out to prevent irritation to the skin.

Wearing shoes that fit is very important, since ill-fitting footwear is a major cause of foot ulcers. People who have not lost the protective sensation in their feet can choose off-the-shelf shoes. Shoes should have some room, preferably ½–⅝ inch, between the front of the shoe and the longest toe. The width of the shoe should accommodate the ball of the foot, and the toes should not be cramped. Selecting a store with a certified pedorthist on staff is a good idea, since this person will know the subtle differences between various styles. It is best to select shoes toward the end of the day, when feet are at their largest.

People who have lost the protective sensation in their feet due to neuropathy or those who have peripheral vascular disease, foot deformities, calluses, ulcers, or other special circumstances should discuss getting customized shoes with their physician.

The skin you're in

A large part of keeping your skin healthy involves maintaining practices that are good for your whole body, such as eating a balanced diet, drinking plenty of water, managing stress, and controlling your blood glucose level. Good diabetes management is especially important, since many skin conditions are related to complications resulting from high blood glucose. By sticking with healthy habits and keeping an eye on your skin, you can avoid many common ailments and be happy with the skin you're in. □

HOW TO AVOID ERRORS IN DIABETES CARE

by Patrick J. O'Connor, M.D., M.P.H., JoAnn M. Sperl-Hillen, M.D., and Becky Klein, R.N., C.D.E.

Medical errors generally make the news only when they are particularly dramatic—the wrong leg is amputated, for example—or tragic—someone dies. But less sensational errors take place every day in numerous settings. Some errors happen in hospitals, some in doctors' offices, some in pharmacies, and some in people's homes, when, for example, two drugs are mixed up or a dose is forgotten.

With all of the steps involved in diabetes care, it is perhaps no surprise that about 80% of people with diabetes experience at least one error in their diabetes care over the course of any one year. Knowing about some of the most common sorts of errors in diabetes care can help you learn to avoid them.

Avoiding incomplete care

Controlling blood glucose levels is often the primary focus of diabetes care, but it should not be the only focus. That's because people with diabetes have a high risk of dying from a heart attack or stroke, so reducing that risk—by controlling blood pressure, controlling blood cholesterol, using aspirin when appropriate, and avoiding tobacco—is important, too. Failing to address a person's risk of heart attack and stroke could be called a medical error.

To get a very good idea of whether you are doing all you can do to prevent a heart attack or stroke, ask your doctor the following questions at your next visit:
■ Is my A1C less than 7%? (Your glycosylated hemoglobin level, also called your HbA_{1c} or A1C level, is a measure of blood glucose control over the previous 2–3 months. The lower it is, the lower your chances of developing diabetes complications.)
■ Is my blood pressure less than 130/80 mm Hg?
■ Is my LDL cholesterol ("bad" cholesterol) less than 100 mg/dl? (For people with heart disease, the recommended goal is less than 70 mg/dl.)
■ Should I be taking an aspirin each day to prevent heart problems?
■ Can you help me stop smoking?

If you are able to achieve the recommended goals for blood glucose, blood pressure, blood cholesterol, and smoking cessation and to maintain those goals over a period of five or more years, you can slice your risk of heart attack or stroke by more than half and very likely add several extra "good" years to your life. If you are not currently meeting these goals, ask your doctor what else can be done to lower your risk of heart attack and stroke.

Avoiding medication errors

Many medicines can be used to help control blood glucose levels, but not all are appropriate or safe for everyone with diabetes. In fact, it is estimated that about 10% of people with diabetes are on a medicine that may not be the safest choice for them. The table on page 466, "Avoiding Medication Mistakes," gives some safety guidelines for choosing which drugs to take. Because so many treatment options are now available, and because so many drugs and other substances can interact with one another, it is important that you and your doctor pick out the medicines that are best for you.

To do your part in avoiding medication errors, do the following:
■ Tell your doctor about any prescription or over-the-counter drugs you are taking. Bring a list of all of your medicines to your appointments, or bring the drugs themselves (in their original containers).
■ Fill all of your prescriptions at one pharmacy, if possible. This makes it easier for your pharmacist to detect potential problems.
■ Keep an up-to-date list of your medicines in your wallet or purse. This can be particularly useful if you need emergency medical care.
■ Talk to your doctor before starting any dietary or herbal supplements. Certain ones are known to interact with prescription drugs.
■ When you refill your prescriptions, note whether your pills (or insulin) look different from those you normally take. If they do, check it out with your pharmacist.
■ Don't stop taking a prescribed medicine because you feel better. Many drugs, including those pre-

AVOIDING MEDICATION MISTAKES

Medication mistakes can include taking a particular drug even though you have a contraindication (medical reason not to take it) and failing to take a drug even though your blood glucose, blood pressure, or blood cholesterol levels suggest you could benefit from taking it. Here are some things to consider regarding drugs used to control diabetes.

IF YOU HAVE THIS SITUATION	CONSIDER THIS OPTION	WHY
Congestive heart failure	Replace metformin (brand name Glucophage) with another drug.	If you have heart failure, metformin can build up in the blood and cause lactic acidosis, a very rare but serious condition. Best choice is insulin.
Congestive heart failure another drug.	Replace rosiglitazone (Avandia) or pioglitazone (Actos) with	These drugs may aggravate or worsen congestive heart failure. Best choice is insulin.
Kidney problems, including a serum creatinine level over 1.4 mg/dl in men or 1.3 mg/dl in women	Replace metformin (Glucophage) with another drug.	Metformin can build up in the blood and cause lactic acidosis, a very rare but serious condition. As kidney problems progress, the best choice is insulin.
Peripheral edema (swollen legs)	Talk to your doctor about causes and treatments.	Both pioglitazone (Actos) and rosiglitazone (Avandia) can cause peripheral edema.
Glycosylated hemoglobin (HbA_{1c}) level above 6.9%	Talk to your doctor about increasing your blood-glucose-lowering medicines.	Maintaining an HbA_{1c} level below 7% reduces risk of blindness, kidney failure, and foot amputations.
Blood pressure above 129/79 mm Hg	Start taking a blood-pressure-lowering drug, or increase the dose(s) of those you are already taking. Certain drug classes called ACE inhibitors, ARB's, and diuretics may be particularly advantageous.	Maintaining a blood pressure level below 130/80 mm Hg is a very effective way to prevent strokes, blindness, kidney failure, heart failure, and heart attacks.
LDL ("bad") cholesterol above 99 mg/dl (or above 69 mg/dl if you have heart disease)	Start taking (or increase your dose of) a drug to lower your cholesterol to the recommended goal. Good choices may include generic simvastatin (Zocor), or atorvastatin (Lipitor).	Maintaining an LDL cholesteol level below 100 mg/dl (or below 79 mg/dl if you have heart disease) typically reduces your risk of heart attack by about 35%.

scribed to help with blood glucose, blood pressure, or blood cholesterol control, are needed to maintain desirable levels once they have been attained. Stopping other drugs, such as some antidepressants, abruptly can cause withdrawal symptoms.

To learn more about the medicines you take, read the information sheets given out with prescriptions by your pharmacist, or talk to your doctor, nurse, or diabetes educator about your medicines. Web sites such as www.webmd.com and www.diabetes.org also offer reliable drug information.

Remember, however, that the information you find on any Web site or book is general information, and that you are an individual with your own personal needs and response to medicines. So talk over what you learn, and your questions, with your doctor.

Avoiding complacency

It's tempting to think that once you've gotten things under control, you can just keep on doing what you're doing forever. But diabetes usually progresses over time, and over the years you will most likely need to increase your medicine doses or add additional medicines to reach your blood glucose, blood pressure, and cholesterol goals—even if you are eating right and getting regular physical activity. It would be a mistake for you and your diabetes care team not to pay attention to blood glucose levels that are gradually creeping up or to any other changes that might indicate that your regimen needs updating. Such changes might include rises in your blood pressure, blood cholesterol, or weight or the onset of any diabetes complications.

Even when your blood glucose, blood pressure, and blood cholesterol are at goal levels, you should have regular (annual or as recommended by your health-care provider) eye exams, foot exams, and tests for microalbuminuria (traces of protein in the urine that signal a higher risk for kidney and heart disease) to check for the presence of diabetes complications. When caught early, diabetes complications are much more treatable.

One often-dreaded change to a person's Type 2 diabetes regimen is the advice to start using insulin. The specific source of dread may be different for different people. Some people, for example, fear needles, while others equate insulin use with more severe disease or fear that the use of insulin may actually lead to complications rather than prevent them. Whatever the cause for resistance, the facts are that many if not most people with Type 2 diabetes eventually require insulin and that the use of insulin can lead to improved control and better quality of life.

Optimal diabetes care typically involves frequent adjustments to your regimen for blood glucose, blood pressure, and blood cholesterol control. If your doctor has not adjusted your medicines or doses recently, ask him to review your medicines with a view to keeping you in good control.

As many tried-and-true medicines go generic, updating your drugs may save you money. Review them with your doctor or pharmacist with a view to lowering costs, and consider using combination tablets that contain more than one drug to reduce your co-pays and the number of pills you take each day. Often, it is both cheaper and safer to use older, proven medicines than to use brand-new ones.

Avoiding insulin errors

Nearly 5 million Americans with diabetes use insulin, which has saved or extended the lives of many more millions of people since it was discovered in 1922. The newer insulins offer a degree of flexibility and control that is greater than that of any other blood-glucose-lowering medicine. Yet there are some substantial risks associated with insulin use and some errors that need to be carefully avoided.

Many people who take insulin use more than one type (usually a long-acting insulin and a rapid-acting one), and it's possible to confuse the two types of insulin and take the wrong one at the wrong time. There are a number of ways to avoid such a mix-up:

■ Keep your rapid-acting and long-acting insulins in consistent and different locations.

■ Mark your vials or pens in some way so it's clear which is which.

■ Note whether one of your insulins is cloudy and one clear. (This won't be the case for everyone, but for some people it may be true.)

■ Note whether the vials or pens for both types of insulin are the same or different shapes and sizes.

■ Use a pen for one type of insulin and syringes and a vial for the other.

■ Some people learn to adjust their mealtime doses of rapid-acting insulin based on their blood glucose level before the meal, the number of grams or servings of carbohydrate in the coming meal, and sometimes on any planned exercise. To make sure you are adjusting your doses correctly, be sure to perform regular blood glucose monitoring and to discuss your readings with your diabetes care team.

■ Some other common mistakes are to skip a dose of long-acting insulin at bedtime because of a lower-than-normal reading (a decision that may cause blood glucose levels to run high all of the next day), to not take insulin when ill (also a decision that may result in high blood glucose), to draw up the wrong dose, to use a vial of insulin or pen beyond the number of days recommended by the manufacturer, and to expose insulin to temperature extremes, rendering it ineffective.

■ Have a sick-day plan that you have discussed with your doctor and diabetes educator. It should specify how to maintain blood glucose control while you are ill and also when to call your health-care provider for advice.

■ Read the information that comes with your insulin and be sure you are storing it correctly and are aware of the number of days an opened vial or pen can be used.

Avoiding hypoglycemia

Have you ever had a blood glucose reading of less than 70 mg/dl on your meter? If so, you have experienced the level of blood glucose at which most people are advised to treat for hypoglycemia. How did you feel? What did you do? It is common to occasionally have readings below 70 mg/dl if you are taking good care of your diabetes. Such low blood glucose levels are usually not a threat to your well-being—as long as you recognize the low blood glucose level and respond to it promptly and appropriately.

Ignoring symptoms of hypoglycemia, on the other hand, can be extremely dangerous, particularly if they occur while you are driving. In that situation, you not only endanger your own life and that of any passengers in your vehicle, but also that of other motorists.

The take-home message is this: If you think your blood glucose level is low, address the problem promptly. Stop what you're doing, check your blood glucose level with your meter, and have a snack if necessary, even if you have to stop your car or interrupt a conversation to do it. (If you don't have your meter with you or can't use it for any reason, go ahead and treat your symptoms of hypoglycemia without checking your blood glucose level first.) Chew and swallow four glucose tablets (containing about 4 grams of carbohydrate each) or drink about 5 ounces of orange juice or a regular (not diet) soft drink. Taking glucose tablets is a good way to treat low blood glucose because it helps you to avoid overtreating.

Sometimes, when people have had consistently higher-than-normal blood glucose levels for a long time, they feel symptoms of low blood glucose when their blood glucose level starts to approach normal. For example, a person who has an average blood glucose level of 200 mg/dl might start to feel symptoms of low blood glucose when his blood glucose level approaches 100 mg/dl. This person is not at risk for serious hypoglycemia. The way to know the difference between a potentially serious low blood glucose level and a false perception of low blood glucose is to check your blood glucose with your meter when you first feel the symptoms. However, as stated earlier, if you are not in a position to check your blood glucose level with your meter, the safest response is to assume it is low and treat it promptly.

Severe hypoglycemia is usually defined as a low blood glucose level that you must have assistance to treat (because, for example, you are too confused to eat or have lost consciousness). If you have ever experienced severe hypoglycemia, it is a good idea to have an emergency glucagon kit in your home or workplace (or both). A friend or family member can learn to give you a life-saving shot of glucagon in case you cannot eat or drink to raise your blood glucose level. However, if neither you nor a companion can deal with your low blood glucose level, instruct your companion to call 911. Paramedics can inject a glucose solution that immediately fixes the problem.

It is a good idea for anyone with diabetes to wear a medical identification bracelet indicating that he has diabetes, just in case he is ever unable to speak for himself.

Avoiding monitoring errors

Your blood glucose meter can provide you with some very useful and important information. When used properly, it can help you learn how specific types and amounts of food, physical activity, and possibly stress affect your blood glucose level. This information can help you plan what to eat and when to exercise, so you stay in better control and avoid low or high blood glucose. If you take insulin, your meter readings can guide you in tailoring your short-acting insulin doses to cover favorite meals or snacks.

To provide you with all of this information, however, your meter needs to be in good working order, and you need to know how to use it correctly. Here are some questions to ask yourself to help determine whether you're using your meter correctly for the most accurate results:

■ Does your meter need to be cleaned periodically? Some do, so check the instruction manual that came with your meter.

■ Do you use control solution occasionally to check the accuracy of your meter?

■ Are the date and time set correctly on your meter? This may be less important if you always record your blood glucose readings immediately by hand in a log, but if you rely on your meter's memory to keep track of your numbers, you need the correct date and time to observe trends in your blood glucose levels.

■ When you start a new batch of test strips, do you need to enter a code in your meter? Some newer meters no longer require this step, but many still do. Those that do will not give accurate results if this step is skipped.

■ When you check your blood glucose, do you get your blood samples from approved body areas? Some meters can be used with blood samples from areas other than the fingertips (such as the palms or forearms), but some meters can only use blood from the fingertips.

■ Are you familiar with general procedure for checking your blood glucose level? Using a blood glucose meter requires that you perform numerous steps, from washing your hands to applying the blood sample to the right spot on the strip. Forgetting a step or performing steps out of order could result in an inaccurate result.

If you have any questions about the correct use of your meter, check your instruction manual, call the meter company's customer service number, or speak with your diabetes educator or another member of your diabetes care team. Your pharmacist may also be able to answer questions about the correct care and use of your meter.

How often and at what times of day you should check your blood glucose depends on many things, including what medicines you take, how much risk you have for developing hypoglycemia, and whether blood glucose information would be helpful to allow you to self-adjust your insulin doses. Many people who take multiple insulin shots (and their doctors) find that occasionally checking their blood glucose level about two hours after meals, in addition to before meals, can help them match their insulin doses to their eating habits and activity levels. Ideally, your blood glucose level two hours after a meal should be no more than 40 mg/dl higher than it was before the meal.

Some people check far more often than is necessary, while others don't check often enough. Discuss with your health-care provider how often to check your blood glucose, when to check, and what to do with your results.

Avoiding errors in the hospital

It's not unusual to be admitted to the hospital at some point in life, so when you have diabetes it makes sense to have some knowledge ahead of time about how your treatment plan could be affected by a hospitalization. Often, oral diabetes drugs are stopped at the time of hospitalization or surgery and insulin is used instead. Insulin has many advantages when you are in the hospital because it allows for a rapid response to changing blood glucose levels.

Typically, nurses will check your blood glucose level for you about four times a day. You can participate in your in-hospital diabetes care by knowing what your readings are and by making sure your meals are designed to accommodate your diabetes control plan. If you feel too ill to speak up on your own behalf, ask a friend or family member to speak up for you.

If possible, talk to your doctor ahead of time about which medicines to continue taking and which to stop (and when) before you enter the hospital. If you are having surgery, it's also a good idea to ask who will be in charge of your diabetes control while you are having surgery and recuperating from it.

If you are in the hospital to give birth, you may be able to retain control over your diabetes management tasks. Depending on the hospital's rules, some women are able to continue using an insulin pump during their stay and to do their own blood glucose monitoring. It's important to find out what's allowed ahead of time, however, so you know what's possible and what isn't.

Your diabetes control plan may change after a serious illness, surgery, or childbirth. Before you leave the hospital, make sure you have in writing what your medicines and doses should be when you arrive home. If some of the medicines you were taking before hospitalization are not on the list, ask why. Also, ask your usual pharmacist to check your new combination of medicines for potential drug interactions or anything that you may be allergic to.

Communication is key

Not all diabetes management errors can be prevented, but many can, especially when you know about the types of errors that are likely to occur. One of the keys to preventing errors is communication with the members of your diabetes care team. If you are not sure how to carry out parts of your diabetes regimen or are not getting the results you expect from your efforts, speak to your doctor or diabetes educator. Regular adjustment of diabetes medicines is the norm as your needs change over time. If you notice changes in your blood glucose, blood pressure, or blood cholesterol levels over time, speak up so that adjustments can be made early and you can stay in the best health possible. □

Women's Health

Tips 773–862 473

Expecting the Best 478
Diabetes, Pregnancy, and Blood Glucose Control

Pregnant and Pumping 484
Great Expectations

Managing Diabetes While Breast-Feeding 490

Vaginitis 493
What Every Woman Needs to Know

Menopause 497
The Latest on Hormone Therapy

Top 10 Health Tips for Women Over 65 503

12

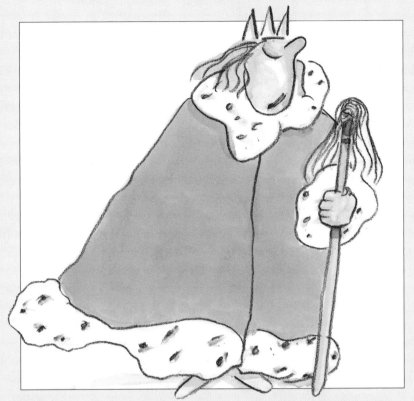

Women's Health Tips

773–862

773. Good blood glucose control before and during pregnancy will minimize all risks to the mother.

774. Ideally, you should strive for near-normal blood glucose levels for at least three months prior to pregnancy.

775. One advantage to using an insulin pump during pregnancy is the ability to make very small insulin dose adjustments.

776. One of the risks of pump use is that if the infusion of insulin is disrupted for any reason, high blood glucose can occur quickly since only rapid-acting insulins are used in pumps.

777. The calorie needs for pregnancy range from 2400 to 2800 calories per day for most physically active pregnant women.

778. Carbohydrate counting is an excellent method of meal planning during pregnancy.

779. Consuming an adequate and consistent amount of carbohydrate helps to keep blood glucose levels in the recommended target range.

780. The normal hormone production and weight gain that occur during pregnancy increase insulin resistance, causing a woman's insulin needs to change during the pregnancy.

781. During the last six months of pregnancy, basal and bolus insulin doses may need to be increased every 7–10 days.

782. To keep tabs on increasing insulin requirements during pregnancy and facilitate adjustments, blood glucose self-monitoring should be done 7–10 times daily.

783. "Starvation" ketones may occur when there isn't enough glucose in the bloodstream to meet the energy needs of both mother and baby.

784. Because the skin has a tendency toward dryness during pregnancy, pregnant women may be more likely to experience irritation at their insulin pump infusion sites.

785. Typically, insulin requirements decrease to 0 at the onset of active labor.

786. While labor leading to a vaginal delivery may lower a woman's blood glucose level, a cesarean section can be stressful to the body and may raise the blood glucose level.

787. Because of the major changes that occur in a woman's body with the delivery of a child, insulin pump basal rates and bolus amounts must be recalculated afterward.

788. Insulin pump therapy can offer flexibility when juggling an infant's feeding schedule with your own meal plan.

789. While having diabetes can make breast-feeding more challenging, diabetes is not considered a medical reason not to breast-feed.

790. Mothers who breast-feed generally have a faster postpartum recovery.

791. The challenges of breast-feeding with diabetes can include more frequent episodes of low blood glucose (hypoglycemia).

792. The composition of breast milk changes constantly, both over time to meet a baby's growing needs, and over the course of each feeding.

793. Both inadequate insulin and low blood glucose can interfere with milk production.

794. The more you nurse, the more milk you will make, and the sooner it will come in.

795. Certain blood pressure and cholesterol-lowering drugs, as well as aspirin, are not recommended for use during breast-feeding.

796. Babies born to mothers with any type of diabetes are prone to hypoglycemia for about 48–72 hours after delivery.

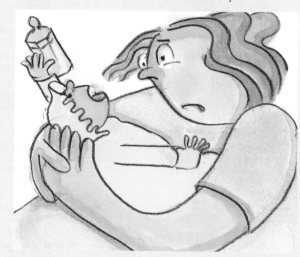

797. A baby who has gotten used to a bottle may have difficulty making the transition to breast-feeding.

798. Insulin is considered safe to take when pregnant or breast-feeding, and there have been no reported cases of adverse effects in babies.

799. Pregnant women should check for ketones every morning before breakfast and any time their blood glucose level exceeds 250 mg/dl. Pregnant women who have ketones in the morning should eat more carbohydrate in the late evening or during the night.

800. Ketones can pass through breast milk and increase the workload for a baby's developing liver.

801. Providing breast milk for one baby requires about 500 additional calories per day.

802. Most women with diabetes experience few problems maintaining a good milk supply.

803. A fetus that is constantly exposed to high levels of glucose can become too large, a condition known as macrosomia.

804. The blood glucose goals suggested by the American Diabetes Association for preg-

nant women are lower than those for the general population with diabetes.

805. Daily urine ketone testing is often advised for pregnant women with diabetes.

806. Diabetic ketoacidosis may develop rapidly and at lower blood glucose levels in women who are pregnant than in those who are not.

807. The rate of miscarriage in women with preexisting diabetes is reduced by keeping blood glucose levels as close to normal as possible in the first trimester.

808. In most cases, gestational diabetes disappears after delivery, but women who have had it have a higher risk of developing Type 2 diabetes later in life.

809. Hormone therapy has been used since the 1960's to alleviate both the short-term symptoms and some of the long-term consequences of menopause.

810. Natural menopause is the result of the cessation of both ovulation and associated hormone (estrogen and progesterone) production.

811. Perimenopause is used to describe the transition period that women go through from their reproductive years to menopause.

812. Diabetes seems to negate the protective effects of estrogen, so women with diabetes are up to four times more likely to develop cardiovascular disease than women who don't have diabetes.

813. In older women who were not previously on hormone therapy, the start of hormone therapy is probably not protective against heart disease and may be harmful. However, in younger women, hormone therapy has not been found to be harmful and is probably protective.

814. Estrogen administered orally or through the skin is an effective tool to prevent and treat osteoporosis by slowing or preventing bone breakdown.

815. As women age, there is an increase in insulin resistance and, to a lesser degree, a decrease in insulin secretion.

816. Hormone therapy is currently approved for the relief or treatment of menopausal symptoms such as hot flashes and vulvovaginal atrophy as well as the prevention of osteoporosis.

817. Estrogen affects brain functions such as body temperature regulation, sleep, and memory.

818. Women who have a blood clotting disorder, a history of previous stroke or heart attack, or cardiovascular disease may be advised not to use hormone therapy.

819. Taking estrogen carries a possible increased risk of blood clots; however, the increase in risk is very small.

820. Estrogen or hormone therapy may cause vaginal bleeding, breast tenderness, bloating, and pelvic cramping. However, these side effects may be temporary.

821. Most studies show that taking estrogen results in an improvement in insulin sensitivity.

822. Women with diabetes are often prescribed micronized progesterone for hormone therapy because it appears not to increase insulin resistance.

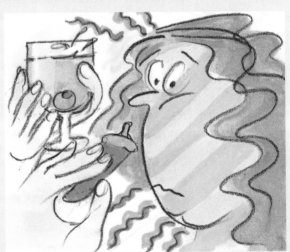

823. For some women, spicy food, alcohol, and caffeine trigger hot flashes.

824. For many women, diabetes is a disease that, perhaps ironically, leads to a longer, healthier life.

825. If you have Medicare Part B, some sessions with a dietitian are covered with a physician's referral.

826. To slow bone loss after menopause, women are advised to get 1500 milligrams of calcium a day.

827. For your body to be able to absorb calcium properly, you also need to get an adequate amount of vitamin D.

828. Make education a priority so that you're informed and knowledgeable about your diabetes care.

829. Skipping doctor visits, exams, or tests to save money could end up costing you a bundle in the future.

830. Preventive measures you can take include getting screened for diabetes complications, cancer, and other conditions; getting immunizations; and taking precautions to prevent falls and injuries.

831. Pneumonia and the flu can be more serious and cause more complications in older people.

832. Doing aerobic, weight-bearing, and stretching exercises can help prevent falls because they strengthen your muscles, increase your range of motion, and improve your balance.

833. Talk to your doctor if you have feelings of sadness or emptiness that last for more than two weeks and are accompanied by any other symptoms of depression.

834. In generalized anxiety disorder, a person feels constantly and excessively anxious. Treatment options include antianxiety medicines, psychotherapy, and relaxation techniques.

835. Getting regular exercise can help you fend off fatigue by giving you more energy during the day and helping you sleep better at night.

836. Get a checkup before you start exercising or increase the amount of exercise you do.

837. Keeping a week's medicines in a pill box that has a separate compartment for each day can help you remember to take them.

838. Don't leave the doctor's office or the pharmacy without being sure when and how often to take your medicines and whether to take them with food or on an empty stomach.

839. Never stop taking a medicine without consulting your doctor first.

840. Some medicines require that you get periodic tests to evaluate whether the drug is working properly.

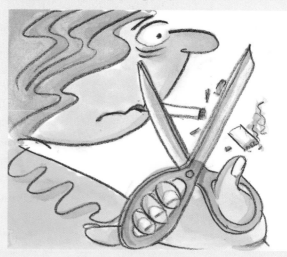

841. Quitting smoking has proven health benefits, even for older people.

842. Catching eye problems early makes it easier to treat them successfully and prevent vision loss.

843. As friends and family members die or move away over time, it's important to make new friends and contacts to avoid social isolation.

844. Some ways to increase your social interaction include volunteering, taking a class, joining a book club, or attending meetings of a diabetes support group.

845. Vaginitis is an inflammation of the lining of the vagina or the vulva that causes itching, burning, unusual discharge, and/or an unpleasant odor.

846. Hormonal changes during menopause or the menstrual cycle and high blood sugar can contribute to vaginal irritation.

847. Bacterial vaginosis, or an overgrowth of harmful bacteria in the vagina, is the most common cause of vaginitis in women of childbearing years.

848. The most common detectable symptom of bacterial vaginosis is abnormal vaginal discharge, often described as thin and grayish-white with a fishy odor.

849. A small amount of yeast occurs normally in the vagina.

850. Yeast overgrowth can occur with use of antibiotics, certain types of birth control pills, hormone replacement therapy, steroid therapy, or even physical or mental stress.

851. Common symptoms of a vaginal yeast infection include itching in the vagina or vulva, as well as burning, painful urination, and pain during sexual intercourse.

852. Studies have shown that as many as two-thirds of all over-the-counter drugs sold to treat vaginal yeast infections were used by women without the disease.

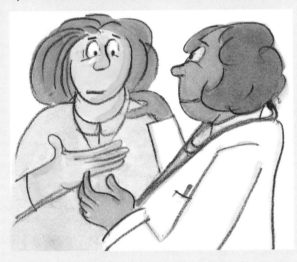

853. A visit to the doctor is the only way to have a vaginal infection diagnosed and treated accurately.

854. Trichomonas vaginalis is a protozoan parasite that causes the sexually transmitted disease trichomoniasis, sometimes called "trich."

855. Many women with trichomoniasis do not notice any symptoms, and infected men are even less likely to have symptoms.

856. Women with diabetes, particularly those with less than optimal blood glucose control, have an increased risk of vaginitis.

857. Vaginal dryness can raise the risk of developing an infection.

858. High blood glucose promotes growth of the fungus that causes vaginal yeast infections.

859. Practicing good hygiene and keeping blood glucose levels under control can help stave off vaginal infections.

860. Feminine deodorants and vaginal sprays can both cause irritation and delay the diagnosis of a vaginal infection if they mask the odor of an infection.

861. Douching can contribute to a vaginal infection by changing the acidity of the vagina. It can also aggravate an existing infection by pushing the organisms deeper into the vagina.

862. Keeping your blood glucose levels under control is beneficial for your vaginal health.

EXPECTING THE BEST

DIABETES, PREGNANCY, AND BLOOD GLUCOSE CONTROL

by Laura Hieronymus, R.N., M.S.Ed., C.D.E.,
and Patti Geil, M.S., R.D., L.D., C.D.E.

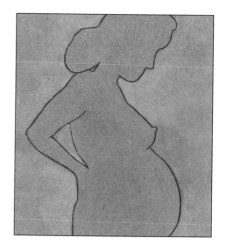

Pregnancy can be a special and exciting time in a woman's life. The anticipation begins as soon as you hear the words, "You're expecting a baby." Once you've gotten used to the amazing news, you may wonder about such things as whether the baby will be a boy or girl, when the baby is due, and, perhaps most important, what you need to do in the meantime to make sure the baby stays healthy and develops normally.

All women feel a certain amount of anxiety and sometimes even fear about how pregnancy will affect them and whether their baby will be healthy and normal. Women with diabetes are no different, but they do have one more thing to be concerned about: maintaining control of blood glucose levels. This is true whether a woman has Type 1 or Type 2 diabetes before becoming pregnant or whether she is diagnosed with a condition called gestational diabetes during pregnancy. The good news is that if a woman who has diabetes (of any type) learns as much as she can about managing her blood glucose and puts that knowledge into practice, she can have a healthy pregnancy and a healthy baby.

Blood glucose control essential

Optimal blood glucose control is important throughout pregnancy, both for the mother's health and the baby's. Glucose in a mother's blood crosses the placenta to her baby, affecting the baby's blood glucose level. (The *placenta*, a flat, circular organ, links the unborn baby to the mother's uterus to provide oxygen, nutrients, and elimination of wastes.) The baby begins making its own insulin around 13 weeks gestation. If the baby is constantly exposed to high levels of glucose, it is as if the baby were overeating: The baby produces more insulin to absorb the extra glucose, resulting in weight gain and an increase in size. Under these conditions, the baby can become too large, a condition known as *macrosomia*. Macrosomia is associated with difficult vaginal delivery, which can lead to birth injury and/or *asphyxia*, a condition in which the baby doesn't get enough oxygen.

Another reason that blood glucose control is important right up to the day of delivery is that if an unborn baby has high levels of insulin on a consistent basis or if the mother's blood glucose level is high during labor, the baby may experience hypoglycemia (low blood sugar) or other complications when the umbilical cord (and the maternal blood supply) is cut.

The details of managing blood glucose levels during pregnancy may be different for women who already have either Type 1 or Type 2 diabetes before pregnancy and for those who are diagnosed with diabetes during pregnancy, or gestational diabetes. (These differences are covered later in this article.) The recommended blood glucose goals, however, are the same.

It is important to note that the blood glucose goals suggested by the American Diabetes Association (ADA) and the American Association of Clinical Endocrinologists (AACE) for pregnant women are lower than those for the general population with diabetes. (See "Plasma Glucose Goals" on page 479.) In addition, the ADA suggests that pregnant women check their blood glucose levels up to eight times per day: once before each meal, again one hour after each meal, at bedtime, and once in the middle of the night. (Any woman who is taking insulin or certain kinds of blood-glucose-lowering pills would need to do additional checks before driving and if she experienced any symptoms of low blood sugar.) Your health-care team may recommend a somewhat different monitoring schedule depending on the type of diabetes you have and how you treat it. However, frequent self-monitoring is needed to ensure that blood glucose levels remain within the recommended range.

In addition to blood glucose monitoring, daily urine ketone testing is often advised for pregnant women with diabetes. Ketones are acid substances that collect in the bloodstream if the body is unable to break down glucose for energy. This can occur if there is not enough insulin to break down glucose in the bloodstream or if there is not enough glucose available to meet energy needs. In either case, the body begins to use stored fat for energy, a process that yields the acidic by-products called ketones. If the body is unable to get rid of the ketones fast enough (via the lungs and urine), they build up and can cause a potentially deadly condition called ketoacidosis.

Ketones in the blood during pregnancy are associated with decreased intelligence in the baby, and an episode of ketoacidosis during pregnancy greatly increases the risk of the fetus dying in the uterus. Diabetic ketoacidosis may develop rapidly and at lower blood glucose levels in women who are pregnant than in those who are not. The best approach for preventing this outcome is to closely monitor blood glucose levels outside the recommended range for pregnancy and to promptly treat elevated blood glucose levels, as directed by your diabetes management team. Notify your diabetes health-care team immediately if you detect ketones in your urine and have a high blood glucose level.

Ketones that occur when there isn't enough glucose in the bloodstream are called "starvation ketones." They may occur in women with gestational diabetes as well as in those with Type 1 or Type 2 diabetes. A woman with starvation ketones would typically have a blood glucose reading in the normal range or lower than normal. If you are getting starvation ketones, your medical team may advise you to increase the amount of calories and carbohydrate in your meals and snacks.

During your pregnancy, if you are not already seeing an endocrinologist, your obstetrician may refer you to one. Most likely, you would see the endocrinologist at least once monthly during the first and second trimesters (approximately the first six months of pregnancy) and every two weeks in the third trimester (the last three months). In addition to your scheduled appointments, you should discuss specific guidelines for prompt follow-up if blood glucose levels are not staying within recommended ranges. Your obstetrician will likely evaluate the growth and condition of your baby throughout your pregnancy with tests such as ultrasound to monitor your baby's size and the non-stress test, which measures a baby's heart rate in response to his or her own movements. Additional

PLASMA GLUCOSE GOALS

The plasma glucose goals published by the American Diabetes Association (ADA) and the American Association of Clinical Endocrinologists (AACE) for pregnancy are lower than the goals recommended for the general population with diabetes. The values shown below are plasma glucose values, the readings given by most meters.

TIME OF DAY	ADA	AACE
Fasting	69–104 mg/dl	60–90 mg/dl
Premeal	69–121 mg/dl	
1 hour after meals	115–138 mg/dl	< 120 mg/dl
2 AM–6 AM	60–120 mg/dl	69–138 mg/dl

testing to monitor your baby's health or yours may be recommended by your obstetrician or by members of your diabetes health-care team.

Insulin needs during pregnancy

During any pregnancy, a woman's insulin needs change, because the normal hormone production and weight gain that occur during pregnancy increase insulin resistance. (See "Insulin Requirements During Pregnancy" on page 480.) In women who do not have or develop diabetes, blood glucose levels remain stable because the pancreas is able to produce more insulin to accommodate the increased demand. In women who have preexisting diabetes or who develop gestational diabetes, the pancreas cannot keep up with the increased demand, so blood glucose levels rise unless steps are taken to lower them.

In women with preexisting diabetes, insulin needs during the first several weeks of pregnancy are not usually that different from those before conception. However, in the latter part of the first trimester, women with preexisting diabetes may have a higher risk of hypoglycemia because of an increase in sensitivity to insulin, rapid fetal growth, and a reduction in eating associated with morning sickness. Around the 16th week of pregnancy,

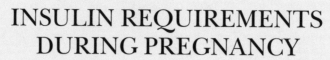

INSULIN REQUIREMENTS DURING PREGNANCY

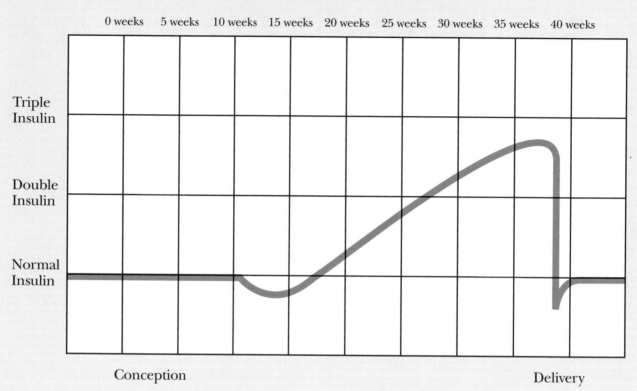

insulin needs gradually increase due to increasing levels of hormones, including human placental lactogen (hPL), a form of "growth hormone" for the baby.

All women with Type 1 diabetes and most with Type 2 either inject or infuse insulin during pregnancy. Women with gestational diabetes also have to take steps to control their blood glucose level, but not all have to inject insulin. Some women with gestational diabetes can keep their blood glucose at recommended levels with changes in diet and moderate exercise. Many, however, must eventually use insulin.

Control before conception

In women with Type 1 or Type 2 diabetes, optimal blood glucose control is essential prior to conception, because it's hard to be absolutely certain of when conception takes place. The incidence of fetal malformations is reduced significantly in women who have near-normal glycosylated hemoglobin (HbA_{1c}) levels before they become pregnant. The rate of miscarriage in women with preexisting diabetes is also reduced by keeping

blood glucose levels as close to normal as possible in the first trimester.

Ideally, you should strive for a near-normal HbA_{1c} test result at least three months prior to pregnancy. It is important to discuss any plans to become pregnant with your diabetes health-care team, particularly if you have vascular complications related to your diabetes such as eye or kidney disease. In this situation, pregnancy is a potential risk to your health. For women with no vascular complications, a thorough physical exam, good nutrition (including a folic acid supplement), and excellent blood glucose control before you become pregnant will help minimize any health risks to you and your baby. Be sure you are using a reliable method of birth control as you work toward optimal blood glucose levels.

Gestational diabetes

Gestational diabetes is a form of glucose intolerance, or difficulty metabolizing glucose, that is first recognized during pregnancy. It affects almost 7% of all pregnancies. Factors that may contribute to a high risk of gestational diabetes include overweight, a history of gestational diabetes with a prior pregnancy, glycosuria (glucose in the urine, which would be found in a routine urine test), and a strong family history of diabetes. In addition, women who are African-American, Hispanic, or from certain Native American groups, as well as women with polycystic ovary syndrome (PCOS) have shown a higher risk for gestational diabetes.

Screening tests should be recommended between 24 and 28 weeks gestation for any woman considered at risk for gestational diabetes by her obstetrician. These tests usually involve drinking a premeasured glucose solution, then having blood samples drawn and checked for glucose level to determine if the body tolerates the glucose load normally. Test levels that are out of range may indicate that the mother's blood glucose levels are likely to rise as the pregnancy progresses.

If you are diagnosed with gestational diabetes, your obstetrician may refer you to a diabetes educator or to an endocrinologist (or both) for help managing your diabetes and your pregnancy. Because blood glucose control is essential during pregnancy, weekly follow-up with the health professional managing your diabetes is usually recommended.

Most cases of gestational diabetes disappear after delivery because two of the primary factors that contribute to insulin resistance and high blood glucose levels are either diminished (the extra weight gained during pregnancy) or gone (the hormones produced by the placenta). If your blood glucose levels were normal prior to pregnancy, they will most likely return to normal after delivery. However, once you have had gestational diabetes, you are likely to develop it again in another pregnancy. You also face a higher risk for developing Type 2 diabetes later in life.

Tools for control

The tools used to maintain blood glucose control during pregnancy are the same as those used to control any case of diabetes. They include a meal plan, an exercise plan, and possibly an insulin plan. **Meal plan.** Whether you have preexisting diabetes or gestational diabetes, you should work with a registered dietitian to design an individualized meal plan for your pregnancy. The plan should focus on foods that provide good nutrition for you and your baby and that help keep your blood glucose level in the desired range. Because carbohydrate has the most immediate impact on blood glucose levels, your meal plan should specify how much carbohydrate to eat and when to eat it. Carbohydrate is found mainly in foods such as breads,

WEIGHT GAIN DURING PREGNANCY

Ever wonder why pregnancy usually involves gaining at least 25 pounds, when a baby weighs only 7 or 8? Here's a breakdown of what accounts for the other 17 or more pounds:

WHAT	POUNDS
Developing unborn baby	7–8
Placenta	1–2
Amniotic fluid	2
Uterus	2
Increase in blood volume	3
Breasts	1
Body fat	5 or more
Increased muscle tissue and fluid	4–7
TOTAL:	*25 or more*

cereals, pasta, starchy vegetables, fruits, and sweets. Frequent blood glucose monitoring will help you determine the appropriate amount and timing of carbohydrate.

Your dietitian can also suggest how many calories you need each day based on your recommended weight gain. The amount of weight you should gain during pregnancy depends on your weight before pregnancy. In general, a woman at a healthy weight before pregnancy should gain 25 to 35 pounds during her pregnancy. Your health-care team may advise you to gain more if you are underweight or less if you are overweight. Keep in mind, however, that pregnancy is definitely not a time to try to lose weight. Most mothers require about 100 extra calories per day during the first trimester and an additional 300 calories per day during the remainder of the pregnancy to ensure the ideal weight gain for the mother and birth weight for the baby. ("Weight Gain During Pregnancy" above illustrates how pregnancy weight gain is distributed.)

In most cases, your dietitian will recommend that you eat three meals a day with two to four between-meal snacks. An evening snack is particularly important to prevent hypoglycemia during the night and urine ketones or nausea in the morning.

EATING FOR TWO

Eating enough of the right foods is one of the most important things you can do to ensure that your baby is healthy. Although nutrient needs increase during pregnancy, most women can meet these needs by eating a balanced diet that includes a variety of foods. However, for some women, prenatal vitamin and mineral supplements, particularly iron, may be necessary. When planning your meals during pregnancy, pay special attention to the following nutrients:

Protein. Pregnant women require an extra 10 grams of protein daily (or a total of 60 grams daily) for a healthy baby and placenta. A three-ounce serving of meat provides approximately 20 grams of protein.

B vitamins. The requirements for B vitamins increase during pregnancy; B vitamins help to metabolize the energy from food and help protein to make new body cells. Getting adequate amounts of a B vitamin called folate, or folic acid, is particularly important in the first three months of pregnancy. Consuming enough folate before pregnancy and in the early stages may lower the risk of neural tube birth defects (birth defects that involve the spinal column) in the baby. Pregnant women require 600 micrograms of folate daily. A half-cup serving of boiled navy beans provides 125 micrograms of folate.

Calcium. Calcium is critical for preserving a mother's bone mass while the baby's skeleton develops. Pregnant women need 1,000 milligrams of calcium daily. An eight-ounce glass of milk provides 300 milligrams of calcium.

Iron. Iron is essential in making hemoglobin, a blood component that carries oxygen through the body to the placenta. It can be difficult to get enough iron in the diet because it is not well absorbed from food, and many women start pregnancy with low iron stores. Pregnant women require 27 milligrams of iron daily. A three-ounce serving of lean beef has almost 3 milligrams of iron.

You may be concerned about the safety of consuming sugar substitutes during pregnancy. At this time, research shows that the four most commonly used sugar substitutes (acesulfame-K, aspartame, saccharin, and sucralose) are safe to use in moderation during pregnancy. Some of these sweeteners do cross the placenta and can reach the baby, but there is no evidence they cause ill effects. If in doubt, follow the advice of your obstetrician.

For more specifics on the components of a well-balanced diet during pregnancy, see "Eating for Two" above.

Physical activity. Regular physical activity is essential to diabetes control and to general health and well-being. Your health-care team can help you determine a safe level of exercise for you during pregnancy. If you have always exercised in the past, you may be able to continue to exercise at a more moderate level while you are pregnant. If exercise was not part of your prepregnancy routine, check with both your obstetrician and endocrinologist before you start, and choose an activity such as brisk walking or swimming to incorporate into your daily routine. Because exercise usually lowers blood glucose, be alert to the symptoms of hypoglycemia, and check your blood glucose level before and after you exercise.

Insulin management. Insulin is the most common medicine used for blood glucose control during pregnancy. Blood-glucose-lowering pills are used much less often because of a lack of data on their safety. However, at least one recent study concluded that glyburide (brand names DiaBeta, Glynase PresTab, or Micronase), when taken by women with gestational diabetes during the last six months of pregnancy, did not change fetal outcome.

Women with Type 1 diabetes may prefer to stick with their usual insulin delivery method during pregnancy, or they may decide to try something new such as insulin pump therapy. For some, using a pump during pregnancy allows them to fine-tune their insulin requirements.

Women with Type 2 diabetes who take pills as part of their diabetes treatment plan are usually advised to switch to insulin during pregnancy. In fact, many health-care practitioners recommend that women with Type 2 diabetes switch to insulin therapy before becoming pregnant. This may help them adjust to insulin therapy and possibly allow them to bring their blood glucose levels into the ranges recommended during pregnancy before they become pregnant.

As mentioned earlier, women with gestational diabetes usually start by seeing how well dietary changes control their blood glucose levels and then add insulin if blood glucose levels do not stay within recommended ranges. Women who must learn to use insulin because of gestational diabetes may find that using an insulin pen is easier than using a syringe. Using premixed insulins, rather than mixing your own, may also simplify your diabetes management.

The most common side effect of insulin therapy is hypoglycemia. Once insulin enters the body and begins working, blood glucose levels may drop lower than recommended if you do not eat to balance the effects, or if you exercise too much. Women using insulin during pregnancy should make sure they receive information about the warning signs and treatment of hypoglycemia. In addition, they should be aware that hypoglycemia unawareness (the inability to detect early signs of low blood sugar) may be more common in pregnant women, especially those with Type 1 diabetes.

Labor and delivery

Most physicians prefer that women with diabetes deliver as close to their due date as possible. Babies delivered after their due date tend to be larger and risk more complications. If natural labor is not timely and a woman plans to deliver vaginally, a hormone called oxytocin can be given, usually intravenously, to induce labor. If a woman is scheduled for a cesarean section, oxytocin is not necessary.

Many women with diabetes are able to deliver vaginally. A cesarean delivery may be needed if a baby is too large (macrosomic), if a woman's pelvis is too small, or if a woman has vascular complications or blood pressure problems. A cesarean delivery may also be required if a baby is in the breech position (when a baby's feet or buttocks enter the birth canal first).

Labor is an intense, active process which can lower a woman's blood glucose level. A cesarean delivery, on the other hand, may raise a woman's blood glucose level because the surgical procedure is a stress on the body. If you have Type 1 or Type 2 diabetes, your doctor may have you on insulin intravenously during labor and delivery. The IV apparatus continually infuses quick-acting insulin and may allow for smoother blood glucose control since adjustments can be made as necessary. The goal is to keep blood glucose levels as normal as possible to prevent hypoglycemia in your newborn. Most women with gestational diabetes do not require any insulin during the labor and delivery process.

After delivery, continuing to maintain blood sugar levels in a near-normal range facilitates the healing process.

MORE READING ON PREGNANCY

For more information on diabetes and pregnancy, you may find the following resources helpful.

Books

Books published by the American Diabetes Association can be purchased through the Internet (http://store.diabetes.org) or by calling toll-free (800) 232-6733.

DIABETES AND PREGNANCY:
WHAT TO EXPECT
American Diabetes Association
Alexandria, Virginia, 2000
$9.95

GESTATIONAL DIABETES:
WHAT TO EXPECT
American Diabetes Association
Alexandria, Virginia, 2000
$9.95

Brochures

These brochures can be read online or ordered by phone, using the toll-free numbers listed below.

Diabetes and Pregnancy
Juvenile Diabetes Research Foundation
http://www.jdrf.org/index.cfm?fuseaction=
home.viewPage&page_id=C7184E81-2A5E-
7B6E-1DC66F56545BF299
To order, call the JDRF at (800) 533-2873.

What I need to know about Gestational Diabetes
National Diabetes Information Clearinghouse
http://diabetes.niddk.nih.gov/dm/pubs/
gestational/
To order, call the NDIC at (800) 860-8747.

Recovery

If you have Type 1 or Type 2 diabetes, your insulin requirements may return to what they were before your pregnancy within a few weeks of delivery. Check your blood glucose levels frequently, and make adjustments in your insulin dosage as needed.

If you had gestational diabetes, it is likely that your blood glucose level will return to normal almost immediately after your baby is born. But since gestational diabetes puts you at increased risk for developing Type 2 diabetes in the future, you should have your blood glucose level measured at your first postpartum checkup (usually 4 to 6 weeks after delivery) and yearly thereafter. To minimize your risk of developing Type 2 diabetes, eat a balanced diet, exercise regularly, and keep your weight at a reasonable level.

Breast-feeding

Diabetes is no barrier to breast-feeding. Breast milk provides the ideal source of nutrition for babies as well as antibodies that fight certain infections. Breast-feeding also promotes weight loss in the mother, may help protect the baby from developing diabetes in the future, and may help to establish a special mother–baby bond.

If you decide to breast-feed, speak with a registered dietitian about the foods you need to eat so that you get enough calcium, fluids, and protein. Breast-feeding in-creases a woman's caloric needs and, because it takes energy, may increase her risk of developing hypoglycemia. Episodes of hypoglycemia are more likely to occur within an hour after breast-feeding, so this is an important time to check your blood glucose level. Napping after meals and snacks is also recommended to lower the risk of hypoglycemia. You may need to adjust your insulin dosage, particularly overnight, to prevent your blood glucose level from dropping during late-night feedings.

Women with Type 2 diabetes who switched from oral pills to insulin during pregnancy are generally encouraged to stay on insulin for at least a month after delivery. For many of the newer diabetes drugs, little or no research has been done on their use in breast-feeding women.

Tough job, big rewards

Managing your diabetes during pregnancy means paying extra attention to your lifestyle during these important months. Though you may feel overwhelmed at times, your health-care team is available to answer your questions and help you attain excellent blood glucose control. The commitment you make now will pay off with the best results in the future: a healthy, happy baby, and a healthy you! □

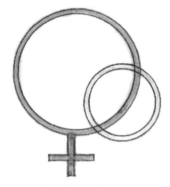

PREGNANT AND PUMPING
GREAT EXPECTATIONS

by Laura Hieronymus, M.S.Ed., A.P.R.N., B.C.-A.D.M., C.D.E., and Patti Geil, M.S., R.D., L.D., C.D.E.

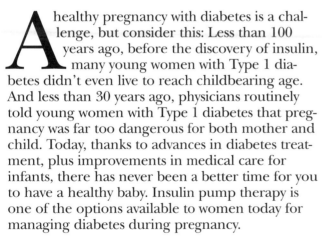

A healthy pregnancy with diabetes is a challenge, but consider this: Less than 100 years ago, before the discovery of insulin, many young women with Type 1 diabetes didn't even live to reach childbearing age. And less than 30 years ago, physicians routinely told young women with Type 1 diabetes that pregnancy was far too dangerous for both mother and child. Today, thanks to advances in diabetes treatment, plus improvements in medical care for infants, there has never been a better time for you to have a healthy baby. Insulin pump therapy is one of the options available to women today for managing diabetes during pregnancy.

Challenges of pregnancy

Pregnancy with diabetes presents a variety of challenges for you and your diabetes management team far beyond the routine morning sickness, fatigue, and strange food cravings experienced by many women who are expecting. The length of time you've had diabetes as well as the course of your disease influences the seriousness of medical risks during your pregnancy. For example, if you have mild retinopathy, it may progress during pregnancy. Your kidney status could worsen. Women with diabetes are at higher risk for frequent and severe hypoglycemia (low blood glucose) during pregnancy because glucose crosses the placenta to provide nutrition for the growing baby. The pregnancy state also tends to allow diabetic ketoacidosis—a dangerous condition usually accompanied by very high blood glucose—to develop quickly. Having a thorough medical evaluation prior to pregnancy is extremely important for determining your individual situation and management solutions. Good blood glucose control before and during pregnancy will minimize all risks to the mother.

Risks to the baby are also a consideration when a woman has diabetes. Most birth defects in infants born to mothers with diabetes are directly related to the mother's degree of high blood glucose at the time of conception. Infants of mothers with poorly controlled diabetes have an increased rate of congenital malformations of the heart, skeleton, and nervous system. Spontaneous abortion, or miscarriage, is also known to occur more often in women with high blood glucose. Additional potential problems include macrosomia, which means the baby is larger than normal for its developmental age, low blood glucose in the baby at birth, and respiratory distress syndrome.

Because the fetal organs are largely developed within the first eight weeks of pregnancy, which may be before you even realize you are pregnant, optimal blood glucose control before conception should be your primary goal. The good news is that if you can maintain normal blood glucose levels before conception and during your pregnancy, you can reduce the risks to yourself and your baby to those of women who don't have diabetes.

Prepregnancy planning

When you have diabetes, it's critically important to plan for pregnancy before conception. For women with no immediate desire to start or expand their family, that includes finding a reliable method of birth control to prevent an unplanned pregnancy.

If you would like to become pregnant within the next year, you should meet with your obstetrician to determine your overall health, stamina, and ability to conceive and carry a pregnancy to term. Genetic counseling may also be beneficial. A diabetes educator can provide intensive education to help you understand the effects of pregnancy on diabetes, as well as work toward optimal blood glucose control for diabetes and pregnancy. Ideally, you should strive for near-normal blood glucose levels for at least three months prior to pregnancy. During this time, be sure to use a reliable method of birth control, and use this time to make sure you have the personal commitment, along with family support, to sustain you through frequent medical and obstetrical visits during the nine months of pregnancy.

Blood glucose control during pregnancy

Regardless of the type of diabetes you have, a goal of optimal blood glucose control is essential for a healthy pregnancy. The blood glucose control goals suggested by the American Diabetes Association and the American Association of Clinical Endocrinologists are lower for pregnant women than for the general population with diabetes. (See "Plasma Glucose Goals" on page 479.) Since your blood glucose goals also depend on the type of meter you use for self-monitoring, be sure you know whether your meter gives whole blood or plasma glucose values. Most health-care professionals prefer the use of a meter that gives plasma-correlated glucose values during pregnancy, if possible.

The following are some strategies for maintaining optimal blood glucose control before and during pregnancy:

Management by a diabetes team. Working with a health-care team that specializes in pregnancy and diabetes is vital to your well-being. Diabetes management team members include a physician to manage your diabetes (such as an endocrinologist); your obstetrician; certified diabetes educators, including a registered nurse and registered dietitian; as well as a pediatrician/neonatologist and perhaps a social worker. Support specialists such as an ophthalmologist and perinatologist may also be members of your health-care team. A reliable health-care team can provide care and support through the process of planning a pregnancy so that when pregnancy occurs, you have help managing both your diabetes and your pregnancy.

Nutrition. If you are planning a pregnancy, meeting with a registered dietitian who specializes in diabetes is recommended. Nutrition assessment generally focuses on calorie and carbohydrate needs for ideal body weight and optimal blood glucose control. A folate supplement to reduce the risk of neural tube defects is recommended for all women of childbearing age.

Physical activity. A good, safe exercise plan that enhances physical fitness assists you with meeting goals for optimal blood glucose control. Physical activity can also be helpful in relieving stress.

Blood glucose self-monitoring. Typical recommendations include frequent blood glucose monitoring during pregnancy, on a schedule of once before each meal, one to two hours after each meal, at bedtime, and once in the middle of the night, for a total of at least eight checks per day. Your diabetes management team may individualize your monitoring schedule to meet your specific needs.

Medication. The medicine most commonly used for blood glucose control during pregnancy is insulin. Women with Type 1 diabetes always require insulin as part of their treatment plan. Women with Type 2 diabetes who take oral medicines as part of their diabetes treatment plan will usually find that insulin, rather than pills, is recommended during pregnancy. With a physician's guidance, a woman with Type 2 diabetes contemplating pregnancy may switch to insulin therapy prior to becoming pregnant. Using insulin may allow a woman to control her blood glucose levels as tightly as possible both prior to and during the early weeks of pregnancy.

The types of insulin used during pregnancy and the method of delivering the insulin should be decided on by a physician with the expertise to manage diabetes. Insulin can be delivered with a syringe, an insulin pen device, or an insulin pump. This article focuses on the use of insulin pump therapy in pregnancy.

Insulin pump therapy

Insulin pump therapy has become an increasingly popular option for diabetes management in the past decade. In fact, the number of insulin pump users grew from 6,600 users in 1990 to approximately 350,000 in 2006. The growing numbers of pump users include women with diabetes who choose to use pump therapy as a means to obtain and maintain the tight blood glucose control necessary for a healthy pregnancy.

An insulin pump is a computerized device about the size of a pager. It pumps rapid-acting insulin at a preprogrammed basal rate, and the pump wearer programs in a bolus amount of insulin at meals and snacks based on the amount of carbohydrate in the food to be eaten. While pump therapy has been used safely and successfully in pregnant women with Type 2 and gestational diabetes, it is *most commonly* part of a pregnancy treatment plan for women with Type 1 diabetes.

Benefits. One advantage to using an insulin pump during pregnancy is the ability to make very small insulin dose adjustments; for example, some pumps allow adjustments in $\frac{1}{10}$-unit increments. In addition, the basal rate of insulin infusion can be changed hourly (or even every half hour, if necessary), allowing the user to closely match insulin delivery with insulin need. These features may be particularly useful as pregnancy progresses, hormone levels change, and insulin needs change accordingly.

Risks. One of the risks of pump use is that if the infusion of insulin is disrupted for any reason, high blood glucose can occur quickly since only rapid- insulins are used in pumps. High blood glucose is always a concern for people with diabetes, but it is especially so during pregnancy when the health of the baby is also at stake.

Low blood glucose, or hypoglycemia, is a risk with any type of insulin therapy, including pump therapy. However, it may be less of a risk with pump therapy. A study published in the journal *Diabetes Care* in 1996 involving 55 people with Type 1 diabetes showed that the incidence of severe hypoglycemia declined more than sixfold during the first year of insulin pump therapy as compared to previous management on multiple daily insulin injections.

Weight gain is another possible risk of insulin pump therapy. It is usually the result of at least one of the following:

■ Improvement in blood glucose control. When blood glucose is high, calories are eliminated in the urine. When blood glucose is brought into the normal range, those calories are instead absorbed by the body.

■ Delivery of too much insulin, leading to hypoglycemia, leading in turn to consuming carbohydrate to raise blood glucose.

■ Managing high-calorie foods or large portions of food with larger or more frequent boluses of insulin.

Working closely with your diabetes management team can help you to minimize any risks associated with pump use.

Self-management requirements

Careful and constant attention to diabetes self-management tasks is essential for any pregnant woman with diabetes. Those who want to use a pump during pregnancy must also be familiar with how to operate a pump and how to troubleshoot if pump problems arise.

Healthy eating. Eating for two doesn't mean eating twice as many calories each day. The calorie needs for pregnancy range from 2400 to 2800 calories per day for most physically active pregnant women. This translates into approximately 300 extra calories a day—the amount found in a snack of cheese and crackers or yogurt with a piece of fruit.

Because your baby's health is so closely tied to your food intake, you should strive to pack the most nutrition power you can into the foods you eat. It's important to eat a healthy variety of foods from all the food groups. The table on page 487, "Healthy Eating," is a guide to the minimum number of daily servings from each food group to meet the needs of women following a 2400-calorie-per-day diet. The food groups marked with an asterisk (*) are sources of carbohydrate; your intake of these foods should be individualized based on your blood glucose levels.

Carbohydrate counting is an excellent method

HEALTHY EATING

This table shows the minimum number of daily servings from each food group
needed to meet nutrient requirements on a 2400-calorie-per-day diet.

FOOD GROUP	SERVING SIZE	SERVINGS PER DAY
Grains, beans, and starchy vegetables*	1 slice bread ⅓ cup cooked beans ½ cup cooked cereal	6 or more
Vegetables*	1 cup raw vegetables ½ cup cooked vegetables ½ cup vegetable juice	4
Fruits*	1 small apple ½ medium banana ½ cup apple juice	3
Milk*	1 cup milk 1 cup yogurt	3
Meat and others	2 to 3 ounces of cooked lean meat, poultry, or fish ½ cup tofu	2
Fats, sweets, and alcohol*	Variable	Consume fats and sweets sparingly. Do not drink alcohol during pregnancy.

* The number of servings of these carbohydrate-containing foods should be individualized based on blood glucose monitoring results.

of meal planning during pregnancy. Carbohydrate is the primary nutrient that affects postprandial (after-meal) blood glucose level; fat and protein have less of an immediate effect. Consuming an adequate and consistent amount of carbohydrate helps to keep blood glucose levels in the recommended target range and is important in promoting a healthy pregnancy outcome. Food sources of carbohydrate include grains, vegetables, fruit, milk, and sweets. Work with your registered dietitian to plan a diet that has the correct amount of carbohydrate for your pregnancy. *Generally, 40% to 45% of your total calories* should come from carbohydrate, although that amount depends on your individual food needs, preferences, and blood glucose levels. A dietitian can determine the target amounts of carbohydrate you need at each meal and snack throughout the day.

Equally important to learning which foods are sources of carbohydrate is learning how to measure out proper portion sizes—to make sure you're eating enough but not too much. You will also need to know how to make adjustments in your insulin doses based on the amount of carbohydrate you choose to eat. A typical insulin-to-carbohydrate ratio is 1 unit of fast-acting insulin for each 10–15 grams of carbohydrate consumed. However, this number is individual and can vary throughout your pregnancy. Self-monitoring of your blood glucose levels is key to using carbohydrate counting as a meal planning method while you are pregnant and pumping.

Changing insulin needs. The normal hormone production and weight gain that occur during pregnancy increase insulin resistance, causing a woman's insulin needs to change during the pregnancy. As the graph on page 480 illustrates, insulin needs during the first several weeks of pregnancy are usually not different from those before conception. However, in the latter part of the first trimester, you may have a higher risk of hypoglycemia because of an increase in sensitivity to insulin, rapid fetal growth, and a reduction in eating associated with morning sickness. Around the 16th week of pregnancy, insulin requirements gradually climb because of increasing insulin resistance (due to weight gain) and increasing levels of hormones, including human placental lactogen (hPL), a form of "growth hormone" for the baby. During the last six months of pregnancy, basal and bolus insulin doses may need to be increased every 7–10 days.

Blood glucose monitoring. To keep tabs on increasing insulin requirements and facilitate adjustments, blood glucose self-monitoring should be done 7–10 times daily. Fasting, premeal, and bedtime blood glucose values can assist in evaluating basal insulin infusion requirements. Checking blood glucose values 1–2 hours after eating can determine the adequacy of your bolus amounts. Many women find that as pregnancy progresses they are up going to the bathroom at least once per night; some take advantage of that time to check their blood glucose. Too-high or too-low blood glucose levels in the middle of the night may signal a need for a basal rate adjustment.

Checking for ketones. In addition to blood glucose monitoring, *many* pregnant women with diabetes are usually advised to do a urine ketone check every morning before eating and additionally if blood glucose is high (above 200 mg/dl) or if they are ill. Ketones are acid substances that collect in the bloodstream when the body is unable to break down glucose properly and begins using fat for energy. If the body cannot get rid of the ketones, they build up and can cause a condition called ketoacidosis. Ketones in the blood during pregnancy are associated with decreased intelligence in the baby. The best approach to preventing and treating ketones is to treat elevated blood glucose levels aggressively, to check for ketones when blood glucose is high, and to promptly use the treatment recommended by your diabetes management team if ketones are present.

Ketones may also occur when there isn't enough glucose in the bloodstream. These so-called starvation ketones may happen to women with preexisting diabetes as well as to those with gestational diabetes. If there is not enough food (glucose) in your system to meet your needs and those of your baby, the body will resort to using fat for energy and consequently produce ketones. In this case, your medical team may advise you to increase the amount of calories and carbohydrate in your meals and snacks.

Prompt troubleshooting. As mentioned earlier, if insulin delivery by an insulin pump is disrupted for any reason, high blood glucose can occur quickly. In this case, prompt action is needed. An injection of rapid-insulin is usually needed to lower blood glucose until delivery of insulin with

IS PUMP THERAPY RIGHT FOR YOU?

For the best results, you should meet the following criteria before starting insulin pump therapy:

■ You should be strongly motivated to improve your blood glucose control.

■ You should be willing to work with your health-care provider as an active member of your diabetes-care team.

■ You should be willing to assume substantial responsibility for your day-to-day care.

■ You should understand and demonstrate correct use of the insulin pump.

■ You should be willing and able to frequently perform blood glucose self-monitoring.

■ You should know how to adjust your self-care routine based on your blood glucose self-monitoring results.

the pump is resumed. The insulin pump should never be disconnected for any significant length of time unless under specific direction from the physician. Frequent blood glucose monitoring is helpful to quickly detect any otherwise undetected interruption in insulin infusion.

Hypoglycemia also requires prompt treatment. Symptoms of hypoglycemia include weakness, shakiness, sweating, and dizziness. If these symptoms occur, ideally you should check your blood glucose level to verify that it is low. If hypoglycemia is not corrected promptly, the blood glucose level may continue to drop, preventing your brain from functioning efficiently and in some cases leading to seizures or unconsciousness.

Treatment for hypoglycemia (typically recommended when blood glucose is 60 mg/dl or less) is usually the consumption of 15 grams of carbohydrate, the amount in about three glucose tablets, one tube of glucose gel, or 4 ounces of fruit juice. A hormone called glucagon, which is given by injection, is available by prescription to treat severe hypoglycemia when a person is unable to eat or drink a carbohydrate source. Discuss proper indications and use of glucagon with your diabetes management team.

Infusion site considerations

Because the skin has a tendency toward dryness during pregnancy, you may be more likely to experience irritation at your infusion site, possibly as a result of the adhesive material at the infusion site, or simply leaving a set in too long. Because irritation can lead to infection, meticulous care of the infusion site is necessary. You should change your infusion site every 24–48 hours and always use it as an opportunity to observe your skin at the site. If skin irritation occurs, work with your diabetes team to determine the cause and treatment. As your pregnancy progresses, you may want to try an infusion site other than your abdomen, or you may want to try an infusion set requiring a different angle of insertion from your usual set.

When the baby arrives

Ideally, you should discuss blood glucose control during labor and delivery—both target goals and method of insulin delivery—with your endocrinologist before you go into labor. Because blood glucose in excess of 120 mg/dl will stimulate the fetal pancreas to produce insulin, making hypoglycemia in the baby a possibility after he or she is born, it is important that your blood glucose level be kept in a lower range. To free you from the responsibility of managing your insulin pump during this time, your endocrinologist may recommend disconnecting your insulin pump and starting an intravenous insulin drip instead. Insulin delivery via an insulin drip can be modified based on blood glucose readings. Typically, insulin requirements decrease to 0 at the onset of active labor. An intravenous glucose infusion can be used to maintain caloric requirements.

Insulin requirements generally remain very low or decrease immediately after delivery. However, the amount of insulin needed immediately after delivery may depend on the type of delivery. Labor leading to a vaginal delivery is an intense, active process that can cause lowering of blood glucose level in the mother. A cesarean section,

on the other hand, is a surgical procedure, which can be stressful to the body and may raise the blood glucose level. In either case, a substantial weight loss occurs at delivery, and the pregnancy hormones that have raised blood glucose levels are diminished, so insulin pump basal rates and bolus amounts must be recalculated at that time. Talk with your physician about this process so you know what to expect. Frequent blood glucose monitoring is recommended to assist with individualizing pump rates and to accommodate other factors such as breastfeeding following delivery.

Breast-feeding has numerous benefits for infants, so unless there is a compelling reason not to, it is recommended for new mothers. Insulin pump therapy can offer flexibility when juggling an infant's feeding schedule with your own meal plan. For one thing, it allows you to safely delay your own meals (and boluses) if the baby needs feeding when you usually eat. It also allows you to use a temporary (usually lowered) basal rate during feedings to avoid hypoglycemia, if necessary.

Are you a candidate for pump therapy?

Day-to-day diabetes management is largely up to you. Having an insulin pump does not relieve you of your diabetes self-management responsibilities. Consider the criteria for trying insulin pump therapy on page 488. If you choose an insulin pump, it is ideal to begin the therapy prior to becoming pregnant. This allows for learning and mastering the use of the pump while working to achieve optimal glycemic control before you become pregnant. If you are interested in using an insulin pump for diabetes management, work with your health-care team to assure you have a full understanding if pump therapy is right for you. □

MANAGING DIABETES WHILE BREAST-FEEDING

by Christine Bradley

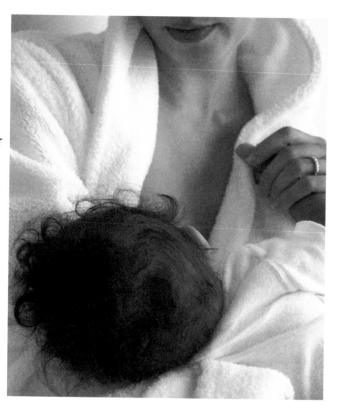

Like all new mothers, those with diabetes face the important decision of whether or not to breast-feed their baby. The benefits of breast-feeding for both mother and infant are well established, and while having diabetes can make breast-feeding more challenging, diabetes is not considered a medical reason not to breast-feed. With the right information and support, mothers who wish to breast-feed can overcome the hurdles that having diabetes may place in their paths and enjoy all of benefits that breast-feeding has to offer.

Benefits and challenges for the mother

Mothers who breast-feed generally have a faster postpartum recovery, faster return of the uterus to its prepregnant size, higher likelihood of returning to their prepregnant weight, delayed resumption of menstrual cycles, and reduced risk of breast, uterine, and ovarian cancer later in life. Breast-feeding can also contribute to feelings of attachment between mother and child.

The challenges of breast-feeding with diabetes can include more frequent episodes of low blood glucose (hypoglycemia). Because breast-feeding burns a lot of calories, a new mother may need to lower her insulin doses (or doses of oral diabetes drugs) and/or eat more food to prevent hypoglycemia.

Benefits for the baby

Breast milk is the perfect baby food. It is packed with live immune cells, immunoglobulins, proteins, fats, carbohydrates (mainly in the form of lactose), various enzymes, vitamins, minerals, and fluid. Breast milk contains an ideal balance of nutrients for an infant and is easy to digest.

The composition of breast milk changes constantly, both over time to meet a baby's growing needs, and over the course of each feeding. The milk produced at the start of a feeding, called foremilk, is watery and not as dense in calories as milk that comes later in the feeding. Foremilk quenches a baby's thirst early in the feeding.

The milk that follows is called hindmilk, and it is rich, creamy, and dense in calories. A baby's suckling stimulates the release of the hormone *oxytocin,* which triggers the milk-ejection reflex, often referred to as the "let-down" reflex. The milk-ejection reflex releases hindmilk, which provides a baby with enough calories to grow and to feel satisfied at the end of a feeding.

In addition to providing the basic nutrients a baby needs to grow and stay healthy, breast-feeding may have some lifelong benefits. Research indicates that breast-feeding may be associated with a lower incidence of Type 1 diabetes in children and possibly of Type 2 diabetes and obesity.

All about lactation

Lactation, or the secretion of milk, is usually divided into three phases: lactogenesis I, lactogenesis II, and lactogenesis III. Lactogenesis I occurs at approximately 16 weeks gestation, when breast tissue has developed to the point where the woman is fully capable of lactation. At this point the breasts contain *colostrum,* a clear yellow substance rich in nutrients. The breasts continue to produce colostrum until a few days after delivery.

Lactogenesis II refers to the significant increase in milk production that occurs 2–3 days after delivery. This stage is often referred to as the milk "coming in." A woman knows she is expressing milk rather than colostrum because the milk looks white or yellowish-white and has a milky consistency. Colostrum is golden yellow and much thicker.

Lactogenesis III is just the continuation of lactation until weaning occurs and the mammary glands cease to secrete milk.

In women with Type 1 diabetes, lactogenesis II may be delayed by as much as two or three days. Women with Type 2 diabetes may also experience a delay, but usually a shorter one. If lactogenesis II is delayed, a woman may still produce small amounts of colostrum, but it may not be enough to hydrate and nourish a baby that is hypoglycemic or has jaundice, a condition in which the skin and eyes appear yellow because there is too much of a substance called *bilirubin* in the blood. Bilirubin is formed when red blood cells break down.

There are several possible reasons for the delay in lactogenesis. One is that breast tissue is very sensitive to insulin levels and requires insulin to produce milk. In effect, the breasts are competing with the rest of the body for available insulin. Inadequate insulin, therefore, can cause lowered or delayed milk production.

Low blood glucose can also interfere with lactogenesis, because when a person becomes hypoglycemic, the adrenal glands release *epinephrine,* which reduces milk production and milk let-down. Also known as adrenaline, epinephrine is a stress hormone that causes many of the symptoms of hypoglycemia.

Dealing with a delay

There are several things to keep in mind when you're waiting for your milk to come in. The first is that nursing frequently is extremely important to long-term breast-feeding success. It is important for all babies to be breast-fed at least every 2–4 hours, but for mothers with diabetes, this is especially important. Frequent nipple stimulation triggers a hormonal positive feedback system that results in an increase in milk production. The more you nurse, the more milk you will make, and the sooner it will come in.

Nursing frequently will also ensure that your baby gets plenty of colostrum, which is exactly what your baby needs at this time. In addition, frequent nursing will give you and your baby the opportunity to practice positioning and latch-on, so that when your milk does come in, your baby will be a pro at effective suckling.

A second thing to be aware of is your body's changing insulin needs. Because a woman's body uses up large amounts of glucose to produce milk,

lactation has an insulin-sparing effect, so that mothers who take insulin may need less of it.

If you have Type 2 diabetes and take oral drugs to lower your blood glucose levels, your doses may similarly need to be adjusted. Women with Type 2 diabetes sometimes experience decreased insulin resistance with breast-feeding, possibly as a result of weight loss associated with breast-feeding or possibly due to some other metabolic change. Whatever the reason, frequent blood glucose monitoring can help you to establish a new food and medicine routine to keep your diabetes under control. Work with your endocrinologist or obstetrical care provider to come up with a plan that works well with your body.

Certain blood pressure and cholesterol-lowering drugs are not recommended for use during breast-feeding. If you take such drugs, speak to your doctor about the safety of continuing them while you nurse. Taking aspirin is also generally not recommended during pregnancy or breast-feeding. If you were previously advised to take aspirin regularly to lower your risk of heart attack, speak to your doctor about alternative means to protect your heart health during this time.

Care of the baby

Babies born to mothers with any type of diabetes are prone to hypoglycemia for about 48–72 hours after delivery. Hypoglycemia is particularly likely if a mother's blood glucose levels were consistently high during pregnancy, causing the fetus to produce a high level of insulin. (A high birth weight, which is also more common among babies born to women with diabetes, is an indicator that a baby may have been exposed to high levels of glucose in the uterus.) After birth, the baby continues to produce a high level of insulin, but its source of glucose is gone, resulting in hypoglycemia.

The nursery staff will monitor your baby's blood glucose levels closely and watch for signs of hypoglycemia such as a low body temperature. Once a mother's milk has come in and the baby is nursing, or if the baby is given formula, hypoglycemia is usually no longer a concern.

In the first few days after delivery, your baby's pediatrician and nurses may urge you to feed your baby formula until your milk comes in to stabilize your baby's blood glucose levels. There are some pros and cons to this. Maintaining hydration and a normal blood glucose level through the help of supplementation can help your baby to maintain his body temperature and be more awake and less lethargic so that when he does nurse, he is alert.

The downside is that introducing artificial nipples before breast-feeding has been established can cause *nipple confusion,* in which an infant has difficulty latching on to and suckling a human breast after exposure to a pacifier or bottle. The sucking technique used to get milk out of a bottle is different from that used to get milk from a breast, and a baby who has gotten used to a bottle may have difficulty making the transition to breast-feeding. Also, the early exposure to formula may increase the baby's risk of developing an allergy to cow's milk protein, especially if there is a family history of milk allergy.

A good compromise if you choose to supplement with formula is to feed your baby through a finger feeder or a supplemental nursing system. A finger feeder is a feeding system that allows you to put breast milk or formula into a small container or syringe that has tubing connected to it. You hold the container in your hand and place the tubing on your finger so that the baby takes both the tubing and the finger into his mouth to nurse. A supplemental nursing system (one popular brand of which is Lact-Aid) works similarly except that the container hangs on a cord around your neck and the tubing is placed on your nipple, so that your baby latches on to your breast as if he were breast-feeding, but he receives the nutrition he needs through the tube.

If you are concerned about cow's milk allergy, speak to your pediatrician about using a protein hydrolysate formula (often called a "hypoallergenic" formula). The cow's milk proteins in these formulas have been broken down in a process that mimics digestion, so they are less likely to cause an allergic reaction. Protein hydrolysate formulas are more expensive than regular formulas, but you may consider it worth the extra cost if you're only going to be supplementing for a few days until your milk supply is established.

A common concern among mothers with diabetes is that insulin will pass through breast milk and lower their baby's blood glucose level. Regular insulin does not appear in breast milk. Studies have yet to show whether insulin analogs, such as lispro (Humalog), aspart (NovoLog), glulisine (Apidra), glargine (Lantus), or detemir (Levemir), appear in breast milk. However, insulin is considered safe to take when pregnant or lactating, and there have been no reported cases of adverse effects in babies.

On the other hand, if you have insufficient insulin in your system and start producing ketones, they can pass through breast milk and affect your baby's health. Ketones are produced when the body breaks down fat for energy. This typically happens when a person doesn't have enough insulin on board to enable glucose to enter the cells. Ketones increase the workload for your baby's developing liver, which can aggravate hyperbilirubinemia and worsen jaundice.

Nutrition during lactation

Good nutrition during lactation is an important part of managing your diabetes. Interestingly, while the foods you eat can cause some slight variations in the content of your breast milk, diet does not have a huge impact on breast milk composition. In fact, you usually can't change your milk content drastically by what you eat. For example, consuming a low-fat diet won't give you skim milk. Widespread studies have found that women from all different parts of the world and from different economic situations have pretty much the same quality of breast milk.

However, the foods you eat still affect your body and your diabetes management. Providing breast milk for one baby requires about 500 additional calories per day. While working on weight-loss goals, meet with a dietitian to find a gradual weight-loss plan that allows you to continue eating healthy foods. Keep in mind that breast-feeding women use about 200 calories per day of their own fat stores to produce breast milk and may lose weight more rapidly than women who do not breast-feed.

Never consume less than 1800 calories a day. Keep the ratio of carbohydrate to fat to protein roughly the same as you did before your pregnancy, but remember that you may need additional carbohydrate at times to prevent or treat hypoglycemia. To avoid big fluctuations in blood glucose levels, choose foods with a low glycemic index or low glycemic load, such as milk, apples, nuts, and carrot sticks.

Dealing with a low milk supply

Other than the initial delay in lactogenesis II, most women with diabetes experience few problems maintaining a good milk supply. Some possible causes of low milk supply in women with either Type 1 or Type 2 diabetes can include prolonged or frequent hypoglycemia, dehydration, stress, and illness. If you think your milk supply may be low, nurse more frequently, or use a breast pump between feedings to stimulate your nipples. In addition, drink plenty of fluids, and rest. It can also help to consult a lactation consultant for guidance or just for reassurance that you're doing the right things.

If you would like to try a dietary supplement to increase your milk supply, talk to a lactation consultant. The supplement most commonly used for this purpose is fenugreek, but it may not be the best choice for women with diabetes. Fenugreek has historically been used to lower blood glucose and cholesterol levels, and there is some modern scientific evidence that it is effective for these uses. If a woman with diabetes were to develop hypoglycemia as a result of taking fenugreek, she could actually worsen her milk supply by causing an increased epinephrine release.

Another botanical supplement traditionally used to increase milk supply is an herb called blessed thistle. However, there have been no large scientific studies examining either its safety or effectiveness.

Your doctor can also prescribe drugs to help increase your milk supply if you have been using the above methods for a couple of weeks with little results.

Worth the challenge

The decision about whether or not to breast-feed is a personal one that only you can make after consulting your doctor and your baby's pediatrician.

Unless there is a medical reason not to nurse, the choice of whether to breast-feed is ultimately up to you, and your health-care provider should support you in whichever feeding method you choose.

If you decide that breast-feeding is right for you, educate yourself ahead of time so that you will be prepared for the changes that your body will go through during lactation. Attending a breast-feeding class or a La Leche League meeting as well as reading a good book about breast-feeding such as *The Womanly Art of Breastfeeding*, by the La Leche League International, can be of help. Having a solid foundation of general breast-feeding knowledge, and seeking the help of a lactation consultant, dietitian, and endocrinologist, as necessary, will help prepare you for situations that may arise. While the first few weeks of breast-feeding can be a challenge, many women with Type 1, Type 2, and gestational diabetes are eventually able to breast-feed successfully for as long as they wish to continue. □

VAGINITIS
WHAT EVERY WOMAN NEEDS TO KNOW

by Laura Hieronymus, M.S.Ed., A.P.R.N., B.C.-A.D.M., C.D.E.,
and Kristina Humphries, M.D.

Chances are that most women reading this article have experienced or will experience a case of vaginitis at least once in their lifetime. In fact, vaginitis is the number-one reason why American women visit their doctor; it accounts for over 10 million office visits annually. Given the prevalence of this condition, one would think women would be well informed about it. Unfortunately, misconceptions about vaginal health abound, and some women may not have heard of vaginitis, let alone know how to deal with it properly.

Vaginitis is an inflammation of the lining of the vagina or the vulva, the exterior part of a woman's genitals, that causes itching, burning, unusual discharge, and/or an unpleasant odor. Most often, the irritation is caused by an infection, although there are other possible causes, such as tumors, certain drug therapies, radiation therapy, foreign objects in the vagina, vaginal contact with fecal matter, or irritants in soaps, douches, spermicides, or other ingredients in barrier contraceptives. In

addition, hormonal changes during menopause or the menstrual cycle, high blood sugar, poor personal hygiene, or restrictive underwear may contribute to the problem. Women with HIV, who have a compromised immunologic status, are at increased risk for some types of vaginitis.

This article focuses on the three infections that most commonly cause vaginitis: bacterial vaginosis, vulvovaginal candidiasis (yeast infection), and trichomoniasis. While it was once thought that vaginal infections were generally harmless, there is evidence that some types of infection can have serious consequences if they go untreated, including complications during pregnancy or infertility. Symptoms usually resolve quickly with medication, but determining which infection is causing them is necessary for effective treatment.

Bacterial vaginosis

This type of infection, the most common cause of vaginitis in women of childbearing years, occurs when there is an overgrowth of harmful bacteria in

WHAT KIND OF VAGINITIS IS IT?

While the amount and consistency of a woman's normal vaginal discharge varies slightly throughout the menstrual cycle, a significant increase or change in the appearance of the discharge may indicate an infection. If you notice abnormal discharge or odor as described in the chart below, don't try to self-diagnose your condition, but call your doctor to discuss your symptoms.

Diagnostic Criteria	Normal (no vaginitis)	Bacterial vaginosis	Trichomoniasis	Candida vulvovaginitis
Discharge	White, thin, fluffy	Thin, white, gray	Yellow, green, frothy	White, curdy, "cottage cheese-like"
Typical odor	None	Fishy	Fishy	None

the vagina. In the United States, as many as 16% of pregnant women experience bacterial vaginosis. A healthy vagina is slightly acidic and is host to both protective and harmful bacteria, yeast, and other microorganisms. If the normal balance of bacteria in the vagina changes and the vagina becomes less acidic, the harmful bacteria can flourish, and bacterial vaginosis can result. Although this infection is usually associated with sexual activity, it can also occur in women who are not sexually active.

Symptoms. An estimated 50% of women with bacterial vaginosis have no symptoms, but the most common detectable symptom is abnormal vaginal discharge, described as thin and grayish-white with a fishy odor. Many women complain that the odor is particularly strong following sexual intercourse or at the time of menstruation. Itching or soreness is rarely associated with this condition.

Detection. Because of the potential lack of symptoms, diagnosis of bacterial vaginosis needs to be confirmed by microscopic evaluation of vaginal discharge for the presence of "clue cells," which are cells coated with the bacteria that cause the infection. These cells, along with a decrease in the acidity of the vagina, the absence of certain beneficial bacteria in the vaginal secretions, and the characteristic odor, are all indicative of bacterial vaginosis.

Treatment. The most commonly prescribed treatment for bacterial vaginosis is an antibiotic regimen. Metronidazole, available as an oral medicine or as a topical gel, or clindamycin, which can be taken orally or as a suppository, are the treatments of choice for most women with positive laboratory analysis of the infection. These drugs are available by prescription from a doctor, and the treatment typically lasts seven days. It is important to note that metronidazole should not be combined with alcohol, as severe nausea and vomiting can result. Because studies show there is some correlation between bacterial vaginosis and premature delivery and low-birth-weight babies, the U.S. Centers for Disease Control and Prevention recommends that all pregnant women who have previously delivered a premature baby be screened for bacterial vaginosis, whether or not they have symptoms of the condition. In addition, some physicians recommend that all women undergoing a hysterectomy or abortion be treated for bacterial vaginosis prior to the procedure, regardless of symptoms, to reduce their risk of developing pelvic inflammatory disease. Male sexual partners do not generally require treatment for this infection.

Vulvovaginal candidiasis

Vulvovaginal candidiasis, or vaginal yeast infection, is the vaginal infection that women most often hear about and the one women with diabetes may have the most trouble with. It occurs at least once a lifetime in approximately three out of four women. Like bacteria, a small amount of yeast occurs normally in the vagina. However, when yeast growth becomes excessive, it can cause symptoms that can be quite uncomfortable. Yeast overgrowth can occur with use of antibiotics, certain types of birth control pills, hormone replacement therapy, steroid therapy, or even physical or mental stress. Women who are pregnant, are obese, or have HIV or poorly controlled diabetes may be more susceptible to yeast infections.

Symptoms. Most women complain of itching in the vagina or vulva that can be constant and quite irritating. Other symptoms may include burning, painful urination, or pain during sexual intercourse. Vaginal discharge is usually heavier than normal, and its appearance varies from a thin whitish-gray to a thick cottage-cheese-like consistency. Usually this discharge is odorless.

Detection. A microscopic analysis of the vaginal secretions for yeast overgrowth is necessary for an accurate diagnosis. Your doctor will take into consideration both your symptoms and your medical history to determine the cause of the infection.

Treatment. Because yeast infections are caused by a fungus, successful treatment entails an antifungal medicine, such as fluconazole, ketoconazole, or terconazole. These prescription drugs are usually delivered intravaginally, in the form of vaginal tablets, creams, or suppositories, although pills are also available. Generally, topical or intravaginal antifungal treatments have fewer side effects and may begin to work faster than oral medicines. Women with diabetes who use a sulfonylurea (such as Amaryl, DiaBeta, Glucotrol, Glynase, or Micronase) may have an increased risk of hypoglycemia if they use an oral antifungal drug.

In addition to prescription drugs, there are several over-the-counter (OTC) remedies for yeast infections. While these treatments can be effective, it's important to see a doctor before using an OTC product. Many vaginal infections are caused by bacteria, not yeast, but women tend to assume that any symptoms of vaginitis indicate a yeast infection.. Studies have shown that as many as two-thirds of all OTC drugs sold to treat vulvovaginal candidiasis were used by women without the disease.

Self-treating with the wrong medicine is counterproductive and can allow an existing infection to become more serious. If you have been evaluated by your doctor and treated for a yeast infection at least twice and feel you can recognize the symptoms, he may advise you to treat recurring infections on your own. However, if you are having frequent yeast infections, see your doctor. He may be able to determine the underlying cause and address the infection with specialized treatment.

If you use a topical treatment, be aware that oil-based creams and suppositories may weaken latex condoms and diaphragms. Check with your pharmacist regarding this potential problem. Male partners do not generally experience symptoms or need treatment, although some report developing a rash or a burning sensation if a condom is not used during sexual activity.

Trichomoniasis

Trichomonas vaginalis is a protozoan parasite that causes the sexually transmitted disease trichomoniasis, sometimes called "trich." It can occur in both women and men and affects up to 7.4 million Americans annually. The vagina is the most common site of infection in women, although the urethra may be infected in both men and women.

Symptoms. In women, symptoms may include a thick, yellowish-green or gray discharge from the vagina, pain or discomfort during sexual intercourse or urination, and a fishy vaginal odor. Other possible symptoms are itching or irritation of the vaginal area and lower abdominal pain. Many women with trichomoniasis do not notice any symptoms, and infected men are even less likely to have symptoms (burning or irritation after urination or ejaculation), which makes it easy for this infection to be passed back and forth between partners, leading to chronic reproductive or urinary complications.

Detection. If trichomoniasis is the cause of the infection, microscopic analysis will show the presence of trichomonads in the vaginal secretions. In addition, a blood test may show an elevated white blood cell count with trichomoniasis.

Treatment. Because the infection is sexually transmitted, both partners should be treated, and sexual intercourse should be avoided until both partners are infection-free. The prescription drug metronidazole is typically used to treat trichomoniasis. This drug may be administered in a single oral dose or taken in smaller doses for a week. Combining this drug with alcohol can result in severe nausea and vomiting. In those who take an anticoagulant, metronidazole—or any other antibiotic—may increase the risk of bleeding.

Diabetes and vaginitis

While all women are susceptible to the infections above, women with diabetes, particularly those with less than optimal blood sugar control, have an increased risk for vaginitis. One reason for this is vaginal dryness, which may occur if the nerves in the vagina are damaged as a result of frequent or prolonged high blood glucose levels. Vaginal dryness can contribute to pain and irritation during and after sexual activity and can raise the risk of developing an infection. Many doctors recommend a water-based lubricant gel or a vaginal cream with estrogen to relieve irritation from vaginal dryness.

When blood glucose levels are not well controlled, women tend to see an increase in the frequency of vulvovaginal candidiasis infections. In fact, recurrent or stubborn yeast infections are one of the clues that can help doctors to detect diabetes in undiagnosed women. High blood sugar promotes growth of the Candida albicans fungus that causes the infection. Because yeast thrive on sugar, they can exceed normal levels, causing recurrent infections if better blood sugar control is not

FOR FURTHER INFORMATION

While a visit to the doctor is the only way to have a vaginal infection diagnosed and treated accurately, information from the following resources can help you to recognize symptoms of infections, understand treatment options, and get answers to other reproductive health concerns.

NATIONAL CENTER FOR INFECTIOUS DISEASES, CENTERS FOR DISEASE CONTROL AND PREVENTION
www.cdc.gov/ncidod/diseases/index.htm
The Centers for Disease Control and Prevention provides national health statistics and data, health information and updates on disease outbreaks for travelers, and fact sheets on a range of health topics. For information on vaginal infections, look up the specific infection in the infectious disease index or use the CDC search feature.

THE NATIONAL WOMEN'S HEALTH INFORMATION CENTER
www.4woman.gov
Run by the Office on Women's Health, a division of the Department of Health and Human Services, this is the official federal Web site on women's health issues. The site provides recent health news of interest to women, resources for support, and links to reliable health information. A site-wide search for vaginitis brings up a list of federal and nonfederal Web sites with information on common vaginal infections.

NATIONAL INSTITUTE OF ALLERGY AND INFECTIOUS DISEASES, NATIONAL INSTITUTES OF HEALTH
www.niaid.nih.gov/publications
Click on "Sexually Transmitted Diseases" or "Women's Health" for information on vaginal infections and many other topics. For a free fact sheet on vaginitis due to vaginal infections, write to NIAID Office of Communications and Public Liaison, NIH, Building 31, Room 7A50, 31 Center Drive, MSC 2520, Bethesda, MD 20892-2520.

AMERICAN DIABETES ASSOCIATION
www.diabetes.org
The ADA Web site explains how diabetes affects a woman's sexual health, covering such topics as vaginitis, menopause, birth control, pregnancy, and sexual dysfunction. From the home page, open "All About Diabetes", click on either "Type 1 Diabetes" or "Type 2 Diabetes," scroll down to "Women and Diabetes".

AMERICAN COLLEGE OF OBSTETRICIANS AND GYNECOLOGISTS
www.acog.org
While this site is primarily aimed at health-care professionals, visitors can access reproductive health news, publications, , and a physician referral service. Free patient education pamphlets can be ordered online or by calling (800) 762-2264.

attained. Finally, higher-than-normal blood glucose impairs the body's ability to fight infection. This may increase the chances of getting an infection, as well as prolong the duration of the condition.

Defending yourself

The best strategy against vaginitis is a good defense. Practicing good hygiene, keeping blood glucose levels under control, and eliminating potential irritants can help stave off unpleasant infections. The following preventive steps are important to vaginal health:

Wear absorbent, loose, dry clothing. Tight, restrictive clothing can trap moisture and increase irritation in the vaginal area. Wearing cotton underwear and pantyhose with a cotton crotch can help air to circulate and keep the area cool and dry. Avoid wearing wet clothing, as it can generate warmth and moisture and promote the growth of certain bacteria or yeast. Change out of sweaty workout clothes and underwear immediately after exercise.

Eliminate chemical irritants in the vaginal area. Perfumed or medicated soaps or bubble baths may contain chemicals that can alter the acid balance of the vagina, causing irritation and leading to infection. Glycerin soap appears less likely to cause vaginal irritation. Items such as feminine deodorants and vaginal sprays should be avoided; not only can they cause irritation, but they may also mask the odor of a vaginal infection, delaying a diagnosis. Scented sanitary napkins, certain detergents, and some spermicides may also be suspect if an infection occurs. If the onset of vaginitis coincides with use of a new detergent, soap, or hygiene product, discontinue using the item for a few days to see if the discomfort lessens.

Avoid douching. Don't douche, even with warm water. Douching changes the acidity of the vaginal area, causing overgrowth of yeast or bacteria or killing off the protective organisms. Douching may also aggravate an existing infection by pushing the organisms deeper into the vagina.

Always wipe from front to back. Wiping from front to back after using the toilet, and especially after a bowel movement, helps to prevent the spread of germs from the rectum to the vagina, where they could lead to infection.

Practice safe sex. Ask your partner to maintain good genital hygiene and to use a condom to prevent any transfer of bacteria. Keep clean any item that comes in contact with the vagina, including a cervical cap or diaphragm.

Maintain optimal blood glucose control. Keeping your blood sugar levels under control is beneficial for plenty of reasons, and your vaginal health is one of them. Good blood glucose control helps keep the nerves in the vaginal area healthy and reduces the sugar that yeast thrive on, decreasing your chances of vulvovaginal candidiasis and other infections. Perhaps most important, good blood sugar control can strengthen your immune system and help your body to prevent and fight infections.

Talk with your diabetes team. Keep up with your health. Stay focused on optimal blood glucose control and ask questions if you have concerns about your vaginal health. Remember that vaginal infections often occur without symptoms. Cultures performed at the time of your PAP smear may be the first clue.

When in doubt...

A small amount of vaginal discharge is normal, and its consistency changes over the course of the menstrual cycle. But if you suspect that you have symptoms of an infection—even if you are not sure—discuss your concerns with your health-care provider right away. If you have an infection, take all your medicine as prescribed. Symptoms can disappear quickly, but it doesn't mean that the cause of the infection is gone. Finally, there are times when an infection can linger despite aggressive medical treatment. If you continue to have symptoms or problems related to vaginitis, it is a good idea to check back with your doctor.

Stay healthy

Vaginitis can occur for a variety of different reasons, and it takes a professional to diagnose and treat it. But you're in charge when it comes to protecting your vaginal and overall health. When you have diabetes, regular exercise, adequate sleep, stress management, a healthful diet, and good blood glucose control are vital to help prevent infections, enhance healing, and keep you feeling your best. □

MENOPAUSE
THE LATEST ON HORMONE THERAPY

by Helen L. Ross, M.D.

Today the average life span of women in the United States is about 80 years. That means most women spend at least 25 years, or more than one-third of their lives, during the menopause years. An estimated 52.4 million women were in the perimenopause (transition to menopause) or menopause years (age 45 or older) in 2000. With so many women reaching this age group (36.5% of women), increased attention has been placed on research studies that focus on these women and their health. Along with the growing body of information about menopause, there has been a significant increase in the number of prescription drugs, over-the-counter drugs, health-care devices, vitamins, and supplements aimed at the menopausal woman.

Hormone therapy (HT) is a medical option used since the 1960's that can alleviate both the short-term symptoms and some of the long-term consequences of menopause. The much-publicized initial results of the WHI (Women's Health Initiative) study published in the summer of 2002 suggested that HT may significantly increase the risk for cardiovascular events and breast cancer. Since those initially reported findings of the WHI study, the use of HT by perimenopausal and menopausal women has plummeted. But more recent publications from the WHI are tempering those initial findings. Therefore, a perimenopausal or menopausal woman and her health-care provider need to consider her individual risk factors before starting HT.

This article discusses the benefits, risks, and alternatives to HT for women with diabetes.

What is menopause?

Physicians define natural menopause as that time after a woman has not had a menstrual period for one year. Natural menopause is the result of the cessation of both ovulation and associated hormone (estrogen and progesterone) production, which results in the cessation of cyclic menstrual periods.

Menopause may also be *induced,* meaning a woman's loss of ovarian function is due to medical intervention (chemotherapy, radiation therapy, or ovulation blockers such as GnRH agonists) or surgery. If a woman has her two ovaries removed prior to natural menopause, she has undergone surgical menopause. However, if a women has a hysterectomy (surgical removal of the uterus) prior to menopause but maintains one or both of her ovaries, she has not gone through menopause. She does not have further menstrual periods, but her ovaries continue to ovulate and make hormones, so she does not reach menopause until the cessation of ovulation and hormone production by the ovaries.

At birth, a girl has about 1–2 million follicles (potential eggs). The average woman ovulates (releases an egg) 480 times in her reproductive lifetime; the vast majority of the follicles degenerate in a process called *atresia.* Follicles remaining just prior to the time of menopause tend not to respond to ovulation-stimulating hormones. This often results in irregular menses, and the normally cyclic nature of estrogen and progesterone release is lost.

Before menopause, estrogen is produced mainly by the ovaries in a form called estradiol. Another type of estrogen, estrone, is created by the conversion of other hormones in adipose (fat) cells. Production of estrogen fluctuates during perimenopause and then decreases after menopause.

Perimenopause is used to describe the transition period that women go through from their reproductive years to menopause. *Climacteric* is an older term you may have heard that refers to the transition from the reproductive phase to the nonreproductive phase, or about the same time as perimenopause. Generally, perimenopause begins during a woman's 40's and lasts from four to seven years, but it can last for as long as 10 years.

Although menopause can occur in a woman's 40's or early 50's, the average age of menopause is 51 years. Spontaneous or natural menopause prior to age 40 is called *premature menopause.* The age of

menopause tends to be familial; women tend to experience menopause at about the same age as their mother or sisters. However, smoking is thought to decrease the age of menopause by one to two years. It has been suggested that other factors, such as the number of births, age of first menses, use of oral contraceptives, and race, may affect the age of menopause, but research has not proven these to be significant factors.

Around age 40, the ovaries start decreasing in size, partly due to atresia of the follicles and partly to a decrease in the supporting ovarian tissue. Fertility decreases prior to menopause; however, women can still conceive during the transition and should use birth control for at least one year following their last menses.

During the perimenopause period, women may experience abnormal bleeding (heavier or lighter menses, irregular menses, intermenstrual spotting), mood swings, hot flashes, and night sweats, as well as other symptoms (such as vaginal dryness, headaches, and sleep disturbances). Often symptoms disappear after perimenopause. Only 10% of women have a complete stop in menses with no abnormal bleeding beforehand. Long-term effects of menopause, such as osteoporosis and vulvar and/or vaginal atrophy, are usually seen later.

Common symptoms of perimenopause and menopause

Not all women experience the same symptoms with menopause, but the following are quite common:
Hot flashes. Hot flashes are experienced at some point by 75% of women during perimenopause. A hot flash is the result of a drop in estrogen. With the erratic estrogen levels in perimenopause, hot flashes can be quite common. Night sweats are hot flashes during the night. Hot flashes vary in the number in a day, the number of years they last, and severity. Symptom management can range from having a cool drink, applying cool washcloths, and dressing in layers, to medical treatment with drugs such as estrogen. Taking estrogen helps 80% to 90% of women with hot flashes. Other treatment options include lifestyle changes and alternative therapies (see below), in addition to other medical options. Progestogens were used in the past by women who couldn't take estrogens. Clonidine (Catapress), originally marketed as an antihypertensive, is also being utilized by some women for hot flashes. Antidepressants, including the selective serotonin reuptake inhibitors (SSRIs, such as fluoxetine [Prozac]) and the serotonin-norepinephrine reuptake inhibitors (SNRIs, such

as venlafaxine [Effexor]) have also been utilized in the treatment of hot flashes. More recently, gabapentin (Neurotin) has been used to help with hot flashes.

Vulvovaginal dryness and atrophy. Some women experience vaginal dryness during perimenopause or menopause, but others never do. Some women also experience atrophy (thinning, loss of elasticity) of the vulva (a woman's external genitalia) and vagina. Avoiding antihistamines, drinking plenty of water, and using vaginal moisturizers such as Replens or water-based lubricants such as K–Y Silk-E and Astroglide can be of benefit. One should not use oil-based or petroleum-based lubricants such as Vaseline, which can irritate vaginal tissue, become a home to bacteria, and break down the latex in condoms, creating leaks. Local estrogens, including creams, rings and a vaginal pill, can assist with vaginal dryness and vulvovaginal atrophy.

Mood swings. Some of the emotional effects linked to perimenopause and menopause may actually be the result of other menopausal symptoms. For instance, hot flashes may be accompanied by heart palpitations, which can feel like anxiety. Night sweats and sleep deprivation can result in memory problems and mood changes. The changes in estrogen levels during perimenopause are known to affect mood just as changing hormone levels do in postpartum depression and PMS (premenstrual syndrome), and puberty. If mood swings interfere with the performance and enjoyment of daily activities and relationships, one should consider seeking medical treatment. Treatment options include hormones, such as oral contraceptives and HT, as well as "mood stabilizers," such as the SSRIs fluoxetine and sertraline (Zoloft) and the SNRIs venlafaxine and duloxetine (Cymbalta).

Long-term consequences of menopause

The loss of hormone production by the ovaries at menopause may raise the risks of certain medical conditions for women, including heart disease, osteoporosis, and vulvovaginal atrophy.

Heart disease. Up until menopause, women who don't have diabetes are less likely than men of their age to develop cardiovascular diseases. After menopause and the loss of the protective effects of estrogen, a woman's risk increases until it matches that of a man. Diabetes seems to negate the protective effects of estrogen, so women with diabetes are up to four times more likely to develop cardiovascular disease than women who don't have diabetes.

Studies have shown that when menopausal women take estrogen, it decreases levels of low-density lipoprotein (LDL) cholesterol (the "bad" cholesterol) and increases high-density lipoprotein (HDL) cholesterol levels (the "good" cholesterol). Other studies have shown that estrogen may have a beneficial effect on blood vessel walls and reduce blood pressure. Scientists are not sure if one or more of these beneficial effects are responsible for the lower rate of cardiovascular disease seen in women who have not yet entered menopause.

Several years ago HT was commonly utilized for the prevention of heart disease. However, the HERS (Heart and Estrogen/Progestin Replacement Study, published in 1998) and the WHI study changed that basic practice. Results of the HERS study led us to reevaluate the thinking that HT prevented heart disease. This study revealed that HT did not result in a secondary prevention of heart disease in women who had already had a stroke or heart attack. During the summer of 2002 this the beneficial cardiovascular effects of HT was questioned with the much-publicized halt of a subgroup in the WHI study. The study arm of women taking combined estrogen-progesterone hormones was stopped in part because of an increase in cardiovascular events. This resulted in a dramatic decrease in perimenopausal and menopausal women taking HT. More recent data from the WHI study confirm that in older women who were not previously on HT, the start of HT is probably not protective and may be harmful. However, in younger women, HT was not found to be harmful and is probably protective. These findings are more consistent with our basic knowledge of menopause and the effects of HT as well as previous clinical studies in these areas.

Osteoporosis. Osteoporosis is a progressive disease in which the bones lose density and become extremely fragile, which can lead to fractures, disability, and even death. Osteopenia, thought to be a precursor of osteoporosis, is a decrease in bone density but not to the extent of osteoporosis. Bones form the framework of the body, but they are also dynamic structures that are constantly being built up and broken down. In a woman's 30's, bone density starts to decline as bone breakdown outpaces bone buildup. After menopause, loss of estrogen accelerates this decline. Treating osteoporosis is thus accomplished by slowing or stopping bone breakdown and/or promoting bone formation.

The currently available treatments stop or slow bone breakdown and/or increase bone formation. Estrogen administered orally or through the skin is an effective tool to prevent and treat osteoporosis by slowing or preventing bone breakdown.

Other drug therapies include calcitonin, selective estrogen receptor modulators (SERMs), and bis-phosphonates. Weight-bearing exercise, calcium supplements, and vitamin D supplements are also used to treat and prevent osteoporosis.

Effects of menopause on diabetes

As women age, there is a decrease in tissue sensitivity to insulin (insulin resistance) and to a lesser degree a decrease in insulin secretion. In addition, with the decrease in estrogen in menopause there is an increase in insulin resistance. Recently, a postmenopausal "metabolic syndrome" has been described that is probably the result of the decreased estrogen and subsequent increased insulin resistance. In addition to the insulin resistance, this syndrome is characterized by increased triglycerides, decreased HDL cholesterol, and an increase in central fat distribution.

Women with diabetes (both Type 1 and Type 2) have an increased risk of bone fractures. Women with Type 1 diabetes have a decrease in bone density. Women with Type 2 diabetes tend to have a normal or increased bone density. The increase in bone fractures in women with Type 2 diabetes is thought to be secondary to diabetic complications (for instance, neuropathy) and falls.

Hormone therapy

HT is currently approved for the relief or treatment of menopausal symptoms such as hot flashes and vulvovaginal atrophy as well as the prevention of osteoporosis. Hormone therapy in menopause can consist of just estrogen (called estrogen therapy, or ET) or both estrogen and a progestogen (HT). Women who still have a uterus need to take both estrogen and a progestogen. In addition, some women also take testosterone.

Estrogen. Estrogen influences many organs of the body. It helps maintain the elasticity of the skin and affects hair growth. Estrogen affects brain functions such as body temperature regulation, sleep, and memory. It is also thought to be protective against macular degeneration and colon cancer.

Estrogen is also beneficial to the pelvic organs. Estrogen maintains the integrity, moisture, and elasticity of the vulva, vagina, and supporting structures, as well as the bladder and its support. Often with menopause (and no estrogen), tissues atrophy and become thin, easily bruisable, and dry. Supporting ligaments loosen, and the result is pelvic relaxation and urinary incontinence. A lack of estrogen also contributes to recurrent urinary

tract infections and vulvovaginal infections such as yeast infections.

Estrogen is available in several different formulations for various routes of administration (pills, skin patches, vaginal preparations), and in combination with progestogens or testosterone. Transdermal (patches, lotions) forms of ET/HT may provide the maximum benefits with the least negative side effects (such as an increase in triglycerides).

Progestogens. Progestogens (progesterone or a progestin) are taken to protect the uterine lining against endometrial cancer. Progesterone is secreted by the ovaries and adrenal glands and, during pregnancy, by the placenta. Progestins are drugs that have similar effects to progesterone. There are several forms of progestins available for HT. The type of progestin prescribed can depend on the woman's symptoms, the potential side effects of each particular progestin, and the woman's medical risk factors such as diabetes. For instance, some progestins reduce the beneficial lipid effects of estrogens; others may increase mood swings.

Progestins can be given orally, transdermally, and via an IUD. They can be given cyclically or continuously. Cyclic regimens involve giving progestogens for 12–14 days a month and usually result in menses when they are withdrawn. In continuous regimens, progestogens are taken each day in small doses.

Continuous regimens may result in breakthrough spotting initially; this is considered normal for up to one year. Approximately 50% of women stop this bleeding by the sixth month, and 80% stop bleeding by a year. Adjusting the HT regimen can usually stop the breakthrough bleeding. Nonprescription progestogen creams and over-the-counter tablets are not protective against endometrial cancer and should not be used for this reason.

Testosterone. Testosterone, which is commonly thought of as a male hormone, is also produced in women by the ovaries and adrenal glands. It is sometimes prescribed in addition to ET or HT when menopausal symptoms are still present. Sometimes women with early or surgical menopause are given testosterone. Side effects of testosterone include hirsutism (increased body hair) and voice changes. Testosterone also has a negative effect on blood lipids, decreasing HDL cholesterol. It may also cause glucose intolerance (the inability of the body to clear glucose from the blood efficiently).

Risks and side effects

Hormone therapy is not for everyone. There are some women who should not use it, and there are risks associated with hormone therapy for all women.

Contraindications. Contraindications to (reasons not to use) HT may include a blood clotting disorder and a history of previous stroke, heart attack, or cardiovascular disease. A history of breast cancer or endometrial cancer may also be considered a contraindication. However, many physicians will prescribe hormones if a woman has been cancer-free for five years because of the benefits derived from HT. Other conditions that may preclude HT include liver disease, abnormal bleeding that has not been evaluated by a medical professional, and pregnancy. Changes in menses can be caused by cancer or precancerous changes of the endometrium, benign conditions such as leiomyomas (muscle growths) or polyps, and hormone imbalances such as thyroid and prolactin abnormalities and should be evaluated prior to the start of HT.

Risks. The risks associated with HT include the following:

■ Blood clots. Taking estrogen carries a possible increased risk of blood clots. However, the risk of a normal women who doesn't take estrogen having a blood clot is 1 in 10,000; taking estrogen increases her risk to 2–3 in 10,000, which is still very small.

■ Endometrial cancer. The risk of endometrial cancer is two to ten times higher for a women taking "unopposed" estrogen if she still has a uterus. ("Unopposed" means she is not also taking a progestogen.) Adding a progestogen to the estrogen decreases that risk to less than that of a woman not on hormones.

■ Breast cancer. This is a controversial subject. If there is an increased risk of breast cancer it is thought to be small. One theory is that HT does not "cause" breast cancer but may increase the growth of breast cancer, if the breast cancer is already present. Women who are diagnosed with breast cancer while on hormone therapy usually have less aggressive cancers and a lower mortality rate than women who do not use hormone therapy.

■ Ovarian cancer. In the past, it was suggested that HT increased the risk of ovarian cancer. More recent evidence suggests that HT may not increase the risk of ovarian cancer.

Side effects. Estrogen or hormone therapy may cause the following side effects:

■ Bleeding. Women may experience cyclic or irregular bleeding or spotting when starting hormone therapy. Regimens can be changed to decrease or stop the bleeding.

■ Breast tenderness. Some women experience breast tenderness initially; this usually decreases after a few months of therapy. Other temporary

---

TIPS FOR GOOD HEALTH

Whether or not you choose to use hormone therapy, following these tips can help you stay in good health.

■ Eat a well-balanced, low-fat, high-fiber diet.

■ Take 1,200 to 1,500 milligrams of calcium a day and consider taking vitamin D.

■ Exercise for 20–30 minutes a day.

■ Moderate your alcohol consumption.

■ Don't use tobacco.

■ Practice stress-reduction techniques.

■ Have yearly physical exams, including pelvic and breast exams as well as preventive health care (mammogram, colonoscopy, bone density, vaccinations, etc.).

■ Continue to use a form of birth control (if you are sexually active) until you have gone at least one year without a menstrual period (unless you've had a hysterectomy).

■ See your health-care provider if you have any abnormal bleeding, including irregular periods, heavier bleeding with your periods, and bleeding or spotting between your periods.

■ Talk to your health-care provider about menopausal symptoms (hot flashes, mood swings, etc.) that are interfering with your daily activities and relationships.

---

symptoms can include bloating and pelvic cramping.

■ Gallbladder disease. There may be an increase in gallbladder problems in women taking HT orally.

Effect of hormone therapy on diabetes

Most studies show estrogen from ET or HT results in an improvement in insulin sensitivity. Estrogen therapy has been associated with lower fasting insulin levels, independent of a woman's age, weight, or type of ET. Women with Type 2 diabetes who take HT have been shown to have lower glycosylated hemoglobin (HbA_{1c}) levels than women with diabetes who are not on HT.

It is thought that progestogens in general have little effect on glucose metabolism. However, some types of progestins (including medroxyprogesterone acetate and levonorgestrel) may increase insulin resistance. Other progestins (norethindrone acetate, micronized progesterone) do not affect insulin resistance. Because of these side effects from progestins, women with diabetes are often prescribed micronized progesterone for hormone therapy.

In women who inject or infuse insulin, taking hormones may change their insulin requirements, so blood glucose levels should be monitored and insulin amounts adjusted as needed. There is no clinically significant interaction between oral diabetes medicines and estrogen or progestogens. However, because estrogen and some oral diabetes medicines are metabolized in the liver, some doctors recommend taking estrogen via a transdermal route instead of a pill to avoid any possible interaction in the liver.

Despite the benefits of HT, its usage among women who have diabetes is half that of women who don't have diabetes. One study showed that 16.7% of menopausal women without diabetes were using HT compared to 8.6% of menopausal women with diabetes. This may be because HT may increase the risk for high triglycerides, endometrial cancer, and gallbladder disease, conditions for which women with diabetes are already at increased risk.

HT in women with diabetes also remains controversial because of the possible effect on cardiovascular risks, including increased lipids and blood clots. Several recent studies have looked at these concerns. The studies are continuing to show a decrease in fasting glucose and total cholesterol in women with diabetes taking HT. One study looking at estradiol and the progestin norethindrone showed no adverse effects on glucose concentration, trigyceride levels, and C-reactive protein (a marker for cardiovascular disease). Transdermal routes of HT are showing a beneficial effect on insulin resistance and lipids (although slightly less than the oral route) and don't increase the risk of clotting.

Alternative treatments

For women who can't or are reluctant to use HT, other therapies may help to alleviate some of the symptoms and secondary effects of peri-menopause and menopause.

Lifestyle adjustments. Hot flashes may be more tolerable with a cool drink, a cool washcloth, and dressing in layers. Some women reduce hot flashes by avoiding triggers, which may include spicy food, alcohol, and caffeine. For some women, breathing techniques can decrease the intensity and duration of hot flashes if used at the start of a flash. In one recent study, exercise had no effect on hot flashes, but weight loss did. Acupuncture may also help

some women. As previously mentioned, weight-bearing exercise, calcium and vitamin D supplementation, preventing falls, stopping smoking, and limiting alcohol consumption help decrease osteoporosis and fractures. Water-based moisturizers and lubricants can help with vaginal dryness.

SERMs. SERMs (selective estrogen receptor modulators), now termed estrogen agonists/antagonists, include raloxifene (Evista) and tamoxifen. Tamoxifen is currently used to treat and prevent breast cancer but is not approved to prevent osteoporosis. Raloxifene has been shown to prevent bone loss and bone fractures with no increased risk of breast cancer or endometrial cancer. Recently, raloxifene has also been shown to have beneficial effects on lipids, decreasing LDL cholesterol. However, it does not increase HDL cholesterol, and it may increase the risk of blood clots. In addition, raloxifene does not help with hot flashes, mood swings, or prevention or treatment of vaginal dryness and vulvovaginal atrophy. There is no need for an added progestogen with raloxifene.

Calcium and vitamin D. Calcium is needed to maintain bone health. A menopausal woman taking estrogen should be getting 1,200 mg of calcium a day. A menopausal woman who is not on estrogen should be getting 1,500 mg of calcium a day. Vitamin D may be taken in combination with calcium or separately. The recommended dietary allowance of vitamin D is 400 IU (international units) for women ages 51–70 years and 600 IU per day for women over age 70. Levels of vitamin D up to 800 IU per day (taken as a supplement) are considered safe.

Bisphosphonates and calcitonin. Bisphosphonates inhibit bone resorption (breakdown) and increase bone formation. Currently, risedronate (Actonel), alendronate (Fosamax), and ibandronate (Boniva) are approved for use in the United States. Side effects include irritation of the stomach and/or esophagus. Newer preparations with weekly and monthly dosing cut down on the frequency of these side effects. Calcitonin, a hormone produced in the parathyroid, is available in a nasal spray and also helps prevent bone breakdown. These agents have no beneficial effects on tissues other than bone.

Commonly used supplements. In general, herbal remedies are not well studied for efficacy, safety, or side effects, nor are they controlled by the FDA. If you choose to use herbs or other over-the-counter supplements, tell your physician. Some herbs have known side effects and drug interactions. In addition, herbal products are not tested or regulated individually to see if they contain what is claimed and lack impurities. Independent testing has found great variance in ingredient type and amounts from bottle to bottle of some herbal supplements. If you're going to consider these, become well educated on the herb and pick a well-known brand. Cost should also be considered; often people spend a small fortune on herbs when prescription drugs may have been both safer and cheaper.

■ Soy and isoflavones. Soybeans contain soy protein and isoflavones, which are estrogen-like chemicals. A diet high in soy foods has been shown to decrease LDL cholesterol and triglycerides and to increase HDL cholesterol, which makes soy foods reasonable additions to the diet. However, recent studies suggest that dietary soy does not help prevent bone loss or alleviate hot flashes.

Soy supplements contain high levels of isoflavones, much higher than the levels found naturally in foods. The risks of these high levels of isoflavones are unknown. However, isoflavones alone do not affect cholesterol and may increase the risk of breast cancer.

■ Black cohosh. Black cohosh is actually a regulated product in Germany and available in the United States as Remifemin. Although research is needed on its mechanism of action and side effects, it seems to help with menopausal symptoms. Appropriate and safe doses have not been determined. It does not seem protective against bone loss or cardiovascular disease. Germany's regulatory body for herbs, Commission E, recommends that black cohosh not be used for more than six months and that it not be taken in addition to HT/ET.

Weighing your options

All perimenopausal and menopausal women should review their symptoms and weigh the benefits and risks of all types of HT with their health-care provider. Because of our rapidly expanding knowledge and experience with perimenopause and menopause and HT, women with diabetes should address these issues with their health-care provider on a regular basis. HT may not be for everyone, but it might be right for you. □

TOP 10 HEALTH TIPS FOR WOMEN OVER 65

by Helen L. Sloan, R.N., C.S., D.N.S., and Anne White Robinson, R.N., D.N.S.

An ancient Chinese proverb says, "One disease, long life; no disease, short life." For many women, diabetes is that one disease that, perhaps ironically, leads to a longer, healthier life. That's because a big part of the treatment for diabetes is adopting a healthy lifestyle: following a nutritious diet, getting regular exercise, not smoking, drinking only in moderation, finding ways to cope with stress, and simply paying attention to one's body. Maintaining a healthy lifestyle gets no less important with age. In fact, it may get more important, since diabetes is a progressive disease. Here are our top 10 tips for women over 65 who want to take charge of their health and stay healthy, strong, and independent in the years to come.

Eat right

If you don't already follow a meal plan, work with a dietitian to design one that helps you achieve your blood glucose goals, lowers your risk of complications, and includes foods that you like to eat. If you have Medicare Part B, some sessions with a dietitian are covered with a physician's referral. You may receive up to three hours with a dietitian in your first year of nutrition therapy and two hours each subsequent year.

The American Diabetes Association recommends eating a variety of high-fiber foods such as whole grains, fruits, and vegetables to get the vitamins, minerals, and other nutrients you need to maintain your overall health. A diet that's low in fat, saturated fat, cholesterol, and sodium will help

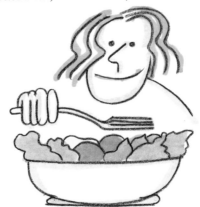

you keep your cholesterol and blood pressure levels in a healthy range and thus lower your risk of heart disease, stroke, and other complications.

A particular concern for women is preventing osteoporosis. As we get older, we gradually begin to lose bone mass. Estrogen helps to maintain bone mass, so after menopause, women can begin to lose bone very rapidly, and this bone loss can lead to osteoporosis. To slow bone loss, women must get an adequate amount of calcium, a mineral the body uses to build bone. The National Institutes of Health recommend that post-menopausal women get 1500 milligrams (mg) of calcium a day. Some calcium-rich foods include milk, yogurt, cheese, collard greens, fortified orange juice, and fortified soy products. If you don't get enough calcium from your diet, you may consider taking supplements.

For your body to be able to absorb calcium properly, you also need to get an adequate amount of vitamin D. For many women, the easiest way to get vitamin D is to get some sun—the body produces vitamin D when the skin is exposed to the sun's ultraviolet rays. However, for people in northern climates, the sun may not be strong enough, and there's evidence that our bodies don't produce vitamin D from sunlight as easily when we get older. It's a good idea to try to get your vitamin D from food sources such as fortified milk. But if you don't drink milk, vitamin D supplements are available; aim for 400–800 international units (IU) a day. Some calcium supplements have vitamin D in them, but you don't need to take calcium and vitamin D at the same time to get the benefits.

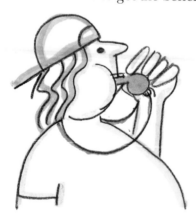

Be the captain of your team

If your health care is the ship, you are the skipper; your primary-care physician and the rest of your health-care team are there to help out and make recommendations, but ultimately it's you who decides what course to steer. Take charge of your medical care in the following ways:

■ Remember that you provide most of your care. You're the one who's responsible for taking your diabetes medicine, monitoring your blood glucose, carrying out your physical activity plan, and deciding what foods to eat. But you can only do it if you know how, so make education a priority. Ask your health-care providers questions, take diabetes education classes, participate in a support group that brings in expert speakers—do whatever it takes to keep yourself informed and knowledgeable about your diabetes care.

■ Communicate with your health-care team about what works and what doesn't in your diabetes care plan. Treatments that work for one person may not work for another, and the only way your health-care team will know if your treatment is working for you is if you tell them. If the medicines you use are causing unpleasant side effects, say so, and ask what can be done about it. If your meal plan leaves you feeling unsatisfied, ask your dietitian to help you work in more foods that you like. Remember, you're the best judge of how you feel.

■ Don't be penny-wise and pound-foolish. Skipping doctor visits, exams, or tests to save money could end up costing you a bundle in the future. If you let a problem go undetected and untreated, it can become more difficult and more expensive to treat later. Take all the recommended preventive care measures now, and attend to small problems before they become big problems.

■ Trust your common sense and don't buy into unfounded diabetes treatments. If a product or treatment sounds too good to be true, odds are it is. Be wary of "breakthrough," "miracle," or "secret" cures and remedies. Don't trust products that claim to cure a wide variety of ailments or promise instant, effortless results. If you hear about an alternative product or method that sounds interesting, talk to your doctor before you try it to find out whether it's safe, effective, and appropriate for you and to make sure it doesn't interfere with the treatment you're currently using. If your doctor thinks the therapy is safe and worth trying, he'll help you work it into your current diabetes plan. Whatever you do, don't abandon your current treatment plan to pursue an unproven alternative.

Practice preventive medicine

A good way to stay healthy is to detect and treat medical problems early—or, better yet, to prevent them altogether. Preventive measures you can take include getting screened for diabetes complications, cancer, and other conditions; getting immunizations; and taking precautions to prevent falls and injuries.

An important concern for women with diabetes is screening for and preventing cardiovascular disease. Having high blood cholesterol and/or high blood pressure raises your risk of heart disease, so you should have your cholesterol checked once a year (or as recommended by your doctor) and your blood pressure checked every time you visit your doctor. You should also get tested once a year for microalbuminuria, or protein in the urine, an early sign of kidney disease and a risk factor for heart attack and stroke. In addition, you should have your HbA_{1c} level checked two to four times each year to get an idea of how well you're controlling your blood glucose level. Keeping your blood glucose as close to normal as possible helps you reduce your risk for diabetes complications.

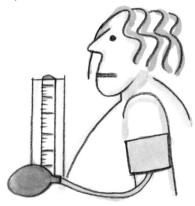

According to the National Cancer Institute (NCI), 1 in 8 women will develop breast cancer at some point in her life, and 1 in 17 will develop colorectal cancer. Detecting these types of cancers early makes treating them more likely to be successful. The NCI recommends that women over 40 get a mammogram (a screening test for breast cancer) every one to two years. Several tests can detect cancer of the colon or rectum, and the American Cancer Society recommends that all people over 50 have either a fecal occult blood test once a year and flexible sigmoidoscopy every five years, a colonoscopy every 10 years, or a barium enema every 5–10 years. In addition, getting regular pelvic exams and Pap smears can help detect cervical, vaginal, and other gynecological cancers.

Another wise precaution to take is getting immunized against pneumonia and influenza. Cases of pneumonia and the flu can be more serious and cause more complications in older people—in fact, pneumonia and influenza are the fifth leading cause of death for people 65 and older. Having diabetes also raises your risk of flu complications, including pneumonia. The Centers for Disease Control and Prevention (CDC) recommends that people over 65 get a flu shot every

September or October; it can greatly reduce your chances of contracting the flu. It is possible to get the flu even after getting a flu shot, but your case will be milder than if you had not been immunized. The CDC also recommends the pneumonia vaccine for all people 65 and older. Most people need just one shot, but some people, including those who had the shot more than five years ago and were under 65 when they got it, need an additional dose. If you haven't had a pneumonia or flu shot, talk to your doctor about getting them.

Medicare helps pay for many different preventive measures and screening tests. If you have Medicare Part B, you can get one flu shot each year and one pneumonia shot in your lifetime. You may also receive one pelvic exam, clinical breast exam, and Pap smear every two years (or every year if you're at high risk for gynecological cancer). One mammogram is covered every year, as is one fecal occult blood test. Other colorectal cancer screening tests are also covered; you can get a flexible sigmoidoscopy or barium enema once every four years or a colonoscopy once every 10 years (unless you have had a sigmoidoscopy in the last four years). If you're at high risk for colon cancer, you can get a colonoscopy every two years. If you don't have Medicare, contact your insurance provider to find out what your plan covers.

Another concern for older women, particularly for those who have osteoporosis or are at high risk of developing it, is preventing falls and bone fractures. Hip fractures in particular can be quite serious: According to the American Association of Orthopedic Surgeons, nearly one in four older people die within a year of fracturing a hip, and about 40% are unable to live independently after their hip fracture. Most serious falls occur in the home, so take steps to make your house fall-proof, such as tacking down rugs, cleaning up clutter, and putting nonslip mats in your shower and by your bathroom and kitchen sinks. Doing aerobic, weight-bearing, and stretching exercises can also help prevent falls because they strengthen your muscles, increase your range of motion, and improve your balance.

Take care of your feet

Having diabetes raises your risk of getting foot infections, so it's important to pay attention to foot care. A common complication of diabetes is neuropathy, which can lead to a loss of sensation in the feet. If you can't feel a cut, scrape, or blister on your foot, you may not treat it, and it may develop into an ulcer. An untreated ulcer can become infected, and, if the infection is serious enough, amputation can be necessary.

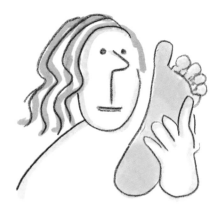

To help prevent foot ulcers and infections, follow these foot-care steps:

- Check your feet once a day for cuts, sores, blisters, or calluses.
- Wash your feet with warm water and mild soap every day.
- Moisturize the tops and bottoms of your feet every day.
- Choose comfortable shoes that don't pinch or place a lot of pressure on any single part of your foot (for example, avoid high heels).
- Have your primary-care physician or podiatrist examine your feet at least once a year.

To really stay on top of the condition of your feet, check them at home for loss of sensation. The Lower Extremity Amputation Prevention Program (LEAP) offers a free screening kit to do just that. (See page 509 for contact information.) The kit includes a device called a monofilament that you or someone else touches to the bottom of your foot in several places. If you don't feel the touch, tell your doctor.

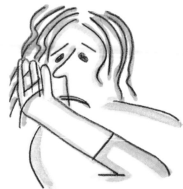

Attend to your mental health

Mental-health problems such as depression and anxiety are not uncommon in older women, but they often go undiagnosed and untreated. Women may dismiss symptoms of depression or anxiety as normal feelings of sadness or worry that they just have to "get over." Health-care providers similarly may not recognize depression or anxiety for what

it is. The fact is, however, that clinical depression and anxiety disorders are not simply passing moods, nor are they a normal part of aging, and they can be treated effectively with medication, counseling, or a combination of both.

Women are twice as likely as men to have depression, and people with diabetes are twice as likely to have it as people who don't have diabetes. Of course, we all go through periods of sadness or grief now and then, but you should talk to your doctor if your feelings of sadness or emptiness last for more than two weeks and are accompanied by any of the following symptoms:

- Loss of interest in things you normally like to do.
- Trouble sleeping or sleeping more than usual.
- Difficulty concentrating or remembering things.
- Weight loss or gain.
- Lack of energy.
- Feelings of hopelessness.
- Withdrawal from your family and friends.
- Thoughts of death or suicide.

Many women experience one of several anxiety disorders. The most common type is generalized anxiety disorder, in which a person feels constantly and excessively anxious. Often, people with generalized anxiety disorder don't know why they are worrying, and sometimes they can't stop worrying even if they realize that their anxiety is exaggerated. In addition to persistent anxiety, symptoms may include trouble sleeping, muscle tension, headaches, hot flashes, and difficulty concentrating. Many people with generalized anxiety disorder also have depression. If you have any of these symptoms, talk to your doctor. Treatment options include antianxiety medicines, psychotherapy, and relaxation techniques.

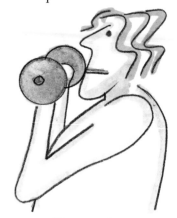

Exercise

Exercise is a beneficial activity for all women, including those who are past menopause. In fact, an individualized exercise program should be part of any treatment plan designed to help control diabetes. Exercise can help lower blood glucose levels and increase insulin sensitivity, or the body's ability to use insulin efficiently. Some people who exercise regularly are able to take less insulin and/or oral diabetes medicine. Exercise can also help you lose weight and maintain weight loss.

The benefits don't stop there. Exercise can also help prevent diabetes complications. Having diabetes makes a woman two to four times more likely to develop cardiovascular disease or have a stroke, but regular physical activity can lower these risks by strengthening the heart, reducing cholesterol levels, and lowering blood pressure.

Exercise is also good for your bones. Weight-bearing activities such as brisk walking, stair climbing, and weight lifting can help maintain bone mass and lower your risk of developing osteoporosis, a condition in which bones become porous and fragile. In addition, by strengthening muscles and improving balance and flexibility, regular physical activity can help you reduce your risk for falls and bone fractures.

And there's more. Getting regular exercise can help you fend off fatigue by giving you more energy during the day and helping you sleep better at night. When you exercise, your body produces chemicals called endorphins, which can act to improve your mood and even relieve the symptoms of anxiety and depression.

According to most recent exercise guidelines from the U.S. Surgeon General, you should aim for at least 30 minutes of moderate-intensity physical activity each day. Jogging or walking at a brisk pace, bicycling, and swimming all qualify as moderate-intensity physical activity, and so can other activities, such as raking leaves, gardening, and washing your car. You don't have to do all 30 minutes at once; you can exercise in several shorter bouts throughout the day. For example, you may spend 20 minutes working in the garden in the morning and then take a 10-minute walk after dinner.

If you don't already exercise regularly and would like to begin or if you would like to increase the amount of exercise you do, pay a visit to your doctor first. It is important to get a thorough physical examination to make sure that exercising will be safe for you. Your doctor will check for complications, including cardiovascular disease, peripheral arterial disease (the hardening of the arteries in the legs and feet), retinopathy (eye disease), nephropathy (kidney disease), and neuropathy (nerve damage). Having one of these complications doesn't mean you can't exercise, but it does mean that certain exercises may be safer for you

than others. For example, if you have proliferative retinopathy, you should avoid high-impact aerobics, heavy weight lifting, and anything that involves straining or jarring movements. If you have neuropathy with loss of sensation in your feet and legs, you should limit weight-bearing exercise and stick to activities such as swimming, bicycling, rowing, and chair exercises. Repetitive activities that place pressure on the feet, such as using a treadmill, walking long distances, jogging, and doing step exercises, may lead to foot ulcers and fractures. If you have nephropathy, it's a good idea to avoid high-intensity or strenuous exercises.

In addition to discussing what types of exercise are appropriate for you, ask your doctor how your blood glucose level may be affected during and after exercise and how to handle any changes you experience.

Manage your medicines

The older you get, the more medicines you're likely to take. In fact, older people spend an estimated $3 billion annually on medicines, and the average older person takes six or seven prescription and over-the-counter medicines a day. That's a lot to keep track of. To help you keep them all straight, make a checklist that includes the names of all the medicines and the times at which you should take them. As you take each dose, check it off the list. Keeping the week's medicines in a pill box that has a separate compartment for each day can also help you remember to take them.

Be sure to follow the directions for taking your medicines. Don't leave the doctor's office or the pharmacy without being sure when and how often you should take your doses and whether to take them with food or on an empty stomach. Also be sure to find out what you should do if you ever forget to take a dose. With some medicines, it's OK to take a missed dose when you remember it—as long as you remember fairly soon after you were supposed to take it. However, if it's nearly time for the next scheduled dose, you may be better off skipping the forgotten dose altogether. Taking two doses of insulin too close together, for example, could cause serious hypoglycemia. If you miss a dose of your medicine and aren't sure what to do, call your doctor or pharmacist.

Many drugs can cause side effects. Some side effects, such as intestinal gas or mild nausea, might be annoying but not medically serious. (In addition, such side effects often subside over time.) Others, however, such as light-headedness or hypoglycemia, can have serious consequences, such as, in this case, falling or having a car accident. Make sure to ask about the possible side effects of the medicines you're taking so you know what to expect and what to do if you experience severe symptoms. Never stop taking a medicine without consulting your doctor first. Stopping some medicines, such as antibiotics and corticosteroids, before you're supposed to can be quite harmful. However, if you think you're having an allergic reaction to your medicine (characterized by hives, itching, swelling, or difficulty breathing), contact your doctor immediately.

Some medicines require that you get periodic tests to evaluate whether the drug is working properly. For example, if you take warfarin (brand name Coumadin) to reduce your risk of having a heart attack or stroke, you need to get regular blood tests to make sure you're getting the right dose. Oral diabetes medicines in the thiazolidinedione class, including pioglitazone (brand name Actos) and rosiglitazone (Avandia), also require certain blood tests because they have the potential to cause liver damage. If you take one of these drugs to control your blood glucose, read the package insert and talk to your doctor to make sure you're getting the tests you should have.

Last but not least, many medicines can interact with other ones. An interaction can increase or decrease the effectiveness of one of the drugs or cause unwanted side effects. To prevent drug interactions, make sure that your doctor and your pharmacist know about everything you're taking—that means all prescription drugs, over-the-counter drugs, herbs, and supplements. It helps to buy all your prescription drugs at one pharmacy, so the pharmacist has a complete list at his fingertips. In addition, once a year, bring all your drugs and supplements to a doctor's appointment and ask him to check for possible interactions.

Stop smoking

Smoking is the leading preventable cause of death in the United States; the American Lung Association estimates that it's responsible for one in seven

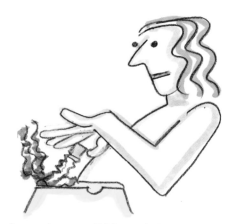

deaths each year. Older adults are reported to be less likely to have tried to quit, possibly because many believe that smoking does not harm their health. The fact is that smoking does harm your health—and that quitting smoking has proven health benefits, even for older people. Smoking raises your risk for lung disease and cancer, and, because it narrows your blood vessels, it also increases your chances of developing heart disease or having a stroke. When you stop smoking, your circulation improves immediately, and your lungs begin to repair damage from the tar and toxic substances contained in cigarette smoke. One year after quitting, the added risk of heart disease that comes with smoking is reduced by one half, and over time, the risk of stroke, lung disease, and cancer also decrease.

If you currently smoke and are ready to stop, talk to your doctor. You and he can discuss ways to quit successfully. Quit-smoking programs through organizations such as the American Lung Association or the American Heart Association may be available in your community. You can find the phone numbers of your local chapters of these organizations in the phone book.

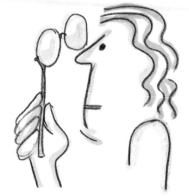

Keep an eye on eye care

Older people often experience vision problems such as cataracts (cloudy or hazy spots on the lens of the eye), macular degeneration (the breakdown

FOR MORE INFORMATION

To learn more about some of the topics raised in the accompanying article, check out these resources.

"Alternative Therapies: Part I. Depression, Diabetes, Obesity"
American Family Physician
Vincent Morelli, M.D., and
Roger J. Zoorob, M.D., M.P.H.
September 1, 2000
www.aafp.org/afp/20000901/1051.html
This article examines some of the complementary and alternative medicine options for treating depression, diabetes, and obesity. It also includes a list of links to Web sites devoted to alternative and complementary medicine.

CENTERS FOR MEDICARE & MEDICAID SERVICES
www.cms.hhs.gov
Find information about Medicare, Medicaid, and other health programs and services.

THE CENTER FOR MENTAL HEALTH SERVICES
www.mentalhealth.org
Find mental-health services in your area with this site's "Services Locator."

HEALTHWISE FOR LIFE
Medical Self-Care for People Age 50 or Better
Molly Mettler
Healthwise, Inc.

Boise, Idaho, 2007
This book for older adults provides information on common conditions, including prevention, home treatment, and when to call a medical professional.

LEAP PROGRAM
(888) 275-4772
http://hrsa.gov/leap
Learn how to check your feet for neuropathy with the LEAP Program. You can get a free screening kit by calling or filling out a form on the Web site.

MEDLINE PLUS HEALTH INFORMATION
www.nlm.nih.gov/medlineplus/nutrition.html
This National Library of Medicine Web site has general tips and information on nutrition as well as the latest news in food research.

NATIONAL IMMUNIZATION PROGRAM
www.cdc.gov/vaccines
Information about all kinds of vaccines, including pneumonia and flu shots can be found on this Web site hosted by the Centers for Disease Control and Prevention.

TOBACCO INFORMATION AND PREVENTION SOURCE
www.cdc.gov/tobacco/index.htm
This Web site hosted by the Centers for Disease Control and Prevention offers information about tobacco and health and, most important, tips on quitting smoking.

---

of the part of the retina that gives us sharp, central vision), and glaucoma (a condition in which pressure builds up in the eye and damages the optic nerve). These conditions can lead to impaired vision or vision loss, which can interfere with your quality of life and increase your risk of falls and fractures. Having diabetes can affect your eyes as well. It doubles your risk for glaucoma, and it can cause a condition called retinopathy, in which damage to the retina causes vision loss.

You can help prevent diabetes-related eye problems by keeping your blood glucose level as close to normal as possible. The next best thing to prevention is early detection; catching eye problems early makes it easier to treat them successfully and prevent vision loss. Because glaucoma and retinopathy often show no symptoms until you start to lose vision, it's important to get

screened for them regularly. The American Diabetes Association recommends having a dilated eye exam every year, even if you don't notice any changes in your vision. If you do notice vision changes, especially sudden ones, don't wait for your annual exam—let your health-care provider know right away. Medicare Part B covers one dilated eye exam each year for people with diabetes. If you don't have Medicare, check to see what your plan covers.

Socialize

Having a social network is important to the body, mind, and spirit. People who are socially active tend to be healthier, happier, and less likely to become depressed. Yet many women have less contact with other people as they get older, sometimes because of a disability that makes getting out of the house difficult, sometimes because friends and family members die or move away over time. If women don't make new friends and social contacts, they may experience social isolation, which can lead to feelings of loneliness and affect their sense of well-being.

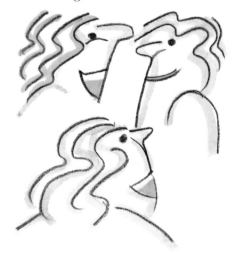

To stay socially active, make a point of getting out of the house. Make dates with your friends to go out to lunch or to the mall. Better yet, make plans to exercise regularly with a friend or group of friends. Exercising with others is usually more fun than exercising on your own, and it can help you stick with your exercise program.

Some other ways to increase your social interaction include volunteering at a school, library, museum, park, or nonprofit organization; participating in a church group or choir; taking a class at a community college; and joining a book club through your public library or a nearby bookstore. Contact your local senior center to see if it serves lunch, shows movies, or offers dance, exercise,

craft, or other kinds of classes. You can also check with your senior center to see if your town has a reminiscence group that you can take part in. Attending a diabetes support group is a good way to meet and socialize with other people who have diabetes and may be facing the same challenges as you are. Check with your senior center or local hospital to see if it offers one. If you live in a retirement community, take advantage of the social and recreational activities offered.

If transportation is a problem for you, see if your senior center offers rides to its events. You can also have family and friends come to you—invite them to your house for parties, meals, or card nights. And don't forget about using the phone, e-mail, or letters to stay in touch with friends and loved ones—whether they live close by or far away.

All too often, older women with hearing problems are reluctant to socialize because they find it difficult or embarrassing to try to communicate with others. If a hearing impairment is keeping you from socializing with others, talk to your doctor. You may benefit from using hearing aids.

Counting to 10

The more you do to stay healthy, the better you will feel. And now that you're equipped with these ten tips you know just what to do. But don't try to change everything at once. Begin with small changes to your routine—such as devoting a few minutes each day to foot care, scheduling more social outings with your friends, or remembering to get your flu shot—and work up to the bigger ones, such as stopping smoking. Incorporate the advice we've given into your routine tip by tip until you follow all 10. The payoff could be a healthier, happier life in the years to come. □

For Parents

Tips 863–1,001 513

Sending Your Kid to Camp 520

Preventing Obesity in Your Child 523

Be Aware of Hypoglycemia Unawareness 527

When Kids Falsify Their Numbers 530

Helping Young Children Succeed With Diabetes Care 534

Getting Eating Habits on a Healthy Track 538

Dental Care for Kids 541

When Your Child Needs Surgery 544

Getting Ready for College 547

13

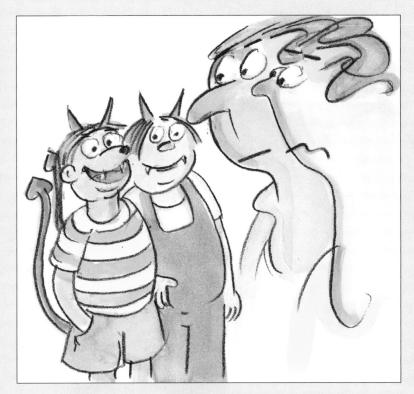

For Parents
Tips

863–1001

863. Taking full responsibility for diabetes at college is easier if the student is already handling the bulk of his care before he leaves home.

864. Before your teen leaves for college, make sure he knows how to communicate with his health-care providers while he is away.

865. Your teen may need to establish a new health-care team in his college environment.

866. Parents should help their teen develop a plan for keeping up with supplies while at college, whether at a local pharmacy or by mail.

867. Parents may choose to continue to han-

dle health insurance paperwork for their college student to guarantee continued insurance coverage.

868. Students should check with the campus health center to find out how to dispose of sharps on campus.

869. Since college living is altogether different from living at home, a student is likely to have some fluctuations in his diabetes control as he adjusts.

870. If a student is pulling an all-nighter, he should eat one carbohydrate choice (15 grams of carbohydrate) for every two hours he is awake after his normal bedtime snack.

871. For safety reasons, your teen should inform at least some of his new friends at college about his diabetes and about how to spot and treat hypoglycemia.

872. It is especially important for your teen to wear medical identification while at college in case of an emergency.

873. Eating cafeteria food for every meal can wreak havoc on blood glucose levels.

874. Ultimately, it's up to the student to learn to make good food choices while at college.

875. It is very important for college athletes with diabetes to educate coaches and teammates about diabetes, especially how to spot and treat hypoglycemia.

876. Researchers think that low blood glucose may continue to affect thinking and performance for an hour or so after it has been treated, so the period right after an episode of low blood glucose may not be the best time to take an important exam.

877. It is important for parents to address the issues of alcohol, drugs, and smoking before a student leaves home.

878. Alcohol lowers blood glucose level anywhere from 6 to 36 hours after the last drink, depending on the amount of alcohol consumed.

879. Some people think that college is a good time to transition from pediatric to adult diabetes care services.

880. It is very important that a college student have a physician available near to campus in case of an emergency.

881. If you can get the school lunch menu in advance, you and your child can review the food choices and decide together which days to buy lunch and which days to pack a lunch.

882. Attempting to force a child to try new foods rarely works.

883. Some children need to be exposed to a new food as many as 15 times (or more!) before they will try it.

884. With young children, it works better to simply make the food available and allow them to decide whether to eat it or at least play with it.

885. When a child is allowed to proceed at his own pace, he may in time begin to eat the foods you want him to eat.

886. One way to introduce new foods to the family menu is to prepare foods that no one has tried before and agree that everyone will take at least a bite.

887. No single food is necessary for good health; many foods provide the same nutrients.

888. The more involved children are in planning and preparing meals, the more likely they are to eat them.

889. Kids are more likely to eat fruits and vegetables if they are readily available when hunger strikes.

890. If there is something that you do not want your child to eat, not buying it is the first step.

891. Having several small meals and snacks a day can help with blood glucose control and prevent overeating for people of all ages.

892. Obesity in children is perhaps the fastest growing disease in the United States.

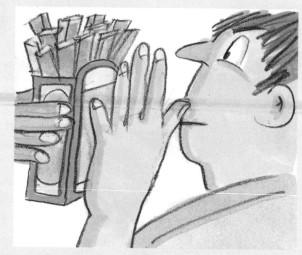

893. Simply skipping the French fries can go a long way toward cutting the fat, calories, and sodium in a fast-food meal.

894. Being overweight can lead to Type 2 diabetes and can also make Type 1 diabetes more difficult to control.

895. To maximize the health and fitness of your children, first love and accept them as they are.

896. Don't forget that children need the unconditional love and acceptance of their parents to succeed and be happy.

897. Don't let Saturday morning cartoons have more influence over your children than you do.

898. Having an assortment of healthful foods available at home is a must.

899. Kids are just like adults in that food tastes better when they're hungry.

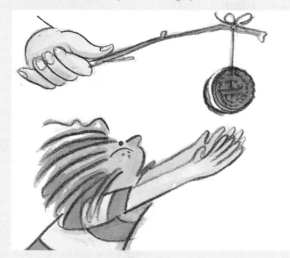

900. Food should not be used as an incentive, a form of punishment, a reward for doing something good, or a way of showing love.

901. Setting limits on sedentary activities like watching TV or using the computer may be a painful but necessary intervention to get your kids more physically active.

902. Don't expect something from your kids that you are not willing to do yourself.

903. Mild hypoglycemia can cause a person to feel uncomfortable and can interfere with his normal functioning.

904. Severe hypoglycemia can cause seizure, loss of consciousness, and coma.

905. Regular blood glucose monitoring can help your child avoid hypoglycemia, and so can paying attention to how he feels.

906. A person with hypoglycemia unawareness either can no longer recognize his lows or his body no longer exhibits the early warning symptoms of low blood glucose.

907. Hypoglycemia unawareness can occur in children as well as adults.

908. By about age six, most children can be expected to recognize symptoms of low blood glucose and understand that what they are feeling is related to low blood glucose.

909. While each person generally has the same symptoms each time he has low blood glucose, it's possible to occasionally have other symptoms.

910. Doing poorly in school can be a sign of undetected hypoglycemia.

911. Even when children experience their usual symptoms of hypoglycemia, they may not notice them if they are very involved in an activity.

912. Ignoring episodes of mild low blood glucose too frequently can lead to hypoglycemia unawareness.

913. Parents may need to remind children of all ages of the importance of treating low blood glucose quickly.

914. Most diabetes professionals recommend checking a child's blood glucose level a minimum of four times a day.

915. If a child has a history of severe low blood glucose during the night, it may be advisable to check blood glucose levels at midnight and at 3 AM routinely once a week.

916. Teens who are learning to drive should be instructed about the importance of checking their blood glucose level before they get behind the wheel.

917. Sticking to a meal schedule makes good sense, both for avoiding hypoglycemia and for avoiding getting too hungry and then getting cranky or overeating when the meal finally takes place.

918. Learning how to make adjustments to insulin doses is another important part of maintaining blood glucose control and preventing hypoglycemia.

919. All children with diabetes should have a readily available source of carbohydrate

with them at all times to treat hypo-glycemia.

920. Easily portable sources of carbohydrate include glucose tablets or glucose gel, LifeSavers, small (4-ounce) juice boxes, and raisins.

921. If a child is having symptoms of low blood glucose but cannot verify it with his meter, he or his caregiver should assume he is low and treat accordingly.

922. Sometimes a falling blood glucose level will produce symptoms of low blood glu-cose even if the level never goes below 70 mg/dl.

923. If a child cannot safely swallow or chew, passes out, or has a seizure because of low blood glucose, it will be necessary to use glucagon to raise his blood glucose.

924. Glucagon generally increases a person's blood glucose level within 5 to 15 min-utes.

925. If a person does not respond to a glucagon injection within 15 minutes, emergency help should be summoned.

926. As your child grows, the recommended dose of glucagon to raise blood glucose will increase.

927. Instead of just throwing out expired glucagon kits, practice mixing and draw-ing it up so you will be well trained when or if glucagon is ever needed.

928. If you have to give your child glucagon, contact his diabetes team afterward to discuss what happened.

929. If your child develops hypoglycemia unawareness, there are steps that can be taken to help him regain his usual feel-ings of low blood glucose.

930. Parents living with diabetes must make time to take care of themselves if they are going to be healthy enough to do the job of being a mother or father.

931. Both mothers and fathers with diabetes may experience many sources of anxiety as a result of having a newborn, and this type of stress can raise blood glucose.

932. Mothers and fathers with diabetes may find it helpful to do some extra blood glucose monitoring as they adjust to hav-ing a new baby.

933. Other areas of life, such as housecleaning or yardwork, may need take a backseat for a while so that parents have time to take care of a new baby and attend to their own health needs.

934. A parent newly diagnosed with diabetes may need to rely on his partner to take over the majority of parenting responsi-bilities for a while as he adjusts to his new diabetes care routine.

935. It is critical for families to acknowledge that when one family member has dia-betes, it affects every member of the family.

936. Families with a newly diagnosed member may want to seek out local diabetes sup-port groups or meet other families who have more experience living with diabetes.

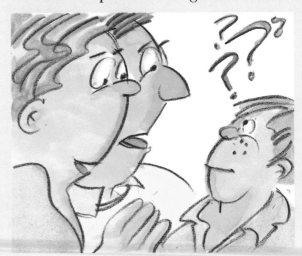

937. When it comes to talking with your kids about diabetes, there truly are no stupid questions.

938. When young children see a parent per-forming diabetes self-care tasks, they nat-urally become curious.

939. It's usually easy for parents with diabetes who have children with diabetes to empathize with their children's experi-ence, but it's also easy for them to forget that diabetes affects each person a little differently.

940. Parents with diabetes need to step back and look at the ways in which their

child's diabetes—and the child's attitude toward it—may differ from their own.

941. In the United States, there are over 100 summer camps that have been developed for the purpose of serving children with diabetes.

942. Diabetes camps are diverse, offering a variety of outdoor activities, arts and crafts, and other forms of recreation.

943. Camp is a big change in routine and a learning experience.

944. While parents of young, first-time campers will probably be most comfortable if their child attends a diabetes camp, older, more independent teens can do well at a traditional summer camps with no diabetes focus.

945. Make sure the camp you are considering is accredited by the American Camping Association.

946. If you choose a traditional camp, be prepared to tell the camp director and nurse precisely what accommodations your child needs while he is at the camp.

947. Be sure you understand the camp's policy on accepting phone calls from parents.

948. Temperatures in cabins, tents, or backpacks can get very high, so insulin should be stored in a refrigerator while at camp.

949. In anticipation of the likely increase in physical activity, many families choose to decrease their child's insulin dose by about 10% at the beginning of camp.

950. While adults with diabetes typically find insulin injections more tolerable than fingersticks, young children often find fingersticks easier to take than injections.

951. Preschool and young school-age children may be disturbed by "holes" being made in their skin by needles or concerned about running out of blood.

952. Injections encroach on a child's personal space, while fingersticks feel less invasive because they can be done with the child holding his hand out several inches away from his body.

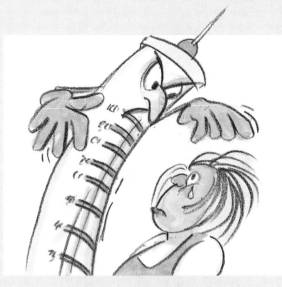

953. You can help your child with diabetes cope by acknowledging his pain rather than telling him that injections or fingersticks don't hurt much.

954. Children are greatly influenced by parental anxiety, so try to remain as relaxed as possible when performing diabetes care tasks.

955. To lower your child's anxiety about injections, choose one area of the house to do most injections, and establish at least one "safe zone" where injections never occur.

956. Writing out a schedule for injections and blood glucose monitoring shows a child that diabetes care is part of a routine and not punishment for something he did.

957. Adults should avoid engaging in lengthy negotiations with their child once the syringe or lancet is out and ready to be used.

958. Distraction is the most practical and effective tool families can use to minimize pain and distress for children.

959. Distraction activities include blowing bubbles, squeezing a soft ball, searching for specific items in a photo or in the room, or saying the alphabet out loud.

960. Some children may find comfort in icing the skin for 10–20 seconds prior to injections.

961. Having diabetes raises the risk of developing periodontal disease, and having periodontal disease is a risk factor for developing Type 2 diabetes.

962. Periodontal disease negatively affects blood glucose control in any type of diabetes.

963. The American Academy of Pediatric Dentistry recommends a first dental visit at age 1 for children who are "at risk" for dental disease; that group includes children with diabetes.

964. Sugary beverages are at the top of the list of foods that promote tooth decay.

965. As soon as a child's first tooth erupts, a parent should brush the tooth twice a day with a soft toothbrush.

966. No fluoride toothpaste is necessary until age two.

967. The use of fluoride-containing toothpaste should always be supervised by a parent or caregiver because of young children's tendency to swallow much of the toothpaste on their brush.

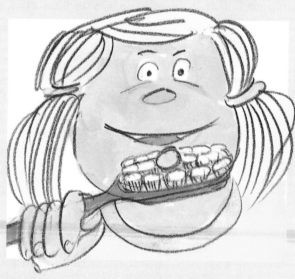

968. Only a pea-size amount of toothpaste is necessary on a child's toothbrush.

969. Teeth should be flossed if they are touching or appear to touch one another.

970. Electric toothbrushes are a great instrument to get kids to brush more thoroughly and longer.

971. Children who have a bedtime snack should brush after the snack.

972. The frequency of office visits for professional cleanings and checkups will vary from child to child.

973. For children whose diabetes is under control, dental visits twice a year may be sufficient.

974. Sealants, or protective plastic coatings for the chewing surfaces of teeth that have deep pits or grooves, are highly effective at preventing tooth decay.

975. Signs and symptoms of oral fungal infections include a milky-white, "cheese curd"–like coating on the inside surfaces of the mouth.

976. Chronic gingivitis, or early periodontal disease, is quite common among children.

977. Smoking is strongly associated with gingivitis.

978. When a person with diabetes undergoes surgery, the anesthesia provider maintains control of his blood glucose level by administering intravenous Regular insulin and glucose as necessary.

979. The amount of anesthetic that is administered to a child is based on his weight.

980. According to the American Society of Anesthesiologists, anesthesia has never been safer.

981. A recent history of upper respiratory infection is one of the most common reasons that elective surgery in children is rescheduled.

982. A person who is undergoing anesthesia will be asked to refrain from eating for a period of time prior to elective surgery.

983. Surgery stresses the body, leading to the release of stress hormones and raising blood glucose levels.

984. One of the most common oral drugs for Type 2 diabetes, metformin (brand name Glucophage and others), normally is not taken for 24 hours prior to surgery.

985. Some hospitals can accommodate the child's favorite toy or other item in the operating room.

986. Most institutions have policies against allowing parents in the operating room except in highly unusual circumstances.

987. It is not uncommon for children to be disoriented after anesthesia, and crying or other expressions of distress are to be expected.

988. If your child complains or seems unusually restless after surgery, pain may be the cause.

989. Teenage girls seem to be at particularly high risk of nausea after surgery.

990. Blood glucose levels can fluctuate considerably after surgery, particularly in the case of major surgeries.

991. Falsification of blood glucose numbers is a common problem among children—and adults—with diabetes.

992. Even doctors who don't have diabetes will admit that they would have trouble doing the monitoring required by diabetes if they had to do it.

993. Feeling overwhelmed by the demands of diabetes care or simply not being able to keep up—and not wanting anyone to know about it—are common reasons for children and teens to falsify numbers.

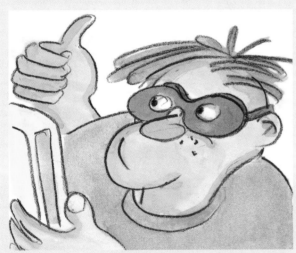

994. If your child or teen knows that you become upset when his numbers are high or low, he may try to protect you by giving you numbers that make you happy, even if they aren't his real ones.

995. If you respond to out-of-range numbers by accusing your child of bad behavior or punishing him in some way, he may give you false numbers to protect himself.

996. One way parents can encourage honesty in their children is to learn to react less emotionally to blood glucose readings.

997. Kids whose parents are able to see mistakes as inevitable and also as learning opportunities are better able to let their parents know when they've slipped up and need help getting back on track.

998. Children with diabetes may test the boundaries by not monitoring or by not following other parts of their diabetes plan.

999. Even motivated children and teens are usually not mature enough to carry out their daily diabetes care tasks without the involvement and supervision of a responsible adult.

1,000. Even if your child is responsible and you trust him, stay involved in his diabetes management. The idea is to be supportive and interested, not punitive.

1,001. Rules that seem arbitrary or that don't clearly result in better health or better diabetes control are unlikely to be followed.

SENDING YOUR KID TO CAMP

by Karen Riley, R.N.

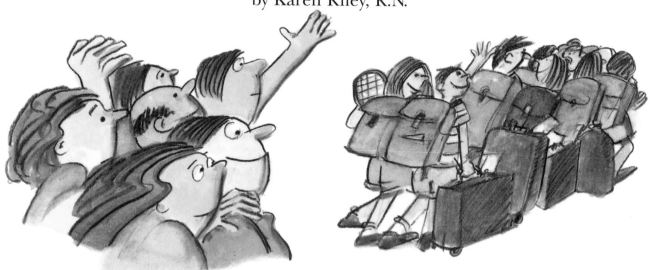

So you're thinking of sending your child to summer camp. What a great idea! Camps are wonderful places—without parents—where children can experience the great outdoors, learn new skills, make friends, meet positive role models, become more independent, and most of all, have fun. Because your child has diabetes, you may be unsure what type of camp is best for him, or you may be reluctant to send him to camp at all for fear that his diabetes will not be managed by the camp staff. However, a little research can help you choose the right camp for your child, and some planning and direction on your part can minimize your fears. You simply need to know the capabilities of the camp's staff and resources so that you can plan accordingly.

There are two general types of camps from which to choose: diabetes camps and traditional camps. Diabetes camps have medical professionals with diabetes-care experience on staff, and most incorporate diabetes self-management education into camp activities. Traditional camps are just that: regular summer camps with no diabetes focus and possibly no medical professionals on staff. Either can be a good choice for a child with diabetes.

Diabetes camps

In the United States, there are over 100 camps that have been developed for the purpose of serving only children with diabetes, though a few also take siblings or friends as partners. Some of the camps have been in existence for many decades, before self-monitoring of blood glucose was even possible, when a diabetes camp was the only safe option for the child who wanted a camp experience. Back then, a diabetes camp was one of the only sources of diabetes education as well.

Today, diabetes camps are diverse, offering a variety of outdoor activities, arts and crafts, and other forms of recreation. All have access to (and should follow) the American Diabetes Association guidelines for the proper care of diabetes at camp. The camp medical staff may consist of physicians, nurses, dietitians, and often, pediatric residents, medical students, nursing students, and social workers. The counselors usually have diabetes too, and many are former campers. These counselors are terrific role models and probably have more of an influence on the campers than the medical staff does.

The goals of most diabetes camps are to incorporate good diabetes management decisions into the camper's daily life and to foster the outlook that a kid with diabetes can accomplish anything he wants. (Do not, however, expect a week or two of "perfect" blood sugar control. Camp is a big change in routine and a learning experience.) Some campers have never even met another child with diabetes before. For these children, camp is especially valuable. It can give them a sense of belonging that they don't have back home.

Traditional camps

Sending a child to a traditional summer camp is a lot like sending him to school: It takes planning. Because traditional summer camps don't usually have staff trained in diabetes issues, parents need to be very involved in familiarizing the camp staff with diabetes care. Just as you did with school staff, you will need to start with the very basics of diabetes management and emphasize what the camp staff needs to do to keep your child safe. Keep in mind that traditional camp staff will likely have even less diabetes experience than school personnel. Do not assume that there is a camp nurse or that the camp nurse will have diabetes knowledge.

Which type of camp to choose?

In choosing a camp, think about your child's interests (such as sports, music, or art) and about how independently he manages his diabetes. He may want a particular sports camp, a Boy Scout camp, or a church camp that his youth group is attending. You may see value in your child meeting other kids with diabetes and learning about self-management.

As you consider all the possibilities, ask yourself the following questions: Is it the first time away from home for a child who doesn't yet check his own blood glucose, or who doesn't want to stop playing when it's time for his snack? Or do you have a teen who has been dependable and quite capable in all aspects of his diabetes care? Is your child easily influenced by peers, so that diabetes care takes a back seat? Does your child seek out adult help when he needs it? Does he hate to tell people he has diabetes?

Parents of young, first-time campers will probably be most comfortable if their child attends a diabetes camp. Kids who need a lot of help and direction in their blood glucose self-monitoring, insulin injections, and food choices would definitely benefit from a diabetes camp.

Pragmatically, your decision may be most influenced by availability and cost. The earlier you apply to a camp, the greater your chances of getting a spot. Most diabetes camps give full or partial scholarships, or "camperships," based on financial need, so ask for information about financial aid before you rule out a camp that seems expensive.

Make sure the camp you are considering is accredited by the American Camping Association. Accreditation ensures the camp takes certain safety measures, which include meeting cleanliness standards, having a high staff-to-camper ratio, hiring credentialed program staff (such as lifeguards), and performing background checks on staff, among many others.

Preparing for camp

Most diabetes camps will provide information or a manual about how diabetes will be managed at camp. Parents can also call the director to talk about any particular concerns. Talking to the par-

ent of a child who has attended the camp can also be arranged.

Preparing for a traditional camp experience will require more advance planning. Parents must be advocates for a safe, fun experience for their camper. Start by asking your child's diabetes team for help and suggestions, then set up a meeting with the camp director. If possible, include the camp nurse if there is one. The camp nurse at a traditional camp is most likely the only medical professional at camp. The nurse may have no Type 1 or Type 2 diabetes experience and may not be on duty 24 hours a day. Find out what you have to work with. Another staff member may need to be involved in your child's diabetes care. If the camp nurse is not available at this first meeting, arrange another time, but don't plan on meeting during camp check-in; it's too busy then.

Be prepared to tell the camp director and nurse precisely what accommodations your child needs while he is at the camp. First, see if you can find a way to work within the system the camp has in place. For instance, it may be simple to move your child's breakfast time 45 minutes to coincide with camp breakfast time. However, insist on accommodations when necessary. For example, your child must carry treatment for low blood glucose at all times, whether food is normally allowed in tents or cabins or not.

After the meeting, put all the information the camp staff needs about your child's diabetes care in writing and provide many copies for them to keep handy. Meet with your camper's cabin counselor at check-in and go over everything again. List the situations in which you want to be called and those in which your camper's physician or diabetes team needs to be called. Be sure you understand the camp's policy on accepting phone calls from parents. Phoning in to camp is handled differently at each camp, and some camps strongly discourage parents from phoning.

Here's a rundown of the areas in which you'll need to plan ahead, whether that means educating the camp staff or packing extra supplies. Make sure you cover each one of these following areas, even if your child is quite independent.

Blood glucose and ketone testing. To make sure your child's blood glucose level is checked as often as it should be while he's at camp, the following questions need to be answered before camp starts: Who will be responsible for monitoring and recording if he cannot do it himself? If the camper does monitor himself, who will make sure it's done on time? If you determine that a check needs to be done at midnight or 3 AM, who will be responsible for that? Where will the meter and strips be kept? (They must be available at all times.) How will used strips and lancets be disposed of?

Make sure the camp staff knows when to check for ketones. If urine or blood ketones are positive, direct that you or the child's physician be called immediately.

Low blood glucose. All camp staff in contact with your camper must be able to recognize hypoglycemia and know what to do if he has a low. Make a list of the symptoms of low blood glucose that your camper usually gets. List more unusual symptoms as well, just in case. Include "seizure" on your list even if your child has never had one. Include a list of the situations in which low blood glucose is more likely to occur.

List the appropriate treatments for lows that occur just before a meal and lows that occur between meals. Make sure glucose tablets and other treatment for lows are carried by either your child or the counselor who is with him at all times. Explain what to do if your child resists treatment, and give direction for rechecking blood glucose after a low. Make sure you and the camp staff answer the following questions before check-in: How will treatment be recorded? Whom will it be reported to? When will it be reported? Is there someone at camp who can give glucagon, if necessary? Where will it be kept? In an emergency, who will call an ambulance? How far is it to the nearest hospital?

Insulin administration and adjustment. Make a plan for insulin storage, injections, and dose adjustments. At camp, insulin should be stored in a refrigerator, even if you normally store opened vials at room temperature at home. Temperatures in cabins, tents, or backpacks can get very high, causing insulin to lose potency. Most camp infirmaries or health centers should have a refrigerator.

If your child cannot draw up insulin or give himself an injection, designate a camp staff member to take care of it. (Again, do not assume the nurse will be available at all times.) An older teen experienced with giving himself injections or using an insulin pump may have confidence to administer and adjust insulin on his own. However, all campers, even independent ones, should have some staff oversight to make sure that injections or boluses are given; it's too easy to forget in the excitement of camp activities. Ask that a staff member keep an eye on your child's insulin administration, and make sure your child understands that this will be the procedure while at camp.

A word of caution to the experienced and the

inexperienced: In anticipation of the likely increase in physical activity, many families choose to decrease their child's insulin dose by about 10% at the beginning of camp (if this reduction is too much, the dose can be increased the next day). If your camper can't make insulin dose changes by himself, you need to answer the following questions: Do you want the staff to follow your camper's home dose schedule? Do you use a scale for raising and lowering doses that depends on your child's premeal blood glucose level? How will decisions about insulin doses be communicated to you? You may want to designate a time that camp staff can call you at home.

If your child uses an insulin pump, make sure you send a back-up pump (if you have one), supplies for insulin injections, and both short-acting and long-acting insulin. If your camper is not completely independent in all aspects of pump use and programming, sending him to traditional camp is probably not a good idea. A diabetes camp would be a better choice.

Meals and snacks. Get the camp's menu ahead of time, as well as the times meals and snacks will be served. Ask if there are frequent last-minute changes to the menu and if meals are usually on time. This can be a problem at traditional camps. Insist that your camper have easy access to food. Usually camps have a "no food in cabins" rule; if so, this rule must be relaxed for your camper. Because of the high activity level at camp, it's very important that your camper have an evening snack, and it's likely he'll need a larger snack than he usually eats at home.

Go over the menu with your camper and make sure that for each meal there is something he will eat. If not, arrange a substitute. The camp may allow foods from home. Campers may have access to vending machines, or they may be able to buy treats at the canteen. Prepare your camper to make the right decisions about when to eat such treats and how much to have.

Diabetes supplies. Make a list of all the supplies your camper would possibly need for the duration of his camp stay and double it. This is true even for insulin vials, which can easily break. If your camper uses a pump, pack twice the amount of set changes you expect him to need. Don't forget extra food, glucose tablets, and other treatments for low blood glucose. For a diabetes camp, check your parent manual or camp communication before packing, as most diabetes camps provide some or all of the diabetes supplies through generous contributions by manufacturers.

Now, just relax

For many parents, camp time is a great opportunity to take a break from the responsibility of diabetes care. Just remember that Boy Scout motto: "Be prepared." If all the bases are covered, your camper can have a safe and enjoyable experience—and you can relax and enjoy your freedom, too. Whether you choose a camp specializing in caring for children with diabetes or a traditional camp program, good planning and preparation will ensure that your child returns home healthy and filled with memories that will last a lifetime. □

PREVENTING OBESITY IN YOUR CHILD

by Nicholas Yphantides, M.D., M.P.H.

It's been over seven years since the day I straddled two medical-quality scales and discovered the monumental challenge that lay ahead of me. I weighed 467 pounds, and I was living a life of profound hypocrisy. As a physician, I gave medical advice every day that didn't jibe with my own overweight, out-of-shape body and unhealthy lifestyle. In other words, I was telling my patients, "Do as I say, not as I do."

It's not that I didn't recognize I was severely overweight; there were daily reminders. A 60-inch waist makes for a very limited wardrobe. I couldn't fit into an airplane seat, wear shorts, or climb a flight of stairs without becoming winded.

I dreaded going to an unfamiliar restaurant, worrying I might not fit into the booth or chairs. I was aware that diabetes and high blood pressure were likely consequences of the way I was living. I knew I needed to make a change, but I kept making excuses and rationalizing the error of my ways.

Finally, a bout with testicular cancer (unrelated to my excess weight) forced me to confront my own mortality for the first time in my life. As a result, I suddenly saw my physical health as a precious gift that I could no longer take for granted and that I was now eager to take much better care of. When I recovered from the cancer, I decided I could no longer go on killing myself with an avalanche of calories and a lack of physical activity.

My approach to weight loss was unconventional in some respects but conventional in others. I decided to take a "radical sabbatical," during which I visited every state in the continental United States and all 30 Major League ballparks, including those in Canada. I enjoyed over 110 baseball games, but rather than feasting on junk food in the stands, I stuck to an aggressive, medically supervised meal plan that reduced my caloric intake while still providing me with the basic and essential nutrition I needed. Through following that diet and performing consistent and intense daily exercise, I lost a total of 270 pounds. And so far, I've kept it off.

Today, exercise and healthy eating are a major part of my life. I'm enjoying focusing on my personal fitness and encouraged by the slow but steady improvement in my body's shape and composition. Whatever pleasure I lost from overeating has been replaced many times over by the blessings and opportunities that have resulted from my transformation. The old saying really is true: "Nothing tastes as good as healthy feels."

As the new father of a precious little girl, I am eager to share these principles of health and well-being with her. And while I may have at times gotten away with proclaiming "Do as I say, not as I do" as a physician, as a parent, there is no such option. Telling my child to do one thing while I do another would go over like a lead Twinkie. It is now the intent and purpose of my life to proclaim, "Do as I say and as I am doing!" I hope that the story of my personal transformation will inspire other parents to aspire to do the same.

The big picture

We all know that American children are exercising less and eating more than they should. Obesity in children is perhaps the fastest growing disease in the United States: Estimates are that there are over 9 million children in the United States who are overweight or obese. Even more sobering is the likelihood that over 75% of these children will grow up to be overweight or obese adults. Many public health experts are seeing evidence—for the first time in over 100 years—that children today may actually have a shorter anticipated life expectancy than their parents.

But life span is not the only issue. The low self-image and emotional trauma that often go along with being obese undermine the quality of the affected child's life as well.

Implications for diabetes

Although there are plenty of reasons to be alarmed by the increasing number of overweight kids, none is more concerning than the dramatic rise in the diagnosis of Type 2 diabetes in kids, which was once very rare in children. Numerous studies have linked the two conditions. Unlike Type 1 diabetes, in which the immune system attacks and destroys the insulin-producing beta cells in the pancreas so that it can no longer produce insulin, Type 2 diabetes occurs when the body loses the ability to respond to the insulin it does produce, a condition known as insulin resistance. As weight increases, insulin resistance generally does, too. The potential complications of either type of diabetes include blindness, heart and kidney disease, and poor circulation to the limbs.

Being overweight is a concern for children with Type 1 diabetes, too. Children with Type 1 diabetes who are significantly overweight also develop insulin resistance, making their diabetes more difficult to control and consequently raising their risk of developing complications down the line.

Diabetes is not the only health risk related to extra weight. Overweight children (with diabetes or not) have an increased risk for asthma, sleep apnea, and all the emotional trauma and pain that can result from poor body image and societal bias and discrimination.

But there is hope! The great news is that Type 2 diabetes and the associated insulin resistance are reversible by applying the same principles that I used to lose over 250 pounds without gastric surgery or any fancy gimmicks. For kids, however, parents must be involved in making the lifestyle changes necessary for good health. It is my hope and expectation that the following principles will equip you with the tools you need to begin that process.

The seven parental pillars of good health

Keeping kids healthy is a family affair. By following the guidelines set out here, you can maximize the health and fitness of your children—and probably yourself, too.

1 Love and accept your children as they are

You must affirm and confirm your children, no matter what their weight may be. This is not about conditional love or pressuring our kids to measure up to our own standards or preconceptions. Never be critical or hostile about your child's weight or you will crush his tender spirit. Your child's physical appearance should not be the issue. In fact, how your children look should almost be irrelevant to you. Your desire is for them to live long, healthy, productive, and fulfilling lives. This may seem like common sense, but as a practicing physician, I have observed parents both in my office as well as out in the community who seem to forget at times that children need the unconditional love and acceptance of their parents.

2 Remember that you're the parent

Please allow me to put on my white lab coat for a moment and speak a little tough love. Listen, kids are your responsibility. You are your kid's mom, your kid's dad. Don't let Saturday morning cartoons have more influence over your children than you do. There is a tug of war going on today for your children's hearts and attention, and you have to step up to the plate and take the position of influence and privilege that you have as their parent. From supervising and ensuring the timely and consistent use of their medicines to influencing the choices and quantity of the time they spend in front of a computer or television, having your appropriate influence as their parent is your responsibility.

If you have excuses and rationalizations about your inability to provide them with the loving supervision and direction they need, what can you expect of them? This is not about imposing harsh rules on your kids or manipulating them but rather lovingly and wisely taking the steps required to positively influence their behavior and choices.

3 Fill the fridge with the right stuff

Kids have a way of eating what's in the kitchen, and what's in the kitchen usually gets there by way of your shopping cart. So what are you filling your shopping cart with? Treats wrapped in plastic? Aluminum cans filled with sugary sodas? Cartons of fat-laden and sugar-packed ice cream? Frozen pizzas? I'm not suggesting that you have to shop at a health-food store or fill the refrigerator with Brussels sprouts and tofu, but having an assortment of healthful foods available at home is a must.

Since kids are born to snack, consider peeling and slicing various kinds of produce so they're readily available and convenient to eat when your kids are hungry. Remember that snacks should be snacks and not extra meals that are packed with calories. Kids who are not overfed on snacks are

IS MY CHIILD OVERWEIGHT?

Concerned parents often ask what their child should weigh. It might seem like a simple question, but it's not. Children have different body types and growth histories, so there is no single weight that's right for every child of a certain age or height.

However, it is possible to find out if your child is in a generally healthy weight range for his height. Your child's health-care provider can tell you whether that's the case, or you can use a growth chart or body-mass index (BMI) chart for children. BMI, which is an indirect measure of body fat, does not account for everything, but it can be used as a guide. Charts are available on the Web site of the Centers for Disease Control and Prevention at www.cdc.gov/growthcharts.

A BMI in the 85th to 95th percentile means a child is considered at risk for being overweight. A child ranking above the 95th percentile for his height and weight is considered overweight and possibly obese.

The American Diabetes Association currently recommends screening children for Type 2 diabetes when a child's BMI or body weight is above the 85th percentile and he also has at least two risk factors for diabetes, such as a family history of Type 2 diabetes, a racial or ethnic background that raises his risk of diabetes, or signs or symptoms of insulin resistance such as high blood pressure or high cholesterol. Type 2 diabetes also occurs more frequently in children of women who have had gestational diabetes.

more likely to eat more nutritious food at mealtimes. After all, kids are just like adults in that food tastes better when they're hungry.

Parents may soon be getting a helping hand from the Walt Disney Company in interesting their children in fresh produce. Various cartoon characters, including Mickey Mouse, SpongeBob, and the Tasmanian Devil are now appearing on fruit and vegetable packaging in stores across the United States in an effort to catch the attention of young customers. This is an exciting and long overdue move in the right direction as society collectively is coming around to recognize the role and responsibility it has in this issue.

4 Eat at home more often

I know that the realities of our hectic, modern-day lives make this a tough one. I'm not suggesting that you and your family abstain from fast food or eating out for the rest of your lives, but I am asking you to try to strike an appropriate balance. From strategic use of leftovers to ready-to-go food in the freezer to making food prep part of your family's daily routine, somehow we need to find more time to sit down and eat healthy meals together at home.

Asking your children to help out with meal preparation will give them an appreciation of different foods and of the effort it takes to serve healthy and delicious meals. If time is truly too short to cook on some days, make an effort to identify local restaurants that have healthy and affordable options, so you're not stuck with fatty, unhealthy foods.

Eating at home may do more than just help prevent obesity. Meals eaten together can promote family togetherness, foster communication, and have a remarkable impact on children. Social research studies have even shown that teenagers who regularly eat with their parents are less likely to take drugs or be depressed and are more likely to be motivated students.

5 Use food for fuel

Food provides nutrition. It should not be used as an incentive program, a form of punishment, a reward for doing something good, or a way of showing love.

I used to eat for all the wrong reasons, so learning and accepting this principle was one of the most important steps of my own personal journey toward healthy living. This is not to say that there aren't important cultural and lifestyle components to food, but in general, we should try to use food primarily to nourish our bodies.

Parents play a critical role in creating an environment where food is not used inappropriately. I know it is a rare parent who hasn't bought his child an ice cream cone as a reward. But that should be the exception and not the daily routine. Try to limit rewarding good behavior or punishing undesirable behavior by using food as the tool. In addition, be deliberate about modeling the appropriate use of food and not using it yourself as a reward, companion, or way to deal with pain, loneliness, or boredom.

Patterns of behavior established in childhood often last a lifetime. As parents, we need to ensure that we don't inadvertently teach our children to rely on food to satisfy needs that go beyond the primary nutritional purpose of food.

6 Regular physical activity is an absolute must

Lack of physical activity is a significant contributor to children being overweight and out of shape. As complex as this whole issue is, it's also very simple: Calories consumed need to balance calories spent. When we consume more calories than we burn, we add extra weight in our body's fuel storage tank of fat. To lose extra weight, we have to burn off more calories than we put into our bodies.

It would be nice to be able to count on kids getting regular exercise through physical education classes at school, after-school programs, and time spent playing outside after school and on the weekends. Unfortunately, many schools have had to cut back on gym classes and other programs, and many neighborhoods are unsafe or not conducive to walking, bike riding, and outdoor play. Kids today also tend to have more access to television, computers, and video games than their parents had, and the net result of less activity and more screen time is our current physical inactivity disaster.

Getting off the couch and helping our kids get exercise by making activity fun is an essential parental role. Setting limits on sedentary activities like watching TV or using the computer may be a painful but necessary intervention. I don't believe in a one-size-fits-all approach, but most professionals strongly suggest that screen time be limited to less than 60–90 minutes a day.

Making physical activity fun and giving it a positive spin is a critical part of getting kids to be active on a regular basis. Finding ways of encouraging kids to play hard at activities they enjoy for at least 30–60 minutes a day would be wonderful and very beneficial. From making vacations physically active to walking rather than driving to getting a dog that will drag your child around on a leash, there are many ways of creating an association between fun and physical exertion.

7 Model it

There is no room for parents to consistently say one thing and do another. Not only is our credibility on the line but, more important, how can we expect something from our kids that we are not willing to commit to ourselves? The message has to be "Do as I say AND as I do!"

This is not to say that perfection is required, but for the most part, we have to live by the principles that we are trying to instill in our kids. I can't tell you how many times parents have dragged their kids in to see me and asked for help with modifying their child's behavior, and I have had to bite my tongue instead of asking the parents if they've looked in the mirror recently. (Trust me, the issue gets addressed, but not in a way that undermines parental credibility and authority in the exam room.)

As a parent, I am eager for my child to thrive, be vibrant, and experience all that life has to offer. I don't want to deprive her of having me around as long as possible, so I am no longer depriving myself of healthy living by consuming an abundance of calories while I waste away on the couch. In many ways, my own personal commitment to maintain my health and fitness is now one motivated by love. And while I demonstrate my love by the way I care for my own body, I also strive to provide her with an environment and upbringing that will help ensure her own healthy state of body, mind, and spirit.

While there are no guarantees and unexpected health issues can always occur, I want to do all I can to live life in a way that sets the right tone and example. I love being healthy and am eager to ensure that my child has that same opportunity. It's about walking the talk. For your children to be healthy, you have to have a healthy family. You have to be a healthy parent by setting a healthy example. You, too, can then proclaim with enthusiasm and integrity, "Do as I say, and as I do!" □

BE AWARE OF HYPOGLYCEMIA UNAWARENESS

by Karen Kelly, R.N., B.S.N., C.D.E., and Amy Gilliland, R.N., M.S.N., C.D.E.

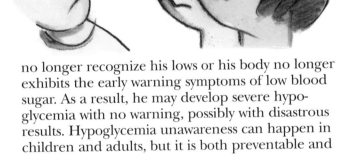

Anyone whose child uses insulin has no doubt been warned of the dangers of hypoglycemia (low blood sugar) and the need to treat it promptly. Mild hypoglycemia can cause a person to feel uncomfortable and can interfere with his normal functioning. Severe hypoglycemia can cause seizure, loss of consciousness, and coma. To prevent severe hypoglycemia, most people with diabetes are advised to treat for hypoglycemia—by ingesting some carbohydrate—when their blood sugar level is 70 mg/dl or lower. At bedtime or during the night, treatment is recommended when blood sugar is below 80 mg/dl.

Regular blood sugar monitoring can help your child avoid hypoglycemia, and so can paying attention to how he feels. Any symptoms of hypoglycemia should prompt you or him to check his blood sugar level and treat for hypoglycemia if necessary.

Not treating for hypoglycemia when blood sugar is low can have some serious consequences, among them severe hypoglycemia and, over time, the development of hypoglycemia unawareness. A person with hypoglycemia unawareness either can no longer recognize his lows or his body no longer exhibits the early warning symptoms of low blood sugar. As a result, he may develop severe hypoglycemia with no warning, possibly with disastrous results. Hypoglycemia unawareness can happen in children and adults, but it is both preventable and treatable.

Clueing in to signs and symptoms

Typical symptoms of hypoglycemia include sweating, shaking, weakness, having a headache, dizziness, and hunger. Hypoglycemia can also cause emotional symptoms such as irritability or, in some cases, giddiness. In young children, signs of low blood sugar may include crying, lethargy, pallor, glassy eyes, sleepiness, or a lack of coordination. Generally, a child will exhibit the same symptoms each time he has low blood sugar.

Since infants and very young children cannot identify signs of hypoglycemia or verbalize their symptoms to their caregivers, it's important for parents and caregivers to notice these signs and act accordingly. Although they may be unaware of a symptom's significance, some toddlers will verbalize symptoms by saying, for example, "I want juice" or "I'm hungry." A preschooler may say he feels tired or that his stomach or legs feel funny. By about age six, most children can be expected to recognize symptoms of low blood sugar, understand that what they are feeling is related to low blood sugar, and understand that they need to take some action to feel better.

If your child does not verbalize any symptoms when he has low blood sugar, you can help him start to recognize symptoms by asking if he noticed any different or funny feeling just before you checked his blood sugar after a low has occurred. This sort of discussion can help even small children make the connection between their feelings and low blood sugar and can reinforce the importance of their saying something when they have symptoms.

While each person generally has the same symptoms each time he has low blood sugar, it's still possible to occasionally have other symptoms. For example, nightmares, restless sleep, slow reaction time, and numbness around the mouth can be unusual signs of low blood sugar. Even doing poorly in school can be a sign of undetected hypoglycemia.

Mark, a junior high school student, had always done well in math, but suddenly he was struggling and his grades were slipping—even though he was putting in as much effort as he always did. His diabetes educator suggested that he check his blood sugar level for several days just before the math class. To his surprise, he found that he was low before class three days in a row, but he hadn't noticed any of his usual symptoms at these times. Once his insulin dose was adjusted to correct the lows, his grades improved, and the experience served as a reminder that blood sugar can be low with no symptoms or with only very subtle symptoms that are easy to ignore.

But a symptom of hypoglycemia doesn't have to be unusual to go unnoticed. Even when children experience their usual symptoms, they may not notice them if they are very involved in an activity. Children also sometimes ignore the signs and symptoms of low blood sugar so they can continue with their chosen activity, or they may not speak up because they feel too embarrassed to let someone know that they are low. This sometimes happens when they are with people they do not know very well or are at school. The trouble is, if they ignore the low too long, it can turn into a severe low, resulting in loss of consciousness or seizure. And if they ignore even mild lows too frequently, they can develop hypoglycemia unawareness.

Preventing hypoglycemia

When a person has frequent episodes of hypoglycemia, his body becomes accustomed to being low, and he no longer experiences symptoms of hypoglycemia at the same blood glucose level. In other words, he develops hypoglycemia unawareness. The first step toward preventing hypoglycemia unawareness, therefore, is to prevent even mild episodes of hypoglycemia.

For parents of young children, prevention efforts include explaining the importance of letting an adult know quickly about any signs or symptoms of low blood sugar. It may be necessary to repeat this information more than once to reinforce it. Parents of older children and teens may also need to remind their children of the importance of treating low blood sugar quickly, since diabetes may not come at the top of a child's or teen's list of priorities.

One of the most important tools for preventing low blood sugar is frequent blood sugar monitoring. Most diabetes professionals recommend monitoring a child's blood sugar a minimum of four times a day—before each meal and at bedtime. In addition, checking before, during, and after exercise is important to see how exercise affects a child's blood sugar level. It may be necessary to add a snack before or after exercise or alter a child's insulin doses on the days he exercises to prevent hypoglycemia.

Who checks a child's blood sugar level—parents, another caregiver, or the child himself—will depend on a child's age and maturity level, among other things. Even if a child can check his own blood sugar level, it works best if parents remain involved, offer emotional support, help with insulin adjustments and other tasks when needed, and generally make sure blood sugar monitoring gets done.

For some children, middle-of-the-night blood sugar monitoring is recommended in addition to regular daytime monitoring. If a child has a history of severe low blood sugar during the night, it may be advisable to check blood sugar levels at midnight and at 3 AM routinely once a week. This is a challenging task for parents, but it can help a lot to see patterns and to determine whether treatment adjustments are working. It is also a good idea to check nighttime blood sugar levels after a day of heavy exercise or physical activity, because a child may have delayed hypoglycemia several hours after exercise has ended. Middle-of-the-night blood sugar levels should also be checked if your child is low at bedtime. Rechecking allows you to see whether treatment of the bedtime low (with a snack) was sufficient.

Teens who are learning to drive should be instructed (and reminded) about another important time to check their blood sugar: before they get behind the wheel of a car. Since most teens value the freedom that having a driver's license represents, reminding them that their license may be revoked if they fail to practice safe driving may help this important lesson sink in.

Another strategy to help prevent hypoglycemia is to keep meal and insulin times consistent, with no more than half an hour of difference for insulin injections and mealtimes from one day to the next. This may be less important for children who use an insulin pump (since a bolus can be delayed until food is ready to be eaten) or inject insulin glargine (brand name Lantus), which has no peak. But sticking to a meal schedule makes good, common sense for other reasons, including avoiding getting too hungry and then getting cranky or overeating when the meal finally takes place. It is also usually recommended that meals have about the same amount of carbohydrate from day to day to help with blood sugar control.

Learning how to make adjustments to insulin doses is another important part of maintaining optimal blood sugar control and preventing hypoglycemia. Adjustments may be needed at mealtimes if, for example, a child refuses to eat, a high-fat meal such as pizza is served, or a child was very active earlier in the day. It may be necessary to lower a morning dose of medium-acting insulin if, for example, a late-afternoon sports event is scheduled. If you are unsure when and how to adjust your child's insulin doses, consult your doctor or diabetes educator.

Treating hypoglycemia

Because of the importance of treating even mild hypoglycemia quickly, all children with diabetes should have a readily available source of glucose with them at all times, and parents (or caregivers) and children alike should know how to treat lows. The recommended steps are as follows:

■ Check blood sugar level with a meter.
■ If it is 70 mg/dl or lower, consume 15 grams of carbohydrate, preferably a source of carbohydrate with little or no fat or fiber. Easily portable sources of carbohydrate include glucose tablets or glucose gel, LifeSavers, small (4-ounce) juice boxes, and raisins. Beverages such as orange juice, regular soda, and nonfat milk may also be used.
■ Wait about 15 minutes, then check the blood sugar level with the meter again. If it is still low

(under 70 mg/dl), consume another 15 grams of carbohydrate. (A child planning to engage in physical activity should consume another 15 grams of carbohydrate if his blood sugar is still below 80 mg/dl.)
■ Wait another 15 minutes, then check again.
■ If the next meal is more than half an hour away, another 15 grams of carbohydrate should be eaten to prevent blood sugar from falling again.

If a child is having symptoms of low blood sugar but cannot verify it with his meter, he or his caregiver should assume he is low and treat accordingly. However, if a child feels low but according to his blood glucose meter is not low, he should not consume any carbohydrate but should check again in 15 minutes. As long as symptoms continue, he should recheck his blood sugar every 15 minutes but only treat if his blood sugar has dropped below 70 mg/dl. Sometimes, a falling blood sugar level will produce symptoms of low blood sugar even if the blood sugar level never goes below 70 mg/dl.

Keep in mind that these are general recommendations that may be individualized by your child's diabetes team. You may be advised to treat your child for hypoglycemia at a higher blood glucose level, for example, or to administer more than 15 grams of carbohydrate if his blood sugar level is below a certain level.

How and when to use glucagon

If a child cannot safely swallow or chew, passes out, or has a seizure because of low blood sugar, it will be necessary to use glucagon to raise his blood sugar. Glucagon is a hormone produced in the pancreas that helps to maintain blood sugar levels by causing the release of glucose from the liver. It can also be given by injection to a person with severe hypoglycemia who is unable to consume a source of carbohydrate to his raise blood sugar level. Glucagon rapidly increases a person's blood sugar, generally within 5 to 15 minutes. If a person does not respond within 15 minutes, emergency help should be summoned.

Even if you have been instructed on how to use glucagon, it is a good idea to review how to mix and give it periodically, especially because as your child grows, the dose will change. The following are the recommended doses for glucagon based on age:
■ 0.25 cc for children under 2 years
■ 0.50 cc for children 2 to 5 years
■ 1.0 cc for children older than 5 years

Glucagon is only available by prescription, and a kit should be kept at school and at home. The kit includes a prefilled syringe and a vial of powdered glucagon. Place all of the diluent (the liquid in the prefilled syringe) into the vial, mix until the glucagon is dissolved, then draw out the dose according to your child's age. Glucagon usually expires after one year, so a new kit is needed yearly. Instead of just throwing out expired kits, practice mixing and drawing it up so you will be well trained when or if glucagon is ever needed.

Glucagon should be given based on a child's symptoms, not his blood sugar level. It's possible for a child to have a seizure or pass out when his blood sugar is around 50 mg/dl one time but to seem fine on another occasion when his blood sugar is closer to 30 mg/dl. No matter what his blood sugar level, do not try to give anything by mouth if your child is having a seizure or is unconscious, because he is at risk of inhaling or choking on the food or liquid. Inject glucagon instead. On the other hand, if your child's blood glucose meter says 22 mg/dl but he is able to drink juice, give him the juice.

Even though glucagon raises blood sugar rapidly, it should not used routinely to treat low blood sugar in children capable of eating or drinking or in situations where parents are having a hard time getting juice into their child. If glucagon is given too frequently, it can lose its effectiveness.

If you have to give glucagon, make sure to contact your child's diabetes team afterward. They will want to adjust your child's insulin doses and talk through the days' events prior to the severe low to see if there's anything that can be done differently next time to prevent it from happening again. Your child may experience nausea and vomiting after receiving glucagon. If he does, you will need to lower his insulin doses and follow his sick-day guidelines until he has recovered.

Dealing with hypoglycemia unawareness

Hypoglycemia unawareness is best prevented, but if your child develops it, there are steps that can be taken to help him regain his usual feelings of low blood sugar. Most likely, his diabetes team will recommend adjusting his target blood glucose range to a higher level for a period of weeks. During this time, it will be more important than ever to avoid any episodes of hypoglycemia. To do this, he or you will need to check his blood sugar level more than the minimum of four times a day to catch undetected lows, and nighttime checks may need to be done routinely.

Hypoglycemia unawareness can be scary, but with persistence and teamwork, it can be reversed and prevented. □

WHEN KIDS FALSIFY THEIR NUMBERS

by Jean Roemer, R.N., M.N., C.P.N.P., C.D.E.

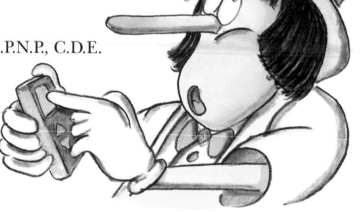

Laura is a bright "almost" thirteen-year-old with freckles, auburn hair, and Type 1 diabetes. She has just finished seventh grade and is a good student. She and her parents come to their medical appointments regularly and are diligent in her diabetes care. At their last visit, her HbA$_{1c}$ (the blood test that indicates the level of blood glucose control over the previous two to three months) was 8.1%, higher than her usual 7.3%. They had explained that family life had been a bit crazy and that she had been sick, which often raises blood glucose levels.

At today's appointment, Laura's mother is certain that Laura's HbA$_{1c}$ level will be lower because

Laura's blood glucose levels have been "nice," and indeed, the logbook they have brought with them shows most of her monitoring results to be in the desired range. But when the nurse educator takes a look at the hospital's lab report and shares the results, Mom and Dad are shocked. Laura's HbA_{1c} is up to 9.0%! Laura's mother looks distressed, and Laura looks at the floor.

"How can that be?" Laura's father asks, sounding worried.

"Could her hormones be causing it to go up now that she is a teenager?" asks her mother.

"That is a possibility," replies Laura's nurse educator, "But she is already on enough insulin for her weight. Also, it is puzzling that her blood glucose monitoring numbers look pretty normal."

"Maybe our meter is off," suggests Dad.

"The meter is OK. It's within 15% of our lab value for glucose." (When the lab drew blood for Laura's HbA_{1c} test, the technician also did a blood glucose test and compared it to a reading using Laura's meter to check the meter for accuracy.)

"I know she's been snacking more," says Mom, "but we've tried to cover it with insulin. Could we have missed something?"

"That's a possibility," replies the nurse educator, "But we'd expect her to gain weight if she were eating too much, and she hasn't. And that still doesn't explain where the high numbers are coming in."

"Well I don't understand!" says Mom. "What do you think the problem is?"

Laura's nurse educator chooses her words carefully. "I'm not sure yet, so let's start with the basics. Could I see Laura's meter, please? Is it all right if I check the memory?"

"Sure. Laura, give her your meter."

Laura replies, "I left it in the waiting room."

"Well, please go get it." Laura reluctantly leaves the room and returns without her meter.

"I can't find it."

"Well go back and look. We just had it two minutes ago."

Laura finally brings in the meter but does not hand it over to the educator; instead she starts playing with the buttons herself. Her dad takes it from her and hands it to the nurse educator, who glances at the logbook and begins to scroll through the memory. Laura hovers and starts pacing back and forth, asking distracting questions.

"Can you tell me where the numbers on your written record came from?" the educator asks, "because I'm not finding any of those in your meter. Who writes these down?"

"I do!" Laura's mother says. Laura looks relieved.

"How do you know what numbers to write down?" the educator asks.

"Laura does her test, and I ask her what it was, and I write it down. We haven't set the time for a while, so maybe the dates are off."

"Do you ever go back and look at the memory in the meter?" asks the educator.

"I haven't. Why?" says Mom.

"Well, here is a 124 on the page for yesterday at dinner, but 324 is in the meter. There is a 118 on the page and 418 in the meter. Here's a 543 in the meter and nothing on the record. And there are a lot of other times that there is nothing in the meter but a number on the page. Does Laura have another meter?"

"Yes, but she only uses it for school."

At this point Laura speaks up, "I think the memory is broken and the dates and times are all messed up. My blood sugars aren't in there. I don't know where those came from!"

Suddenly Laura's mom's brows knit together and her face slowly flushes as she begins to understand that she has been deceived by her daughter. "Laura!" she says. "What is going on here?" Laura's dad is quiet, but he looks angry.

Laura's chin wobbles, but she has nothing to say. Mother is shocked, disappointed, frightened at her child's ability to deceive, frightened about what this means for her health, and embarrassed that her daughter could and would falsify numbers. Laura is relieved to have it out in the open but is afraid she has hurt her mother, knows she is in trouble, and feels like a failure. Laura's nurse educator, however, is not surprised.

Falsification of blood glucose numbers is a common problem among children—and adults—with diabetes. Health professionals experienced in diabetes management recognize when it occurs, but many parents are taken by surprise. This article attempts to help parents understand why it happens and learn how to create a home environment that minimizes the likelihood of falsification.

Sources of trouble

Diabetes management is an all-day, every-day, "24/7" burden of responsibility. It's inconvenient for adults and children alike, and having to prick a finger or other body part four or more times a day for blood glucose monitoring is not fun despite all the modern technology that makes doing so less painful than in years past. Even doctors who don't have diabetes will admit that they would have trouble doing the monitoring required by diabetes if they had to do it. So it's not surprising that even when teenagers are physically and intellectually capable of carrying out all the tasks of their diabetes self-care, they are still not always able to meet the demands placed upon them by their health-care professionals and parents.

Feeling overwhelmed by the demands of diabetes care or simply not being able to keep up—and not wanting anyone to know about it—are common reasons for children and teens to falsify numbers. Some other reasons are the following:

The desire to please. Children and teens vary in their understanding of how blood glucose levels affect their health, either immediately or long-term, but they do understand that their levels are important to their parents, and they respond to parental reactions to blood glucose readings. If parents react with pleasure to in-range readings but with fear and anxiety to high readings, they may be inadvertently steering their child toward falsifying numbers.

That's because children generally want to please their parents, not disappoint them. Meeting expectations so as not to disappoint parents is a strong motivator for many teens, too. If your child or teen knows that you become upset when his numbers aren't what they should be, he may try to protect you from that distress by giving you the numbers that make you happy, rather than the real ones. Alternatively, if you respond to out-of-range numbers by accusing your child of bad behavior or punishing him in some way, he may give you false numbers to protect himself.

People lie to health-care professionals about their diabetes care for similar reasons: to please them and to avoid "getting in trouble." The problem is that these people don't get the help they need to stay in better control. In some cases, their health-care providers may even prescribe changes to their self-care regimen that result in worse control since they're basing their advice on false information.

One way that parents can encourage honesty in their children is to learn to react less emotionally to blood glucose readings. Instead, they can adopt the attitude that all blood glucose readings—high, low, or in-range—provide useful information. The key is knowing how to respond to that information, and that's where a child's health-care provider can help. Parents should be clear about which blood glucose levels require action and what that action should be. They should also be aware of the many factors that can affect blood glucose levels, such as illness or stress. And they should remember that kids with diabetes are human and will inevitably make mistakes. Kids whose parents are able to see mistakes as inevitable and also as learning opportunities are

better able to let their parents know when they've slipped up and need help getting back on track.

Testing boundaries. Boundary testing is a normal part of childhood and the teen years. However, children and teens also desire clear boundaries that help them feel structured and secure. Most teens will test those boundaries to see what they can get away with, how invested the adult is in maintaining the boundary, and whether consequences will result from breaking the rules. Children with diabetes may test the boundaries by not monitoring or by not following other parts of their diabetes plan. (Usually the result is elevated HbA_{1c} test results, angry parents, and embarrassment.)

How a parent can or should respond to boundary testing depends on the child and the situation. In some cases, it may be enough for a parent to restate the rules, supervise the child's diabetes care more closely, and praise him for carrying out diabetes tasks. In others, particularly if a child refuses to perform diabetes care tasks or is having trouble in other areas such as school or socializing, professional counseling may be in order.

Creative exploration. Years ago, when blood glucose monitoring still required obtaining a large, hanging drop of blood and rinsing and blotting the test strip before it could be read, I was privileged to facilitate a focus group for adolescents with diabetes. Over the course of the conversation, there evolved a discussion about how various shades of nail polish painted on test strips would create various blood glucose levels. Some kids had even "tested" substances such as grape jelly, syrup, or milk to see what they could do to obtain high, low, and normal values.

To some degree, these kids may have been looking for a way to produce in-range numbers to please their parents. But they also may have been just having fun experimenting with their meters. Many of the newer meters are able to discern blood from other substances, but some kids will still experiment to see what works and what doesn't. (Parents may need to remind their child that test strips are expensive and not to be wasted and that meters are not toys.)

Desire for independence. It is normal and natural for a child to want greater freedom and independence as he gets older, and most parents are pleased when a child expresses an interest in taking more responsibility for his diabetes care. However, parents must remember that even motivated children and teens are usually not mature enough to carry out their daily diabetes care tasks without the involvement and supervision of a responsible adult whose presence will help them be accountable for their actions. A child or teen who knows that no one will be asking about his monitoring results or reviewing his meter memory is more likely to write down any old number in his logbook if he happens to miss a blood glucose check or two.

Even if your child is responsible and you trust him, stay involved in his diabetes management. Ask him how his numbers are running, and ask how he's coping with his blood glucose monitoring, carbohydrate counting, and other tasks. Offer to help if he's having trouble keeping up or during stressful times such as final exams. In addition, check his meter memory from time to time (once a week, for example), and look for timing, accuracy, and patterns of monitoring. Check to make sure the meter's date and time are correct. The idea is to be supportive and interested, not punitive.

If you have a software package that analyzes blood glucose monitoring results, considering transferring your child's meter memory to the computer periodically. Go over the charts or graphs that the software generates with your child.

"Cheating culture." Many people believe that cheating has become more common in our culture. Who hasn't read a newspaper article recently about workplace theft, cable fraud, music piracy, auto insurance fraud, academic cheating, lying on resumes, or cheating on income tax? While falsifying blood glucose readings has no economic benefits, it could be seen as a way to "succeed" easily and quickly without putting in the hard work of controlling blood glucose levels.

How can a parent dissuade this kind of thinking? For one thing, it helps for both parents and kids to understand why health-care providers recommend blood glucose monitoring, counting carbohydrates, and all of the other diabetes tasks that are sometimes painful and often time-consuming. Rules that seem arbitrary or that don't clearly result in better health or better diabetes control are unlikely to be followed. Parents who aren't sure why a particular diabetes task is advised or don't feel they can adequately explain it to their child in an age-appropriate way should ask their child's health-care provider for help.

It also helps for parents to behave the way they'd like their children to behave—in other words, to set a good example. Parents who continue to pursue goals that are important to them in spite of setbacks demonstrate the value of hard work to their kids and also demonstrate that slipping up doesn't have to mean giving up. Slipping up may be disappointing, but it's also an opportunity to rethink how you're doing things and to find a better way.

A fresh start

Back at the nurse educator's office, Laura was tearful and trying hard to maintain her composure. Her parents were quiet. The educator spoke.

"Laura, first of all, you need to know that you are not the only person to make up blood sugar numbers. It happens. Kids and even some adults do it for all kinds of reasons. It would help me to know a little bit about how you got to the point of making up numbers. Can you describe what was going on?"

Laura looked at her feet and didn't answer.

The educator softly said, "This is hard isn't it, Laura?" Laura nodded. "Are you tired of doing the fingersticks?"

Laura nodded yes.

"It's hard to do them all the time, isn't it?" the educator suggested, thinking that maybe Laura simply felt burned out.

Laura shook her head no, then burst into sobs. "It's not that so much. I don't mind doing the sticks, mostly, that is. I mean, yes, sometimes it's a big pain to do, especially when I have to test when I'm out with friends or something. But it started because sometimes I ate dessert at lunch and knew I shouldn't, but everybody was eating it and I wanted to, or sometimes somebody gives me candy on the bus and then I know my blood sugar will be high. And when it's high everyone gets all upset and grills me." Laura looked at her mother accusingly, "You get all mad at me and ask me what I ate and don't let me eat all of my snack when I'm high, and you are always both so happy when my number is normal. And Daddy, you always tell me I'm going to lose my legs and eyes, and that just doesn't help!" Laura sobbed, and her father rose from his chair to put his arm around his child and give her a hug. Mom's eyes filled with tears, feeling her daughter's pain with insight into the situation.

The educator tried to summarize what Laura said. "So sometimes you know why your blood sugar is high (because you ate dessert or candy) and it is easier to keep the peace in your family by not letting them know. You are trying to protect your parents from distress and keep yourself out of the hot seat, so to speak?"

Laura nodded yes.

The nurse educator continued, "Laura, no one is perfect at this. Everyone, whether they have diabetes or not, is tempted to eat sweets or snacks at times. We can fit these foods into your meal plan, but we have to cover them with insulin so your blood sugar doesn't go too high.

"Also, just so you know, now that you're a teenager, your hormones are causing your insulin not to work as well, and you may have high numbers when you didn't do anything outside your plan. We can adjust your plan for this, too, but only if we know that you're getting high numbers."

Laura nodded, but she looked somewhat skeptical.

The nurse educator continued, "Would it be helpful to you if your mom didn't 'freak' and withhold food when your numbers are high and your dad didn't lecture you?"

Laura nodded yes.

The educator looked at Mom and Dad and asked "What do you think? Do you think you can do that?"

Mom said, "I'll do my best, but I worry."

"I'm sure you worry. It's hard not to. But try not to put a value on Laura's numbers for the time being. In other words, there are not good numbers and bad numbers, but instead, high numbers and low numbers. I think if you look at them that way, it may help."

Dad sighed. "I don't know. Those high numbers just worry me!"

The educator nodded and said, "I'm sure that you will be anxious, but perhaps you could refocus that energy on trying to problem-solve with Laura when her numbers are high. Help her figure out what to do next."

To Laura she said, "I think it would be a good idea for your parents to go back into the memory of your meter at least once a week to look over your numbers. This way, you know that they will be helping you get back on track."

To Laura's parents she said, "This is simply an exercise so that Laura knows you are behind her, helping to keep her accountable, and stepping in to help if she has trouble."

Once their emotions had cooled, Laura, her parents, and the nurse-educator put together a plan. They worked out a way for Laura to eat some extra carbohydrate occasionally and take extra insulin to cover it. Laura admitted that she didn't always want dessert or candy but sometimes ate it because everyone else was eating. The educator tried role-playing with her to help her develop some skills for saying no if she didn't want food. They also acted out some scenarios for how Laura would tell her mom if she had eaten candy on the bus and might have high blood glucose because of it.

Listening to all of this, Mom and Dad began to realize how important it was for Laura not to feel different from her friends and that their own fears and anxieties had contributed to the problem. They vowed to pay more attention to what they said to Laura and how they reacted to Laura's blood glucose monitoring results.

Finally, Laura was able to smile and seemed relieved. She had a fresh start. It had been a difficult yet understandable situation, and everyone learned from it. □

HELPING YOUNG CHILDREN SUCCEED WITH DIABETES CARE

by Alisha Perez, M.S., C.C.L.S.

One afternoon, at the close of a children's support group session, I gathered the kids around for an activity. I sketched a tree trunk on a roll of butcher paper and gave each child two green paper leaves. On one, I asked them to write or draw something that they thought was hard about taking care of diabetes, and on the other, to write or draw something they thought was easy about taking care of diabetes. I had intended the exercise to be a simple expressive outlet, but as I read through their responses, I realized I was getting a loud, clear, and somewhat surprising message from the young people I was caring for.

Not just small adults

Ask adults with diabetes which they find more tolerable, insulin injections or fingersticks, and most will choose injections. The newest insulin needles are so fine and short that they cause very little discomfort. Adults will swear that fingersticks are far worse. There are, in fact, many more sensory receptors in the fingertips, and lancets are much thicker than insulin needles.

I was hearing the opposite story, however, from the young children. When I had gathered all their responses, I was left with 104 hard leaves and 103 easy leaves. The 104th belonged to a five-year-old boy who simply stated, "Nothing about diabetes is easy" and firmly shoved his blank second leaf back into my hand. Fair enough.

I read each leaf and sorted them by topic. While about 10 different topics appeared repeatedly, the two diabetes care tasks mentioned most frequently were fingersticks and injections. Fifty-two percent of the hard leaves bore pictures or words about insulin injections, while only 9% of the hard leaves identified aspects of blood glucose monitoring. Conversely, 51% of the easy leaves showed drawings or told stories of lancets, tiny drops of blood, and meters, and only 10% of the easy leaves mentioned injections.

Understanding their experience

Most of the children who contributed leaves were preschool-age or school-age. To better understand why they identified hard and easy tasks the way they did, it is worth considering some of the characteristics of this developmental stage.

As children enter the preschool years and move into early school-age years, their use of language and symbols increases rapidly, and magical thinking emerges. Magical thinking describes a child's tendency to believe that he has the ability to cause (or prevent) outcomes with his thoughts, actions, or words. For example, a child may believe that the snow began to fall simply because he wished for it to happen.

The concept of *conservation* is also a challenge for children in the preschool and early school-age years. Conservation is the preservation of a physical quantity in spite of a change in shape or some other transformation. For example, a cup of water looks different when poured from a short, wide glass to a tall, thin glass, but it is still the same amount of water. However, a preschool-age child who has not grasped this concept may complain that his sister has more to eat than he does if her sandwich is cut into two pieces and his is left whole. Or a child who refuses to eat mashed potatoes because she hates white food will swear they taste much better when a drop of red food coloring is added.

Children also develop physically during this stage, acquiring both gross and fine motor skills that enable them to play with more complex toys as well as carry out tasks, such as brushing their teeth, that previously someone else had to do for them. Power struggles with parents are common when young children try to assert their newly acquired skills and independence. An example is the three-year-old who insists on dressing himself. His mother, who is already late for work, tries to help speed the process along and is met with a hand shove and a loud, "I can do it myself!"

All of these aspects of development play a role in how young children understand and respond to diabetes care. For example, magical thinking may lead a young child to believe his injections will cure his diabetes or possibly that his injections are punishment for misbehavior or inappropriate thoughts. Family power struggles may emerge around diabetes care as a child becomes able to perform some of his own diabetes care tasks, such as doing fingersticks, and also begins to want more control over what happens to his body. However, while some children can monitor their own blood glucose at an early age, parents are still responsible for, and encouraged to remain closely involved in, all aspects of diabetes management.

Children in this age range tend to be concerned about how health-care experiences and procedures will affect their bodies. They may be disturbed by "holes" being made in their skin by needles or concerned about running out of blood.

A lack of understanding about conservation may help explain why children often prefer fingersticks to insulin injections. From an adult's perspective, insulin needles and lancets are both sharp metal objects that cause a pricking or painful sensation. From a child's perspective, however, there are some important differences. An insulin syringe has a naked needle on the end, which, no matter how short, is still clearly a needle. Lancets, however, are neatly hidden within the lancing device. Even though children may watch the lancet being inserted into the lancing device, they will often not be as focused on the lancet once it is hidden.

The issue of outward appearances, combined with limitations in logical reasoning, may also help to explain why young children often protest larger doses of insulin. The more insulin that's in the syringe, the larger its physical appearance. A syringe that is filled with insulin can be as long as 5 inches from the top of the plunger to the tip of the needle. If getting insulin is thought of as scary or painful, more insulin may seem worse.

Injections also encroach on a child's personal space. The closer to the midline or center of the body, the more threatening the procedure may seem to the integrity and safety of the body. This probably explains why young children tend to be much more resistant to rotating injections on their bellies than on their legs or arms. Fingersticks, on the other hand, feel less invasive because they can be done with the child holding his hand out several inches away from his body.

Young children will often share their thoughts and perceptions of injections through play. Recently, a four-year-old child sat on the clinic playroom floor pretending to give insulin with a needle-less syringe to a baby doll. She pulled the plunger back as far as it would go.

"This baby is gonna get a big shot. He's crying," she said. I followed her script and made soft crying sounds on behalf of the doll.

"She needs more," the girl said as she pretended to refill the syringe, this time only pulling the syringe back a few units. I continued the soft crying for the doll, thinking I was still following her lead.

"No! The baby's not crying. It's just a little shot," she said, as if it were obvious that a small amount of insulin would not cause the baby to cry the way a large amount did.

Another typical playroom scenario involves the dolls receiving injections in the face, neck, or chest. The children will often look toward an adult immediately after an injection as if to ask, "What are the chances of that happening to me?" My response to this type of play is always supportive and reassuring: "We can pretend to give the baby his insulin there, but real children would never get an insulin shot in those places."

The problem of pain

Understanding cognitive ability is only the first step in grasping the children's message about their experiences with injections and fingersticks. The second is accepting the existence of pain in diabetes management. It seems less harsh and more comforting to tell parents and children that it really doesn't hurt at all. When children do report pain, adults may say it's "just anxiety" or that the child is "seeking attention" or "trying to gain control." While these emotional and behavioral issues are likely to play an important role in pain perception, they are not separate from actual pain.

I continue to hear health-care professionals and parents referring to "psychological" pain. People are forever pointing their fingers at this pesky, imaginary perpetrator that allegedly causes children to yell, flail, and physically resist the tiniest needle stick.

This idea of a separate, psychological pain is not quite accurate, according to the latest pain theories. The pain-sensing system can be influenced by cognitive, emotional, behavioral, and contextual variables. This means that the *same* child, experiencing the *same* amount of tissue damage, on the *same* area of the skin, is likely to report *different* levels of pain depending on factors such as how anxious he is, the setting in which he experiences the

painful stimuli, and his understanding of what is happening. Yes, there is a psychological component to pain, but it often causes actual changes in pain perception.

The concept that pain perception is influenced by external factors is far less grim than the idea that the intensity of pain is strictly related to the amount of tissue damage, because it implies that there is an opportunity to reduce pain by changing the variables that influence it.

Helping children cope better

Children are resilient beings, and eventually, most learn to cope well with the routine of diabetes management. Health-care providers and parents can facilitate coping for young children with the following tips.

Acknowledge your child's fears. Understand that injections and fingersticks may be scary to children and that kids may experience real discomfort. Refrain from telling your child that his claims of discomfort from shots or fingersticks are wrong. Responses such as "You didn't feel that" can be embarrassing and frustrating if the child truly did experience pain. A more helpful response to a child who says, "That really hurt!" might be, "I can tell you had some pain. Let's try and find a way to make it easier next time."

Reduce anxiety-provoking factors. Because some children may be less apprehensive if needles are hidden, families may want to try using an injecting device such as the Inject-Ease, made by BD, which encases the syringe and needle. Be aware, however, that the device may have the opposite effect on children who dislike large injection devices.

Provide your child with one minute of preparation time per year of age for injections or fingersticks rather than abruptly interrupting his activity. For example, if your child is three years old, give him a cue three minutes before injection; if he is five years old, give the cue five minutes prior.

Adults should try to remain as relaxed as possible. Children are greatly influenced by parental anxiety. Talk softly and slowly. Try not to escalate the tone or speed of your speech if your child begins to cry or resist.

Everyone involved in blood glucose monitoring or injecting insulin may want to practice controlled breathing. Instruct your child to take a deep, slow breath, hold for three seconds, and exhale slowly. Do this two to three times together. Time the insulin injections with the last breath, and have your child blow out as the needle is being inserted, as if he were blowing away the pinch.

When possible, find a quiet place to do injections. In the home, families may want to choose one area of the house to do most injections. This may help the child feel less anxious by setting a clear, physical boundary for where injections happen. If using one area of the home is not possible, then try to pick at least one area to be a "safe zone" where injections never occur.

Make a schedule. Using a doll or child-friendly chart, create a rotation schedule that your child can understand easily. Families can mark the appropriate injection sites on a cloth or vinyl doll and then write the day and time insulin injections are due in that site. Some children may prefer a simple calendar chart with days, times, and sites written out. Either type of schedule will provide a clear sense of where injections will go and when they will happen, reassuring the child that diabetes care is part of a routine and not a punishment for something he did.

Offer limited choices. For children who like to take part in their own diabetes management, parents may find it helpful to set a clear limit on what choices are available rather than posing broad questions such as, "Where do you want to put the shot today?" Instead, allow your child to choose one of only two possible injection sites or fingers.

Work quickly. All choices should be offered and discussions finished before the injection or blood glucose monitoring supplies are out of their storage place. Adults should avoid engaging in lengthy negotiations with their child once the syringe or lancet is out and ready to be used. Looking at the syringe or lancet while discussing its use often creates more anticipatory anxiety.

Use distraction. Distraction is the most practical and effective tool families can use to minimize pain and distress for children. The use of cognitive distraction and touch distraction is based on the theory that cognitive activities and stimulation of the skin by stroking, rubbing, or applying pressure create impulses that travel to the brain and spinal cord quickly and interrupt the pain impulses that travel through the same pathways, reducing pain perception. Several recent studies suggest that both cognitive and touch distraction may be quite effective in reducing pain during immunization injections.

Cognitive distraction activities include blowing bubbles or a party-blower, squeezing on a soft ball, searching for specific items in a colorful photo or in the room, doing simple math equations out loud, counting, or saying the alphabet. Touch and pressure distraction may be helpful for children who are too upset to effectively engage in a cognitive activity during injections. The easiest way to use this technique is to apply pressure to the injec-tion site with the thumb for 10 seconds just prior to the injection. People often use this technique in reverse when they experience pain. For example, a person bumps his shin and immediately rubs the injury to reduce the pain.

Another technique involves gently stroking the skin within an inch of the injection site as the insulin is being administered, using the fingers that are not being used to pinch up the skin. This may take some coordination and practice. If a second person is available to assist with injections, he can softly stroke the skin near the site as the injection is given. There is also a small, plastic device available called the ShotBlocker that helps create pressure distraction around the injection site.

Reduce pain where possible. Families may seek the advice of their medical team in choosing the smallest, shortest needles and lancets for their child. Some children may also find comfort in icing the skin for 10–20 seconds prior to injections. This can help by desensitizing the receptors in the surface of the skin.

Help older kids, too. Be available to support school-age and adolescent children as they become more competent at completing diabetes management tasks independently. Older children may still experience some anxiety or discomfort around diabetes tasks. Children are more likely to engage in coping behaviors with an adult acting as a coach than they might on their own.

Follow-up and support

Fear and distress over needles are appropriate responses to the management of diabetes for many children. In most cases, parental efforts to reduce anxiety and improve coping will be sufficient. However, some situations merit closer attention by a mental health professional, such as if a child frequently remains upset for more than 10 minutes after an injection or fingerstick. Similarly, if insulin is not being properly administered or there is great difficulty in following the blood glucose monitoring schedule recommended by your health-care team due to your child's distress, seek immediate support from your child's diabetes care team.

Kids have a remarkable capacity to learn to cope with a variety of stressors, especially with the support of caring adults. The coping strategies described here require consistent practice to be effective, but not all need be used at once. I encourage families to start slowly by choosing one or two techniques to work on over a few weeks. It's important to give any one technique a few tries before giving up. Eventually, the child and family will discover which strategies work best for them. □

GETTING EATING HABITS ON A HEALTHY TRACK

by Amy Sullivan, R.D., L.D.N., C.D.E.

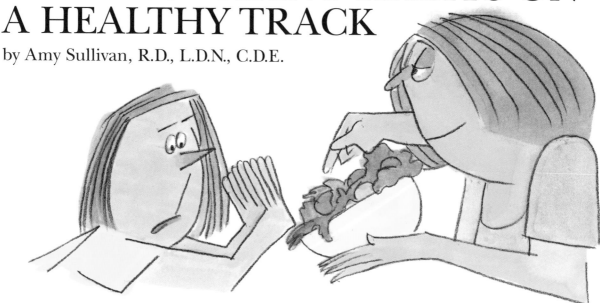

As you walk down the aisle of the grocery store, you realize two things: The store is devoting more and more shelf space to boxed meals and convenience foods, and more and more of those items are ending up in your cart. You know that many of these products are high in sodium and fat and low in other nutrients, and you wonder how your grocery list got this way.

Is it because you're always too busy to cook these days? Is it because your kids demand the foods they see on television and refuse to eat the foods you cook? Or is it something else?

Whatever the reason, you vow that from now on, good nutrition has to take priority, and you are determined to get your whole family eating more healthfully.

Barriers to healthy eating

Families face many barriers to healthy eating these days. Some parents aren't sure what good nutrition is. Some have trouble saying no to children who would like to subsist on sweets or fast foods. Some parents are well aware of what makes a balanced meal but never have a moment to prepare one. And some kids are so busy they never seem to eat at home.

Eating at school. Making healthy food choices at school can be tough for your child if the school has vending machines with soft drinks and foods such as potato chips, cookies, and candy bars. The choices in the school's cafeteria may not help promote healthier eating habits either. These days, it's not unusual for schools to serve nachos, pizza, snack foods, and desserts for lunch every day, in addition to the more conventional school cafeteria food.

The good news is that more parents, teachers, and lawmakers are realizing that the high-fat, high-calorie foods kids are eating at school are contributing to the rise in obesity among school-age children, and they're doing something about it. Some school districts are changing the choices in the vending machines in schools, while others are turning off the vending machines during lunch hours in hopes of promoting better choices and healthier eating habits. So far, Arkansas, California, and West Virginia have enacted laws to help with the vending machine situation, and other state legislatures have introduced bills laying out guidelines for their school districts.

If you can obtain the school lunch menu in advance, you and your child can review healthy food choices and decide together which days to buy lunch and which days to pack a lunch. Most schools can provide this information monthly, and schools must do so if it is part of the child's medical care plan.

Fast food. According to the National Restaurant Association, Americans spend more of their total food spending on foods eaten away from home than those eaten at home. The average adolescent visits a fast-food restaurant at least twice a week. Fast food is notoriously high in fat and sodium (while low in fruits, vegetables, and fiber), and restaurant portions are notoriously large, making it very easy to overeat.

There may be times when eating out is your

only option, but there are ways to make healthier choices even at fast-food restaurants. Most fast-food chains now have menu items such as grilled chicken sandwiches and salads with low-fat dressings. Simply skipping the French fries can go a long way toward cutting the fat, calories, and sodium in a meal. You may need to take the time to educate your children about what's in the food they're eating and to negotiate about acceptable fast-food choices.

Picky eaters. Young children are often resistant to trying new foods, but even some older children and adults are picky about what they eat, and this can make it difficult to introduce new foods to the family table. Compounding the problem may be the techniques parents have used to try to encourage their child to try new foods. Attempting to force a child to try new foods, for example, rarely works. Making a big deal about a child's eating habits is also not helpful. In general, the more that is made out of a child's not eating a food, the more that child will not eat it. Once mealtimes have become stressful power struggles, it's hard to turn the tide.

Overcoming pickiness

Getting your children to try new foods may require both accepting that a certain amount of resistance to trying new things is normal and acknowledging the influence parents have over what their child will try. For example, when a parent makes a face or remarks that a food is bad, the child is not likely to want to eat it either. On the other hand, if a child sees a parent eating a food with enjoyment, he may want to imitate that parent. He may also take a cue from a parent who bravely tries a food he doesn't think he'll like or that he disliked in the past.

Even with no negative parental messages, some children need to be exposed to a new food multiple times (as many as 15 or more) before they will try it. Pressuring a child to try a food will not speed up the process. With young children, it works better to simply make the food available and allow them to decide whether to eat it or at least play with it, which can make them more comfortable with it. They may need to play with a new food many times to become comfortable with it. Once a child is comfortable playing with a food, he may be willing to put his finger on the food then lick the finger. This is an easy way for a child to get a small taste of a food without actually eating it. Once that becomes familiar, a child may be willing to pick the food up and put it in his mouth. When a child is allowed to proceed at his

own pace, he may in time begin to eat the foods you want him to eat.

Older children should similarly not be forced to eat foods they don't like, but they may be more willing to at least try a bite. One possibility for introducing new foods to the family menu would be to prepare a food that no one in the family has tried before. That way, everyone tries it at the same time, and no one is singled out. It may take preparing a new food several different ways before finding one the family likes. A household rule may have to be that everyone must try the new food regardless of whether they think they'll like it. Start with a tablespoon of the new food and then work in more as the acceptance of the new food increases. They don't have to love the new food, just be willing to have a small taste or have a very small portion of the food.

As your family experiments with new foods and finds which they like and don't like, keep in mind that no single food is necessary for good health. If your child doesn't like cauliflower, for example, he may be willing to eat kale, which provides many of the same nutrients. If he doesn't like tomatoes, he can get his vitamin C from oranges. The goal is an overall healthy diet, not acceptance of any particular food.

Tips for making the transition

Making any lifestyle change is usually easier if it is done gradually, a step at a time. As you work on changing your family's eating habits, therefore, pace yourself, and remember that there is no perfect diet.

One new food at a time. When preparing a meal, add one new food to the meal and keep the other components of the meal familiar. Adding the unknown to the known can help your family members accept a new food. Also, you don't have to serve new foods every day; including something new at a couple of meals each week is sufficient.

Let your child help. Another way to help the likelihood that your child will eat new foods is to have him help with planning and preparing of the meal. The more involved children are in these decisions, the more they are willing to try something that is new.

Make changes gradually. If your kids are used to drinking whole milk and eating white rice, it may be unrealistic to expect them to switch to skim milk and brown rice overnight. However, in the case of milk, you may be able to get them to switch first to reduced-fat (2%) milk, then to low-fat (1%) milk, and finally to skim milk. If you meet resistance along the way, you can try mixing two types of milk (reduced-fat with low-fat, or low-fat with skim) and gradually reducing the proportion of the higher-fat milk. If your children will only drink flavored milk, do the same thing by gradually reducing the amount of flavored milk in the glass.

This same technique can be used with foods such as whole wheat pasta and brown rice, although it obviously takes more effort to cook two pans of rice than to mix two types of milk. Rather than mixing rices, you might try serving very small portions of brown rice to introduce it gradually. Homemade pancakes or muffins, though, can be made into whole-grain pancakes or muffins without a lot of extra work.

Snack on fruits and vegetables. Kids are more likely to eat fruits and vegetables if those items are readily available when they're hungry (and snacks like chips and crackers are not). Anticipate the demand for snacks by cutting up some vegetables and washing some fruit in advance. When dinner is being prepared and the kids are hungry, offer them an apple or some carrot sticks or sliced cucumbers with a little low-fat dip to help curb their hunger until dinner is ready. Mixing fruit with cottage cheese or yogurt may give it even more appeal— and add nutrients to the snack as well.

Allow "junk food" in moderation. Suddenly telling a child he can no longer have his favorite snack food is likely to make him want it even more—and set you up for a parent–child control struggle. Unless there's an absolute need to rule out a food completely (because of a peanut allergy, for example), you may have more success changing your child's eating habits by continuing to allow moderate amounts of "junk food." You might decide that your child can have one serving of his desired snack once a day, at a time he chooses. A rule like this gives your child some control over what he eats, but you are still setting limits to keep his overall diet a healthy one.

Follow the pyramid

What if you need some help figuring out which foods you and your family should be eating? One helpful tool is the USDA Food Pyramid, which can be found on the Internet at www.MyPyramid.gov. The site provides basic information about the various food groups, including the amounts of each food group needed according to age, sex, and level of physical activity. You can also use the MyPyramid Tracker to assess your current food intake and get some tips on improving it.

In general, the new pyramid encourages replacing processed grains with whole grains and adding more legumes (such as lentils and dried beans),

NUTRITIOUS SNACKS

Young children normally eat frequent, small meals. A child's stomach is small and cannot hold or digest a lot of food at one time. Even for older kids, though, having several small meals and snacks a day can help with blood glucose control and prevent overeating since they won't come to meals starving. Snacks don't have to be unhealthy. Here are some nutritious snacks to offer to your kids and eat yourself:

- Carrots, celery sticks, or any other vegetable with low-fat dip
- Popcorn (plain or low-fat)
- Trail mix (with or without nuts)
- Apple with peanut butter
- Yogurt with fruit or granola
- Hummus with whole wheat pita bread
- Whole-grain cereal with low-fat milk
- Baked tortilla chips with salsa
- Cheese with whole wheat crackers

fruits, and vegetables to the diet. It offers suggestions on choosing leaner meats and heart-healthy oils. No foods are ruled out altogether, but certain ones are emphasized. For example, while all vegetables are good for you, dark-green and orange vegetables such as broccoli and sweet potatoes contain higher amounts of vitamins and minerals than paler vegetables.

Many other organizations' Web sites offer nutrition information as well, including the American Diabetes Association (www.diabetes.org). A particularly good resource with nutrition information and recipes for both parents and children is www.KidsHealth.org, a Web site of the Nemours Foundation.

Put parents in charge

Learning to say no to a child's demand for a popular cereal or snack food can be tough, but when grocery shopping or planning meals and snacks, the parents should ultimately decide what is available in the house. If there is something that you do not want your child to have, not buying it is the first step. If it is not in the house to eat, it's not a temptation to your child.

But what if *you* want foods you'd prefer your child not eat? To preserve family harmony, eat those foods only outside the home, and request that other adults or teens in the household do likewise. Similarly, if you have relatives who bring over treats you'd prefer your family not eat, talk with those relatives privately and explain politely that you're trying to improve your family's eating habits.

Shortcuts

Every cook needs an arsenal of shortcuts for when time is short or energy low. Here are some ideas:

■ Buy frozen vegetables, precut vegetables, or prepackaged salads for quick and nutritious vegetable side dishes.

■ Cook larger batches of food on weekends so there are leftovers during the week.

■ Use a microwave to bake potatoes or sweet potatoes in minutes.

■ Learn which whole grains cook quickly. Quinoa and kasha, for example, take only about 15 minutes on the stovetop.

■ Keep some cans of beans in the cupboard for quick bean salads or dips. Canned low-fat refried beans make quick burritos, and canned low-fat chili with lentils or beans makes a quick meal.

Working together

Although the desire to have your family eat healthier may start with you, your school-age or teenage children may surprise you by getting on board rather than resisting your plan. They may be learning about nutrition at school or simply developing an interest in health and fitness on their own. Young athletes, in particular, may be receptive to the idea that good nutrition can improve their game. And young chefs may welcome the opportunity to experiment in the kitchen.

Even if your plan meets with opposition, however, the fact that you are setting a good example and setting limits on the types and amounts of food that come into your home is likely to influence your family's eating habits in a positive way in the long run. □

DENTAL CARE FOR KIDS

by Brian S. Martin, D.M.D.

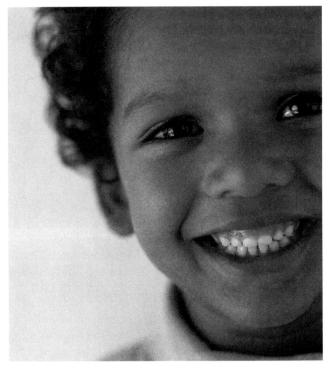

Periodontal disease, a chronic infection of the gums and bone structure of the mouth, has been called the "sixth complication" of diabetes because of the link between the two diseases. Having diabetes raises the risk of developing periodontal disease, and having periodontal disease is a risk factor for developing Type 2 diabetes. Periodontal disease negatively affects blood glucose control in any type of diabetes.

The good news for kids with diabetes is that periodontal disease is less common among children than among adults. But the time to take preventive steps against it and to establish good dental health habits is in childhood.

The American Academy of Pediatric Dentistry recommends a first dental visit at age 1 for children who are "at risk" for dental disease. Children with diabetes fit into this category. Education of the child's parents or caregivers is a critical part of the dental team's mission to promote good oral health care for children.

First dental visits

The focus of the age 1 dental visit is largely to provide anticipatory guidance to the child's parents or caregivers. It should include a comprehensive review of the child's current oral health status, noting the presence or absence of cavities; the condition of the soft tissues, including the tongue, insides of the cheeks, and gums; and overall growth and development. Any signs of *xerostomia,* or a reduced flow of saliva, should be closely monitored, since a reduction in saliva is associated with an increased incidence of cavities.

The child's diet should also be reviewed. Sugary beverages such as fruit juices, soft drinks, sweetened iced tea, and chocolate and strawberry-flavored milk are at the top of the list of foods that promote tooth decay. Because sweetened beverages also raise blood glucose levels, they are often not a big part of the dietary habits of children with diabetes, but if they are, parents should be aware of their role in causing cavities.

Home oral hygiene practices are another area that should be reviewed at the age 1 dental visit. Before a child's teeth erupt, the mouth is largely self-cleaning. However, parents can use a wet washcloth to wipe the mouth if they wish. As soon as the first tooth erupts, the parent should brush the tooth twice a day with a soft toothbrush. No fluoride toothpaste is necessary until 2 years of age, and the use of fluoride-containing toothpaste should always be supervised by a parent or caregiver because of young children's tendency to swallow much of the toothpaste on their brush. Only a pea-size amount of toothpaste is necessary on a child's toothbrush, and teeth should be brushed twice a day. Toothbrushes should be replaced approximately every 3–4 months, or when the bristles become frayed.

Teeth should be flossed if they are touching or appear to touch one another. A good rule of thumb is that if a toothbrush bristle cannot smoothly pass between two teeth, flossing is needed. Floss should be used daily. Over time, kids will learn to like having their teeth flossed!

Research has shown that kids do not do a very good job of brushing their own teeth until age 8 or 9, so it is probably safe to assume the same applies to floss. Electric toothbrushes are a great instrument to get kids to brush more thoroughly and longer, and there is very little if any risk associated with their supervised use.

In addition to twice-daily brushing, children who have a bedtime snack should brush after the snack. Going to bed without brushing allows the bacteria that cause cavities to feast on the bedtime snack particles, raising the risk of tooth decay. There is also less saliva in the mouth during sleep, which also increases the risk of tooth decay.

As a child grows older

From the dentist's perspective, office-based preventive care appointments for children with diabetes are very similar to those for children who don't have diabetes. Slight modifications to appointment times may be appropriate, as early morning appointments for younger children may result in better behavior and increased attention

TREATING NIGHTTIME HYPOGLYCEMIA

It's not uncommon for kids with diabetes (particularly those who use insulin) to develop low blood glucose, or hypoglycemia, during the night. Parents often try to prevent it by giving their kids juice, milk, or crackers during the night. If low blood glucose develops, these same foods, glucose tablets, or candy are commonly used to treat it. However, kids are typically hard to wake up at night (and often don't remember it in the morning), so brushing their teeth after treating for hypoglycemia is usually not practical. Yet eating or drinking in the middle of the night does raise their risk of cavities.

To prevent tooth decay without middle-of-the-night toothbrushing sessions, it may help to have kids use a nightly fluoride gel or rinse at bedtime in addition to their regular toothpaste. In addition, a quick swish or swallow of plain water after the snack should go a long way toward preventing decay.

span. "Tell, show, and do" techniques should be employed by the dental team to put the child at ease and provide a positive experience in the dental office.

The frequency of office visits for professional cleanings and checkups will vary from child to child. For children whose diabetes is under control, a biannual examination, cleaning, fluoride treatment, and anticipatory guidance visit with the dental team is often appropriate. But it is not uncommon for a dentist to recommend visits more frequently than every six months, particularly if a problem is discovered or if the child's medical history dictates closer follow-up. As the child grows older, visit frequency should be tailored to his individual needs.

If dental surgery is needed, a consultation with the child's endocrinologist is necessary, particularly if the child will be instructed to have nothing by mouth (no food or drink) for a period of time prior to treatment. In dentistry, this is commonly the case prior to sedation or a general anesthetic. Teenagers with diabetes are often admitted to the hospital for surgical removal of their third molars, or wisdom teeth. Not only will they and their parents need presurgical counseling, but the importance of good blood glucose control following removal of a wisdom tooth should be reviewed as well. Poor blood glucose control following surgery can contribute to impaired or delayed healing of the soft and hard tissues of the mouth.

Tackling dental problems

In the adult diabetes population, periodontal disease is the greatest oral health risk. In children with diabetes, cavities and fungal infections (candidiasis) are more common.

To help prevent cavities, some dentists recommend sealants, which are protective plastic coatings for the chewing surfaces of teeth that have deep pits or grooves. They are highly effective in preventing decay (although regular brushing, flossing, and avoiding sugary foods are still important even with sealants).

Children with braces or other forms of orthodontia may need a reminder that it is very, very important to maintain excellent oral hygiene throughout orthodontic treatment. Lack of proper oral hygiene can result in cavities, which will need to be repaired when the braces are removed.

Signs and symptoms of oral fungal infections include a milky-white, "cheese curd"–like coating on the inside surfaces of the mouth. The gums or other soft tissues may also appear red. An oral fungal infection is usually not painful and rarely interferes with eating. It is treated with topical antifungal medicine (commonly the drug nystatin), which is very effective.

While advanced periodontal disease is more common in adults than children, chronic gingivitis, or early periodontal disease, is quite common. Gingivitis causes gum tissue to swell, turn red, and bleed easily when brushing or flossing. Treating it may require more frequent professional cleanings and greater attention to home care.

Smoking and piercing

Dentists see firsthand the damage done by smoking and the use of other tobacco products. Smoking is known to be strongly associated with gingivitis, an early stage of periodontal disease that can lead to advanced stages. While kids may not be too concerned about eventual tooth loss or other health concerns related to smoking later in life, they may be receptive to hearing that tobacco makes them smell bad, look bad, have brown teeth, and have no money right now. Don't hesitate to enlist your dentist's help in encouraging your child to stop smoking or using tobacco.

Dentists also see the damage done by tongue and lip piercings. While not all piercings lead to trouble, some do, and they can cause lip and gum scarring and even loss of teeth, either by breaking the teeth themselves or by destroying the gum tissue, ligament, and bone that holds the teeth in the mouth. When permanent teeth are lost, it is a life-long issue. A $75 piercing can add up to thousands of dollars in dental work down the road.

Part of the whole

Oral health is increasingly recognized as a critical component of systemic health. However, it is generally understood that fewer than 50% of the U.S. population seek regular, preventive dental care. This lack of preventive care sets the stage for episodic, emergency-based care, which does little to ensure the long-term oral health of an individual. Deeply rooted cultural prejudice regarding dentistry and oral health care play a role in the low use of preventive dental care, as does personal finance and insurance coverage status. However, advances in dental technology, anesthesia, and care delivery now allow dental practitioners to practice "pain-free" dentistry with good cosmetic outcomes.

Because of the significant impact that dental and oral complications can have on the quality of life of a person with diabetes, taking advantage of what dentistry has to offer is crucial for people with diabetes. Start your child off on the right foot with a professional examination, regular follow-up care, and good home oral hygiene. With the right information and regular care, it is possible for a person with diabetes to have a healthy mouth for a lifetime. □

WHEN YOUR CHILD NEEDS SURGERY

by Edward Scott Vokoun, M.D.

Surgery can be a frightening proposition for anyone. But when the person having surgery is your child, the anxiety can be especially hard to deal with.

I have a friend whose young daughter recently needed abdominal surgery. She recounts feeling "scared and overwhelmed. I had complete confidence in the doctors and staff. The hospital was wonderful too. But I just couldn't help feeling unbelievably frightened."

Unfortunately, your child's diabetes can make a challenging situation like surgery even more intimidating. It is therefore especially important for you to understand how diabetes affects the *perioperative period* (the time leading up to, during, and following surgery) to ensure the best possible outcome for your child.

Understanding the surgical process

While it is natural to feel nervous about a process over which you have no control, learning about that process can help ease the anxiety. Controlling your own apprehension can also help your child control his anxiety—kids are often much more in tune with adults' state of mind than we give them credit for.

There are many common reasons a child may need surgery. Young children may need abdominal surgery, such as hernia repairs; ear, nose, and throat surgery, such as tonsillectomies or placement of ear tubes (tubes that allow air into the middle ear, helping prevent infection); or ophthalmologic procedures, such as the correction of *amblyopia*, or a "lazy eye." They may also require anesthesia for dental work or imaging exams, such as *MRI* (magnetic resonance imaging) or *CT* (computed tomography) scans, that require a person to lie still. Older children frequently need to have appendectomies, orthopedic surgery, or tooth extractions. There are also a variety of less common reasons a child may require surgical treatment.

For many people, the most anxiety-provoking part of surgery is the use of anesthesia. Many people question its safety. However, according to the

American Society of Anesthesiologists, anesthesia has never been safer. Since the early 1980's, the number of all deaths related to anesthesia has decreased from one in 10,000 to one in 250,000.

A child who is undergoing surgery will be under the supervision of an anesthesiologist or an anesthetist throughout the perioperative period. Anesthesiologists are physicians certified by the American Board of Anesthesiology to provide anesthetic care. Similarly, Certified Registered Nurse Anesthetists are nurses licensed to provide such services. Both certifications require years of training.

Anesthesiologists and anesthetists have a number of roles in caring for a person who is undergoing surgery. These health-care professionals are trained to produce the sleeplike state called anesthesia and are also in charge of the prevention and treatment of pain. Anesthesia providers are also experts in how conditions such as diabetes affect the body, and they provide treatment for these conditions during the perioperative period. For instance, in someone with diabetes, the anesthesia provider maintains control of the blood glucose level during surgery by administering intravenous Regular insulin and glucose as necessary. He also may check blood glucose levels before, during, and after the operation.

In effect, the anesthesiologist or anesthetist is the representative for your child's primary-care provider during surgery, so communicating with him can help smooth the surgical process and provide you with more peace of mind.

Before surgery

Once it has been determined that a child with diabetes needs surgery, the anesthesiologist or anesthetist will require certain information so that he can address the special needs of the child. Important information for parents to provide includes any allergies or other medical issues the child has, current medicines the child is taking, past surgeries the child has had, if any, the child's history of response to anesthesia, and any family history of response to anesthesia. The child's current weight is also crucial, since the amount of anesthetic to be administered is based on weight.

Providing a history of recent upper respiratory infection is important as well. Undergoing anesthesia is generally safe, but a history of respiratory symptoms in the month leading up to surgery can lessen the margin of safety. In fact, a recent history of upper respiratory infection is one of the most common reasons that elective surgery in children is rescheduled. Signs of respiratory infection, which include a cold, runny nose, fever, wheezing, or coughing, should be mentioned to the anesthesia provider.

Most medical centers have a system for handling preoperative medical screenings. As part of the screening, the child's medical history should be reviewed by the anesthesia provider. In some cases, especially when the child has a complicated medical history, a face-to-face interview between the child's parents and the anesthesia provider may be appropriate, while in other cases a phone call may be sufficient.

The anesthesia provider, in conjunction with the child's parents or guardians and the surgeon, will determine the best technique for administering the anesthetic. *General anesthesia* is a state similar to sleep. Because the body loses control of its ability to breathe independently while under general anesthesia, respiratory support must be provided. *Regional anesthesia* can take a number of forms, including blocks of nerve bundles that communicate with an extremity such as an arm or leg, and *epidural* (spinal) anesthetic injections that create a loss of sensation in a specific area of the body. *Local anesthesia* may take the form of injections of anesthetic directly at the surgical site. The various techniques may also be combined. Regardless of which technique is agreed upon, the anesthesia provider should explain the plan and obtain the informed consent of the child's parents or guardians.

Diabetes and surgery

Surgery stresses the body, leading to the release of stress hormones. These hormones normally raise blood glucose levels and with them, insulin requirements. It is this stress response that makes people with diabetes require more insulin during an illness, and it can similarly complicate blood glucose control during and after surgery.

A person who is undergoing anesthesia will be asked to fast for a period of time prior to elective surgery. This requirement helps to ensure that the person has an empty stomach, reducing the likelihood that he will vomit and inhale his stomach contents into his lungs. For simplicity's sake, many institutions instruct people preparing for surgery to fast after midnight the day of surgery. According to guidelines published by the American Society of Anesthesiologists, people who are about to have surgery should abstain from fatty meals for eight hours prior to surgery; light carbohydrate meals, infant formula, and fatty or pulpy liquids for six hours prior to surgery; breast milk for at least four hours prior to surgery; and clear fluids, including fruit juice without pulp, for at least two hours prior to surgery.

Needless to say, the effects of surgery and its preparation present a challenge for children with diabetes, and those who take insulin must adjust their insulin regimens accordingly. One common way to adjust a typical insulin regimen in preparation for surgery is to halve the amount of long-acting insulin the child usually takes the evening before surgery and to skip any short-acting insulin the morning of surgery. This maintains some background insulin but reduces the risk of hypoglycemia (low blood glucose) while fasting. If the child uses an insulin pump, the basal delivery of insulin is typically continued while the bolus doses are not given. A child's blood glucose level should also be checked more frequently during the perioperative period. Insulin dosing and blood glucose monitoring should be discussed as part of the preoperative screening process. Blood glucose should be checked the morning of the surgery with a plan for administering glucose if blood glucose levels are low or for insulin if levels are high.

Children with Type 2 diabetes who take only oral medicines also have special needs when having surgery. One of the most common oral drugs, metformin (brand name Glucophage and others), normally is not taken for 24 hours prior to surgery. Other oral diabetes drugs may or may not be taken depending on the child's needs. Because it is common for acid reflux (heartburn) to accompany Type 2 diabetes, it is important to inform your child's anesthesia provider of any history or symptoms of this condition, since controlling stomach acid (to prevent it from entering the lungs) is one of the goals of anesthetic care during surgery.

The day of surgery

The day of surgery is not going to be a normal day. Working parents may have to take the day off. Day-care arrangements may be necessary for brothers and sisters. Everyone may be awake much earlier than usual. Your child may have to skip breakfast. And there may be long waits before, during, and after surgery. Amidst all this, there will be plenty of opportunities for parents, the child having surgery, and other family members to feel anxious.

However, there are several strategies for helping your child deal with anxiety. First, do your best to keep yourself calm. Tell your child as much as possible about what to expect ahead of time. Oral medicine to reduce anxiety, ease the stress of separation, and provide *amnesia* (loss of memory) may also be an option for your child. Be sure to ask if the hospital has a special waiting area for children and whether it can accommodate the child's favorite toy or other item in the operating room.

In young children, general anesthesia is typically brought about with a mask using anesthetics in gas form. Older children who are able to tolerate the insertion of an intravenous (IV) line while awake can be put under anesthesia with intravenous medicine. The advantage of intravenous anesthetics is an increased margin of safety. However, many people report that the placement of an IV line is among their most stressful experiences during surgery. More mature children may be able to tolerate the procedure if you discuss it with them beforehand. Techniques to reduce the pain of inserting an IV line, including using topical creams and local anesthetic, can be helpful as well.

The operating room is a busy place. When a patient arrives, it can feel like a NASCAR pit crew is working on him. It is not a good place for a parent. Most institutions have policies against parental observation except in highly unusual circumstances. These policies are instituted with the safety of the child in mind; anxious parents who misunderstand what is going on may take unwise actions that place their child at risk. Parents can be reassured that with modern anesthetic techniques, it is unlikely their child will remember anything from the operating room.

Recovery

After surgery, a child is normally brought into a recovery area (called the Post-Anesthesia Care Unit [PACU] by most hospitals) where he is cared for by highly trained staff. A parent may be given the opportunity to see his child at this time. It is not unusual for children to be sleepy after anesthesia, but this effect generally wears off within hours. It is also not uncommon for children to be disoriented while recovering, and crying or other expressions of distress are to be expected.

Some common postoperative issues include pain and nausea. Options for pain control range from narcotics and anti-inflammatory drugs to Tylenol. The good news is that children recover much faster from surgical procedures than adults do.

If your child complains or seems unusually restless, pain may be the cause. It is perfectly appropriate to ask for better pain control for your child, but it's also important to understand that there may be side effects that come with too much pain medicine, such as lethargy and nausea.

Surveys of adults have shown that they rank nausea as one of the most unpleasant aspects of recovery from surgery, even ahead of pain. Teenage girls seem to be at particularly high risk of nausea. However, management of postoperative nausea and vomiting has advanced considerably in recent years with the introduction of many highly effective drugs.

Blood glucose levels can fluctuate considerably after surgery, particularly in the case of major surgeries. Lack of a desire to eat, stress, and nausea related to the surgery can also affect blood glucose levels. With frequent blood glucose checks, insulin regimens can usually be restarted right away. Oral medicines can normally be restarted as soon as the child is able to resume eating and drinking.

Final thoughts

Nothing can replace the natural protective instinct that we feel for our children, and a certain amount of presurgery anxiety is to be expected. But a healthy dose of education, planning, and vigilance can help make the experience of surgery much better for both you and your child. □

For Parents

GETTING READY FOR COLLEGE

by Amy Gilliland,
R.N., M.S.N.,
and Linda Siminerio,
R.N., Ph.D., C.D.E.

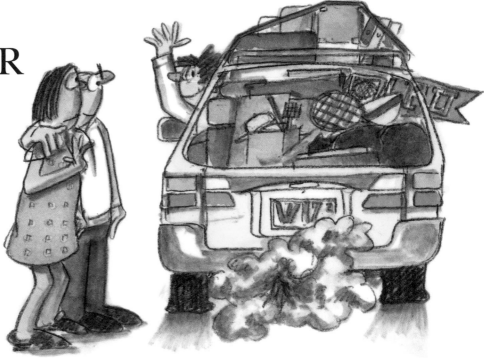

Maybe you have been preparing for this since your son or daughter was in kindergarten, or maybe it sneaked up on you all of a sudden: Your teen has graduated high school and is preparing to start college. You feel proud and excited to see him taking this big step toward adulthood, yet you may also be feeling a little anxious.

Most graduating seniors and their parents share mixed feelings of apprehension and excitement before college begins, but teens with diabetes and their parents often have some added concerns. Since the college-bound student will soon have full responsibility for his day-to-day diabetes care, both student and parents want to feel confident that the student can handle his diabetes on his own and fit his self-care routine into college life.

This article offers tips and suggestions on making the transition from high school to college easier on the whole family. By creating a plan of action, parents and young adults can lighten their anxiety and be ready for this important period of growth and change.

Leaving the nest

Although having full responsibility for diabetes care may seem daunting at first, young adults can and do successfully manage their diabetes and thrive in college on their own. It helps a lot, however, if the student is already handling the bulk of care before he leaves home.

From experience, you know that managing diabetes is a balancing act. Not only is it necessary to balance food with activity and insulin, but your

family has also balanced the responsibilities for your teen's diabetes care. Ideally, the process of shifting more diabetes care responsibility to your teen happened gradually as he progressed through high school. Over time, he probably began monitoring his own blood sugar, learning how to determine the amounts of insulin he needs to take, and balancing meals and exercise. Usually during high school, parents still need to remind their son or daughter to monitor regularly, take insulin, or carry supplies. In college, however, the student is on his own to remember and carry out diabetes care.

If a teenager is not handling most of his diabetes responsibilities prior to high school graduation, a good time for him to start is during the summer months before the fall college semester begins. This way the young person is able to have responsibility for care while he still has the safety net of parents in place.

Before your teen leaves for college, make sure he knows how to communicate with his health-care providers and educators while he is away. Most likely he will have access to e-mail or to a fax machine. However, if continuing communication with his health team at home will be difficult, your teen may need to start a new team in his college environment.

Despite their worries, most parents find that college students manage their diabetes quite well on their own. During semester breaks, parents are often pleasantly surprised by the growth and development that has happened while their son or daughter was away. The teenager they may have struggled with in high school usually grows nicely into adulthood during his time away at college. Taking an interest in diabetes often goes along with this maturity.

Keeping up with supplies

As surprising as it may seem to some college freshmen, diabetes supplies will not magically appear in their dormitory room the way they may have at home. Keeping up with supplies is important to avoid last-minute runs to the pharmacy. At college, running out of supplies can be a big problem if the pharmacy is far from the campus and parents are not around to pick up supplies in a pinch.

Parents should help their teen develop a plan for keeping up with supplies. When they first arrive on campus, parents and student may want to establish a relationship with the local pharmacy, just as they have done at home, so the student knows where prescriptions can be dropped off and how to restock when he needs supplies.

Another way to handle supplies is through a mail-order pharmacy service. Supplies can be delivered directly to the student or sent home so that parents can keep track of orders and payment. Mail-order services usually distribute supplies in three-month increments, eliminating monthly visits to the pharmacy for refills. However, most mail-order pharmacies re-quest notification two weeks prior to the actual date of delivery. Noting reorder dates on the calendar can help you and your teen keep track of when to call for refills. If you plan to have supplies delivered to your home at the start of the fall college semester, your reordering schedule should roughly coincide with semester breaks. This will allow the student to restock his supplies while at home on visits.

Another convenient way for students to order their supplies is online. Internet access is readily available on most campuses, and many pharmacies and mail-order houses have Web sites that are set up for online orders. However, it is a good idea to keep copies of written prescriptions at school so the student can go to a local pharmacy and get supplies if there is a problem with delivery of his online order.

Students should be responsible for keeping up with their supplies or at least notifying parents when they are running low. Dealing with insurance issues and completing the paperwork, however, is something that parents may want to continue to handle to guarantee insurance coverage.

Storing and disposing of supplies safely is important, since casually leaving needles or lancets around can be dangerous. Students will need to work out an arrangement with roommates on where diabetes equipment should be stored in the dormitory room, apartment, or fraternity house.

Students should check with the campus health center to find out how to dispose of sharps (needles and lancets) and syringes. (Loose lancets, needles, and syringes should never be thrown in the trash or in a recycling bin.) Different campuses may have different regulations. Some colleges may require the student to use a sharps container, while others may say it's OK to use a coffee can or detergent bottle with a secure lid. Likewise, some campuses may want the student to drop off full containers at the health center, while others may allow the student to tape the container shut and throw it in the regular trash.

Dealing with highs and lows

Since college living is altogether different from living at home, your teen's blood glucose levels are likely to vary until he adjusts to his new surroundings. Don't be overly upset about it; this readjustment happens at first to almost everyone who leaves home. Give your teen support and encouragement as he finds a way to stabilize his blood glucose levels.

The day-to-day variation of class schedules, meal times, and stress and activity levels will influence your teen's diabetes control. Classes may be scheduled during morning hours one day and not until the afternoon the next. Consequently, your teen may be eating breakfast and taking insulin at 6 AM one day and not until 11 AM the next. This type of variation will affect his blood sugar level.

Psychological stress can take its toll, too. Being away from home is easy for some and hard for others. Many students get homesick, especially if this is their first time away. The stress of adjustment to college life along with all of the other changes can make moods swing and blood sugar control go haywire.

If your teen's blood sugar level is bouncing wildly from day to day, encourage him to look at patterns to determine what is making it high or low. Maybe the cafeteria pizza has a bigger effect on his blood glucose than the pizza he ate at home. Maybe low blood sugar is simply the result of the extra walking or biking that he is doing to get from one end of campus to the other. The old regimen from home simply may not work at college.

Here are some blood sugar control rules of thumb for the student to keep in mind as he finds his way:

- Depending on the type of insulin used, there should be no more than four hours between meals and snacks.
- If a student is pulling an all-nighter, he should eat one carbohydrate choice (15 grams of carbohydrate) for every two hours he is awake after his normal bedtime snack.
- Always be prepared to treat hypoglycemia by carrying a source of carbohydrate at all times.
- Keep hypoglycemia treatment options in the dorm room at all times.

For safety reasons, your teen should inform at least some of his new friends at college about his diabetes and about how to spot and treat hypoglycemia. It's important that he describe his typical symptoms of low blood sugar so they won't be misinterpreted. If his friends know that he becomes irritable and grumpy when his blood glucose level is low, for example, they will be more likely to understand and help.

Having an informed roommate or buddy could also be a potential lifesaver. Although emergencies are unlikely, your teen should be prepared for them. Even if he has never needed glucagon to treat very low blood sugar, he should ask key people to learn how to use glucagon, just in case.

It is especially important for your teen to wear medical identification while at college in case of an emergency. He is new to the college community, and most people will not know about his diabetes. He could end up in a situation where low blood sugar is mistaken for drug or alcohol abuse, which could be dangerous as well as embarrassing to him.

A change in the menu

Another challenging aspect of college life, particularly for a freshman, is adapting to cafeteria food. Although most students are familiar with school menus, eating cafeteria food for every meal can wreak havoc on blood sugar levels.

Weight gain and high blood glucose can develop because of the high-fat and high-carbohydrate choices offered by cafeterias. However, many college cafeterias have made a concerted effort to offer a variety of meal choices, including healthier options such as salads, baked entrees, and fruits and vegetables. Nonetheless, making appropriate meal choices can be challenging when you have ample availability of food and no adult looking over your shoulder. Away from home and the close supervision of parents, some freshmen find it easy to throw their meal plan out the window. This can be frustrating for parents, but ultimately it's up to the student to learn from his mistakes and control what he eats.

OFF-TO-COLLEGE CHECKLIST

This checklist will help teens remember what to pack for college as well as which places to go to and which people to see once they're on campus.

PACKING LIST:
Batteries
Emergency phone contacts
Extra insulin, strips, pump supplies
Pharmacy phone numbers
Set of prescriptions
Sharps container

PEOPLE WHO SHOULD KNOW ABOUT A STUDENT'S DIABETES:
Coaches and/or professors
Friends
Health center staff
Resident assistant
Roommates

LOCATE AND VISIT THE FOLLOWING:
Local hospital emergency room
Local pharmacy
Local physician
Student health center

To help the young adult handle the challenge of eating at college, parents and student may want to make an appointment with the dietitian prior to the start of the fall semester to update his meal plan and review exchanges and carbohydrate counting.

Most campuses allow students to rent or purchase a refrigerator and/or microwave for their room. You and your teen may want to look into this so he can store some healthy alternatives if the cafeteria menu doesn't suit his meal plan.

Educating friends and teachers

Deciding who in the college community should know about your teen's diabetes is an individual choice. If your family has lived in the same community throughout high school, your teen probably has a group of key people—friends, neighbors, school staff, and coaches—who know about his diabetes. But going away to school opens up a whole new world, along with a fresh group of friends and acquaintances. He will again need to decide who to inform about his diabetes.

Important people to tell are roommates and resident assistants. These people need to understand what diabetes is and, most important, understand the signs, symptoms, and treatment of hypoglycemia. They will also need to be told that diabetes supplies such as needles and lancets will be kept in the room.

Other people who should know are friends your teen will be spending a lot of time with. He will probably find that most people are interested and supportive if he is frank and honest with them. If your teen has had negative experiences in the past in telling friends, keep in mind that he was probably dealing with younger, less mature individuals. Typically, fellow college students will be receptive and eager to help.

It is very important for college athletes with diabetes to educate coaches and teammates about diabetes, especially on the treatment of hypoglycemia. Sharing diabetes information with professors is probably not necessary unless the professor has specific rules about eating in the classroom. If this is the case it would be a good idea to let the professor know that it may be necessary to eat in case of hypoglycemia. However, researchers think that low blood glucose may continue to affect thinking and performance for a while (perhaps an hour or so) after it has been treated. So the period right after an episode of low blood glucose may not be the best time to take an important exam, run a race, or give a presentation. If a student has just had a severe incident of hypoglycemia or thinks that patterns of low blood sugar are affecting his academic performance, he may want to discuss his diabetes with professors while trying to get his blood glucose levels under better control.

The school's health center should also be informed about your teen's health history and current diabetes regimen. Learning where the health center is located is one of the first things you should do. Parents and the student should also find out how health services are provided on campus and if facilities like hospitals and emergency rooms are accessible.

Drugs and drinking

It is likely your teen will be exposed to alcohol, drugs, and smoking on campus, so it is important to address these issues before he leaves home. Not only are drugs such as marijuana and cocaine illegal, they also can cause emotional, physical, and psychological problems. If you add diabetes to the mix, it can make matters worse.

While smoking cigarettes may seem less danger-ous than using illicit drugs, smoking is the leading preventable cause of death in the United States today. In addition to the long-term health consequences of smoking, such as lung cancer, high blood pressure, heart disease, and stroke, in the short term, smoking reduces teens' lung capacity and rate of lung growth, hampers sports performance, increases the resting heart rate, and causes respiratory problems. Teens who smoke are also much more likely than nonsmokers to use alcohol and other drugs.

Many drugs, including cigarettes, affect appetite, causing the user to either overeat or undereat. For a person with diabetes, an alteration in appetite can greatly affect blood glucose level. Drugs can also change the user's mental state, which can result in the person forgetting to eat or, in the case of a person with diabetes, to check his blood sugar level or take his insulin.

The same problem can occur with alcohol use. Even though in most states alcohol is legal for people 21 and over, it is still considered a drug. Alcohol can cause confusion, forgetfulness, and changes in blood sugar level. If your young adult decides to drink alcohol, he should be aware of some precautions to take, because drinking too much or drinking at the wrong time of day can be dangerous for someone who has diabetes. It is a good idea for parents to sit down and talk with their young adult before he leaves for college so that he has a better understanding of what could happen to him if he drinks and to formulate some guidelines for safe experimentation.

Alcohol lowers blood sugar level. This effect can last anywhere from six to 36 hours after the last drink, depending on the amount of alcohol consumed. Since alcohol can also mask the symptoms of hypoglycemia, anyone with diabetes should check his blood sugar level during and after drinking alcohol to make sure he is not hypoglycemic. To counter the blood-glucose-lowering effect of alcohol, it helps to eat while drinking. And of course, drinking in moderation is safer for everyone.

Choosing adult diabetes care

Continued diabetes care and follow- up is very important during the young adult years. Many pediatricians and pediatric diabetes centers will provide continued follow-up care for their patients throughout college. Most, however, will refer the young person to adult services once he graduates college.

Whether a student continues diabetes care with a pediatrician or pediatric endocrinologist throughout college is an individual choice. Some feel that the young college student is dealing with so many changes that adjusting to new health-care services simply complicates matters. Others think that the transition to college is a good time to change to adult care services. The decision should be discussed with the doctor and be based on what is most comfortable for the student.

It is very important, however, that the student have a physician available near to the campus community in case of an emergency, illness, or any other health-care issue that arises during the year. If the campus health center does not seem to meet your teen's needs, a local physician can offer more individual or comprehensive care.

Routine visits to the teen's usual health-care provider can be scheduled for college breaks to eliminate the need for special trips home. With busy college schedules, it is easy to forget or neglect routine checkups. At this time probably more than ever, keeping up with diabetes care is extremely important.

As your family takes this important step forward, it is wise to schedule an education appointment with a diabetes educator before your teen goes off to college. Often, diabetes education is directed to the parents, especially if the teen was diagnosed with diabetes at a young age. Now is a good time for a refresher course that includes special emphasis on how to fit good diabetes care into campus life.

New life phase

Starting college can be challenging for both young adults and their parents. Sometimes parents worry about their son or daughter being away from their care and supervision. It is also natural for families to go through the "empty nest" syndrome for a while. Everyone misses the college student and feels that there is a space left behind.

However, most families adapt quickly. Some parents soon find that they, too, have newfound freedom. If there are no younger siblings at home, parents may find that they do not need to wake up as early in the morning or that weekend nights don't entail waiting up for the teen to come home. They may have more time for friendships and activities that they may have put on the back burner while their teen was growing up. And they can take pride in watching their college student grow into adulthood.

With careful planning and preparation, the transition to college life can be a positive experience for everyone in the family. □

14

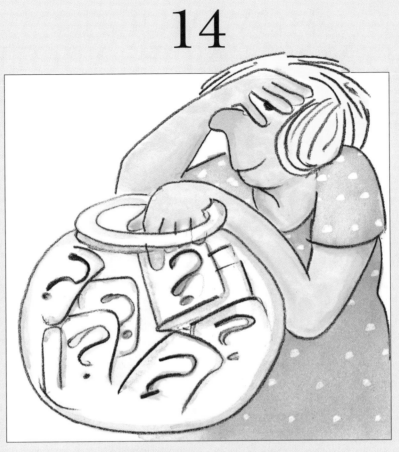

Quizzes

How Much Do You Know About
Blood Glucose Monitoring? 554

How Much Do You Know About
Storing Insulin? 556

How Much Do You Know About
Handling Sick Days? 558

How Much Do You Know About
Routine Medical Tests? 560

How Much Do You Know About
Diabetes and Your Eyes? 562

How Much Do You Know About
Chronic Kidney Disease? 564

How Much Do You Know About
Heart Disease Risk? 566

HOW MUCH DO YOU KNOW ABOUT BLOOD GLUCOSE MONITORING?

by Virginia Peragallo-Dittko, R.N., B.C.-A.D.M., M.A., C.D.E.

Blood glucose monitoring is the quintessential tool for diabetes self-management. The numbers provide you with vital information for making decisions and solving problems. Take the following quiz to find out how much you know about this critical self-care tool.

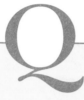

1. What are the target ranges for blood glucose before and after meals?
   A. 70 to 110 mg/dl before a meal, less than 150 mg/dl after a meal.
   B. 90 to 130 mg/dl before a meal, less than 180 mg/dl after a meal.
   C. Below 200 mg/dl before or after a meal.
   D. 126 mg/dl or higher before or after a meal.

2. If your blood glucose level is high first thing in the morning, which of the following reasons may explain why? (More than one answer may be correct.)
   A. Late-night eating.
   B. Early-morning release of hormones.
   C. Your liver may be releasing a lot of glucose into your bloodstream overnight.
   D. You need an adjustment in your dose of insulin or oral medicine.

3. You should not use alternative-site monitoring if you think your blood glucose is low.

   TRUE   **FALSE**

4. Which of the following techniques can help you get enough blood from your finger for an accurate reading?

   A. Set the lancing device to puncture more deeply.
   B. Wash your hands with warm water first.
   C. After lancing, gently massage your finger until a droplet forms.
   D. Rotate to different fingers or sites so that you don't develop calluses.

5. You can get reimbursed for a new blood glucose meter at any time.

   TRUE   **FALSE**

6. How often can a lancet be safely reused?
   A. There's no limit to the number of times a lancet can be reused.
   B. Lancets should be used only one time.
   C. Lancets can be used for one week.
   D. After you clean a lancet with alcohol, it can be used for three days.

7. There is no reason to check your blood glucose level with your meter if you have a glycosylated hemoglobin (HbA_{1c}) test done every three months.

   TRUE   **FALSE**

1. **B.** The American Diabetes Association recommends the following general blood glucose targets for nonpregnant individuals: 90 to 130 mg/dl before a meal, and less than 180 mg/dl one to two hours after the start of a meal. You and your health-care team may modify these targets based on your health and lifestyle.

2. **A, B, C, D.** High blood glucose readings first thing in the morning are common and have many possible explanations.

Many people find that what they eat at night has a large impact on their blood glucose readings the next morning. If you eat a snack before bedtime, try changing your snack choice, the timing of your snack, or the portion. If you eat dinner late in the evening, try eating earlier for a few nights to see whether the timing of your meal may be the culprit. If it is, and if your mealtime can't be changed, medicine may need to be prescribed or adjusted.

Another possible explanation is the dawn phenomenon, or high blood glucose resulting from the body's late-night release of hormones that work against insulin. The dawn phenomenon can be managed with oral medicines or insulin.

Your liver might be releasing a lot of glucose into the bloodstream because the signals telling it to shut off aren't working. If this is the case, the drug metformin may be prescribed, since its main action is to signal the liver to shut off. Insulin has a similar effect.

3. **TRUE.** Blood glucose readings taken from alternative sites such as your forearm, thigh, and upper arm are not always identical to results obtained from your fingertips or palm. Blood flows more quickly to the fingers and the palm of the hand than to the arms and legs. Whenever blood glucose changes quickly, the alternative sites will lag behind the fingers in showing the change. If you suspect low blood glucose, or if you don't have symptoms of hypoglycemia when your blood glucose is low (a condition called hypoglycemia unawareness), the best site to use is a fingertip. Alternative-site monitoring is usually safe to use just before or two hours after a meal.

4. **A, B, C, D.** Several things can make it easier to get a drop of blood from your finger. First, wash your hands with warm water to increase the blood flow to your fingertips. Next, let your hand or arm drop down by your side for a minute before using the lancing device. After lancing, gently massage your finger until a blood droplet forms.

It is best not to use the same site each time. Instead, rotate to different fingers or use alternative sites (if your meter works with blood samples from alternate sites) so that you don't develop calluses.

Check to see if your lancing device has a feature that allows you to adjust the depth of the puncture. Another option is to switch to a blood glucose meter that requires less blood.

5. **FALSE.** Medicare will reimburse you for a new blood glucose meter every five years. If you have private insurance, check with your insurance carrier to see how often your plan allows you to be reimbursed for a new meter. Free meters are often available through your diabetes educator, health-care team, or pharmacy or through health fairs, coupons, or mail-order companies. Before you accept a free meter or switch to a different meter, check with your insurance carrier to see if the strips are covered. Some plans have tiered systems that assign a lower co-payment for certain blood glucose test strips. A meter system listed as "preferred" generally has a lower co-payment.

6. **B.** Lancets are designed and labeled to be used once and then thrown away. While this is the ideal way to use them, there may be circumstances in which you need to use your lancets more than one time. If you choose to reuse, don't wipe the lancet with alcohol, since that will remove the coating that makes the stick less painful; change the lancet if it appears dull or looks bent; wash your hands thoroughly before lancing your finger; don't use an alternative site right after applying lotion; and always check for signs of infection such as redness or swelling at the site.

7. **FALSE.** The glycosylated hemoglobin (HbA_{1c}) test measures your body's exposure to glucose over the preceding three months. It is not an exact average of your blood glucose; rather, it is a weighted average, meaning that roughly half of the result is determined by blood glucose levels in the month before the test. Although the HbA_{1c} test is a very helpful way to see the big picture, and research has supported the benefits of aiming for a target result of 6.5% to 7%, it does not replace daily monitoring. You need your daily blood glucose monitoring to help you make decisions about food or medicine adjustments, prevent low blood glucose, and manage illness. □

HOW MUCH DO YOU KNOW ABOUT STORING INSULIN?

by Virginia Peragallo-Dittko, R.N., B.C.-A.D.M., M.A., C.D.E.

Incorrect storage of insulin can lead to high blood glucose levels, higher prescription costs, and unnecessary inconvenience. However, the storage guidelines for insulin can be confusing, and they differ according to the type of insulin you use. Take the following quiz to find out how much you know about insulin storage so that you can get the most out of this vital treatment.

Q

1. Where or how should a container of insulin be stored once the stopper or seal has been punctured?
   A. It should be stored in the refrigerator.
   B. It should be stored at room temperature.
   C. It should be stored in a kitchen cabinet.
   D. It should be stored on a windowsill.

2. In-use insulin in a pen cartridge or prefilled pen can be kept at room temperature until it is empty..

   TRUE   **FALSE**

3. If the expiration date on a vial of insulin reads January 2008, you can use it until which time?
   A. New Years Day 2008.
   B. End of January 2008.
   C. Until you empty the vial.
   D. March 1, 2008.

4. Which of the following are signs that something is wrong with your insulin suspension of NPH, 70/30, 75/25, or 50/50? (More than one answer may be correct.)
   A. The insulin looks like skim milk after you gently roll the vial, cartridge, or pen.
   B. There are clumps in the vial, cartridge, or pen after a gentle roll.
   C. The vial, cartridge, or pen appears frosted.
   D. Clear fluid is separate from small crystals before you gently roll the vial, cartridge, or pen.

5. When traveling with insulin, which of the following must you do?
   A. Use insulin pens only.
   B. Keep all insulin cool.
   C. Prefill your syringes so that you don't have to bother with refrigeration.
   D. Consider the type of trip planned and the storage guidelines for your insulin.

1. B. Containers of insulin that are in use—or that have had their seal or stopper punctured—can be stored at room temperatures between 59°F and 86°F. (For Apidra, however, the storage guidelines define room temperature as below 77°F.) If the air temperature in your home frequently exceeds 86°F, you should always keep your insulin refrigerated, and you may not benefit from using insulin pens, because they cannot be refrigerated when in use. Unopened insulin should be stored in the refrigerator at a temperature between 36°F and 46°F.

2. FALSE. The in-use storage recommendations for insulin cartridges or prefilled pens vary according to the type of insulin. Here are the current manufacturer guidelines for pen cartridges and prefilled pens:

■ Levemir: 42 days
■ Apidra, Lantus, Humalog, Novo-Log, Novolin R: 28 days
■ Humulin N, Novolin N, Novolin 70/30, NovoLog Mix 70/30: 14 days
■ Humulin 70/30, Humalog Mix 75/25, Humalog Mix 50/50: 10 days

In contrast, vials of all in-use insulin products except Levemir can be kept at room temperature (59°F to 86°F) for 28 days. Vials of Levemir can be kept at room temperature for 42 days. The primary reason for the different in-use recommendations for vials and cartridges or pens is based on the expected use of insulin pens. Because pens are designed to be portable, the insulin in pens is expected to be shaken a bit more and exposed to wider temperature ranges than vials. Pens and cartridges also contain fewer units of insulin than vials, so it is likely they will be used up more quickly.

All manufacturers caution against refrigerating in-use pens or pen cartridges because of the likelihood that condensation will form in the insulin container.

3. B. The potency of the insulin you buy is assured if you use it before the expiration date stamped on the label. Insulin is considered expired at the end of the month stamped on the box. However, insulin may lose its potency before the official expiration date if you continue to use a vial, pen, or pen cartridge beyond the number of days specified by the manufacturer. If you see an unexplained change in your blood glucose patterns, open a new, unexpired vial, pen, or cartridge of insulin. If the insulin's expiration date is approaching, call your supplier before you open the box to see if you can get a replacement supply.

If you get three-month supplies of insulin from a mail-order prescription company, check that the insulin will not expire before you get a chance to use it. Some people routinely order more insulin than they need out of fear and end up with a lot of expired insulin.

4. B, C. Some insulins are supposed to be clear, and some are supposed to be cloudy. You do not have to roll the clear insulins such as Humulin R, Novolin R, NovoLog, Humalog, Apidra, Lantus, and Levemir. You do need to roll the cloudy insulin suspensions such as Humulin N, Novolin N, Humulin 70/30, Novolin 70/30, Humalog Mix 75/25, NovoLog Mix 70/30, Humulin 50/50, and Humalog Mix 50/50. The cloudy insulin suspensions should be gently rolled 10 times and should look like skim milk when you are finished. Do not use the insulin if the container appears frosted or the insulin has small, hard, white clumps in it.

5. D. How to store your insulin when you are traveling depends on the type of trip you are taking. In most cases, it's fine to simply follow the same in-use storage guidelines you use at home and make sure you have extra insulin and supplies in case your stay is extended.

If it is likely that your insulin will be exposed to temperature extremes during your trip—as it might be on a tropical vacation or skiing trip, for example—you may want to purchase an insulin storage kit. Most kits come with a freezable gel or cooler pack and are designed to keep insulin cool. If you are staying in a hotel, you can use an ice bucket filled with ice to refreeze the gel pack, but don't put your insulin in the ice bucket. Insulin cannot be used if it has been frozen. □

HOW MUCH DO YOU KNOW ABOUT HANDLING SICK DAYS?

by Janice Woodrum, R.N., B.S.N.

Having to deal with the flu, a stomach virus, or even a common cold is a drag for anyone. But for people with diabetes, such illnesses can be even more bothersome and potentially hazardous. During an illness, blood glucose levels can be unpredictable, raising the risk of dehydration and other serious complications such as diabetic ketoacidosis. The way to stave off serious problems when you're sick? As usual, it's education, planning ahead, and knowing when to seek help. Take this quiz to see how much you know about handling sick days and how well prepared you are to deal with one.

Q

1. When you're sick, your body produces hormones that can raise your blood glucose to dangerous levels.

   TRUE   **FALSE**

2. People with diabetes should check their urine for ketones on sick days for which of the following reasons?
   A. Sustained high blood sugar can lead to diabetic ketoacidosis (DKA).
   B. DKA can occur if you're unable to keep down any foods or liquids.
   C. DKA can result in coma or even death if not treated promptly.
   D. All of the above.

3. When you are unable to eat regular solid foods, which carbohydrate-containing foods might be more palatable? (More than one answer may be correct.)
   A. ½ cup of fruit juice.
   B. ½ cup of a non-diet, caffeine-free soft drink.
   C. 2 tablespoons of peanut butter.
   D. 1 low-fat ice cream bar, Fudgsicle, or Popsicle.

4. It's OK to omit your oral diabetes medicine or insulin when you're too sick to eat very much.

   TRUE   **FALSE**

5. Which of the following is *not* a sign or symptom of diabetic ketoacidosis?
   A. A blood glucose reading below 70 mg/dl.
   B. Stomach pain, nausea, or vomiting.
   C. Blood glucose readings over 250 mg/dl.
   D. Medium or large amounts of ketones in the urine.

6. Your sick-day kit should include which of the following? (More than one answer may be correct.)
   A. Supplies to check blood glucose level and ketones.
   B. Over-the-counter medicines for headache, fever, nausea, diarrhea, and nasal congestion.
   C. Directions from your health-care provider for when to take extra insulin or diabetes medicines.
   D. Extra insulin.
   E. Sick-day foods and fluids.
   F. All of the above.

1. TRUE. Illness, infection, surgery, and serious injuries are all physical stresses on the body. The body responds to stress by releasing hormones, primarily epinephrine (also known as adrenaline) and cortisol, that cause the liver to release stored glucose, effectively raising blood glucose level. Normally, this would provide cells with extra energy to fight the stress, but without enough insulin in circulation, the glucose simply stays in the blood. When you're sick, therefore, it's important to check your blood glucose level every four to six hours, take insulin or diabetes medicines as prescribed, keep careful records, and call your doctor if your blood glucose level stays above 240 mg/dl for more than 24 to 48 hours.

2. D. When there's not enough insulin in your system to enable your cells to use glucose for energy, your body begins to break down fat for energy instead. When this happens, an acidic by-product of fat metabolism called ketones can build up in the blood and spill over into the urine. Due to frequent urination, you can also get dehydrated, and electrolytes like sodium and potassium can get out of balance. Together with elevated blood glucose level, these factors add up to a condition called diabetic ketoacidosis (DKA), which, if not quickly corrected, can cause coma or even death. Ketones can also build up if you do not take in enough carbohydrate in foods or liquids—even if your blood glucose level is not very high.

During an illness, insulin users should check their urine for ketones several times a day, and everyone should check for ketones if blood glucose is above 250 mg/dl. If there is more than a trace, call your health-care provider for advice.

3. A, B, D. Each of these choices contains about 15 grams of carbohydrate, the amount of carbohydrate you should take in every hour if your blood glucose level is under 180–200 mg/dl. If your blood glucose level is over 200 mg/dl, alternate a carbohydrate-containing food or drink one hour with 8 ounces of a non-caloric liquid the next hour. If your blood glucose level is over 240 mg/dl, drink 8 ounces of noncaloric liquids every hour, but be sure to get at least 10 servings per day of foods or drinks containing 15 grams of carbohydrate. This will help prevent low blood glucose and also keep your body from burning too much fat for energy.

4. FALSE. Even if you eat less when you're sick, you may need more insulin or oral diabetes medicine than usual, because the stress hormones that accompany illness tend to raise blood glucose levels. Unless your health-care provider directs you otherwise, keep taking your usual medicines. However, there is the possibility of your blood glucose level going too low if you are unable to eat, so if you can't stomach solid foods, try eating soft foods or at least drinking carbohydrate-containing liquids to prevent hypoglycemia. If you are having severe vomiting or diarrhea, you should contact your health-care provider for instructions.

5. A. Diabetic ketoacidosis generally begins with signs and symptoms of high blood glucose, including increased thirst and urination, dry mouth, fatigue, and blood glucose readings over 250 mg/dl. As ketones build up in the blood, they usually cause nausea, stomach cramps, and vomiting, and moderate to large amounts of ketones show up in the urine. Signs of more severe DKA include fruity-smelling breath, deep and rapid breathing, and extreme drowsiness or confusion. Left untreated, DKA progresses to coma or even death. Report early signs of DKA to your health-care provider at once; you may be able to reverse the symptoms with more insulin and liquids. Advanced symptoms may require immediate hospitalization.

6. F. When you feel sick, you'll probably feel more like going to bed than running to the store. That's why it's a good idea to always keep some sick-day foods and supplies in your house. Supplies to check your blood glucose level are the first priority, and insulin users in particular should have a supply of urine ketone strips as well. If your health-care provider has given you a sliding scale for how much extra insulin to take when blood glucose or ketone levels are high, be sure to keep a copy of these instructions with your supplies. Its also a good idea to keep some extra insulin in the refrigerator. Even some people who don't regularly use insulin keep quick-acting insulin on hand to take if their blood glucose level goes over 200 mg/dl or so during an illness.

Over-the-counter medicines—for headache, fever, cough, head congestion, diarrhea, etc.—can also help keep you comfortable during an illness. Ask your health-care provider to review and approve your preferred OTC drugs, then keep some on hand for when the need arises. □

HOW MUCH DO YOU KNOW ABOUT ROUTINE MEDICAL TESTS?

by Robert S. Dinsmoor

People with diabetes are advised to have a number of medical tests on a routine basis, both to evaluate how well their current diabetes regimen is working and to detect any signs of complications early, when treatment is most likely to be effective. Yet many people are not fully aware of the purpose behind the tests their doctors order, what desirable results are, or how often certain tests should be performed. Take this quiz to test your knowledge about medical tests commonly used in people with diabetes.

1. What exactly does the HbA_{1c} test measure?
   A. The amount of hemoglobin the bloodstream.
   B. The amount of glucose in the bloodstream.
   C. The percentage of hemoglobin in the bloodstream that is glycosylated.
   D. Heartbeat irregularities.

2. How often should you have your cholesterol checked?
   A. Four times a year.
   B. Once a year.
   C. Once every two years.
   D. Once every five years.
   E. It depends on how well your cholesterol levels have been controlled.

3. Ankle blood pressure measurements can be used interchangeably with blood pressure measurements taken at the arm.

   TRUE   **FALSE**

4. During a dilated eye exam, what condition(s) is your eye doctor screening for? (More than one answer may be correct.)
   A. Diabetic retinopathy.
   B. Macular edema.
   C. Macular degeneration.

   D. Glaucoma.
   E. All of the above.

5. What is a desirable result for a microalbuminuria test?
   A. Less than 30 micrograms per milligram of creatinine for a spot collection.
   B. Less than 30 milligrams per 24 hours for a 24-hour collection.
   C. Less than 20 milligrams per minute for a timed collection.
   D. All of the above.

6. Which of the following is *not* a test doctors use to screen for peripheral neuropathy?
   A. Pinprick test.
   B. Vibration perception.
   C. Temperature test.
   D. Pressure sensation.
   E. Litmus test.
   F. Ankle reflexes.

7. People taking either pioglitazone (brand name Actos) or rosiglitazone (Avandia) should have their liver function tested regularly.

   TRUE   **FALSE**

1. **C.** The HbA$_{1c}$ test, also known as the glycosylated hemoglobin test, measures the percentage of hemoglobin in the bloodstream that is glycosylated, or chemically bound to glucose. Once bound to hemoglobin, glucose molecules remain bound to the hemoglobin for the life of the red blood cell, which is approximately 120 days. By measuring what percentage of hemoglobin is glycosylated, doctors can get a sense of what blood glucose control has been like over the previous two to three months.

People who don't have diabetes typically have an HbA$_{1c}$ of around 5%. The American Diabetes Association (ADA) recommends that people with diabetes strive to keep their HbA$_{1c}$ levels below 7% in general and specifically as close to normal as possible.

2. **E.** According to the ADA, adults with diabetes generally should be tested for lipid disorders at least annually—and more frequently if needed to achieve target lipid levels. In those with low-risk lipid values (an LDL level of less than 100 mg/dl, an HDL level greater than 50 mg/dl, and triglyceride levels less than 150 mg/dl), lipid testing should be repeated every two years.

3. **FALSE.** An ankle blood pressure measurement is used to diagnose peripheral vascular disease, or atherosclerosis affecting the blood vessels outside the heart, such as those of the legs and feet. Blood pressure at the ankle is usually the same as or greater than blood pressure at the arm. However, if the blood pressure measurement taken at the ankle is much lower than the blood pressure measurement taken at the arm, that may be a sign that peripheral vascular disease is present.

4. **E.** Dilating your pupils allows detection of a number of serious eye diseases, including diabetic retinopathy, macular edema, macular degeneration, and glaucoma. In diabetic retinopathy, blood vessels swell and sometimes abnormal new blood vessels form in the retina of the eye. These can hemorrhage and cause scarring and retinal detachment. In macular edema, the macula—the part of the eye responsible for sharp, straight-ahead vision—becomes swollen, causing blurry vision. In macular degeneration, the macula gradually becomes injured, causing wavy or blurry vision. In glaucoma, high pressure within the eye gradually injures the retina and the optic nerve, causing slow loss of vision.

5. **D.** All of the above. The microalbuminuria test, which detects the leakage of small amounts of the protein albumin into the urine, is a screening test for the earliest stages of diabetic kidney disease. It can be performed in one of three ways and also involves checking urinary creatinine levels. (Creatinine is a by-product of normal muscle breakdown.) To monitor your albumin levels, your doctor can order a "random spot collection," which is a one-time in-office check; a 24-hour urine collection (analyzing all of the urine you produce in 24 hours); or a timed collection (analyzing all of the urine you produce over a certain number of hours). A "normal" result depends on the particular method used. In general, a "normal" result is less than 30 micrograms of albumin per milligram of creatinine in the spot collection, less than 30 milligrams per 24 hours in the 24-hour collection, or less than 20 micrograms per minute in the timed collection. To be diagnosed with microalbuminuria, a person has to reach certain levels of albumin on at least two out of three tests over a period of three to six months.

6. **E.** A litmus test is not used in testing for diabetic peripheral neuropathy. Signs of neuropathy or diminished blood circulation in the feet include ulceration, callus formation, cracks in the skin, and hair loss. In addition, doctors can test for sensation using a pin prick. They can use special tuning forks to test your ability to sense vibration. They can test sensation to temperature using a special cold tuning fork or other device. They can also test pressure sensation using graded nylon monofilaments that buckle at specific pressures. This allows doctors to discover a person's threshold for feeling pressure at a given place on the skin. They can also test a person's ankle reflex by tapping a mallet on the Achilles tendon on the back of the ankle. If the ankle fails to jerk normally, that may be a sign of diabetic neuropathy.

7. **TRUE.** The first drug of the thiazolidinedione class to be approved, troglitazone (brand name Rezulin), had to be pulled off the market because of reports of severe liver toxicity. While the currently available thiazolidinediones, pioglitazone (Actos) and rosiglitazone (Avandia), have not been associated with liver toxicity, they are similar to troglitazone, so periodic liver function tests are recommended for anyone taking them. □

HOW MUCH DO YOU KNOW ABOUT DIABETES AND YOUR EYES?

by A. Paul Chous, M.A., O.D.

Most people know that diabetes can damage their eyes and, in the worst-case scenario, result in blindness. In fact, damage to the eye's light-sensitive retina caused by diabetes, known as *diabetic retinopathy,* is the leading cause of legal blindness for American adults under the age of 74 (legal blindness is defined as vision less than 20/200 with use of the best possible lens prescription, or less than 20° of side vision). Diabetic retinopathy is estimated to blind 12,000–24,000 Americans every year. In addition, diabetes can affect many parts of the eye other than the retina, resulting in an array of eye conditions and vision problems. Take this quiz to find out how much you know about the effects of diabetes on your eyes.

1. Which of the following eye conditions or diseases is more commonly found in people with diabetes? (More than one answer may be correct.)
   A. Astigmatism.
   B. Corneal irritation and dry eyes.
   C. Glaucoma.
   D. Cataract.
   E. Double vision.

2. Which of the following most accurately describes diabetic retinopathy?
   A. High blood glucose causes the retina to detach and bleed.
   B. The retina loses its circulation.
   C. Chronic high blood glucose damages retinal blood vessels, leading to leakage of blood and fluid, swelling, and the development of abnormal, new blood vessels.
   D. High internal eye pressure damages the retina and optic nerve.

3. Good visual acuity on an eye chart means that a person with diabetes has healthy eyes.

   TRUE   **FALSE**

4. Most people with diabetic retinopathy should not engage in vigorous physical activity because it may promote retinal bleeding.

   TRUE   **FALSE**

5. People with diabetes should see either an optometrist or an ophthalmologist experienced with diabetes and its effects on the eyes.

   TRUE   **FALSE**

6. People with Type 2 diabetes rarely lose vision because of their diabetes.

   TRUE   **FALSE**

1. B, C, D, and E. High blood glucose levels damage the clear windshield at the front of the eye, the cornea, causing scratchiness, burning, redness, and reflex tearing (excess tear production triggered by dry eyes). Glaucoma, progressive damage to the optic nerve associated with elevated internal eye pressure and resulting in vision loss, is about 50% more common in people with diabetes. Cataract, a common, age-related clouding of the eye's internal lens, occurs at a younger age and progresses more quickly in people who have diabetes. This is due, at least in part, to the hyperglycemic "caramelization," or glycation, of lens proteins, in which sugars react with the proteins, causing them to clump together and form cloudy areas in the lens. High blood glucose can also damage nerves responsible for precisely coordinating the movements of both eyes, resulting in double vision. In addition, people with diabetes are more likely to develop blockage of retinal blood vessels ("retinal vascular occlusion") and stroke of the optic nerve ("ischemic optic neuropathy"). The risk of developing all these conditions can be minimized with tight blood glucose, blood pressure, and lipid (cholesterol and triglyceride) control.

2. C. Diabetic retinopathy comes in three forms: *nonproliferative,* characterized by the formation of microaneurysms (tiny blood vessel outpouchings that look like small red dots), small hemorrhages, and fluid swelling within the retina; *proliferative,* characterized by growth of fragile new blood vessels that break easily, bleed profusely, and lead to scar tissue capable of detaching the retina; and *macular edema,* characterized by significant fluid swelling within the most visually sensitive part of the retina. Macular edema can occur alone or with either of the first two forms of retinopathy.

3. FALSE. Many serious eye diseases do not affect central vision (the ability to see shapes, colors, and fine details, such as small letters on a chart) until late in their course. It is not at all uncommon for people with severe diabetic retinopathy or glaucoma to have 20/20 or better visual acuity at the time they are diagnosed with these conditions. By the time a person has visual symptoms, it is sometimes too late to improve lost vision, and the overall prognosis for preserving vision is poorer.

4. FALSE. Restrictions concerning exercise and retinopathy apply to neither the majority of people with diabetes, nor even to the majority of people with diabetic retinopathy. The only group of people at high risk for retinal bleeding associated with exercise are those with untreated, recently treated, or actively bleeding *proliferative* diabetic retinopathy, because these people have abnormal blood vessels that can be broken quite easily. There is absolutely no ophthalmic reason that people with nonproliferative retinopathy, or those with successfully treated proliferative retinopathy, cannot participate in vigorous physical activity, including moderate resistance (weight) training. However, a person should always check with his eye doctor to be certain of his retinal status before performing vigorous exercise.

5. TRUE. The American Diabetes Association recommends that people with diabetes see either an experienced optometrist or ophthalmologist annually for a dilated eye exam. After four years of postgraduate education, Doctors of Optometry are trained and licensed to diagnose and treat disorders and diseases of the eyes and visual system through nonsurgical means, including the use of prescription eye drops and oral medicines, as well as to detect the ocular manifestations of systemic conditions, such as high blood pressure and diabetes. Ophthalmologists are medical doctors who complete residency training in the medical and surgical management of eye disease. Optometrists routinely work closely with subspecialist ophthalmologists (such as retinal specialists) when people with diabetes require laser or surgical treatment.

6. FALSE. Although it is true that a higher percentage of people with Type 1 diabetes experience small blood vessel diabetes complications, including retinopathy, more people with Type 2 diabetes suffer significant vision loss in terms of absolute numbers. Part of the reason, of course, is that people with Type 2 diabetes outnumber those with Type 1 nine to one. In addition, those with Type 2 are more likely to develop diabetic eye diseases other than retinopathy—in particular, cataract, glaucoma, and ischemic optic neuropathy (poor blood flow to the optic nerve)—as a function of both age and high blood glucose. Diabetes of any type poses substantial risks to your eyes and vision. □

Diabetes and Your Eyes

HOW MUCH DO YOU KNOW ABOUT CHRONIC KIDNEY DISEASE?

by Maria Karalis, M.B.A., R.D., L.D.

People who have diabetes, high blood pressure, or a family history of chronic kidney disease are at higher risk of developing kidney disease. The type of kidney disease most commonly associated with diabetes is called diabetic nephropathy.

Prevention of chronic kidney disease is possible, and early treatment can slow its progression and reduce your chances of developing further complications. Take this quiz to find out what steps you can take to prevent chronic kidney disease or delay its progression if it has already been diagnosed.

1. What do the kidneys do? (More than one answer may be correct.)
   A. Regulate levels of body fluids and important minerals, such as sodium and potassium.
   B. Remove wastes from the blood.
   C. Release hormones important to controlling blood pressure, making red blood cells, and keeping bones strong.

2. How often should people with diabetes be tested for diabetic kidney disease?
   A. Once a year.
   B. Once every two years.
   C. Once every three years.

3. Which of the following ethnic groups are at increased risk for chronic kidney disease? (More than one answer may be correct.)
   A. African-Americans.
   B. Asian-Americans.
   C. Hispanic Americans.
   D. American Indians.

4. Which of these tests are used to screen for chronic kidney disease? (More than one answer may be correct.)
   A. A blood creatinine test used to estimate glomerular filtration rate (GFR).
   B. Blood pressure.
   C. A test for protein in the urine (a marker of kidney damage).

5. If you are at increased risk for kidney disease, there is very little you can do to lower the chances of developing it.
   TRUE   **FALSE**

6. What are other problems that may develop as kidney disease progresses?
   A. Anemia.
   B. Bone disease.
   C. Both anemia and bone disease.
   D. None of the above.

1. A, B, C. Your kidneys do many important jobs to keep you healthy. When their function is impaired, however, you may experience symptoms such as swollen ankles or feet, having to urinate more often (especially during the night), and feeling more tired than usual. Reduced kidney function also means that less insulin is excreted from the body, possibly leading to less need for injected insulin or diabetes drugs in people who have diabetes.

2. A. People with diabetes should be tested once a year for signs of kidney disease. In most cases, the earliest sign of diabetic kidney disease is *microalbuminuria,* or small amounts of the protein albumin in the urine.

3. A, B, C, D. Diabetes, which is the number one cause of chronic kidney disease, is more common in these ethnic groups. Chronic high blood glucose levels damage the blood vessels in the kidneys. Over time, this causes destruction of the *nephrons,* or "filtering units" of the kidneys, which normally remove waste products from the blood. Keeping your blood glucose levels under control can help prevent this kind of damage.

High blood pressure, the second leading cause of chronic kidney disease, is more common in African-Americans. High blood pressure also damages the blood vessels in the kidneys, impairing their ability to filter waste from the blood.

4. A, B, C. All of these tests are used to detect chronic kidney disease. The American Diabetes Association (ADA) recommends that people with diabetes have their blood pressure checked at every doctor visit and that they be tested for microalbuminuria, or protein in the urine, once a year. A blood creatinine test can also be used to figure out your GFR, a measure of how well your kidneys are removing wastes and fluids from your blood. (*Creatinine* is a waste product from muscle activity. When your kidneys are not working properly, creatinine builds up in the blood.) If you have your latest blood test results, you can calculate your GFR easily with a GFR calculator. Go to www.kidney.org/professionals/kdoqi/gfr_calculator.cfm—you will need your blood creatinine result, age, race, and sex.

A GFR of more than 90 millimeters (ml) per minute is usually considered normal for adults. In young adults, however, GFR is about 120–130 ml per minute—this number goes down with age. Chronic kidney disease is defined by the National Kidney Foundation as having a GFR below 60 ml per minute for three or more months.

5. FALSE. Studies have found that controlling your blood glucose levels can help prevent and slow the progression of kidney disease. Keeping your blood pressure under control also helps. Taking large amounts of over-the-counter pain relievers can harm the kidneys, so avoiding heavy or long-term use can also help prevent kidney damage.

6. C. As kidney function declines, the kidneys no longer make enough of the hormones *erythropoietin* (EPO) and *calcitriol.*

EPO stimulates the bone marrow to make red blood cells. Less EPO means fewer red blood cells, or a condition also known as anemia. (Anemia can also result from low hemoglobin levels, which in turn can be caused by insufficient levels of iron and certain B vitamins.) If you have kidney disease, be sure to have your red blood cell and hemoglobin levels checked to see if you are anemic. Your doctor may prescribe injections of a man-made form of EPO to treat your anemia. Many people with kidney disease and anemia also need to take iron supplements.

In people with kidney disease, the kidneys make very little calcitriol, a form of vitamin D that normally helps the body absorb calcium from food. Low levels of calcitriol result in low blood levels of calcium. Kidney disease can also impair the kidneys' ability to filter phosphorus, leading to high blood phosphorus levels. Eventually, these imbalances cause the parathyroid glands to release too much *parathyroid hormone* (PTH), leading to a condition called *secondary hyperparathyroidism* (too much PTH in the blood). A high PTH level causes calcium to be removed from the bones, resulting in a condition known as *renal osteodystrophy,* which causes the bones to become thin and weak and raises the risk of bone fractures. Secondary hyperparathyroidism can also affect other organs and tissues, including your heart and blood vessels.

If you have early kidney disease, your PTH level may be high due to low calcitriol levels. Your doctor may prescribe synthetic calcitriol or another drug to lower PTH. Treatment of both anemia and secondary hyperparathyroidism should begin early to reduce further complications. □

HOW MUCH DO YOU KNOW ABOUT HEART DISEASE RISK?

by Mark Nakamoto

Cardiovascular disease is two to four times more common in people with diabetes than in people without diabetes. It is also the leading cause of death for people with diabetes. Despite these grim figures, there is hope. Making lifestyle changes and taking one or more of an ever-growing arsenal of medicines can help to reduce your risk for cardiovascular disease. Take the following quiz to find out how much you know about your risk for cardiovascular disease and the steps you can take to lower that risk.

Q

1. Although men with diabetes have reason to worry about heart disease, women with diabetes should be more concerned about getting breast cancer.

    TRUE   **FALSE**

2. Whether you exercise every day for 30 minutes at a time or for shorter periods that add up to 30 minutes, you are reducing your risk for heart disease.

    TRUE   **FALSE**

3. Which of the following meets the American Diabetes Association's goals for lowering risks of heart disease and diabetes complications in people with diabetes?
    A. A blood pressure of 135/85 mm Hg.
    B. A low-density lipoprotein (LDL) cholesterol level of 99 mg/dl.
    C. A glycosylated hemoglobin (HbA_{1c}) level of 7.5%.
    D. A high-density lipoprotein (HDL) cholesterol level of 25 mg/dl.

4. Which of the following lifestyle choices will help to reduce your risk for heart disease? (More than one answer may be correct.)
    A. Stopping smoking.
    B. Losing weight if you are overweight.
    C. Making sure that less than 10% of your total daily caloric intake comes from saturated and *trans* fats.
    D. Drinking three glasses of red wine a day.

5. A daily aspirin is recommended for all people with diabetes to prevent heart attacks and strokes.

    TRUE   **FALSE**

6. A diet rich in fruits and vegetables and low in sodium and red meat can be as powerful as a prescription drug in lowering blood pressure.

    TRUE   **FALSE**

7. People with diabetes need to be extra cautious about their heart disease risk factors because of which of the following? (More than one answer may be correct.)
    A. Having diabetes puts a person at the same risk for a heart attack as a person who has already had a heart attack or stroke.
    B. People with diabetes tend to have higher triglyceride levels than others, increasing their risk.
    C. People with diabetes tend to have higher LDL cholesterol levels than others, making them more likely to have a heart attack.
    D. High blood glucose levels can contribute to heart disease.

1. **FALSE.** Although breast cancer is often in the headlines, heart disease is the leading cause of death for women (and men) with or without diabetes. In fact, cardiovascular diseases kill almost twice as many women as all cancers combined. In addition, although cardiovascular disease is less prevalent in premenopausal women without diabetes than in men of the same age, premenopausal women who have diabetes seem to lose this sex-linked protection, putting them at risk levels for heart disease equivalent to that of men. Diabetes also doubles the risk of having a second heart attack in women (but not in men).

2. **TRUE.** The Surgeon General recommends that people engage in 30 minutes of moderate-intensity activity most days of the week, but many people complain that they do not have the time. Studies have shown, however, that getting in 10 minutes of moderate activity here and 15 minutes there can add up and that 30 total minutes of activity gained in this way per day provide similar health benefits to doing 30 minutes of activity all at once. What constitutes moderate activity? Biking, gardening, and brisk walking all fit the bill.

So if you can't fit a block of 30 minutes of exercise a day (or a trip to a gym) into your busy schedule, small steps toward your goal could include a brisk walk on your lunch hour, taking the stairs up to your office rather than the elevators, getting off the bus a stop early, or parking at the far end of the lot at the grocery store.

3. **B.** High blood pressure for adults with diabetes is defined as a systolic blood pressure (the top number) above 130 mm Hg and/or a diastolic blood pressure (the bottom number) above 80 mm Hg. Adults with diabetes are advised to keep their levels of low-density lipoprotein (LDL, or "bad") cholesterol below 100 mg/dl, their levels of triglycerides (another blood fat) below 150 mg/dl, and their levels of high-density lipoprotein (HDL, or "good") cholesterol above 40 mg/dl for men or 50 mg/dl for women. The goal for glycosylated hemoglobin (HbA_{1c}) levels, which indicate a person's average blood glucose level over the previous 2–3 months, is below 7.0% for most people with diabetes. Because an individual may have other health priorities or problems that make attaining some of these goals difficult or dangerous, people must work with their health-care team to set personalized goals and treatment plans.

4. **A, B, C.** If you smoke, stopping smoking is one of the best steps you can take to help your heart, your lungs, and your risk for diabetes-related complications. If you need a little help, your physician can prescribe counseling or certain medicines to help you quit. Overweight and obesity increase risks for heart disease, high blood pressure, and cholesterol abnormalities, and weight loss can reduce these risks. Registered dietitians often design meal plans for people with diabetes in which 25% to 30% of daily calories come from fats. Calories from saturated and *trans* fats (types of fat that can raise a person's level of LDL cholesterol) should be kept below 10% of total daily calories, and people at high risk of heart disease may be advised to cut saturated and *trans* fat intake to less than 7% of total calories. Saturated fats are found in animal-derived products such as meats and dairy products and are also in vegetable oils from tropical nuts such as coconut oil, palm oil, and palm kernel oil. *Trans* fats are chemically altered vegetable oils that are found in foods such as some margarines, commercial baked goods, and fried foods.

Moderate intake of alcohol is OK for some people with diabetes and has been linked in some studies to some benefits for the heart; however, a moderate intake is defined as no more than one drink per day for women or two drinks per day for men, and no national health organization recommends starting to drink alcohol if you do not do so already. One drink consists of 12 ounces of beer, 5 ounces of wine, or 1½ ounces of 80-proof distilled liquor.

5. **FALSE.** A daily aspirin has been shown to reduce risks for heart attack in men by about 30%. However, aspirin therapy is not recommended for everyone, or even everyone with diabetes. As with any drug, aspirin has some side effects, including increased risks for gastrointestinal bleeding and even a form of stroke. People with low risk for developing cardiovascular disease may be more likely to experience bleeding problems than to show much benefit from lowering their already low risk of heart disease. Also, aspirin has not been studied as a preventive treatment for heart disease in people with diabetes under 30 and should not be given to children or teenagers under age 21 who may have the flu or chicken pox because of the risk

of developing Reye Syndrome (a potentially fatal condition). Finally, even some people who do meet the criteria for a daily aspirin regimen may have "aspirin allergy" or be "aspirin resistant"; these people may benefit more from taking other related drugs, such as clopidogrel (brand name Plavix); than from taking aspirin.

6. TRUE. The DASH (Dietary Approaches to Stop Hypertension) eating plan, which emphasizes reducing intake of red meat while increasing intake of fruits, vegetables, whole-grain foods, and low-fat dairy products, has been shown to significantly reduce blood pressure levels as much as a blood-pressure-lowering drug. Its efficacy at lowering blood pressure is enhanced when combined with a decreased sodium intake. The DASH-Sodium study showed that people who followed the DASH eating plan along with a low-sodium restriction (less than 1,500 milligrams of sodium per day) lowered their blood pressure more than people following the DASH plan or a low-sodium restriction alone. The 2005 Dietary Guidelines for Americans recommends limiting sodium intake to less than 2,300 milligrams per day (roughly the amount in a teaspoon of table salt) for many peo-ple and to less than 1,500 milligrams per day for people with high blood pressure, middle-age or older adults, and African-Americans.

To learn more about the DASH eating plan and how it can work with your diabetes meal plan, talk with your physician or a registered dietitian. You can download a PDF description of the plan that includes recipes from www.nhlbi.nih.gov/health/public/heart/hbp/dash. You can also order a copy of the booklet from the Web site or by calling (301) 592-8573 or (240) 629-3255 (TTY).

7. A, B, D. Having diabetes is considered to be the risk equivalent of already having heart disease. People with diabetes tend to have higher triglyceride levels than people without diabetes, and higher triglyceride levels are linked to increased risks for heart disease. People with diabetes do not seem to be more likely to have higher LDL levels than people without diabetes. However, researchers *have* found that people with diabetes tend to have smaller, denser LDL particles that are more apt to cause cardiovascular damage. Over time, high blood glucose levels also increase risks for cardiovascular disease. □

Index

A

Acanthosis nigricans, 462
Acarbose (Precose), 140, 431
ACE inhibitors, 239, 240, 241, 268, 286–287
Adrencorticotropin (ACTH), 102
Aerobic exercise, 68–69, 70, 333, 334, 337, 341
Aerobic exercise machines, 343–344
Aging. *See* Elderly
Albumin, 66, 133, 134, 135, 285, 561
Alcohol consumption
    after bariatric surgery, 379
    and blood glucose levels, 145–146, 158, 550
    of college students, 550
    and HbA$_{1c}$ levels, 136
    and high blood pressure, 238
    and hypoglycemia, 44, 45, 47, 145–146
    moderate intake, 567
    and nutrition supplements, 205
    and osteoporosis risk, 447, 449
    and sleep disorders, 455
Allergic reaction to insulin, 175
Alpha-beta blockers, 239, 240
Alpha-blockers, 239
Alpha-glucosidase inhibitors, 45, 151, 232, 234–235
Alpha-lipoic acid, 223
American Diabetes Association
    blood glucose goals of, 48, 49, 58, 62, 181, 305, 439–440, 478, 479, 555
    blood pressure goals of, 135, 237, 305
    on cholesterol-lowering drugs, 431
    on diet and nutrition, 503–504
    on eye screening, 509, 563
    on fat intake, 391
    on fiber intake, 256
    on foot examinations, 253
    on foot problem risk, 304
    on HbA$_{1c}$ levels, 131, 133, 134, 561
    on ketone testing, 294
    on kidney disease screening, 285, 286, 565
    on protein intake, 393
    on pump therapy, 194
    on retinopathy, 440
    on sodium intake, 391
    Standards of Medical Care, 439
    on vitamin and mineral supplements, 207–208

American Dietetic Association, 95, 256
American Heart Association, 263, 265, 267, 430, 431
Americans with Disabilities Act (ADA), 54
Amernorrhea, 446
Amputation risk, 252, 304, 309, 310
Amylin, 224–226, 233
Analgesics, and kidney disease, 286
Anemia, 136, 216, 268–269, 379, 565
Angiotensin-converting enzyme (ACE) inhibitor, 65, 66, 239, 240, 268, 286–287
Angiotensin receptor blocker (ARB), 65, 66, 239, 240, 268, 286, 287
Antibodies, 23, 30
Antidepressants, 103, 116
Antioxidants, 208, 219–223
Antiseptic, in wound healing, 317
Aspart (NovoLog), 141, 172, 183
Aspirin therapy, 18, 65, 70, 491, 567–568
Assistive devices, 271, 272–273
Atherosclerosis, 67, 68, 266, 270, 281, 305, 429
Autonomic neuropathy, 44, 66, 254–255
Axokine, 371

B

Bacterial infections, 461–462, 493–494
Balance
    disturbances, 351
    exercises, 347–350, 351
    sense of, 345–346, 351
Bariatric surgery, 376–380
Basal insulin, 139, 155, 173, 177, 182–187
Behavior changes. *See* Lifestyle changes
Beta-adrenergic agonists, 25
Beta-blockers, 239, 240
Beta-carotene, 208, 220, 221–222
Beta-cell function, 145, 187–188
Bethanechol (Urecholine), 290
Biguanides, 44–45, 232, 233–234
Bile acid sequestrants, 430–431
Binge eating disorder, 92–96
Bisphosphonates, 449–450, 502
Blindness, 65, 122, 440, 441
Blood glucose levels
    and alcohol consumption,

145–146, 158
    and carbohydrate intake, 157
    during college transition, 548–549
    and complications of diabetes, 133–134
    and exercise, 16, 20, 40, 143–144, 158, 184
    and fiber intake, 257
    fluctuations in, 141–146
    and heart disease risk, 19, 68, 69
    high. *See* Hyperglycemia
    low. *See* Hypoglycemia
    and menstruation, 17
    overnight patterns, 184–185, 186, 542, 555
    postprandial, 140, 146–153, 181, 225–226
    during pregnancy, 478, 479, 480
    and retinopathy, 134, 437, 438, 441–442
    after stroke, 272, 273
    and stress, 70–80, 144
    and surgery, 545, 546
    target goals, 48–49, 58, 63, 69, 134, 137, 155, 439–440, 555
    in Type 2 diabetes, 24, 134
    and weight loss, 24
Blood glucose monitoring
    and alcohol consumption, 550
    alternative-site, 555
    averages in, 138
    basal insulin, 185–186
    of children, 521–522, 528–529
    continuous glucose monitors, 148–149, 160–163
    equipment and supplies, 36–37, 53
    errors, avoiding, 468–469
    false readings, 144–145
    frequency of, 22, 61, 135, 138–139
    and gastroparesis, 288–289
    HbA$_{1c}$ test, 62, 69, 132–136, 231, 286, 439
    during hospitalization, 469
    during illness, 36, 63, 559
    and insulin therapy, 19, 61, 176, 190
    mealtime, 154–155, 159
    pattern of readings, 138–140, 159
    post-meal, 140, 148–149, 181, 184, 289
    during pregnancy, 52, 134, 135, 478–479, 485, 488
    premeal, 180
    at summer camp, 521–522

Blood pressure
  at ankle, 561
  monitoring, 69, 242
  See also High blood pressure
Blood tests
  BUN (blood urea nitrogen), 286
  fasting plasma glucose, 61
  HbA$_{1c}$, 62, 69, 132–136, 231, 286,
    439, 530, 531, 555, 561
  for ketones, 42, 294–295
  oral glucose tolerance, 61
Body image, 86–91
Body-mass index, 269, 525
Bolus insulin
  extending/delaying, 157–158
  insulin pump, 37, 158, 177, 180,
    194, 289
  timing of, 148, 149, 151–152, 153
  two-phase, 177–178
  unused, 180–181
Bone fractures, 446, 500, 505
Bone loss, of osteoporosis, 215,
  445–450, 499–500
Bone mineral density test, 448–449
Brain, and hunger, 370–372
Brain damage, of hypoglycemia, 154
Breast-feeding, 484, 489, 490–493
Breathing exercises, 81, 377–378, 536
Brittle diabetes, 141
Burnout, 115, 122

C

Caffeine
  and bariatric surgery, 379
  and blood glucose fluctuations,
    145
  and sleep disorders, 455
Calcitonin, 450, 502
Calcitriol, 565
Calcium
  absorption, 449, 504
  blood levels of, 565
  food sources of, 379, 401, 446, 448,
    482, 504
  in menopause, 502
  during pregnancy, 482
  recommended intake, 447, 448,
    504
  supplements, 215–216, 217, 377,
    379, 448, 504
Calcium channel blockers, 239, 240
Calluses, foot, 307, 316
Calories
  burning, 333, 336, 369
  daily needs, 390
  on food labels, 391
  low-calorie diet, 369, 524
Candidiasis of the skin, 462
Capsaicin products, 317

Carbohydrate burning, 332
Carbohydrate counting
  basic, 32
  from food labels, 392
  and hypoglycemia, 47
  information sources, 157
  during pregnancy, 486–487
  vegan/vegetarian diet, 405, 411
Carbohydrates, dietary
  on food labels, 391–393
  in gluten-free foods, 27, 32–33
  glycemic index of foods, 149–151,
    152–153, 157, 179
  and hyperglycemia, 50
  and hypoglycemia, 46, 64
  during illness, 35, 559
  low-carbohydrate high-protein
    diet, 21, 39–40
  refined/processed foods, 435
Cardiac autonomic neuropathy,
  254–255, 267
Cardiac rehabilitation, 262–265
Cardiomyopathy, diabetic, 267
Carotenoids, 220, 223
Cataracts, 441, 443, 508, 563
Celiac disease
  complications of, 15, 27–28
  defined, 26–27
  diagnosis of, 28, 30–31
  gluten-free diet for, 15, 28, 31–32
  incidence of, 29–30
  information sources, 29, 30–31
  risk factors for, 28–29
  support groups for, 29
  symptoms of, 27
  with Type 1 diabetes, 32–33
Charcot foot, 307
Children and teens, diabetic
  blood glucose monitoring,
    521–522, 528–529
  in college transition, 547–551
  dental care for, 541–543
  and developmental stages, 535
  diet and nutrition for, 525–526,
    534, 538–541
  fear of injection, 536–537
  and hypoglycemia, 43, 522,
    527–530, 541
  and insulin therapy, 529, 534–537
  and obesity prevention, 368,
    523–527
  and pain perception, 536
  summer camps for, 520–523
  during surgery, 544–546
  Type 1, 26, 32
  Type 2, 25, 524, 525, 545
Chlamydia, 259
Chlorpropamide (Diabinese), 142,
  154
Cholecystokinin, 370

Cholesterol levels
  drug treatment, 64–65, 69–70, 429,
    430–433, 433
  and heart disease risk, 68, 305, 429,
    433
  lifestyle changes for, 68, 430,
    433–436
  monitoring, 69, 505, 567
  and Type 2 diabetes, 135
Chromium, 212–213, 217
Ciliary neurotrophic factor (CNTF),
  371
Claudication, intermittent, 310, 357
Cognitive behavior therapy (CBT),
  103
Combination therapy, 231
Complications, diabetic
  and balance disturbances, 351
  and blood glucose levels, 133–134,
    281, 282, 437–438, 467
  constipation, 255–258
  depression, 102
  and exercise, 507
  eye diseases, 441, *See also*
    Retinopathy, diabetic
  fear of, 121, 122, 123
  gastroparesis, 152, 157, 255,
    288–291
  and high blood pressure, 26, 60,
    135, 237
  and hyperglycemia, 48
  monitoring for, 66–67
  stroke, 270–274
  urinary tract infections (UTI),
    259–262
  See also Heart disease; Neuropathy;
    Nephropathy; Peripheral neu-
    ropathy; Sexual problems
Congestive heart failure, 71
Constipation, 255–258
Continuous glucose monitor,
  148–149, 160–163
Copper, 214
Corns, removal of, 316
Corticotropin-releasing factor (CRF),
  102
Cortisol, 102, 115, 154
Creatinine, 565
Cystic fibrosis, 25

D

DASH (Dietary Approaches to Stop
  Hypertension) plan, 286, 568
Dawn phenomenom, 144, 155, 555
Debridement, of foot ulcers, 311–312
Dehydration, 21, 24, 33, 34, 36, 42,
  182, 335
Denafil (Levitra), 276
Dental care, for children, 541–543

Depression
    and binge eating disorder, 93
    and body image, 89
    diagnosis of, 102–103
    after heart attack, 265
    information sources, 104–105
    and sleep disorders, 455
    and stress response, 102, 115
    symptoms of, 102, 506
    treatments for, 102–105, 116
    yoga for, 338
Dermatitis herpetiformis, 27–28
Dermopathy, diabetic, 463
Detemir (Levemir), 141–142, 183,
    184, 189
Diabetes
    defined, 23
    diagnosis of, 26, 60–61
    information sources, 59
    risk factors for, 25, 60, 432
    symptoms of, 23–24, 25, 61
    treatment. See Drugs, diabetes;
        Insulin therapy
    types of, 25
    See also Type 1 diabetes; Type 2
        diabetes
Diabetes camps, 520, 521
Diabetes Control and Complications
    Trial (DCCT), 49, 133, 134, 136,
    437–438, 439, 440
Diabetes management
    in college, 547–551
    education and training for, 57, 62
    information sources on, 59
    plan for, 57–59
    sick-day plan, 21–22, 34, 36–37, 63
    spousal support in, 111–114
    See also Blood glucose monitoring;
        Diet and nutrition; Exercise;
        Lifestyle changes; Meal planning
Diabetes Prevention Program (DPP),
    343, 444
Diabetes supplies
    for blood glucose monitoring,
        36–37, 53
    in college, 548
    disposal of, 194, 548, 555
    insulin storage, 556–557
    sick-day box, 21, 22, 33–39,
        451–452
    storage of, 557
    at summer camp, 523
    travel with, 194–195
Diarrhea, and dehydration, 34, 36
Diastolic blood pressure, 65, 237, 567
Dietary Reference Intakes (DRI), 206
Diethylpropion (Tenuate), 372
Dietitian, registered, 16, 17, 19, 62,
    68, 95, 175, 264, 314, 377, 436, 481,
    484, 485, 567

Diet and nutrition
    antioxidants in, 222
    for bariatric surgery, 377, 378, 379
    and blood glucose fluctuations,
        142–143
    calcium intake, 379, 446, 448, 482
    carbohydrate intake. See Carbohy-
        drates, dietary
    for cardiac rehabilitation, 264
    for children, 525–526, 534,
        538–541
    cholesterol goals, 433–435
    in college, 549
    counseling, 68, 95, 314
    DASH plan, 286, 568
    fat intake. See Fat, dietary
    fiber intake, 68, 143, 256–258, 392,
        418, 420, 435, 436
    glycemic index of foods, 149–151,
        152–153, 157, 179
    healthy tips, 207
    during illness, 559
    information sources, 32, 62, 540
    ketogenic diet, 42–43
    liquid diet, 288, 291–292, 377, 378
    low-calorie diet, 369, 524
    low-carbohydrate high-protein diet,
        21, 39–40
    meal timing, 142, 155–156, 529
    nutrient requirements, daily,
        206–207, 209, 213, 217
    omega-3 fatty acids in, 104
    and osteoporosis risk, 446–447
    protein intake. See Protein, dietary
    serving size, 389–391, 396–399
    weight loss, 69, 95, 369, 373–375,
        435, 524
    for women, 503–504
    See also Food labels; Gluten-free
        diet; Meal planning; Recipes
Dilantin, 25
Dipeptidyl peptidase-4 inhibitors, 45,
    233, 234–235
Diuretics, 238, 239, 240, 268
Doctors
    anesthesiologists/anesthetists, 544
    for college students, 550–551
    and complications prevention, 465
    and drug therapy, 466
    foot problem specialists, 307–308
    ophthalmologists, 563
    during pregnancy, 479, 485
    in team approach, 61, 444
    weight loss team, 375
Domperidone (Motilium), 290
D-Phenylalanine derivatives, 232, 233,
    234–235
DPP-4 inhibitors, 232
Drugs
    antibacterials, 261

antibiotics, 261–262
antidiarrheal/antivomiting, 36
and blood glucose fluctuations,
    146
and blood glucose level, 51
blood-pressure–lowering, 65,
    69–70, 238–241, 268, 286–287,
    466, 568
blood-pressure–raising, 241
cholesterol-lowering, 64–65, 69–70,
    429, 430–433, 443
for depression, 103, 116
and diabetes risk, 25
for erectile dysfunction, 275, 276
for gastroparesis, 290
for heart disease, 69–70, 466,
    567–568
for heart failure, 268–269
hormone therapy, 497–498,
    500–502
interactions, 508
and nutrient absorption, 206
for osteoporosis prevention,
    449–450
and osteoporosis risk, 447
pain and fever relievers, 35, 378
in sick-day box, 35–36
weight-loss, 368, 369, 370–372, 432
for yeast infections, 495
See also Vitamins and minerals
Drugs, diabetes (oral), 231–236
    during breast-feeding, 491
    classes of, 231–233, 234–235
    combination therapy, 231
    errors, avoiding, 465–467
    exenatide (Byetta), 227–230, 231,
        233
    and hyperglycemia, 50–51
    and hypoglycemia, 44–45, 113,
        154, 226
    and insulin resistance, 24–25
    mealtime, 140, 142
    missed dose, 236
    postprandial, 150–151
    pramlintide (Symlin), 224–226,
        229, 233
    during pregnancy, 233, 236
    sick-day guidelines, 36
    and surgery (children's), 545
Dual energy x-ray absorptiometry
    (DXA), 448
Dyslipidemia, 68, 429, 436

E

Eating disorders
    binge eating, 92–96
    information sources on, 96
Eating out, and trans fat intake, 415
Echocardiograms, 267

Ecthyma, 461
Edema, 284, 466
Elderly
  balance problems of, 351
  calcium supplements for, 215
  exercise for, 336
  and foot problems, 252–253
  and osteoporosis, 446
  vitamin supplements for, 205
Electrocardiogram, 267
Electroconvulsive therapy, 105
Electrolyte imbalance, 33–34
Electrophysiology, 253
Emergency preparedness, 450–453, 549
Emotional issues. *See* Mental health
Employment. *See* Jobs
Endocrinologists, 479, 485, 542
Endoscopy, upper, 289
Environmental triggers, for Type 1 diabetes, 23
Epinephrine, 44, 559
Erectile dysfunction, 274–279
Erythromycin, 290
Erythropoietin (EPO), 565
Escherichia coli, 259
Estrogen, 280, 446, 450, 498, 499, 500
Exenatide (Byetta), 45, 227–230, 231, 233, 371
Exercise
  action plan, 100
  ADA guidelines for, 40
  aerobic, 68–69, 70, 333, 334, 337, 341
  aerobic exercise machines, 343–344
  balance, 347–350, 351
  and bariatric surgery, 377, 379
  benefits of, 62–63, 68, 341–342
  and blood glucose levels, 16, 20, 40, 143–144, 158, 184
  budgeting for, 344–345
  calorie burning during, 333, 336
  in cardiac rehabilitation, 263–264
  for children, 526
  for constipation prevention, 257
  defined, 70, 158
  after eating, 149
  for elderly, 336
  fat burning during, 332, 333, 334
  and foot problems, 314
  and heart disease, 567
  and hyperglycemia, 50
  and hypoglycemia, 45, 158, 336
  interval training, 335–336
  and ketones, 40
  myths about, 332–336
  during pregnancy, 482, 485
  and retinopathy, 357, 507, 563
  and sleeping patterns, 458

  stretching, 352–358
  time of day, 143, 333–334
  and Type 1 diabetes, 63
  walking, 334, 342–343
  weight-bearing, 333, 336, 447, 449, 507
  and weight loss, 334, 336, 524
  yoga, 337–340
Eye examinations, 65–66, 443–444, 466, 509, 561
Ezetimibe (Zetia), 431

F

Family and Medical Leave Act (FMLA), 56
Family therapy, for binge eating disorder, 95
Fast food
  and children, 538–539
  portion size of, 397, 398
  trans fat in, 413
Fasting plasma glucose test, 61
Fat
  burning during exercise, 332, 333, 334
  chemical structure of, 414
  metabolism, 39, 40
  storage of, 334
Fat, dietary
  and blood glucose rise, 143
  and cholesterol control, 64, 68, 433–436, 443, 567
  daily needs, 390
  on food labels, 391, 434
  hydrogenated, 412, 413–414, 434
  recipe modification, 418
  recommended intake, 415
  role in cooking, 417
  saturated fat, 433–434, 435, 436, 443, 567
  trans fat, 64, 412–415, 434, 435, 443, 567
  unsaturated fat, 434
  in vegetarian/vegan diet, 409
Fenugreek, 492–493
Fiber, dietary, 68, 143, 256–258, 392, 418, 420, 435, 436
Fibrates, 431
Fight-or-flight response, 79, 80, 337
Fingersticks, 534, 535
Fish oil, 431, 435, 443
Flavor, in cooking, 418, 420
Fluid intake
  with bariatric surgery, 377, 378, 379
  for constipation prevention, 258
  emergency preparedness, 451
  with exercise, 335, 340
  for urinary regularity, 261
Fluoroquinolones, 261

Flu shot, 19–20, 64, 505
Folic acid (folate), 208, 209, 210
Food and Drug Administration (FDA), 213, 229, 231, 372, 388, 390, 394, 395, 434
Food labels
  health claims on, 395, 396
  ingredients list, 395–396
  nutrition information on, 214, 388–393
  serving size on, 389–391, 398–399
  terminology, 394
  trans fat on, 414, 415, 434
Foot care
  daily inspection, 144, 306, 464
  guidelines/tips, 254, 306, 312–313, 464, 505–506
  over-the-counter products, 315–317
Foot examinations, 66, 253–254, 304, 464, 467
Foot problems
  and amputation risk, 252, 304, 309, 310
  causes of neuropathy, 252–253
  deformities, 307, 310–311
  diagnosis of neuropathy, 253–254, 304
  information sources, 308
  medical specialists, 307–308
  of peripheral vascular disease, 310
  prevention of, 304–306
  treatment for, 67, 254
  types of, 306–307
  ulcers, 252, 254, 304, 306, 309–315, 463
  and yoga, 340
Fractures, 446, 500, 505
Free radicals, 208, 216, 219
Fructosamine test, 135
Fungal infections, 307, 317, 462, 495, 543
Furunculosis, 461

G

Gangrene, 310, 462
Gastric bypass (bariatric) surgery, 376–380
Gastroesophageal reflux disease (GERD), 456
Gastroparesis, 152, 157, 255, 288–291
Gastropathy, 44, 143, 257, 258
Genetics
  and celiac disease, 28
  and heart disease, 67–68
  and osteoporosis, 445
  and Type 1 diabetes, 23
  and Type 2 diabetes, 24
Gestational diabetes, 25, 60, 61, 172, 236, 480–481, 482–483

Ghrelin, 370, 376
Glargine (Lantus), 139, 183, 184, 189, 229
Glaucoma, 441, 508, 563
Glimepiride (Amaryl), 142, 154, 188
Glipizide (Glucotrol), 142, 154, 188
Glomerular filtration rate (GFR), 285–286
Glucagon, 21, 22, 38, 64, 154, 224, 225, 228, 488, 529–530
Glucose metabolism, 442
Glucose tablets/gels, 38
Glucotoxicity, 189
Glulisine (Apidra), 141, 172, 183
Gluten-free diet
    carbohydrates in, 15–16, 27, 32–33
    foods to avoid, 31–32
    foods to eat, 32
    product sources for, 28
    as treatment for celiac disease, 15, 28, 31–32
Gluten intolerance, 27–28, 206
    See also Celiac disease
Glyburide (DiaBeta), 154, 188
Glycemic index of foods, 149–151, 152–153, 157, 179
Glycogen, 43, 187
Glycosylated hemoglobin test.
    See HbA$_{1c}$ test
Glycosylation, 132–133
Granuloma annulare, 462–463
Group therapy, for binge eating disorder, 95

H

Hammertoe (claw toe), 307, 310–311, 463
HbA$_{1c}$ levels
    and chromium supplements, 212
    and complications risk, 63, 133–134, 466
    postprandial, 147
    during pregnancy, 480
    and retinopathy, 441–442
    target goals, 231, 437, 439–440, 561, 567
HbA$_{1c}$ test, 62, 69, 132–136, 231, 286, 439, 505, 530, 531, 555, 561
Health insurance, 136, 139, 195, 438, 439, 548
Heart attacks, 18, 67
    and cardiac rehabilitation, 262–265
    depression after, 265
    silent, 255
    symptoms of, 70–71
Heart disease
    and blood glucose levels, 135
    cardiac autonomic neuropathy, 254–255, 267

and cardiac rehabilitation, 262–265
and cholesterol level, 68, 305, 429
drug therapy for, 69–70, 268–269, 466, 567–568
and exercise, 567
heart failure, 265–270
and high blood pressure, 68, 237, 305
and lifestyle changes, 64, 68–69, 264–265, 342
and postprandial blood glucose levels, 225–226
prevention of, 64–65
risk factors for, 64, 67–68, 147, 265, 266–267, 412–413, 432
surgical treatment of, 269–270
in women, 67, 499, 504–505
Heart-rate variability test, 255
Hemochromatosis, 25, 216
Hemoglobin, 132–133
High blood glucose. *See* Hyperglycemia
High blood pressure
    causes of, 266
    defined, 236–237, 567
    and diabetes complications, 26, 60, 135, 237
    drug treatment of, 65, 69–70, 238–241, 268, 286–287, 466, 568
    and heart disease risk, 68, 237, 305
    and lifestyle changes, 238, 286
    and meal plan, 62, 568
    and nephropathy, 65, 66, 284, 286–287, 565
    and peripheral neuropathy, 305
    and retinopathy, 442–443
    and stroke, 270
    target goals, 237–238
High-density lipoprotein (HDL), 68, 69, 135, 210, 264, 430, 431, 435–436, 499, 500
Homocysteine, 210
Hoodia, 371
Hormones
    appetite-influencing, 370
    and blood glucose fluctuations, 144
    counterregulatory, 154
    and depression, 115
    in growth years, 182–183
    sex, 280, 446
    and stress response, 102, 545, 555
Hormone therapy, 497–498, 500–502
Hospitalization, blood glucose monitoring during, 469
Hot flashes, 498–499
Hunger, 368–372
Hydrogenated fat, 412, 413–414
Hyperglycemia
    causes of, 50–52, 175

defined, 43–44
and eye problems, 563
identifying, 49–50
and nutrient deficiencies, 206
and peripheral neuropathy, 252
postprandial, 147, 225–226
and sexual problems, 281–282
and skin conditions, 460, 461, 462
Somogyi phenomenon, 185, 186
and stress, 17, 51–52
symptoms of, 50
Hyperinsulinemia, 413
Hyperosmolar hyperglycemic state, 52–53, 63, 295
Hypertension. *See* High blood pressure
Hypoglycemia
    and alcohol consumption, 44, 45, 47, 145–146
    causes of, 43, 113, 153–154, 174–175, 190
    in children, 43, 522, 527–530, 542
    delayed-onset, 143, 158
    and drug therapy, 44–45, 113, 154, 226
    and exercise, 45, 158, 336
    and fall prevention, 446
    and insomnia, 455
    overtreating, 143
    during pregnancy, 44, 483, 488
    prevention strategies, 47, 155–159, 468, 528–529
    risk factors for, 44, 45
    at summer camp, 522
    symptoms of, 44, 63–64, 113, 136, 154, 468, 488, 527–528
    treatment of, 46–47, 64, 174, 190, 224, 468, 529, 549
Hypoglycemia unawareness, 45–46, 136, 154, 528, 530, 555
Hysterectomy, 498

I

Immune system
    and celiac disease, 27, 33
    and cortisol, 102
    and Type 1 diabetes, 23
Immunizations, 19–20, 64, 505
Implantable cardioverter defibrillators (ICDs), 269
Infections
    bacterial, 461–462
    and blood glucose levels, 140, 144, 461
    and foot ulcers, 312–313
    fungal, 307, 317, 462, 495, 543
    and hyperglycemia, 53
    and ketone levels, 41
    respiratory, 545

urinary tract, 259–262
vaginitis, 493–495
Influenza vaccine (flu shot), 19–20, 64, 505
Information sources
  biking, 362
  carbohydrate counting, 157
  celiac disease, 29, 30–31
  depression, 104–105
  diabetes management planning, 59
  diet and nutrition, 32, 62, 540
  eating disorders, 96
  emergency preparedness, 452
  employment, 55
  foot problems, 308
  gluten-free products, 28
  insulin therapy, 181
  lifestyle change, 100
  pregnancy, 483
  relaxation techniques, 81
  sexual problems, 278, 282
  sleeping problems, 459
  storytelling, 109
  stretching exercises, 357
  stroke rehabilitation, 271, 273
  summer camps, 522
  vaginal infection, 496
  vegan/vegetarian diet, 410–411
  vitamins and minerals, 218
  weight loss, 374
  women's health, 509
Injection aids, 192
Insomnia, 454–459
Insulin
  absorption rate, 45
  allergic reaction to, 175
  basal, 139, 155, 173, 177, 182–187
  bolus. See Bolus insulin
  role in blood glucose regulation, 24, 137, 139–140, 171, 187
  storage of, 557
  types of, 172–174, 189
  unused, 156–157, 180–181
Insulin injection
  extending/delaying, 157
  fear of needles, 188, 192, 536–537
  fingersticks, 534, 535
  jet injectors, 176, 193, 195
  needle disposal, 194, 548
  and pain, 534, 535
  pens, 142, 176, 192–193, 195, 557
  sites, 175
  at summer camp, 522–523
  syringes, 176, 191–192, 195
  timing of, 189
  vials, 51, 176, 557
  See also Diabetes supplies; Insulin pump; Insulin therapy
Insulin pump
  basal insulin delivery, 139, 183,

185, 194
  bolus insulin delivery, 37, 158, 177, 180, 194, 289
  candidates for pump therapy, 194
  defined, 176, 191
  during pregnancy, 486, 488, 489
  problems with, 142, 183–184
  pros and cons of, 195
  at summer camp, 523
  supplies, 38, 51
Insulin resistance
  defined, 187
  and lifestyle change, 172
  in menopause, 500
  treatments for, 24, 189
Insulin sensitivity factor, 180
Insulin therapy
  and after-meal spikes, 150
  basal-bolus approach, 155
  during breast-feeding, 491
  challenges of, 174–175
  delivery systems, 51, 175–176, 189–190, 191–196
  errors, avoiding, 467–468
  fluctuations in blood glucose level, 141–142
  during hospitalization, 469
  during illness, 559
  information sources, 181
  and meal timing, 142, 155–156, 529
  omission of doses, 52
  during pregnancy, 479–480, 482–483, 485–486, 487–489
  premeal doses, 178–179, 180
  psychological resistance to, 188–189
  rapid-acting insulin, 156, 172, 174, 177–182, 289, 467
  sick-day guidelines, 36, 467
  after stroke, 272
  starting dose, 191
  and surgery (children's), 545
  and weight gain, 190–191
  See also Insulin injection; Insulin pump
Iron
  food sources of, 401
  during pregnancy, 482
  supplements, 205, 216, 217, 379, 565
Ischemia, 310
Isoflavones, 503

J
Jet injectors, 176, 193, 195
Jobs

accommodation, 56
attendance/leave policies, 56
benefits, 53–54
disclosure of diabetes, 55–56
resources for employee rights, 55
responsibilities, 54–55
search, 54
Joint mobility, limited, 311

K
Keratopathy, 441
Ketoacidosis, diabetic (DKA)
  causes of, 40–42, 175, 182, 293, 559
  diagnosis of, 294–295
  during pregnancy, 479, 484
  sick-day plan, 63
  symptoms of, 37, 52, 294, 559
  in Type 2 diabetes, 293–294
Ketone bodies, 39
Ketones
  defined, 21, 39
  excessive, 293
  and exercise, 40
  and low-carbohydrate diet, 39–40, 42
Ketone testing
  blood vs. urine, 42, 294
  guidelines, 36, 42
  during illness, 559
  during pregnancy, 42, 479, 488
  with strips, 37–38, 41, 42
  at summer camp, 521–522
  when to test, 294–295
Kidney disease, diabetic. See Nephropathy
Kidney failure, 285
Kidney function, 44, 283, 284, 565

L
Lactose acidosis, 232
Lactose intolerance, 28, 379
Lancets, 548, 555
Left Ventricular Assist Device (LVAD), 270
Leptin, 370, 371
Lifestyle changes
  action plan for, 99–100
  attainable goals for, 99
  with bariatric surgery, 378–380
  in cardiac rehabilitation, 264–265
  cholesterol lowering, 68, 430, 433–436
  and heart disease, 68–69, 341–342
  and high blood pressure, 238, 286
  for menopause symptoms, 502–503
  motivation for, 98–99, 123
  and self-efficacy, 97–98

smoking cessation, 65, 69, 306, 314, 443, 449, 508, 567
weight-loss strategies, 373–375
See also Exercise; Diet and nutrition
Lipid management, 64–65, 433–436, 443
Lispro (Humalog), 141, 172, 183
Liver, role in blood glucose regulation, 24
Lorcaserin, 372
Low blood glucose. *See* Hypoglycemia
Low-calorie diet, 369, 524
Low-carbohydrate high-protein diet, 39–40
Low-density lipoprotein (LDL)
blood test, 69
and estrogen, 499
and eye disease risk, 443
and heart disease risk, 68, 305, 412, 567, 568
lowering, 64, 135, 264, 429, 430–431, 432–435, 436, 466
and niacin, 210, 431
oxidative damage to, 219
Lycopene, 208, 220, 222

M

Macrovascular disease, 64
Macular degeneration, 561
Macular edema, 561
Magnesium, 214, 217, 446
Magnetic resonance imaging (MRI), 289
Manganese, 216, 217
Mazindol (Mazanor), 372
Meal planning
during breast-feeding, 492
drug timing in, 142, 148–149
and hyperglycemia, 50
and hypoglycemia, 45, 155–156
nutrition intake, 68
during pregnancy, 481–482, 485, 486–487
and recipe modification, 416–418, 420
recipe sources, 417
at summer camp, 523
See also Diet and nutrition; Vegan diet; Vegetarian diet
Mean arterial pressure (MAP), 442–443
Medical exams/tests
blood pressure, 69
bone mineral density, 448–449
for exercise program, 69
eyes, 65–66, 443–444, 467, 509, 561
feet, 66, 253–254, 304, 314, 467
for gastroparesis, 289

for heart failure, 267
for nephropathy, 66, 285–286, 561, 565
for neuropathy, 66, 314–315
for peripheral neuropathy, 253–254, 304, 561
for peripheral vascular disease, 310
physicals, 19, 61, 63
recommended, 66
screening, 504–505
urinalysis, 260
See also Blood tests; Ketone testing
Medical nutrition therapy (MNT), 430
Medicare, 136, 139, 320, 505, 509
Medications. *See* Drugs; Drugs, diabetes (oral)
Meditation, 81, 144
Meglitinides, 232, 233, 234–235
Menopause
defined, 498
health risks of, 499–500
and hormone therapy, 497–498, 500–502
lifestyle changes in, 502–503
symptoms of, 498–499
Menstruation
amenorrhea, 446
blood glucose fluctuation during, 144
cessation of, 498
Mental health
binge eating disorder, 92–96
and body image, 86–91
burnout, 115, 122
and diabetes care team, 63
distress and frustration of diabetes management, 115–117
mind/body medicine, 83
and self-efficacy, 97, 121–122
and spirituality, 83–85
and storytelling, 106–110
See also Depression; Stress
Metabolic syndrome, 25, 237, 429, 432, 433
Metaclopramide (Reglan), 290
Metformin (Glucophage), 24, 210, 228, 232, 269, 431, 438, 466, 545
Metronidazole, 494
Microalbuminuria, 66, 133, 134, 283, 285, 286, 287, 437, 438, 467, 505, 561, 565
Microdialysis, 254
Miglitol (Glyset), 140, 431
Mind/body medicine, 83
Minerals. *See* Vitamins and minerals
MODY (Maturity Onset Diabetes of Youth), 25
Molybdenum, 217
Monotherapy, 231

Monounsaturated fats, 391, 434, 435–436, 443
Multivitamins, 205, 208, 211, 377, 378
Mycoplasma, 259

N

Nateglinide (Starlix), 44, 140, 142, 151, 154
National Institute of Diabetes and Digestive and Kidney Disorders, 59
Nausea and vomiting
and dehydration, 34, 36
of gastroparesis, 288
of gastropathy, 258
in heart attack, 70
of ketoacidosis, 37, 559
of kidney disease, 285
postoperative, 546
Necrobiosis lipoidica diabeticorum, 463
Needles
disposal of, 194, 548
fear of, 188, 192, 536–537
and pain, 534, 535
Nephropathy
and blood glucose control, 133, 438
diabetes as risk factor for, 40
drug therapy for, 466
and high blood pressure, 65, 66, 284, 286–287, 565
and protein intake, 287
screening for, 66, 285–286, 561, 565
stages of, 283–285
Nerve damage. *See* Neuropathy
Neuropathy
anterior ischemic optic, 441, 442, 443
and antioxidant supplements, 223
autonomic, 44, 66, 254–255, 309–310
and bladder infections, 260
and blood glucose control, 134, 437, 438
cardiac autonomic, 254–255, 267
and erectile dysfunction, 275
gastropathy, 44, 143, 257, 258
and sexual problems, 282
and skin dryness, 460
treatment of, 65–66
See also Foot problems; Peripheral neuropathy
Niacin, 208, 209, 210, 431, 433
Nitrofurantoin macrocrystals, 261
Nutrients. *See* Vitamins and minerals
Nutrition. *See* Diet and nutrition
Nuts and seeds, in vegetarian diet, 406, 409

O

Obesity and overweight
  binge eating disorder, 93, 95
  in children, 368, 523–527
  defined, 368, 376, 525
  and diabetes risk, 60
  and heart disease risk, 17, 68,
    266–267
  and hunger, 368–372
  medical costs of, 342
  See also Weight loss
Obstetrician, 479, 484, 485
Occupational therapy, 272, 273
Octreotide (Sandostatin), 290
Omega-3 fatty acids, 104, 431, 435,
  443
Ophthalmologists/optometrists, 563
Oral glucose tolerance test, 61
Orgasm disorders, 281
Orlistat (Xenical), 369, 432
Orthopedists, 307
Orthotics, 306
Osteopenia, 449
Osteoporosis, 215, 445–450, 499–500,
  505
Overweight. *See* Obesity and
  overweight

P

Painful sexual intercourse, 281
Pain management, 67, 378
Pain perception, children's, 536
Pain perception test, 253
Pancreas, role in insulin production,
  24, 25, 26, 33, 137, 139–140, 171,
  187
Pancreatitis, 25
Parathyroid hormone, 450, 565
Parenteral nutrition, total, 289
Parkinson disease, ketogenic diets
  for, 42
Pedorthists, 307, 321–322
Penile implants, 279
Penile injection therapy, 277
Penile splint, 279
Peptide YY, 371
Percent Daily Values (%DV), 206,
  213, 388, 390, 391
Perimenopause, 498
Peripheral neuropathy
  and atherosclerosis, 305
  causes of, 252–253, 309
  diagnosis of, 253–254, 304, 561
  and exercise, 357, 507
  symptoms of, 304–305, 306, 309
  See also Foot problems
Peripheral vascular disease, 310,
  314, 463

Phentermine (Adipex-P), 372
Physical exam, 19, 61, 63
Physical therapy, 271–272, 273, 307
Phytonutrients, 220
Pioglitzone (Actos), 24, 508, 561
Pneumonia vaccine, 20, 64, 505
Polycystic ovary syndrome (PCOS),
  280
Polyunsaturated fats, 391, 434, 435
Postprandial hyperglycemia, 147,
  225–226
Pramlintide (Symlin), 45, 224–226,
  229, 233
Precision Xtra meter, 41, 42
Prediabetes, 23, 24, 25, 48
Pregnancy
  blood glucose levels during, 478,
    479, 480
  blood glucose monitoring during,
    52, 134, 135, 478–479, 485, 488
  drug therapy during, 233, 236
  exercise during, 482, 485
  eye examinations during, 66
  gestational diabetes of, 25, 60,
    172, 236, 480–481, 482–483
  information sources, 483
  insulin therapy during, 479–480,
    482–483, 485–486, 487–489
  ketone levels during, 21
  ketone testing during, 42, 479, 488
  labor and delivery, 483, 489
  meal planning during, 481–482,
    485, 486–487
  medical care during, 479, 485
  nutrient needs during, 205, 482
  planning for, 485
  postpartum care, 483–484
  risks of, 44, 484–485
  and Type 1 diabetes, 172
  and Type 2 diabetes, 172, 236
  urinary tract infection risk,
    259–260
  vaginitis screening during, 494
  weight gain during, 481, 486
  yoga during, 339
Progestogens, 498, 500, 501–502
Protein, dietary
  after bariatric surgery, 379
  on food labels, 393
  and kidney function, 287
  low-carbohydrate high-protein diet,
    21, 39–40
  during pregnancy, 482
  recommended amounts, 393
  in sick-day box, 35
  in vegan diet, 400–401
  and wound healing, 314
Psychotherapy, 95, 103
Pyridoxine, 208, 209, 210

R

Raloxifene (Evista), 450
Recipe modification, 416–420
Recipes
  Asian Noodle Bowl, 408
  Chowder, Corn and Potato, 408
  Macaroni and Cheese, Momma's
    Original, 419
  Macaroni and Cheese, Momma's
    Slimmed-Down, 419
  Pears, Oven-Poached, 407
  Pudding Parfaits, Graham, 407
  Yogurt Sipper, Fruity, 291–292
Recommended Dietary Allowance
  (RDA), 206–207, 213
Rehabilitation, after stroke, 271–274
Relaxation response, 80
Relaxation techniques, 80–82, 123,
  144, 458
Repaglinide (Prandin), 44, 140, 142,
  151, 154
Resistance exercise, 18, 63, 69, 70,
  344
Respiratory infection, 545
Restless leg syndrome, 456
Retinal detachment, 442, 561
Retinopathy, diabetic
  and blindness, 65, 122, 440, 441
  and blood glucose control, 134,
    437, 438, 441–442
  and exercise, 357, 507, 563
  eye examinations, 65–66, 443–444,
    561
  forms of, 563
  and high blood pressure, 442–443
  incidence of, 440–441
  and vitamin supplements, 221
Riboflavin, 208, 209, 210
Rimonabant, 372
Rosiglitazone (Avandia), 24, 466,
  508, 561

S

Salt (sodium), 391, 417, 418, 568
Saturated fat, 412, 433–434, 435, 436,
  443, 567
School lunches, 538
Scleredema adultorum, 464
Selective estrogen receptor modula-
  tors (SERMs), 450, 502
Selenium, 216, 217
Self-efficacy, 97, 121–122
Self-esteem, and body image, 87,
  88–89
Semmes–Weinstein monofilament
  test, 253, 314
Serving size
  controlling, 398–399, 416–417

on food labels, 389–391, 398–399
increase in, 397–398
standard, 398
and weight gain, 396–397
Sex hormones, 280, 446
Sexual hygiene, 261
Sexual problems
diabetes-related, 281–282
erectile dysfunction, 274–279
information sources, 278, 282
types of, 280–281
Shoes
fitting, 252, 254, 321, 464
lacing, 322–323
Medicare program, 320
orthotics, 306
selection criteria, 318–321
therapeutic, 313, 320
unsuitable styles, 321
Sibutramine (Meridia), 372, 432
Sick days
guidelines, 559
planning for, 21–22, 34, 36–37,
63, 144, 467
supplies for, 21, 22, 33–39,
451–452, 559
See also Infections
Sildenafil (Viagra), 276
Skin conditions
bacterial infections, 461–462
diabetes-associated, 462–463
diabetes-related, 463–464
dryness, 307, 460–461
fungal infections, 307, 317, 462
from insulin injections, 175, 190
prevention tips, 464
Sleep apnea, 455–456, 458
Sleep disorders, 454–459
Sleeping patterns
and blood glucose fluctuations,
145
and lifestyle changes, 455, 458
napping, 458
Sleep log, 457, 458
Smoking
and bariatric surgery, 378
cessation, 65, 69, 265, 306, 314,
443, 449, 508, 567
and dental problems, 543
health risks of, 17, 68, 254, 265,
447, 550
and premature death, 20
and sleep disorders, 455
Snacks
nutritious, 525, 540
at summer camp, 523
timing of, 555
trans fat in, 413
Soaps, for foot care, 315–316

Social support
for binge eating disorder, 95
for celiac disease, 29
in college, 548–549
sources for, 59–60
spousal, 111–114, 119
for women, 509–510
Sodium intake, 391, 417, 418, 568
Somogyi phenomenon, 185, 186
Speech-language therapy, 272, 273
Spirituality, 83–85
Spousal support, 111–114, 119
Statins, 64–65, 429, 430, 433, 443
Steroidal drugs, and blood glucose
fluctuations, 146
Storytelling, healing effects of,
106–110
Stress
and blood glucose levels, 70–80,
144
and depression, 102
fight-or-flight response, 79, 80, 337
and heart disease risk, 265
and hyperglycemia, 17, 51–52
of illness, 559
and ketone levels, 41
management tips, 115–117
relaxation techniques for, 80–82,
144
and sleep disorders, 456, 458
yoga for, 337–338
Stretching exercises, 352–358
Stroke, 270–274, 432
Sugar alcohols, 392, 393, 418
Sulfonylureas, 44, 113, 142, 150–151,
156, 187–188, 228, 232–233,
234–235, 438, 495
Summer camps
diabetes management at, 521–523
diabetic vs. traditional, 520–521
information sources, 522
Surgical treatment
bariatric (weight loss), 376–380
of children, 544–546
dental, 542–543
of erectile dysfunction, 279
of heart failure, 269–270
hysterectomy, 498
Symptoms
of autonomic neuropathy, 254
of celiac disease, 27
of depression, 102
of diabetes, 23–24, 25, 61
of gastroparesis, 288
of gastropathy, 258
of heart attack, 70–71
of heart disease, 70
of heart failure, 265, 266, 267
of high blood pressure, 237
of hyperglycemia, 50

of hyperosmolar hyperglycemic
state, 52–53, 295
of hypoglycemia, 44, 63–64, 113,
136, 154, 468, 488, 527–528
of ketoacidosis, 37, 294
of peripheral neuropathy,
304–305, 306, 309
of peripheral vascular disease, 310
of urinary tract infections, 260
Syndrome X, 25, 237
Syringes, 176, 191–192, 195, 548
Systolic blood pressure, 65, 237, 567

T

Tadalafil (Cialis), 276
Tegaserod (Zelnorm), 290
Tempeh, 404, 406
Testosterone, 280, 500
Thiamine, 208, 209, 210
Thiazolidinediones (TZDs), 44–45,
232, 233, 234–235, 431, 508, 561
Tinea, 462
Toenails, 254, 304, 307, 316–317
Toes, hammertoe (claw toe), 307,
310–311, 463
Tofu, 404
Tolazamide (Tolinase), 142, 154
Tolbutamide (Orinase), 142, 154
Tolerable Upper Intake Level (UL),
206, 207, 213
Transcranial magnetic stimulation
(TMS), 105
Trans fat, 64, 412–415, 434, 435,
443, 567
Trauma, healing through story-
telling, 106–110
Travel
blood glucose fluctuations during,
146
insulin therapy during, 194–195
Trichomoniasis, 495
Triglycerides, 68, 69, 135, 429, 431,
435, 568
Trimethoprim, 261
Troglitazone (Rezulin), 233, 561
Type 1 diabetes
blood glucose control in, 133–134
and bone loss, 447
causes of, 23, 25, 137, 171–172
celiac disease with, 32–33
and exercise, 63
and ketoacidosis, 24, 37, 39, 41, 42
and ketone testing, 37
in pregnancy, 172
signs and symptoms of, 23–24, 25
and vitamin B_{12} supplements, 206
Type 2 diabetes
and blood glucose levels, 24, 134
and bone loss, 447–448

causes of, 24, 25, 137, 172
in children, 25, 524, 525, 545
and cholesterol levels, 135
drug therapy for, 24–25, 44–45,
145, 187–188, 230–236
and exercise, 69
and high blood pressure, 135
insulin resistance in, 24, 25, 102,
172, 187, 189
insulin therapy for, 25–26, 145,
187–191
and ketoacidosis (DKA), 293–294
and ketone testing, 37, 42
in pregnancy, 172
progression of, 25–26, 145, 188
and retinopathy, 563

U

Ulcers, foot, 252, 254, 304, 306,
309–315, 463
Urethral suppository, 276
Urinary tract infections (UTI),
259–262
Urinary tract system, 259, 260
Urination, increased, 23, 24, 33, 50,
211
Urine reagent strips, in ketone
testing, 41, 42, 294, 559
Urine test
for ketones, 294, 479
for kidney disease, 286, 561
USDA Dietary Guidelines, 211
USDA Food Pyramid, 540

V

Vacuum devices, for erectile
dysfunction, 278–279
Vaginal dryness, 281, 499
Vaginitis, 493–497
Vaginosis, bacterial, 493–494
Vagus nerve, electrical stimulation
of, 105
Vanadium, 213–214, 217
Vasodilators, 239, 240–241, 268, 276
Vegan diet
ingredients in, 404, 406
menu planning, 403–404
protein in, 400–401
vitamin supplements for, 205
See also Vegetarian diet
Vegetables
snacks, 540
in vegetarian diet, 406, 409
Vegetarian diet
carbohydrate counting, 405, 411
food pyramid for, 401–402
information sources, 410–411
ingredients for, 406, 409–411

menu planning, 402–403
nutrients in, 400–401
recipes, 407–408
See also Vegan diet
Vitamin A, 209, 210, 449
Vitamin B_{12}, 206, 208, 209, 210, 378,
401
Vitamin C, 206, 208, 209, 220,
221–222, 223
Vitamin D, 209, 210, 215, 379, 401,
446, 449, 502, 504
Vitamin E, 208, 209, 220, 221–222,
223
Vitamin K, 209, 446
Vitamins and minerals
antioxidant supplements, 208,
219–223
with bariatric surgery, 377, 378,
379
daily requirements, 209, 217
deficiencies, 27, 206, 210, 211–212
defined, 205, 211
in diabetes treatment, 207–208,
210, 212–216
in diet, 206–207, 209, 217, 218, 222
on food labels, 393
information sources, 218
in menopause, 502
multivitamins, 205, 208, 211, 377,
378
during pregnancy, 205, 482
supplements (mineral), 211,
212–216
supplements (vitamin), 205–206,
207–210
in vegetarian diet, 401
See also specific nutrients
Vulvovaginal candidiasis, 494–495

W

Warfarin (Coumadin), 508
Warts, removal of, 316
Weight
and blood glucose levels, 145
and body image dissatisfaction, 86,
87, 88
body-mass index, 269
healthy, 69
and hypoglycemia, 154, 175
and insulin therapy, 190–191
during pregnancy, 481, 486
set level, 369
See also Obesity and overweight
Weight loss
bariatric surgery, 376–380
and binge eating disorder, 94, 95
and blood glucose levels, 24
and body image, 89
distress and frustration with, 117

drug treatment in, 368, 369,
370–372, 432
and exercise, 18, 334, 336, 524
information sources, 374
low-calorie diet, 369, 524
low-carbohydrate diets, 40
and nutrition, 63
plan, 69, 95
sign of Type 1 diabetes, 23
strategies for, 373–375, 435
and weight training, 333
Weight training, 333, 336, 446, 449
Women
and blood glucose control, 52, 144
body image dissatisfaction of, 88
breast-feeding, 484, 489, 490–493
and celiac disease, 29
folic acid supplements for, 210
health tips for, 501, 503–510
heart attack symptoms in, 70
and heart disease risk, 67, 499,
504–505
and hormone therapy, 497–498,
500–502
labor and delivery, 483, 489
and osteoporosis, 445–446,
499–500
screening tests for, 504–505
testosterone in, 280, 500
and urinary tract infections,
259–260, 261
and vaginitis, 493–497
vitamin supplements for, 205
See also Menopause; Menstruation;
Pregnancy
Wound-care products, 316
Wound dressings, 314
Wound healing, 310, 311–314, 464

X

Xerostomia, 541

Y

Yeast infection, vaginal, 494–495
Yoga, 337–340

Z

Zinc, 215, 401